British Association of Dermatologists' Management Guidelines

British Association of Dermatologists' Management Guidelines

Edited by

Neil H. Cox BSc, MBChB, FRCP (Lond & Edin)
Consultant dermatologist
Cumberland Infirmary
Carlisle
UK

John S.C. English MBBS, FRCP
Consultant dermatologist
Nottingham University Hospital
Nottingham
UK

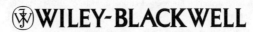
WILEY-BLACKWELL
A John Wiley & Sons, Ltd., Publication

This edition first published 2011, © 2011 British Association of Dermatologists

Blackwell Publishing was acquired by John Wiley & Sons in February 2007. Blackwell's publishing program has been merged with Wiley's global Scientific, Technical and Medical business to form Wiley-Blackwell.

Registered office: John Wiley & Sons, Ltd, The Atrium, Southern Gate, Chichester, West Sussex, PO19 8SQ, UK

Editorial offices: 9600 Garsington Road, Oxford, OX4 2DQ, UK
The Atrium, Southern Gate, Chichester, West Sussex, PO19 8SQ, UK
111 River Street, Hoboken, NJ 07030-5774, USA

For details of our global editorial offices, for customer services and for information about how to apply for permission to reuse the copyright material in this book please see our website at www.wiley.com/wiley-blackwell

Library of Congress Cataloging-in-Publication Data

British Association of Dermatologists.
  British Association of Dermatologists' management guidelines / edited by Neil H. Cox, John S.C. English.
    p. ; cm.
    Includes bibliographical references.
    ISBN 978-1-4443-3552-1
    1. Skin–Diseases–Treatment–Standards.   2. Dermatology–Standards–Great Britain.   I. Cox, Neil H.
II. English, John S. C.   III. Title.
    [DNLM: 1. Skin Diseases–therapy–Practice Guideline.   2. Dermatology–methods–Practice Guideline.
WR 650 B862 2011]
    RL110.B75 2011
    616.5–dc22

                                          2010024518

ISBN: 9780470654552

A catalogue record for this book is available from the British Library.

This book is published in the following electronic formats: ePDF 9781444329872; Wiley Online Library 9781444329865; ePub 9781444329889

Set in 9.25/11.5pt Minion by Aptara® Inc., New Delhi, India
Printed and bound in Singapore by Fabulous Printers Pte Ltd

1 2011

Contents

A tribute to Professor Neil H. Cox

Unfortunately, Neil died suddenly in December 2009. I had known Neil since the mid 1980s when we were both registrars in Glasgow with Professor Rona Mackie. Neil very quickly developed the high degree of skill in writing and editing dermatology papers and book chapters; to a level that I will never achieve. This book was one of his 'babies' as he had contributed more to the BAD guidelines than any other author and so knew them inside out. I hope I have done him and his guidelines justice in helping edit this compendium.

Dr John S.C. English 2010

Introduction

It is with great pleasure that I introduce this compilation of the British Association of Dermatologists guidelines. I was an Honorary Secretary of the British Association of Dermatologists from 1996 to 2000 when the guidelines process was initially developed through the auspices of the then Drug and Therapeutics Committee. As described later in the book, we wanted the guidelines not only to represent best practice but also to reflect a consensus of views of British dermatologists. So we published draft documents in the BAD newsletter for a 3-month consultation before submission to the British Journal of Dermatology.

We hoped that the guidelines might act as a reference source for the development of dermatology education resources for healthcare practitioners, patients and the general public. Hence, when we developed our website they were made freely downloadable.

When I became President of the BAD some 10 years later, it was clear that the guideline process was a great success – a tribute to the innumerable clinicians who took part in their development. The editors of the BJD also told us that they were highly cited articles and reprints were requested internationally.

People enjoy access to information through many routes and it seemed to me that a compilation of the guidelines in a book would make the information available in another useful format.

The hard work of Neil Cox, in particular, along with John English has brought this to fruition. Reading it now, it seems not only a source for knowledge about the management of and therapies used in skin conditions but also an illustration of the evolution of the guidelines process over the last decade; a process in which Neil Cox was intimately involved.

Sadly, as Neil's last work it has also become a tribute to his memory.

I hope you find the book enjoyable and informative.

Dr Colin Holden BSc, MD, FRCP
Past President
British Association of Dermatologists

Preface

The guidelines contained in this publication have mostly been published in the *British Journal of Dermatology* within the last 10 years, and are all available online from the British Association of Dermatologists (BAD) website www.bad.org.uk. In preparing this compendium of the guidelines, we have been aware of three main factors.

Firstly, many of the guidelines have now been updated since they were first published. Most of the updates have given greater prominence to therapeutics, especially with regard to newer approaches, and to areas of controversy. By comparison, the initial versions generally 'set the scene' and contained more text about epidemiology and older treatments than in the updated versions. Therefore, many of these earlier versions still have value as review material, and we felt that references to these should be included.

Secondly, the whole process of assimilating, assessing and extrapolating evidence to be applied in clinical settings has been a rapidly changing field. This is discussed in more detail on pX. Although there is now a preferred style of citation of evidence and recommendations for BAD guidelines (see pX), the style differs somewhat between guidelines. This, in part, reflects styles in use at the time of writing as well as pragmatic issues such as ease of updating and of collaborating with other specialists to produce multidisciplinary guidelines. Additionally, some of the guidelines were produced as consensus documents (British Photodermatology Group) and have a different style.

Thirdly, no evidence is ever perfect, multiply replicated and applicable in all scenarios. Even with good evidence, the strength of a recommendation may vary between individuals who have assessed that evidence. External factors such as different healthcare systems or edicts by government bodies may influence recommendations. Newly emerging evidence needs to be put in context, and some evidence may create as many questions as it answers. Therefore, we have added some editorial comments about each guideline, and some details of recent evidence and of other guidelines and reviews, mostly by use of web addresses.

Finally, guidelines need to be useful. The BAD guidelines are written primarily for dermatologists and other specialists. They have been produced in summary format, capable of being copied and laminated for quick reference. They have also included other tools for the user, such as some suggested audit points. For this compendium, we have tried to extend this usefulness by adding guidelines that may be more applicable to primary care users (e.g. Clinical Knowledge Summaries (CKS) and reference material from the New Zealand DermNet). We have also included some guidance from bodies such as the UK National Health Service (NHS) and the UK National Institute for Health and Clinical Excellence (NICE), as well as material from other national dermatology bodies (such as the American Academy of Dermatology) and a variety of cancer organisations. We have also supplemented each topic, where applicable, with patient information resources that provide Patient Information Leaflets (PILs) or web-based information about specific conditions, prevention of disease, or about treatments.

Thus, for each guideline, in addition to reproducing the published version, we have included a web address for the guideline, some editorial comment, selected additional guidelines or other references for users, web details of the BAD's own PIL and details of additional patient-orientated sources of information.

We hope that these measures will increase the utility of the guidelines beyond the original presentation.

We thank all guideline authors for their dedication to this project, and to current and previous members of the BAD's Therapy Guidelines and Audit Subcommittee who have overseen the production of guidelines throughout the last decade.

N.H. Cox & J.S.C. English
Editors 2009

Background to the British Association of Dermatologists clinical guidelines

The British Association of Dermatologists (BAD) started its programme of writing guidelines over 10 years ago, with impetus from Professors Hywel Williams and Chris Griffiths and the Therapy Guidelines and Audit Subcommittee of the BAD. The process of developing national guidelines began for various reasons, at least partly because of a realisation that many guidelines were being developed by local groups of dermatologists (or others), with varying quality and sometimes with significant input or endorsement from pharmaceutical manufacturers, and it was felt that a national approach, independent from external influence, and produced in a way that would have broad consultation amongst members of the Association, would be preferable. There was also external impetus in that the Royal College of Physicians (RCP) of London wanted all specialist societies to generate some national audit criteria, and it was felt that the strongest suggestions would be achieved by basing them on evidence-based national guidelines.

The guidelines writing and consultation process had some key features [1], some of which have altered with time. The initial plan was to write guidelines 'by dermatologists, for dermatologists' (but with the knowledge that at least some parts of these guidelines would be applicable to primary care and to other disciplines). The guidelines were to be prepared by small groups, including some clinicians working out with academic centres; they would include an evaluation of the strength of the available evidence, and recommendations would be made together with suggestions for possible audit. All draft versions, once approved by the Therapy Guidelines and Audit Subcommittee, which was central to this process, would be circulated to the membership of the Association for a 3-month consultation period, inviting any comments and, thus, acting as a peer review as well as giving a sense of ownership of the guidelines to all members of the BAD. Some aspects have changed slightly over the years, as described below, but the basic aims and methods remain unchanged, and a valuable resource has been built up by clinicians who have put much time and effort into this process.

Although the original aim was primarily to produce disease-related guidelines, it became apparent that there was also a need for guidelines on specific treatments; this has led to guidelines on systemic therapies such as azathioprine and biological agents for psoriasis. One of the major changes that took place over the years was in relation to authorship. In some cases, additional authors were included (for example, because of experience in performing a Cochrane review of a subject), or because of the breadth of some topics; for example, guidelines on biological agents needed to take into consideration the needs for a register of use of such agents and to include authors who would be involved with such a register. Recognising the value of unified guidelines on topics that spanned different specialties led to multidisciplinary guidelines, initially for melanoma (involving the BAD and members of the Melanoma Study Group) and later for Squamous Cell Carcinoma (with Plastic Surgery). An even broader group has been involved with revised Melanoma guidelines, and guidelines for monitoring of isotretinoin have taken a further step by having a lay member representing the relevant (acne) patient support group. Perhaps, the greatest change, and the main subject of the following discussion, has been changes in expectations for guidelines in terms of their validity, independence from any conflicts of interest and in the explicit links between available evidence and the recommendations that are made.

Fairly rapidly, writing guidelines evolved into a 'business', the most pertinent parts of this culture being the production of definitions of what a guideline represents, issues around the legal position of guidelines and the evolution of 'guidelines for guidelines' that dictated certain content aspects, stringency requirements for evidence to be viewed as valid, systems for grading of evidence and the strength of the recommendations that could be drawn from such evidence. The process that had been adopted by the BAD had acknowledged that there were areas of 'normal established practice' that were not supported by high-quality evidence, that there were many areas lacking head-to-head comparisons of treatment, that evaluation of successful treatment was often subjective, and that lack of formal evidence did not necessarily preclude recommending a treatment. Therefore, the link between quality of evidence initially used in the BAD guidelines (stratified in a manner similar to that used by the US Task Force on Preventative Care Guidelines) and the recommendations that were made allowed less easily measurable factors to be taken into consideration. The subsequent shift in expectations for production of guidelines, described below, meant that the recommendations of a guideline would be more tightly limited by the validity of the available evidence on which it was based.

Although future clinical trials were increasingly expected to meet validity criteria, notably those of the CONSORT statement (Consolidated Standards of Reporting Trials) [2], these criteria were proposed some years after the start of the BAD guidelines production process. Whilst they set a new level of expectation for clinical trials, these criteria could not necessarily discredit the conclusions of historical studies where descriptions of trial design were not always recorded to the new level of detail that CONSORT advised. Furthermore, those performing clinical trials needed to be educated in application of these new standards [3, 4] before these standards could become the norm. Whilst many older trials were undoubtedly suboptimal as a basis for evidence in guidelines, the opposite also applied in some instances; some good-quality trials used selected patients, often excluding older patients or those with co-morbidities, and thus, only truly represented a minority of subjects with a particular condition.

As guidelines for guidelines developed further, more objective methods to quantify the validity of guidelines were constructed; the most relevant to the BAD (as it was adopted by the RCP) was the AGREE instrument [5, 6], in which a scoring system for guidelines was suggested based on various aspects such as applicability, stakeholder involvement (in our case, consultation with the membership), robustness of searches for evidence, clear links between strength of evidence and the recommendations, through to statements about editorial independence from any funding bodies or other conflicts on interest and inclusion of 'user tools' (in our case, summary tables and lists of possible audit points). Guidelines for guidelines started to force a direct link between the grading of evidence and the strength of recommendation. Whilst the BAD guidelines were actually complying with many of the suggestions and thus 'scoring points' (for example, there was

no extrinsic funding and there was a consultation process with potential users – the membership of the BAD), space constraints precluded stating all of these points in every guideline. A further publication was produced to explain how many of these 'new' recommendations were already being addressed [7], and the two references outlining the BAD guidelines process [1, 7] were added to subsequent guidelines so that institutions that wished to score guidelines could access the 'process' issues behind each of the BAD guidelines. More recently, large organisations have revisited the issue of guidelines for guidelines in deciding the key components that they wish to see in their own guidelines; the World Health Organization, for example, published a series of 16 articles on guideline development including comparisons of different guidelines for guidelines [8] and how they wished their own guidelines to be structured [9].

More explicit links between quality of evidence and the therapeutic recommendations that could be made have gradually became more widely used [10–12] and were summarised for BAD guidelines authors by Dr Tony Ormerod in 2004 [13]. This publication includes a summary of how to rank evidence, and to make recommendations, that is more rigid than that used in previous BAD guidelines, but more robust (this advice is currently being updated). However, even at this time changes were still being suggested; one study of six systems used by 51 organisations involved in clinical practice guidelines suggested that all of them had important shortcomings [14]. A new scheme for assessing the level of evidence and strength of recommendations was used in the BAD guideline on biological agents for psoriasis, recognising that some recommendations could only be given a low 'D' rating due to lack of evidence, but that such evidence may still be very important (for example, formal consensus of experts would fall into this category) [15]. Yet it remains difficult to apply guidance on how to mix research evidence, expert opinion and patient experience, and how to formalise a consensus recommendation that remains an inevitable element of most guidelines [16].

What does this mean for the reader of the present book? First, it should be appreciated that the main stakeholder group for most of the guidelines is dermatologists, although some guidelines have been written in collaboration with other specialists involved with treatment of a specific disorder. Second, the link between quality of evidence and strength of recommendation has not only involved a subjective component (for example, even if informally, most guidelines have taken costs, availability and convenience into account when making therapeutic recommendations), but has also altered in format with time as new recommendations for writing guidelines have been incorporated. Finally, many of the guidelines may not 'score' well on guideline appraisal systems unless the separate publications documenting the guideline process [1, 7] are also taken into consideration. For this reason, some of the guidelines presented here are formal updated versions of previous publications; in other instances, where rewriting a full guideline with a more modern evidence-recommendation summary would have been unlikely to lead to fundamentally different advice, authors have had an opportunity to add new information or to adjust evidence or recommendation grading in order to ensure that the conclusions are currently applicable.

In some respects, although arguably subjective rather than rigorous (and making assumptions of behalf of patients), our original avoidance of an automatic extrapolation from strength of evidence to grade of recommendation has been vindicated, as current developments in guideline recognise that other factors such as values and preferences of patients, and wise use of resources, are pertinent in making recommendations. The need to consider costs (resource utilisation) in guidelines was recognised some years ago [17]. Thus, for example, guidelines produced by the National Institute for Clinical Excellence (NICE) in the UK [18] include formal cost-benefit analyses – but these include guidelines that are written as much for healthcare commissioners as for clinicians, some that are specific to individual treatments and some that are sufficiently broad-ranging that they are very large and less 'user-friendly' for easy reference than the BAD guidelines. At the time of writing, the recommendations of the Grading of Recommendations, Assessment, Development and Evaluation (GRADE) Working Group have been reviewed in detail and are likely to be adopted as the 'gold standard' for guideline production [19–23], having been and endorsed by many guideline-producing organisations [24]. Obviously, the wide consultation and high costs of some of these measures (such as performing cost-benefit analyses) will have a major impact on the ability of specialty groups to write comparable guidelines; some will feel that succinct guidelines, as currently produced by the BAD, are more suitable for application in clinical situations.

As allude to above, in order to allow simultaneous publication of guidelines that were produced in a staged manner over a period of years, including some that have been formally updated but retained their original evidence and recommendation hierarchies, we have published this group of guidelines largely in the format in which they were originally published. All were subject to methodologies, consultation processes and compliance with reasonably accepted guideline-writing criteria that applied at the time of writing and, as discussed, we have incorporated some updates within this structure. Where appropriate, the editors have added details of other guideline or systematic review resources for additional reading or for comparison. Especially in areas of imminent or rapid change, we have included comments on new data that have become apparent during the proof stages; where necessary for expedient publication, this may be 'stand-alone' rather than integrated within the prose. Finally, we have used our discretion to add an editorial comment in situations where there are issues of inadequate or conflicting evidence or opinion, either within or between guidelines.

This remains a process of evolution; Drs Bell and Omerod discuss the present aspirations of the BAD for its guideline author in pXIV.

Finally, neither this nor any other compendium of guidelines can ever be and remain both comprehensive and up-to-date. We advise readers to supplement these guidelines with additional web resources and textbooks that include guidelines, systematic reviews or other forms of evidence-based medicine [18, 25–29], as well as with guidelines aimed at other user groups. The latter include, in the UK, the Clinical Knowledge Summaries – previously known as PRODIGY guidelines – which contain disease-orientated, evidence-based information for primary care, produced by the Sowerby Centre for Health Informatics at Newcastle (Schin; http://www.schin.co.uk); these include guidelines on several dermatological topics, many with input from authors of guidelines in this book [30]. Guidelines available on websites based in other countries may also be useful [31, 32], and the National Guideline Clearinghouse [33] keeps a database of guidelines that fulfil their specific criteria (although there are not many dermatological guidelines included at present). For those wishing to assess in more detail the evidence that contributes to guidelines, issues about how to find evidence, hierarchy of evidence, systematic reviews and appraisal of studies can be found in standard texts [25, 34].

N.H. Cox & J.S.C. English
Editors 2009

REFERENCES

1 Griffiths CEM. The British Association of Dermatologists guidelines for the management of skin disease. *Br J Dermatol* 1999; 141: 396–7.

2 http://www.consort-statement.org

3 Cox NH, Williams HC. Can you COPE with CONSORT? *Br J Dermatol* 2000; 142: 1–3.

4 Ormerod AD. CONSORT your submissions: an update for authors. *Br J Dermatol* 2001: 145: 378–9.

5 The AGREE Collaboration. Guideline development in Europe: an international comparison. *Int J Technol Assess Healthcare* 2000; 16: 1036–46.

6 Appraisal of Guidelines for Research and Evaluation AGREE Instrument. London: St George's Medical School, 2001 (http://www.agreecollaboration.org/1/agreeguide).

7 Cox NH, Williams HC. The British Association of Dermatologists therapeutic guidelines: can we AGREE? *Br J Dermatol* 2003; 148: 621–5.

8 Oxman AD, Schünemann HJ, Freitheim A; WHO advisory committee on health research. Improving the use of research evidence in guideline development: 1. Guidelines for guidelines. *Health Res Policy Syst* 2006; 4: 13.

9 Oxman AD, Schünemann HJ, Freitheim A. Improving the use of research evidence in guideline development: 14. Reporting guidelines. *Health Res Policy Syst* 2006; 4: 26.

10 Harbour R, Miller J, for the Scottish Intercollegiate Guidelines Network Grading Review Group. A new system for grading recommendations in evidence based guidelines. *Br Med J* 2001; 323: 334–6.

11 http://www.sign.ac.uk/methodology/index.html

12 http://www.nice.org.uk/nhsevidence/

13 Ormerod AD. How to go about writing a clinical guideline for the B.A.D. http://www.bad.org.uk//site/622/default.aspx.

14 Atkins D, Eccles M, Flottorp S, *et al*. Systems for grading the quality of evidence and the strength of recommendations I: critical appraisal of existing approaches. The GRADE Working Group. *BMC Health Serv Res* 2004; 4: 38.

15 Ormerod AD. Recommendations in British Association of Dermatologists guidelines. *Br J Dermatol* 2005; 153: 477–8.

16 Rycroft-Malone J. Formal consensus: the development of a national clinical guideline. *Qual Health Care* 2001; 10: 202–3.

17 Atkins D, Best D, Briss PA, *et al*. Grading quality of evidence and strength of recommendations. *Br Med J* 2004; 328: 1490.

18 www.nice.org.uk

19 Guyatt GH, Oxman AD, Vist GE, *et al*, for the GRADE Working Group. GRADE: an emerging consensus on rating quality of evidence and strength of recommendations. *Br Med J* 2008; 336: 924–6.

20 Guyatt GH, Oxman AD, Vist GE, *et al*, for the GRADE Working Group. GRADE: what is "quality of evidence" and why is it important to clinicians? *Br Med J* 2008; 336: 995–8.

21 Guyatt GH, Oxman AD, Kunz R, *et al*, for the GRADE Working Group. GRADE: going from evidence to recommendations. *Br Med J* 2008; 336: 1049–51.

22 Schünermann AHJ, Oxman AD, Brozek J, *et al*, for the GRADE Working Group. GRADE: grading quality of evidence and strength of recommendations for diagnostic tests and strategies. *Br Med J* 2008; 336: 1106–10.

23 Guyatt GH, Oxman AD, Kunz R, *et al*, for the GRADE Working Group. GRADE: incorporating considerations of resources use into recommendations. *Br Med J* 2008; 336: 1170–73.

24 Kunz R, Djulbegovic B, Schünemann HJ, Stanulla M, Muti P, Guyatt G. Misconceptions, challenges, uncertainty, and progress in guideline recommendations. *Semin Hematol* 2008; 45: 167–75.

25 Williams HC, Bigby M, Diepgen T, Herxheimer, Naldi L, Rzany B (eds). *Evidence-Based Dermatology, 2nd edn*. Oxford: BMJ Books/Blackwell Publishing, 2008.

26 http://www.blackwellpublishing.com/medicine/bmj/dermatology/default.asp

27 Cochrane Skin Group. http://www.csg.cochrane.org.

28 Cochrane Library. http://www.thecochranelibrary.org.

29 NHS National Library for Health. http://www.library.nhs.uk.

30 NHS Clinical Knowledge. http://www.cks.nhs.uk/home.

31 New Zealand Dermatology Guidelines. http://www.dermnetnz.org.

32 American Academy of Dermatology guidelines. http://www.aad.org/research/guidelines/index.html.

33 National Guideline Clearinghouse. http://www.jcaai.org.

34 Bigby M, Williams HC. *Evidence-based dermatology*. In: Burns DA, Breathnach SM, Cox NH, Griffiths CEM (eds). *Rook's Textbook of Dermatology, 8th edn*. Oxford: Blackwell Science, 2010, p 7.1–7.23.

Writing a British Association of Dermatologists clinical guideline: an update on the process and guidance for authors

This advice is aimed at the authors of British Association of Dermatologists (BAD) guidelines.

The idea for developing a new topic for a BAD guideline usually comes from a member of the BAD, but could come from patient representatives or other organizations such as the Royal College of Physicians (RCP).

The intention is that a guideline will be comprehensive and up-to-date, aimed at dermatologists and nurses working in clinical dermatological practice.

Before proceeding, the topic must be agreed by the Therapy and Guidelines Subcommittee (T&G).

Authorship

If the topic suggestion is from a BAD member, they may be involved in writing the guideline. As a bare minimum, authorship should consist of three clinicians with an interest in the area and ideally representing both teaching hospital and district general hospital practices; for consensus-based recommendations a larger group is more effective. The lead author will identify their coauthors with support from the T&G if necessary. Depending on the guideline topic, nursing and patient representatives may be invited to join the guideline development group (GDG) or alternatively they may be involved at the peer review stage. For conditions managed by more than one specialty, the other specialties should be represented in the GDG (e.g. malignant melanoma) and some such guidelines may be developed in collaboration with another body (e.g. RCP for vitiligo). The group can also include specialist registrars for whom involvement in producing a guideline is a worthwhile educational objective.

The process

Over recent years the guideline process has evolved to become increasingly complex with a rigorous methodology, and the amount of work involved should not be underestimated. The first step in the guideline process is identifying the scope and clinical questions that are going to be addressed. It is best if the topic has a limited focus with carefully identified questions. The framework of PICO (Patients, Interventions, Comparators and Outcomes) can assist in focusing the questions. Recommendations are based on evidence drawn from a systematic review of the literature pertaining to these questions. This involves employing a comprehensive search strategy to identify all available evidence, followed by appraisal of the papers and grading of the evidence.

As a result of this comprehensive process there has been a tendency for the most recently produced guidelines to be detailed and lengthy, thereby moving away from one of the original aims to produce concise guidance which the clinician can refer to quickly in the clinical setting. The policy of producing a laminated version for use in the clinic has become difficult to implement. In addition, it is important that the BAD continues to expand the range of patient information leaflets (PILs) and these should concur with information given in guidelines.

Consequently, authors of future guidelines will be encouraged to produce three documents in parallel:
1. A review of the literature (for a guideline update this would be limited to publications since the original was produced) in which a clear synthesis of evidence shows the strength of evidence supporting an intervention and whether the literature agrees or disagrees. Relevant harms and crude relative costs should also be considered where important.
2. A concise clinical guideline, which is clearly linked to the evidence, for use in the dermatology clinic.
3. Relevant PILs in the standard BAD format.
All three documents would be subjected to the usual peer review process and the first two would subsequently be published in the British Journal of Dermatology (BJD).

The concise guideline provides a focus for defining the recommendations, would be suitable for publication in a book of BAD guidelines and would be amenable to adaptation for use by other professionals such as general practitioners and pharmacists.

With each guideline, authors should consider audit points arising from their recommendations. The National Institute for Health and Clinical Excellence (NICE) Technical Manual devotes a chapter to this. Authors would also be well placed to contribute to the Database of Uncertainties about Effects of Treatments (DUETs, Appendix 1).

Peer review

Once a draft BAD guideline has been produced, it is first peer reviewed by all members of the T&G, which includes representatives from the British Dermatological Nursing Group and the British National Formulary. If they have not been involved directly as authors, members of any relevant patient support groups will be invited to review the guideline at this stage.

Comments will be fed back to the authors, appropriate amendments made and the final draft approved by the T&G before being published in the BAD Newsletter. There then follows a consultation period during which the entire membership is invited to return comments. These are collated by the Chair of the T&G and fed back to the authors for final amendments to be made. A final draft is then reviewed by the T&G prior to publication in the BJD and on the BAD website. There is the facility for abridging the paper guideline if there are extensive tables and reproducing these on the BAD website. The steps involved in producing a guideline are summarized in Appendix 2.

British Association of Dermatologists support for guideline authors

In addition to changes that have evolved in the process of guideline development, there are ever-increasing demands on members' time, and the BAD recognizes that authors provide their time and expertise free of charge and should be supported as much as possible. The following support will be available:

Two meetings of the GDG will be offered at Willan House, one at commencement of the process for identifying questions and dividing responsibilities for sections between members, and the other towards the end for pulling the draft document together. Members' travel expenses will be reimbursed and lunch will be provided and a member of the T&G will attend to support and provide consistency.

The T&G administrator/information scientist will organize, attend and record minutes of the meetings and will subsequently play a major role in performing the literature review and supporting the authors with appraisal of papers, grading of evidence (Appendix 3) and production of evidence tables. Members of the T&G will be available for advice and support at all stages in the process.

Identified questions will first be approved by the T&G. A realistic timeline for the guideline development will be sought from the authors and a date for the second meeting set at the first. Guidelines which take too long to develop risk being out of date by the time they are published.

Support will also be provided for guideline updates with a single meeting at Willan House offered where substantial changes to the original document are required. The information scientist will perform a re-run of the original literature search prior to the meeting.

Procedures for updating

Once a guideline is published, the process does not stop. Guidelines should be updated if any new evidence significantly changes the conclusion. Otherwise they need to be reviewed after 5 years and the originally defined search strategy should be re-run to obtain the last 5 years of evidence. Authors are approached by the T&G to undertake this work and produce an updated guideline. This, after the usual peer review process, would appear in the BJD and the text on the website, including the PIL if necessary, would be updated with a renewed date for currency. If original authors are unable to undertake an update it is the responsibility of members of the T&G to seek alternative authors or to perform the task themselves. If the updated literature search reveals that a guideline needs no changes the T&G can authorize a new use-by date of 5 years; however, if a guideline is not updated then it should be removed from the website as potentially it could be misleading.

Appendix 1. Useful resources

Helpful skills in producing guidelines are a grounding in evidence-based medicine and systematic review. Training in these areas is available to Cochrane reviewers (http://www.cochrane.org/resources/training.htm and http://www.cochrane.org/admin/manual.htm).

Parts 1 and 2 of the following publication provide an invaluable resource: Williams H, Bigby M, Diepgen T, Herxheimer A, Naldi L, Rzany B (editors). *Evidence Based Dermatology*. London: BMJ Publishing Group, 2003.

Examples of best practice are to be found on the NICE (http://www.nice.org.uk/page.aspx?o=201982) and the Scottish Intercollegiate Guidelines Network (http://www.sign.ac.uk/methodology/index.html) guideline websites and currently the BAD adopts their approach to evidence tables and grading of the evidence (Appendix 3).

From the outset it useful to be aware of the AGREE instrument (Appendix 4) which is a widely used guideline scoring instrument to rate the quality of the guideline (http://www.agreecollaboration.org/1/agreeguide/).

Current BAD guidelines are published in the BJD and are recognized internationally. They also appear on the BAD website and are linked in with the National Electronic Library for Health (http://www.library.nhs.uk/). They should also meet the selective criteria of the U.S. National Guideline Clearinghouse (NGC) (http://www.guideline.gov/), increasing the audience and benefits of the guideline. Those guidelines that go on to the NGC site have further utility for producing summaries, comparisons and palmtop downloads.

Criteria for a DUETs (http://www.library.nhs.uk/DUETS) uncertainty are as follows: (i) an up-to-date systematic review has shown that there is an uncertainty over treatment effects; (ii) existing systematic reviews are out of date; (iii) there is no relevant systematic review.

There are many patient organizations under the umbrella of the skin care campaign (http://www.skincarecampaign.org/) that can assist in guideline development or review as stakeholders.

Appendix 2. Summary of steps involved in producing a guideline

1 Title suggestion approved by the T&G
2 Lead author and coauthors identified

3 Initial meeting to identify questions, and to produce a scope, a search strategy and selection criteria. Allocation of sections/tasks to GDG members. Timeline and date of second meeting agreed

4 Scope and questions approved by the T&G

5 Data extraction: literature search performed by BAD information scientist (IS) and identified titles and abstracts forwarded to relevant section author

6 Authors with assistance of IS systematically sift and discard those that are irrelevant and scrutinize remaining papers to assess if they meet selection criteria. IS documents the selection process

7 Critical appraisal of the quality of remaining studies by at least two authors against tick lists with a third arbiter for disagreements

8 IS synthesizes the data from eligible studies and produces evidence tables with quantitative pooling of data if appropriate

9 Evidence tables circulated to all authors for comments

10 Getting from synthesis of evidence to a recommendation is not straightforward. There needs to be a dialogue between GDG members at this stage. The process should take into account the body of evidence, i.e. not just one paper

11 Section authors write draft review, concise guideline and PIL and identify potential audit points and DUETs

12 Second meeting to present a synthesis of data, review draft recommendations and establish consensus and implications for practice. IS will summarize recommendations

13 Draft documents collated by authors and IS and finalized

14 Review by T&G, comments fed back to authors and amendments made

15 Publication in BAD Newsletter for wide consultation

16 Redrafting in light of received comments

17 Review by T&G

18 Publication in BJD, BAD website and other sites, e.g. NGC

19 Five-year review: authors contacted by T&G. Literature search re-run by IS. If needed, updated guideline and PIL subjected to usual peer review process. If no update needed, renew web-based document with 5-year expiry date

20 Alternatively, publish updated guideline in BJD and on the website

Appendix 3. Levels of evidence and grades of recommendation (from Scottish Intercollegiate Guidelines Network)

The older format used in previous guidelines is updated in the light of advances in the methods of guideline development.

The published studies selected from the search should be assessed for their methodological rigour against a number of criteria. Checklists may be used to assess the selected studies; these are available in Appendix C–I of the NICE Technical Manual. The overall assessment of each study is graded using a code '++', '+' or '−', based on the extent to which the potential biases have been minimized, as in the Table.

Levels of evidence

Level of evidence	Type of evidence
1++	High-quality meta-analyses, systematic reviews of RCTs, or RCTs with a very low risk of bias
1+	Well-conducted meta-analyses, systematic reviews of RCTs, or RCTs with a low risk of bias
1−	Meta-analyses, systematic reviews of RCTs, or RCTs with a high risk of bias[a]
2++	High-quality systematic reviews of case–control or cohort studies
	High-quality case–control or cohort studies with a very low risk of confounding, bias or chance and a high probability that the relationship is causal
2+	Well-conducted case–control or cohort studies with a low risk of confounding, bias or chance and a moderate probability that the relationship is causal
2−	Case–control or cohort studies with a high risk of confounding, bias or chance and a significant risk that the relationship is not causal[a]
3	Nonanalytical studies (for example, case reports, case series)
4	Expert opinion, formal consensus

RCT, randomized controlled trial. [a]Studies with a level of evidence '−' should not be used as a basis for making a recommendation.

Grades of recommendation

Once a level of evidence has been derived and evidence tables drawn up levels of recommendation can be derived. These are the conclusion of the guideline and it is important that they stand out and stand alone. Often they can be highlighted in a box or a table. The level of the recommendation is determined by the level of evidence although the usefulness of a classification system based solely on this has been questioned because it does not take into consideration the importance of the recommendation in changing practice and it may be that more sophisticated derivations of strength of recommendation will appear in future.

Class	Evidence
A	• At least one meta-analysis, systematic review, or RCT rated as 1++, and directly applicable to the target population, or
	• A systematic review of RCTs or a body of evidence consisting principally of studies rated as 1+, directly applicable to the target population and demonstrating overall consistency of results
	• Evidence drawn from a NICE technology appraisal
B	• A body of evidence including studies rated as 2++, directly applicable to the target population and demonstrating overall consistency of results, or
	• Extrapolated evidence from studies rated as 1++ or 1+

Class	Evidence
C	• A body of evidence including studies rated as 2+, directly applicable to the target population and demonstrating overall consistency of results, or • Extrapolated evidence from studies rated as 2++
D	• Evidence level 3 or 4, or • Extrapolated evidence from studies rated as 2+, or • Formal consensus
D (GPP)	• A good practice point (GPP) is a recommendation for best practice based on the experience of the guideline development group

NICE, National Institute for Health and Clinical Excellence; RCT, randomized controlled trial.

Appendix 4. AGREE and National Guideline Clearinghouse (NGC) criteria

AGREE criteria

Scope and purpose

1 The overall objective(s) of the guideline should be specifically described
2 The clinical question(s) covered by the guideline should be specifically described
3 The patients to whom the guideline is meant to apply should be specifically described

Stakeholder involvement

4 The GDG should include individuals from all the relevant professional groups
5 The patients' views and preferences should be sought
6 The target users of the guideline should be clearly defined
7 The guideline should be piloted among end users

Rigour of development

8 Systematic methods should be used to search for evidence
9 The criteria for selecting the evidence should be clearly described
10 The methods used for formulating the recommendations should be clearly described
11 The health benefits, side-effects and risks should be considered in formulating the recommendations
12 There should be an explicit link between the recommendations and the supporting evidence
13 The guideline should be externally reviewed by experts prior to publication
14 A procedure for updating the guideline should be provided

Clarity and presentation

15 The recommendations should be specific and unambiguous
16 The different options for diagnosis and/or treatment of the condition should be clearly presented
17 Key recommendations should be easily identifiable
18 The guideline should be supported with tools for application

Applicability

19 The potential organizational barriers in applying the recommendations should be discussed
20 The potential cost implications of applying the recommendations should be considered
21 The guideline should present key review criteria for monitoring and audit purposes

Editorial independence

22 The guideline should be editorially independent from the funding body
23 Conflicts of interest of guideline development members should be recorded

Criteria for inclusion of clinical practice guidelines in NGC

1 The clinical practice guideline contains systematically developed statements that include recommendations, strategies, or information that assists physicians and/or other health care practitioners and patients make decisions about appropriate health care for specific clinical circumstances.
2 The clinical practice guideline was produced under the auspices of medical specialty associations; relevant professional societies, public or private organizations, government agencies at the Federal, State, or local level; or health care organizations or plans. A clinical practice guideline developed and issued by an individual not officially sponsored or supported by one of the above types of organizations does not meet the inclusion criteria for NGC.
3 Corroborating documentation can be produced and verified that a systematic literature search and review of existing scientific evidence published in peer reviewed journals was performed during the guideline development. A guideline is not excluded from NGC if corroborating documentation can be produced and verified detailing specific gaps in scientific evidence for some of the guideline's recommendations.
4 The full text guideline is available upon request in print or electronic format (for free or for a fee), in the English language. The guideline is current and the most recent version produced. Documented evidence can be produced or verified that the guideline was developed, reviewed, or revised within the last 5 years.

H.K. BELL (*Chair*) and A.D. ORMEROD (*Immediate Past Chair*)
BAD Therapy and Guidelines Subcommittee, September 2008.

http://www.bad.org.uk/Portals/_Bad/Guidelines/Clinical%20Guidelines/How%20to%20go%20about%20writing%20a
%20BAD%20Clinical%20Guideline%20-
%20BJD%20paper.pdf

REFERENCE

1 Bell HK, Omerod AD. Writing a British Association of Dermatologists clinical guideline: an update on the process and guidance for authors. *Brit J Dermatol* 2009; 160: 725–8.

1 Inflammatory dermatoses

To date the British Association of Dermatologists (BAD) have produced guidelines on seven inflammatory dermatoses. They are: alopecia areata (AA), vitiligo, bullous pemphigoid, contact dermatitis, lichen sclerosus urticaria and pemphigus. For guidance on how to manage other dermatoses, such as eczema and psoriasis, we have listed various resources below. This section incorporates a wide range of conditions, all difficult to treat, and perhaps on occasions, no treatment is warranted as the risk of potential harm may outweigh the disease morbidity. An underlying theme of these guidelines is patient safety and all of them address this in one way or another. Safety of powerful immunosupression treatments is paramount and many of the audit points include areas of patient safety to audit. Unfortunately, a lack of utility for treating some dermatoses such as vitiligo and AA has been unearthed by the guidelines. There is a continuing theme throughout the guidelines that more good quality randomised clinical trials are needed to help inform us of the best treatments for these difficult to treat, disabling diseases.

PROFESSIONAL RESOURCES

BAD guidance for psoriasis

http://www.bad.org.uk/site/769/Default.aspx
http://www.bad.org.uk/Portals/_Bad/Guidelines/Clinical
    %20Guidelines/BAD-PCDS%20Psoriasis
    %20reviewed%202010.pdf

BAD guidance for atopic eczema

http://www.bad.org.uk/Portals/_Bad/Guidelines/Clinical
    %20Guidelines/PCDS-BAD%20Eczema
    %20reviewed%202010.pdf

British Association of Dermatologists' Management Guidelines, 1st edition. Edited by Neil Cox and John English.
© 2011 British Association of Dermatologists.

Guidelines for the management of alopecia areata

S.P.MacDONALD HULL, M.L.WOOD,* P.E.HUTCHINSON,† M.SLADDEN†
AND A.G.MESSENGER‡

Pontefract General Infirmary, Pontefract WF8 1PL, U.K.
*Rotherham District General Hospital, Rotherham S60 2UD, U.K.
†Leicester Royal Infirmary, Leicester LE1 5WW, U.K.
‡Royal Hallamshire Hospital, Sheffield S10 2JF, U.K.

Accepted for publication 17 April 2003

Summary   These guidelines for management of alopecia areata have been prepared for dermatologists on behalf of the British Association of Dermatologists. They present evidence-based guidance for treatment, with identification of the strength of evidence available at the time of preparation of the guidelines, and a brief overview of epidemiological aspects, diagnosis and investigation.

Disclaimer

These guidelines have been prepared for dermatologists on behalf of the British Association of Dermatologists and reflect the best data available at the time the report was prepared. Caution should be exercised in interpreting the data: the results of future studies may require alteration of the conclusions or recommendations in this report. It may be necessary or even desirable to depart from the guidelines in the interests of specific patients or special circumstances. Just as adherence to these guidelines may not constitute a defence against a claim of negligence, so deviation from them should not necessarily be deemed negligent.

Introduction

Alopecia areata is a chronic inflammatory disease which affects the hair follicles and sometimes the nails. The onset may be at any age and there is no known race or sex preponderance. Alopecia areata usually presents as patches of hair loss on the scalp but any

Correspondence: Andrew Messenger.
E-mail: a.g.messenger@sheffield.ac.uk

These guidelines were commissioned by the British Association of Dermatologists Therapy Guidelines and Audit subcommittee. Members of the committee are N.H.Cox (Chairman), A.S.Highet, D.Mehta, R.H.Meyrick Thomas, A.D.Ormerod, J.K.Schofield, C.H.Smith and J.C.Sterling.

hair-bearing skin can be involved. The affected skin may be slightly reddened but otherwise appears normal. Short broken hairs (exclamation mark hairs) are frequently seen around the margins of expanding patches of alopecia areata. The nails are involved in about 10% of patients referred for specialist advice. Data from secondary and tertiary referral centres indicate that 34–50% of patients will recover within 1 year, although almost all will experience more than one episode of the disease, and 14–25% progress to total loss of scalp hair (alopecia totalis, AT) or loss of the entire scalp and body hair (alopecia universalis, AU), from which full recovery is unusual (< 10%).[1,2] One study from Japan reported that spontaneous remission within 1 year occurred in 80% of patients with a small number of circumscribed patches of hair loss.[3] The prognosis is less favourable when onset occurs during childhood[1,4–6] and in ophiasis[6] (alopecia areata of the scalp margin). The concurrence of atopic disease has been reported to be associated with a poor prognosis[3,6] but this has been disputed.[7]

About 20% of people with alopecia areata have a family history of the disease, indicating a genetic predisposition.[8] Associations have been reported with a variety of genes, including major histocompatibility complex, cytokine and immunoglobulin genes, suggesting that the genetic predisposition is multifactorial in nature. The hair follicle lesion is probably mediated by T lymphocytes.[9] The association between alopecia areata and other autoimmune diseases suggests that alopecia areata is itself an autoimmune disease, although this is unproven.

Diagnosis

The diagnosis of alopecia areata is usually straightforward although the following may cause diagnostic difficulties:

- Trichotillomania: this condition probably causes most confusion and it is possible that it coexists with alopecia areata in some cases. The incomplete nature of the hair loss in trichotillomania and the fact that the broken hairs are firmly anchored in the scalp (i.e. they remain in the growing phase, anagen, unlike exclamation mark hairs) are distinguishing features
- Tinea capitis: the scalp is inflamed in tinea capitis and there is often scaling but the signs may be subtle
- Early scarring alopecia
- Telogen effluvium
- Anagen effluvium (drug-induced) may mimic diffuse alopecia areata
- Systemic lupus erythematosus
- Secondary syphilis

Occasionally, alopecia areata presents as diffuse hair loss which can be difficult to diagnose. The clinical course often reveals the true diagnosis but a biopsy may be necessary in some cases.

Investigations

Investigations are unnecessary in most cases of alopecia areata. When the diagnosis is in doubt appropriate tests may include:

- Fungal culture
- Skin biopsy
- Serology for lupus erythematosus
- Serology for syphilis

The increased frequency of autoimmune disease in patients with alopecia areata is probably insufficient to justify routine screening.

Management

An overriding consideration in the management of alopecia areata is that, although the disease may have a serious psychological effect, it has no direct impact on general health that justifies the use of hazardous treatments, particularly of unproven efficacy. In addition, many patients, although by no means all, experience spontaneous regrowth of hair.

Counselling

An explanation of alopecia areata, including discussion of the nature and course of the disease and the available treatments, is essential. Some patients are profoundly upset by their alopecia and may require psychological support. Contact with other sufferers and patient support groups may help patients adjust to their disability. The decision to treat alopecia areata actively should not be taken lightly. Treatment can be uncomfortable for the patient, time consuming and potentially toxic. It may also alter the patient's attitude to their hair loss. Some patients find it difficult to cope with relapse following or during initially successful treatment and they should be forewarned of this possibility. These considerations are particularly important in children where the social disruption and focusing of the child's attention on their hair loss, which may result from active treatment, have to be weighed carefully against the potential benefits. On the other hand, some patients are appreciative that something has been tried, even if it does not work.

Treatment

A number of treatments can induce hair growth in alopecia areata but none has been shown to alter the course of the disease. The high rate of spontaneous remission makes it difficult to assess efficacy, particularly in mild forms of the disease. Some trials have been limited to patients with severe alopecia areata where spontaneous remission is unlikely. However, these patients tend to be resistant to all forms of treatment and the failure of a treatment in this setting does not exclude efficacy in mild alopecia areata. Few treatments have been subjected to randomized controlled trials and, except for contact immunotherapy, there are few published data on long-term outcomes.

No treatment

Leaving alopecia areata untreated is a legitimate option for many patients. Spontaneous remission occurs in up to 80% of patients with limited patchy hair loss of short duration (< 1 year),[3] although the remission rate in patients reaching secondary care is lower. Many patients may therefore be managed by reassurance alone, with advice that regrowth cannot be expected within 3 months of the development of any individual patch.

The prognosis in long-standing extensive alopecia is poor. However, all treatments have a high failure rate in this group and some patients prefer not to be treated, other than wearing a wig if appropriate.

Corticosteroids

Topical corticosteroids (Strength of recommendation C, Quality of evidence III; see Appendix 1). Potent topical corticosteroids are widely used to treat alopecia areata but there is little evidence that they promote hair regrowth. A randomized controlled trial of 0·25% desoximetasone cream in 70 patients with patchy alopecia areata failed to show a significant effect over placebo.[10] Topical corticosteroids are ineffective in AT/AU.[11,12] Folliculitis is a common side-effect of topical corticosteroid treatment.

Intralesional corticosteroids (Strength of recommendation B, Quality of evidence III). Depot corticosteroid injected intralesionally stimulates hair regrowth at the site of injection in some patients. Porter and Burton reported that tufts of hair grew in 33 of 34 sites injected with triamcinolone hexacetonide in 11 patients with alopecia areata and in 16 of 25 sites injected with triamcinolone acetonide in 17 patients. The effect lasted about 9 months.[13] In a study from Saudi Arabia 62% of patients achieved full regrowth with monthly injections of triamcinolone acetonide, the response being better in those with fewer than five patches of < 3 cm in diameter.[14] This method is most suitable for treating patchy hair loss of limited extent and for cosmetically sensitive sites such as the eyebrows. Hydrocortisone acetate (25 mg mL^{-1}) and triamcinolone acetonide (5–10 mg mL^{-1}) are commonly used. Corticosteroid is injected just beneath the dermis in the upper subcutis. A 0·05–0·1 mL injection will produce a tuft of hair growth about 0·5 cm in diameter. Multiple injections may be given, the main limitation being patient discomfort. Intralesional corticosteroids may also be administered by a needleless device (e.g. Dermajet™). The device should be sterilized between patients. Abell and Munro reported that 52 of 84 patients (62%) showed regrowth of hair at 12 weeks after three injections of triamcinolone acetonide using the Porto Jet needleless device compared with one of 15 (7%) control subjects injected with isotonic saline.[15] The results were less favourable in AT than in localized alopecia. Skin atrophy at the site of injection is a consistent side-effect of intralesional corticosteroid therapy, particularly if triamcinolone is used, but this usually resolves after a few months. Repeated injection at the same site or the use of higher concentrations of triamcinolone should be avoided as this may cause prolonged skin atrophy. There is a risk of cataract and raised intraocular pressure if intralesional corticosteroids are used close to the eye, e.g. for treating eyebrows.[16] There is a single case report of anaphylaxis in a patient receiving intralesional triamcinolone acetonide for treatment of alopecia areata.[17] Intralesional corticosteroids are not appropriate in rapidly progressive alopecia nor in extensive disease.

Systemic corticosteroids (Strength of recommendation C, Quality of evidence III). Long-term daily treatment with oral corticosteroids will produce regrowth of hair in some patients. One small partly controlled study reported that 30–47% of patients treated with a 6-week tapering course of oral prednisolone (starting at 40 mg daily) showed > 25% hair regrowth.[18] Unfortunately, in most patients continued treatment is needed to maintain hair growth and the response is usually insufficient to justify the risks.[19] There are several reports of high-dose pulsed corticosteroid treatment employing different oral and intravenous regimens (intravenous prednisolone 2 g,[20] intravenous methylprednisolone 250 mg twice daily for 3 days,[21,22] oral prednisolone 300 mg once monthly,[23] dexamethasone 5 mg twice weekly[24]). The differences in treatment protocols and patient selection make it difficult to compare these studies directly, and none was controlled. Overall, about 60% of patients with extensive patchy alopecia showed a cosmetically worthwhile response to pulsed corticosteroids, whereas fewer than 10% of those with ophiasiform disease and AT/AU responded. The oral and intravenous routes of administration appear equally effective. Significant side-effects have not yet been reported with pulsed administration of systemic corticosteroids in alopecia areata. However, short- and long-term hazards of systemic corticosteroids are well known and potentially severe, and in view of these dangers it is not possible to support their use until there is better evidence of efficacy.

Contact immunotherapy (Strength of recommendation B, Quality of evidence II-ii)

Contact immunotherapy was introduced by Rosenberg and Drake in 1976.[25] The contact allergens that have been used in the treatment of alopecia areata include 1-chloro-2,4-dinitrobenzene (DNCB), squaric acid dibutylester (SADBE) and 2,3-diphenylcyclopropenone

(DPCP). DNCB is mutagenic against *Salmonella typhimurium* in the Ames test[26] and is no longer used. Neither SADBE nor DPCP are mutagenic. One DPCP precursor is mutagenic[27] and batches should be screened for contaminants by the supplier. DPCP is more stable in solution and is usually the agent of choice.

The protocol for contact immunotherapy using DPCP was described by Happle *et al.*[28] The patient is sensitized using a 2% solution of DPCP applied to a small area of the scalp. Two weeks later the scalp is painted with a weak solution of DPCP, starting at 0·001%, and this is repeated at weekly intervals. The concentration is increased at each treatment until a mild dermatitis reaction is obtained. Some clinicians treat one side of the scalp initially to distinguish between a treatment response and spontaneous recovery if hair regrowth occurs. Once hair regrowth is observed, both sides of the scalp are treated. In patients with severe long-standing alopecia, in whom spontaneous recovery is unusual, this precaution is unnecessary. Opinions are divided on whether patients should be allowed to treat themselves.

Once a maximum response is achieved most practitioners reduce the frequency of treatment. In patients in whom full regrowth of hair is obtained treatment can be discontinued. Subsequent relapses will usually respond to further contact immunotherapy, although this cannot be guaranteed.

A review of all the published studies of contact immunotherapy concluded that 50–60% of patients achieve a worthwhile response but that the range of response rates was very wide (9–87%).[29] Patients with extensive hair loss are less likely to respond.[30,31] Other reported adverse prognostic features include the presence of nail changes, early onset and a positive family history.[29] In most studies treatment has been discontinued after 6 months if no response is obtained. In a large case series from Canada clinically significant regrowth occurred in about 30% of patients after 6 months of treatment but this increased to 78% after 32 months of treatment, suggesting that more prolonged treatment is worthwhile.[32] The response in patients with AT/AU was less favourable at 17% and this was not improved by treatment beyond 9 months. Relapses may occur following or during treatment. In the Canadian series relapse following successful treatment occurred in 62% of patients.

Two case report series of contact immunotherapy in children with alopecia areata reported response rates of 33%[33] and 32%.[34] A third study found a similar short-term response in children with severe alopecia areata, but < 10% experienced sustained benefit.[35]

Adverse effects. Most patients will develop occipital and/or cervical lymphadenopathy during contact immunotherapy. This is usually temporary but may persist throughout the treatment period. Severe dermatitis is the most common adverse event but the risk can be minimized by careful titration of the concentration. Uncommon adverse effects include urticaria,[36] which may be severe,[37] and vitiligo.[38,39] Cosmetically disabling pigmentary complications, both hyper- and hypopigmentation (including vitiligo), may occur if contact immunotherapy is used in patients with racially pigmented skin. Such patients should be warned of this risk before embarking on treatment. Contact immunotherapy has been in use for 20 years and no long-term side-effects have been reported.

Precautions. Contact immunotherapy is an unlicensed treatment that uses a nonpharmaceutical grade agent. Patients should be fully informed about the nature of the treatment; they should be given an information sheet and give signed consent. Great care must be taken to avoid contact with the allergen by handlers, including pharmacy, medical and nursing staff, and other members of the patient's family. Those applying the allergen should wear gloves and aprons. There are no data on the safety of contact immunotherapy during pregnancy and it should not be used in pregnant women nor in women intending to become pregnant. Owing to these concerns about sensitization and the extent of the measures required to prevent this, and also because of the possible risks in pregnancy, availability of contact immunotherapy is limited and many departments are unwilling to provide this treatment.

DPCP is degraded by light. Solutions should be stored in the dark and patients should wear a hat or wig for 24 h following application.

Phototherapy and photochemotherapy

Ultraviolet B treatment. Although ultraviolet (UV) B erythema has been used in much the same way as other skin irritants there is little documented evidence of efficacy.

Psoralen plus ultraviolet A treatment (Strength of recommendation C, Quality of evidence III). There are several uncontrolled studies of psoralen plus UVA (PUVA) treatment for alopecia areata, using all types of PUVA (oral or topical psoralen, local or whole body UVA irradiation),[40–43] claiming success rates of up to 60–65%. Two retrospective reviews have reported low response rates[44] or suggested that the response was no better than the natural course of the disease,[45] although these observations were also uncontrolled. The relapse rate following treatment is high and continued treatment is usually needed to maintain hair growth, which may lead to an unacceptably high cumulative UVA dose.

Minoxidil (Strength of recommendation C, Quality of evidence IV)

An early double-blind study reported a significantly greater frequency of hair regrowth in patchy alopecia areata in patients treated with topical 1% minoxidil compared with placebo.[46] Subsequent controlled trials in patients with extensive alopecia areata using 1% or 3% minoxidil failed to confirm these results.[47–49] Two of these studies reported a treatment response during an extended but uncontrolled part of the trial.[48,49] In one study comparing 5% and 1% minoxidil in extensive alopecia areata regrowth of hair occurred more frequently in those receiving 5% minoxidil but few subjects obtained a cosmetically worthwhile result.[50] Topical minoxidil is ineffective in AT and AU.

Dithranol (Strength of recommendation C, Quality of evidence IV)

There is a small number of case report series of dithranol (anthralin) or other irritants in the treatment of alopecia areata.[51–53] The lack of controls makes the response rates difficult to evaluate but only a small proportion of patients seems to achieve cosmetically worthwhile results. In one open study 18% of patients with extensive alopecia areata achieved cosmetically worthwhile hair regrowth.[51] The published data indicate that dithranol needs to be applied sufficiently frequently and in a high enough concentration to produce a brisk irritant reaction in order to be effective. Staining of hair limits its use in fair-haired individuals.

Miscellaneous

The dual properties of ciclosporin as an immunosuppressive drug and as a hypertrichotic agent make it a logical choice in treating alopecia areata and this is supported by animal studies. Although there is only a small number of published uncontrolled trials with low patient numbers the evidence that ciclosporin does stimulate hair regrowth in some patients with alopecia areata is convincing.[54] However, as ciclosporin has to be given orally (it is not active topically) side-effects are a major consideration and, in patients with severe alopecia areata, the cosmetically worthwhile response rate is probably too low to justify the risks[55] (*Strength of recommendation D, Quality of evidence III*).

Treatments which were ineffective in controlled trials include oral zinc[56] and isoprinosine.[57] One randomized double-blind trial showed a significant positive effect of aromatherapy.[58] This awaits confirmation.

Wigs

For many female patients with extensive alopecia areata a wig or hairpiece is the most effective solution.[59] Some men also request a wig although male wigs rarely appear as natural. Acrylic wigs are much cheaper than real hair wigs and are easier to look after. However, some patients prefer bespoke real hair wigs, mainly because the better fit allows a wider range of social activities. National Health Service (NHS) charges for wigs are laid out in NHS leaflet HC12 (currently £50·70 for an acrylic wig and £195·40 for a bespoke human hair wig). Information on entitlement to free wigs is given in leaflet HC11.

Summary of recommendations

Alopecia areata is difficult to treat and few treatments have been assessed in randomized controlled trials. The tendency to spontaneous remission and the lack of adverse effects on general health are important considerations in management, and not treating is the best option in many cases. On the other hand, alopecia areata may cause considerable psychological and social disability and in some cases, particularly those seen in secondary care, it may be a chronic and persistent disease causing extensive or universal hair loss. In those cases where treatment is appropriate there is reasonable evidence to support the following:
- *Limited patchy hair loss:* Intralesional corticosteroid (B III).

  Intralesional corticosteroids stimulate hair regrowth at the site of injection. The effect is temporary, lasting a few months, and it is unknown whether the long-term outcome is influenced.
- *Extensive patchy hair loss*: Contact immunotherapy (B II-ii)

- *Alopecia totalis/universalis*: Contact immunotherapy (B II-ii).

Contact immunotherapy is the best-documented treatment in severe alopecia areata but it is not widely available, involves multiple visits to hospital over several months and stimulates cosmetically worthwhile hair regrowth in < 50% of patients with extensive patchy hair loss. It is the only treatment likely to be effective in AT/AU although the response rate in such patients is even lower. It may cause troublesome temporary local inflammation but serious side-effects are rare.

Potent topical corticosteroids and, to a lesser extent, dithranol and minoxidil lotion, are widely prescribed by dermatologists for limited patchy alopecia areata, and are safe, but there is no convincing evidence that they are effective.

Continuous or pulsed systemic corticosteroids and PUVA have also been used to treat alopecia areata. However, in view of the potentially serious side-effects and inadequate evidence of efficacy, none can be recommended at this time.

Children may be treated in a similar fashion to adults. However, intralesional corticosteroids are often poorly tolerated and many clinicians are reluctant to use aggressive treatments such as contact immunotherapy in children.

Patient support

National Alopecia Areata Foundation, PO Box 150760, San Rafael, CA 94915–0760, U.S.A. (This organization supports research and publishes several useful patient information sheets and a regular newsletter.)

Hairline International, Lyons Court, 1668 High Street, Knowle, West Midlands B93 0LY, U.K.

Internet resources

http://www.alopeciaareata.com (National Alopecia Areata Foundation website.)

http://www.ehrs.org (Website of the European Hair Research Society. Links to several alopecia areata sites.)

Conflict of interests

None of the authors has a financial or commercial interest in any of the treatments discussed. A.G.M. occasionally acts as a consultant to pharmaceutical companies who manufacture and market products for the treatment of hair loss disorders.

References

1 Walker SA, Rothman S. Alopecia areata: a statistical study and consideration of endocrine influences. *J Invest Dermatol* 1950; **14**: 403–13.
2 Gip L, Lodin A, Molin L. Alopecia areata. A follow-up investigation of outpatient material. *Acta Derm Venereol (Stockh)* 1969; **49**: 180–8.
3 Ikeda T. A new classification of alopecia areata. *Dermatologica* 1965; **131**: 421–45.
4 Anderson I. Alopecia areata: a clinical study. *Br Med J* 1950; **ii**: 1250–2.
5 Muller SA, Winkelmann RK. Alopecia areata. *Arch Dermatol* 1963; **88**: 290–7.
6 De Waard-van der Spek FB, Oranje AP, De Raeymaecker DM *et al.* Juvenile versus maturity-onset alopecia areata—a comparative retrospective clinical study. *Clin Exp Dermatol* 1989; **14**: 429–33.
7 Sharma VK, Muralidhar S. Treatment of widespread alopecia areata in young patients with monthly oral corticosteroid pulse. *Pediatr Dermatol* 1998; **15**: 313–17.
8 McDonagh AJG, Messenger AG. The pathogenesis of alopecia areata. *Dermatol Clin* 1996; **14**: 661–70.
9 Gilhar A, Ullmann Y, Berkutzki T *et al.* Autoimmune hair loss (alopecia areata) transferred by T lymphocytes to human scalp explants on SCID mice. *J Clin Invest* 1998; **101**: 62–7.
10 Charuwichitratana S, Wattanakrai P, Tanrattanakorn S. Randomized double-blind placebo-controlled trial in the treatment of alopecia areata with 0.25% desoximetasone cream. *Arch Dermatol* 2000; **136**: 1276–7.
11 Pascher F, Kurtin S, Andrade E. Assay of 0.2% fluocinolone acetonide cream for alopecia areata and totalis. *Dermatologica* 1970; **141**: 193–202.
12 Leyden JL, Kligman AM. Treatment of alopecia areata with steroid solution. *Arch Dermatol* 1972; **106**: 924.
13 Porter D, Burton JL. A comparison of intra-lesional triamcinolone hexacetonide and triamcinolone acetonide in alopecia areata. *Br J Dermatol* 1971; **85**: 272–3.
14 Kubeyinje EP. Intralesional triamcinolone acetonide in alopecia areata amongst 62 Saudi Arabs. *East Afr Med J* 1994; **71**: 674–5.
15 Abell E, Munro DD. Intralesional treatment of alopecia areata with triamcinolone acetonide by jet injector. *Br J Dermatol* 1973; **88**: 55–9.
16 Carnahan MC, Goldstein DA. Ocular complications of topical, peri-ocular, and systemic corticosteroids. *Curr Opin Ophthalmol* 2000; **11**: 478–83.
17 Downs AM, Lear JT, Kennedy CT. Anaphylaxis to intradermal triamcinolone acetonide. *Arch Dermatol* 1998; **134**: 1163–4 (Letter).
18 Olsen EA, Carson SC, Turney EA. Systemic steroids with or without 2% topical minoxidil in the treatment of alopecia areata. *Arch Dermatol* 1992; **128**: 1467–73.
19 Winter RJ, Kern F, Blizzard RM. Prednisone therapy for alopecia areata. A follow-up report. *Arch Dermatol* 1976; **112**: 1549–52.
20 Burton JL, Shuster S. Large doses of glucocorticoid in the treatment of alopecia areata. *Acta Derm Venereol (Stockh)* 1975; **55**: 493–6.
21 Friedli A, Labarthe MP, Engelhardt E *et al.* Pulse methylprednisolone therapy for severe alopecia areata: an open prospective study of 45 patients. *J Am Acad Dermatol* 1998; **39**: 597–602.

22 Perriard-Wolfensberger J, Pasche-Koo F, Mainetti C *et al*. Pulse of methylprednisolone in alopecia areata. *Dermatology* 1993; **187**: 282–5.

23 Sharma VK. Pulsed administration of corticosteroids in the treatment of alopecia areata. *Int J Dermatol* 1996; **35**: 133–6.

24 Sharma VK, Gupta S. Twice weekly 5 mg dexamethasone oral pulse in the treatment of extensive alopecia areata. *J Dermatol* 1999; **26**: 562–5.

25 Rosenberg EW, Drake L. In discussion of Dunaway DA. Alopecia areata. *Arch Dermatol* 1976; **112**: 256.

26 Summer KH, Goggelmann W. 1-chloro-2,4-dinitrobenzene depletes glutathione in rat skin and is mutagenic in *Salmonella typhimurium*. *Mutat Res* 1980; **77**: 91–3.

27 Wilkerson MG, Connor TH, Henkin J *et al*. Assessment of diphenylcyclopropenone for photochemically induced mutagenicity in the Ames assay. *J Am Acad Dermatol* 1987; **17**: 606–11.

28 Happle R, Hausen BM, Wiesner-Menzel L. Diphencyprone in the treatment of alopecia areata. *Acta Derm Venereol (Stockh)* 1983; **63**: 49–52.

29 Rokhsar CK, Shupack JL, Vafai JJ *et al*. Efficacy of topical sensitizers in the treatment of alopecia areata. *J Am Acad Dermatol* 1998; **39**: 751–61.

30 van der Steen PH, Baar HM, Happle R *et al*. Prognostic factors in the treatment of alopecia areata with diphenylcyclopropenone. *J Am Acad Dermatol* 1991; **24**: 227–30.

31 Gordon PM, Aldrige RD, McVittie E *et al*. Topical diphencyprone for alopecia areata: evaluation of 48 cases after 30 months' follow-up. *Br J Dermatol* 1996; **134**: 869–71.

32 Wiseman MC, Shapiro J, MacDonald N *et al*. Predictive model for immunotherapy of alopecia areata with diphencyprone. *Arch Dermatol* 2001; **137**: 1063–8.

33 MacDonald Hull SP, Pepall L, Cunliffe WJ. Alopecia areata in children: response to treatment with diphencyprone. *Br J Dermatol* 1991; **125**: 164–8.

34 Schuttelaar ML, Hamstra JJ, Plinck EP *et al*. Alopecia areata in children: treatment with diphencyprone. *Br J Dermatol* 1996; **135**: 581–5.

35 Tosti A, Guidetti MS, Bardazzi F *et al*. Long-term results of topical immunotherapy in children with alopecia totalis or alopecia universalis. *J Am Acad Dermatol* 1996; **35**: 199–201.

36 Tosti A, Guerra L, Bardazzi F. Contact urticaria during topical immunotherapy. *Contact Dermatitis* 1989; **21**: 196–7.

37 Alam M, Gross EA, Savin RC. Severe urticarial reaction to diphenylcyclopropenone therapy for alopecia areata. *J Am Acad Dermatol* 1999; **40**: 110–12.

38 Henderson CA, Ilchyshyn A. Vitiligo complicating diphencyprone sensitization therapy for alopecia universalis. *Br J Dermatol* 1995; **133**: 496–7 (Letter).

39 MacDonald Hull SP, Norris JF, Cotterill JA. Vitiligo following sensitisation with diphencyprone. *Br J Dermatol* 1989; **120**: 232.

40 Claudy AL, Gagnaire D. PUVA treatment of alopecia areata. *Arch Dermatol* 1983; **119**: 975–8.

41 Lassus A, Eskelinen A, Johansson E. Treatment of alopecia areata with three different PUVA modalities. *Photodermatology* 1984; **1**: 141–4.

42 Mitchell AJ, Douglass MC. Topical photochemotherapy for alopecia areata. *J Am Acad Dermatol* 1985; **12**: 644–9.

43 van der Schaar WW, Sillevis SJ. An evaluation of PUVA-therapy for alopecia areata. *Dermatologica* 1984; **168**: 250–2.

44 Taylor CR, Hawk JL. PUVA treatment of alopecia areata partialis, totalis and universalis: audit of 10 years' experience at St John's Institute of Dermatology. *Br J Dermatol* 1995; **133**: 914–18.

45 Healy E, Rogers S. PUVA treatment for alopecia areata—does it work? A retrospective review of 102 cases. *Br J Dermatol* 1993; **129**: 42–4.

46 Fenton DA, Wilkinson JD. Topical minoxidil in the treatment of alopecia areata. *Br Med J* 1983; **287**: 1015–17.

47 Vestey JP, Savin JA. A trial of 1% minoxidil used topically for severe alopecia areata. *Acta Derm Venereol (Stockh)* 1986; **66**: 179–80.

48 Price VH. Double-blind, placebo-controlled evaluation of topical minoxidil in extensive alopecia areata. *J Am Acad Dermatol* 1987; **16**: 730–6.

49 Ranchoff RE, Bergfeld WF, Steck WD *et al*. Extensive alopecia areata. Results of treatment with 3% topical minoxidil. *Cleve Clin J Med* 1989; **56**: 149–54.

50 Fiedler-Weiss VC. Topical minoxidil solution (1% and 5%) in the treatment of alopecia areata. *J Am Acad Dermatol* 1987; **16**: 745–8.

51 Fiedler-Weiss VC, Buys CM. Evaluation of anthralin in the treatment of alopecia areata. *Arch Dermatol* 1987; **123**: 1491–3.

52 Nelson DA, Spielvogel RL. Anthralin therapy for alopecia areata. *Int J Dermatol* 1985; **24**: 606–7.

53 Schmoeckel C, Weissmann I, Plewig G *et al*. Treatment of alopecia areata by anthralin-induced dermatitis. *Arch Dermatol* 1979; **115**: 1254–5.

54 Gupta AK, Ellis CN, Tellner DC *et al*. Cyclosporine A in the treatment of severe alopecia areata. *Transplant Proc* 1988; **20**: 105–8.

55 Shapiro J, Lui H, Tron V *et al*. Systemic cyclosporine and low-dose prednisone in the treatment of chronic severe alopecia areata: a clinical and immunopathologic evaluation. *J Am Acad Dermatol* 1997; **36**: 114–17.

56 Ead RD. Oral zinc sulphate in alopecia areata—a double blind trial. *Br J Dermatol* 1981; **104**: 483–4.

57 Berth-Jones J, Hutchinson PE. Treatment of alopecia totalis with a combination of inosine pranobex and diphencyprone compared to each treatment alone. *Clin Exp Dermatol* 1991; **16**: 172–5.

58 Hay IC, Jamieson M, Ormerod AD. Randomized trial of aromatherapy. Successful treatment for alopecia areata. *Arch Dermatol* 1998; **134**: 1349–52.

59 Cheesbrough MJ. Wigs. *Br Med J* 1989; **299**: 1455–6.

Appendix 1

Strength of recommendations

A There is good evidence to support the use of the procedure

B There is fair evidence to support the use of the procedure

C There is poor evidence to support the use of the procedure

D There is fair evidence to support the rejection of the use of the procedure

E There is good evidence to support the rejection of the use of the procedure

Quality of evidence

I Evidence obtained from at least one properly designed, randomized controlled trial

II-i   Evidence obtained from well-designed controlled trials without randomization

II-ii Evidence obtained from well-designed cohort or case–control analytical studies, preferably from more than one centre or research group

II-iii Evidence obtained from multiple time series with or without the intervention. Dramatic results in uncontrolled experiments (such as the results of the introduction of penicillin treatment in the 1940s) could also be regarded as this type of evidence

III   Opinions of respected authorities based on clinical experience, descriptive studies or reports of expert committees

IV   Evidence inadequate due to problems of methodology (e.g. sample size, or length of comprehensiveness of follow-up or conflicts of evidence).

http://bad.org.uk/Portals/_Bad/Guidelines/Clinical
    %20Guidelines/Alopecia%20Areata.pdf

Comment

Unfortunately, since 2003 there is still a lack of evidence of
efficacy of therapeutic interventions in the management of
AA [1]. A Cochrane systematic review published in 2008
sums up the problem [2] and confirms the therapeutic
nilhism:

> Few treatments for AA have been well evaluated in
> randomised trials. There are no RCTs on the use of
> diphencyprone, dinitrochlorobenzene, intralesional corti-
> costeroids or dithranol although they are commonly used
> for the treatment of (AA). Similarly although topical
> steroids and minoxidil are widely prescribed and appear
> to be safe, there is no convincing evidence that they are
> beneficial in the long-term. Most trials have been reported
> poorly and are so small that any important clinical ben-
> efits are inconclusive. There is a desperate need for large
> well-conducted studies that evaluate long-term effects of
> therapies on quality of life. Considering the possibility of
> spontaneous remission especially for those in the early stages
> of the disease, the options of not being treated or, depending
> on individual preference wearing a wig may be alternative
> ways of dealing with this condition.

One might have expected that the biological therapies
would have helped in AA, but unfortunately, this does not
appear to be the case, as a recently published study reports
that alefacept was not effective in severe AA [3]. As yet,
other studies of other biologics in the management have
not been reported.

REFERENCES

1 MacDonald Hull SP, Wood ML, Hutchinos PE, *et al.* Guidelines for the management of alopecia areata. *Brit J Dermatol*
2003; 149: 692–9.
2 Delamere FM, Sladden MM, Dobbins HM, Leonardi-Bee
J. Interventions for alopecia areata. *Cochrane Database Syst
Rev* 2008; Issue 2: CD004413 (http://www.mrw.interscience.
wiley.com/cochrane/clsysrev/articles/CD004413/frame.html).
3 Strober BE, Menon K, McMichael A, *et al.* Alefacept for
severe alopecia areata: a randomized, double-blind, placebo-
controlled study. *Arch Dermatol* 2009; 145: 1262–6.

Additional professional resources

Alopecia areata, Clinical Knowledge Summaries 2009.
    http://www.cks.nhs.uk/alopecia_areata#.
Garg S, Messenger AG. Alopecia areata: evidence-
    based treatments. *Semin Cutan Med Surg* 2009;
    28:15–18.

BAD patient information leaflet

http://www.bad.org.uk/site/795/default.aspx

Other patient resources

http://www.alopeciaonline.org.uk
http://www.naaf.org
http://www.alopeciaonline.org.uk
http://www.alopecia-awareness.org.uk

Guidelines for the management of bullous pemphigoid

F.WOJNAROWSKA, G.KIRTSCHIG, A.S.HIGHET,* V.A.VENNING† AND
N.P.KHUMALO

Department of Dermatology, Oxford Radcliffe Hospital, The Churchill, Old Road, Headington, Oxford OX3 7LJ, U.K.
*Department of Dermatology, York District Hospital, York YO3 7HE, U.K
†Department of Dermatology, North Hampshire Hospital, Basingstoke, RG24 9NA, U.K.

Accepted for publication 9 January 2002

Summary   These guidelines have been prepared for dermatologists on behalf of the British Association of Dermatologists. They present evidence-based guidance for treatment, with identification of the strength of evidence available at the time of preparation of the guidelines and a brief overview of epidemiological aspects, diagnosis and investigation. The guidelines reflect data available from Medline, Embase, the Cochrane library, literature searches and the experience of the authors of managing patients with bullous pemphigoid in special and general clinics for over 10 years. However, caution should be exercised in interpreting the data obtained from the literature because only six randomized controlled trials are available involving small groups of patients.

Disclaimer

These guidelines have been prepared for dermatologists on behalf of the British Association of Dermatologists and reflect the best data available at the time the report was prepared. Caution should be exercised in interpreting the data: the results of future studies may require alteration of the conclusions or recommendations of this report. It may be necessary or even desirable to depart from the guidelines in the interests of specific patients or special circumstances. Just as adherence to these guidelines may not constitute a defence against a claim of negligence, so deviation from them should not be deemed negligent.

Definition

Bullous pemphigoid (BP) is an acquired autoimmune subepidermal bullous disease in which autoantibodies are directed against components of the basement

Correspondence: Prof. Fenella Wojnarowska.
E-mail: Fenella.Wojnarowska@orh.nhs.uk

These guidelines were prepared for the British Association of Dermatologists Therapy Guidelines and Audit subcommittee. The members are N.H.Cox (Chairman), A.V.Anstey, C.B.Bunker, M.J.D.Goodfield, A.S.Highet, D.Mehta, R.H.Meyrick Thomas and J.K.Schofield.

membrane zone of the skin. Mainly IgG (rarely IgA, IgM and IgE) autoantibodies bind to components of the hemidesmosome adhesion complex, the BP230 and BP180 antigens. The antigen–antibody interaction has been demonstrated to result in subepidermal blister formation in animal models.

Epidemiology

BP is the most common autoimmune blistering disease in the West with an estimated incidence of six to seven cases per million population per year in France and Germany.[1,2] The figures in the U.K. are unknown, but are probably similar or higher. It occurs equally in both sexes and is usually a disease of the elderly (> 70 years) but can also affect younger patients and children. BP has been reported in association with malignancies; however, most large series have concluded that there is no increased incidence of malignancy in patients with BP in western countries compared with age- and sex-matched controls.[3]

Clinical presentation

BP is a non-scarring blistering disease, typically with a flexural distribution of skin lesions. However, the disease may be generalized or may be localized to one site. Mucous membranes are involved in about 50% of patients, with the oral mucosa most frequently affected. Tense blisters arise on either erythematous or normal-appearing skin. Oral lesions consist of small blisters or erosions and are found mainly on the palatal mucosa. The blister formation may be preceded by an urticarial or eczematous rash. The degree of itch varies from none to intense and may precede the appearance of blisters by weeks, months or occasionally years.

Laboratory diagnosis of bullous pemphigoid

The diagnosis is established clinically, histologically and immunopathologically (direct and/or indirect immunofluorescence, IF). All these investigations can be done after treatment has been started,[4] although prolonged treatment will reduce the number of positive IF results.

Biopsy of a fresh blister shows a subepidermal cleft with a mixed dermal inflammatory infiltrate often containing numerous eosinophils. Direct IF of perilesional skin shows linear deposits of IgG and/or C3 at the basement membrane zone (other immunoglobulins may also be present). Indirect IF using serum (blister fluid or urine if no serum can be obtained) demonstrates circulating IgG (sometimes with other immunoglobulins) or C3 binding in a linear pattern at the basement membrane of squamous epithelia (normal skin or monkey oesophagus substrates).

The class of immunoglobulin bound to the basement membrane zone on direct IF distinguishes linear IgA disease (LAD) (only IgA on direct IF) from BP. Indirect IF performed on salt-split skin will differentiate BP from epidermolysis bullosa acquisita (EBA) and from a subgroup of cicatricial pemphigoid (CP). The antibodies are detected at the roof of the artificial blister in BP and at the base in laminin 5-CP and in EBA. However, this is not relevant to most clinical practice, as both CP and EBA are far rarer diseases and none of the published controlled clinical trials in BP has used this method to classify patients.

Differential diagnosis

Other subepidermal autoimmune bullous diseases such as CP, EBA and LAD are the most difficult to differentiate and this is usually done on the combination of the clinical picture (which may evolve with time), direct IF and indirect IF on salt-split skin.

Erythema multiforme, generalized fixed drug eruption, impetigo and acute viral infections (particularly chickenpox in adults) can all be confused with BP on

first presentation. The clinical course, bacterial and viral studies, histopathology and IF studies will all help to achieve a diagnosis.

Treatment

The aim of treatment is to suppress the clinical signs of BP sufficiently to make the disease tolerable to an individual patient (reduction of blister formation, urticarial lesions and pruritus).

The disease is self-limiting and usually remits within 5 years. The mortality rate prior to the use of oral corticosteroids was reported by Lever in 1953 to be 24%;[5] the mortality rates today vary between 6% and 41%.[6] Patients with BP are usually elderly, often on multiple therapies and at high risk of adverse drug reactions and side-effects. High doses of immunosuppressants may put these patients at risk of life-threatening adverse effects more dangerous than the BP.

The treatments available work via different mechanisms. Some aim to suppress the inflammatory process, e.g. corticosteroids, antibiotics (e.g. tetracyclines, sulphones) and other anti-inflammatory drugs. Other immunosuppressive treatments aim to suppress the production of the pathogenic antibodies, e.g. high-dose corticosteroids, azathioprine, methotrexate, cyclophosphamide and cyclosporin. Plasmapheresis removes pathogenic antibodies and inflammatory mediators. Immune-modulating treatments include intravenous immunoglobulins.

There are two approaches to the initial control of the disease, and currently there is insufficient evidence to reject either approach. Some clinicians favour the use of minimum doses of systemic therapy to control the disease, individualizing treatment and accepting that in the occasional patient more aggressive therapy may be needed. Other clinicians believe in controlling all patients with high-dose initial therapy. Treatment is tapered once control of the disease has been achieved. During prolonged maintenance treatment the occasional blister is not an indication for increasing the dose of treatment or changing it. The treatment should be reduced whenever the disease has been well controlled for a month or more. In this way it is possible to ensure that the patient is not being over-treated.

A systematic review of treatments for BP searching Medline, Embase and the Cochrane library identified only six randomized controlled trials (RCTs) with a total of 293 patients.[7] The characteristics and major outcomes of the five relevant studies[8–12] are summarized in Table 1.

Table 1. Randomized controlled trials for the treatment of bullous pemphigoid

First author (follow-up), number of patients treated/randomized, interventions (dose)	Number of patients	Equivalent prednisolone dose in mg daily for a 70-kg patient	Major outcome
Morel[8] 1984 (51 days) 24/26 Pred (0·75 mg kg^{-1}) 22/24 Pred (1·25 mg kg^{-1})	50	52·5 vs. 87·5 mg daily	No significant difference in effectiveness but more side-effects on the higher dose
Burton[9] 1978 (3 years) 13/13 Pred (30–80 mg) 12/12 Azath (2·5 mg kg^{-1} + Pred (30–80 mg)	25	30–80 mg daily (dose per kg body weight not specified)	Lower total dose steroids (45% reduction) in the Azath group
Roujeau[10] 1984 (6 months) 15/17 Pred (0·3 mg kg^{-1}) 22/24 Plasma ex + Pred (0·3 mg kg^{-1})	41	21 mg daily	Lower total dose steroids: 1240 ± 728 mg in the plasma exchange group vs. 2770 ± 1600 mg
Guillaume[11] 1993 (6 months) 31/32 Pred (1 mg kg^{-1}) 36/36 Azath (1·7–2·4 mg kg^{-1}) + Pred (mg kg^{-1}) 31/32 Plasma ex + Pred (mg kg^{-1})	100	70 mg daily	Similar effectiveness in all three groups; severe complications more often noted in the Azath group
Fivenson[12] 1994 (2 & 10 months) 6/6 Pred 40–80 mg 14/14 nicotinamide + tetracycline	20	40–80 mg daily (dose per kg body weight not specified)	Very small numbers, no difference in effectiveness but more severe side-effects and disease recurrence in the Pred group

Pred, prednisolone; Azath, azathioprine; Plasma ex, plasma exchange.

From a systematic review of treatment of BP we can draw three conclusions. Firstly, prednisolone doses higher than 0·75 mg kg^{-1} daily (52·5 mg daily for a 70-kg patient) do not seem to confer additional benefit; doses of systemic corticosteroids greater than 0·75 mg kg^{-1} or prednisolone 30 mg or more daily were all associated with significant mortality.[8,9,11,12] Secondly, the effectiveness of azathioprine and plasma exchange is difficult to assess. Thirdly, tetracyclines and nicotinamide may be effective, but larger trials are needed.

Systemic corticosteroids

The efficacy of systemic corticosteroid treatment in BP was demonstrated in uncontrolled clinical studies and is well established in clinical experience.[13–15] However, few studies are directly comparable because patients differ in severity of disease and there are also differences between treatment regimens, therefore optimum dosage schedules remain a subject for debate.

The corticosteroids most commonly used are prednisolone and prednisone, and dosages relate to these drugs unless otherwise stated. Typical recommendations for widespread disease are for a starting daily dose of about 1 mg kg^{-1} continued until cessation of new blister formation, then gradually decreased according to clinical course.[11,16,17] However, many studies do not closely relate corticosteroid dose to body weight, and tend to use a uniform starting dose, usually ranging between 40 and 80 mg daily, typically 60 mg daily.[14] More recently, lower starting doses of 20–40 mg daily have been recommended.[18]

It is common clinical experience that there is a correlation, albeit approximate, between disease severity and the amount of systemic corticosteroid required for control.[15,19,20] A retrospective study of 23 patients treated with prednisone 1 mg kg^{-1} daily showed a significant correlation between the pretreatment number of blisters and the time needed to achieve control.[16] Aggressive treatment in eight elderly patients with intravenous methylprednisolone 750–1800 mg daily reduced blistering within 24 h, although subsequent morbidity was severe.[21] Systemic corticosteroid therapy seems the best established initial treatment for BP (*Strength of recommendation A, Quality of evidence II*; see Appendix 1).

The introduction of measures for prevention of corticosteroid-induced osteoporosis (guidelines produced by the Bone and Tooth Society of Great Britain and the Royal College of Physicians, 2000) must be considered at the outset of systemic corticosteroid treatment in all patients, and implemented whenever practicable.

Topical corticosteroids

In a study of 10 patients with extensive and generalized BP, treatment with 0·05% clobetasol propionate cream achieved complete healing in all patients within

17 days of treatment. Seven of the 10 patients remained in remission at the time of reporting (1–10 months).[22] Twenty patients with BP (involvement of less than 60% body surface) in a second study were treated with very potent topical corticosteroids: in seven patients BP was completely suppressed and the same number obtained remission with an 11-month follow-up. There were mild side-effects of cutaneous infection and skin atrophy.[23] The use of topical corticosteroids has also been reported in a large number of case reports and smaller series of fewer than five patients.[23–26]

It would seem therefore that topical corticosteroids alone are likely to be most useful for localized and mild to moderate disease (*Strength of recommendation A, Quality of evidence* III). They may be a useful adjunct to systemic treatment.[27] A recent publication by Joly *et al.*[28] also supports the use and benefits of topical corticosteroids as a sole treatment in moderate and severe disease, and highlights the mortality associated with high-dose oral corticosteroids.

Antibiotics and nicotinamide

There is some evidence, one small RCT[12] (Table 1), small uncontrolled trials, and case reports that antibiotics and nicotinamide (niacinamide) should be considered as the first line of treatment for both localized and mild to moderate disease (*Strength of recommendation B, Quality of evidence* II-ii/iii). There are 38 reports (183 patients) of BP treated with tetracycline or erythromycin, often in combination with nicotinamide and sometimes with topical or even oral corticosteroids. Occasional blister formation was accepted in most reports.

There are only two case series involving 11 and 15 patients, and many case reports, of the beneficial effect of erythromycin in children and adults.[29–31] Erythromycin should be considered for treatment, particularly in children (adult dose 1000–3000 mg daily), and perhaps in combination with topical corticosteroids. A beneficial effect may be seen within 1–3 weeks after commencing treatment (*Strength of recommendation B, Quality of evidence* II-iii).

There are several case reports and small series that describe the beneficial effect of tetracyclines, usually in combination with nicotinamide. It was helpful in the majority within 1–3 weeks; however, some patients received topical or even systemic corticosteroids in addition.[12,32–36] There is a small RCT supporting this treatment (see Table 1) and emphasizing the reduction

in side-effects compared with systemic corticosteroids.[12] Tetracyclines and nicotinamide should be considered for treatment in adults, perhaps in combination with topical corticosteroids (*Strength of recommendation B, Quality of evidence* II-ii). The optimum doses are not established. Tetracycline has been used at doses of 500–2000 mg daily, doxycycline at 200–300 mg daily, and minocycline at 100–200 mg daily. Tetracycline should be avoided in renal impairment and doxycycline and minocycline in patients with hepatic impairment. Minocycline should be stopped if hyperpigmentation occurs. A few cases of minocycline-associated pneumonia and eosinophilia are described, necessitating immediate withdrawal of minocycline. Nicotinamide has been used at doses of 500–2500 mg daily; it should be started at 500 mg daily and then gradually increased to 1500–2500 mg daily. When blister formation is suppressed sufficiently the antibiotics and nicotinamide must be reduced slowly, one at a time, over several months to avoid relapse.

Azathioprine

After systemic corticosteroids, azathioprine in doses of up to 2·5 mg kg^{-1} daily is the most commonly used drug in BP. It is mostly employed as an adjunct to systemic corticosteroids for its presumptive 'steroid-sparing' effect. However, the efficacy of azathioprine as a steroid-sparing agent in BP has been addressed in only two RCTs, with conflicting results (Table 1). One RCT reported a 45% reduction in cumulative prednisolone dosage over a 3-year period.[9] Conversely, a larger RCT found no difference in remission rates at 6 months in patients treated with corticosteroids only compared with those receiving combination treatment with prednisolone and azathioprine[11] (*Quality of evidence* IV).

As a sole therapeutic agent, azathioprine has also been reported in very small uncontrolled series to be effective in inducing remission and in maintaining a corticosteroid-induced remission (*Quality of evidence* IV).

Azathioprine dose should be optimized both with regard to efficacy and myelosuppression risk by prior measurement of thiopurine methyltransferase (TMPT) activity, although this test is not universally available. In view of its side-effect profile, it is recommended that azathioprine is only considered as a second-line treatment to prednisolone where response has been inadequate and either the disease is not suppressed or the side-effects are troublesome and unacceptable (*Strength of recommendation B, Quality of evidence* IV).

Dapsone and sulphonamides

There are no RCTs with respect to the use of either dapsone or sulphonamides either as sole treatments or as adjuncts in the management of BP. Four retrospective series covering a total of 110 patients have reported experience with dapsone 50–200 mg daily or (rare cases) with either sulfapyridine or sulfmethoxypyridazine 1–1·5 g daily. These were employed either as sole treatments or in combination with topical corticosteroids. The response rate was around 45% in three series,[37–39] but only 15% in the fourth.[40] Response was slower in onset than with systemic corticosteroids (2–3 weeks) (*Quality of evidence IV*). A single small uncontrolled series reported a possible steroid-sparing effect in patients in whom dapsone was added to existing treatment with prednisolone and azathioprine[41] (*Quality of evidence IV*).

Glucose-6-phosphate dehydrogenase deficiency predisposes to haematological side-effects and should be excluded in predisposed races. The side-effect profile of dapsone and sulphonamides is potentially hazardous in the elderly. These treatments should be considered only if other treatments are ineffective or contraindicated (*Strength of recommendation B, Quality of evidence III*).

Other immunomodulatory treatments

The following treatments may be useful in individual resistant cases.

Cyclophosphamide

Published experience with cyclophosphamide is very limited. In three individual cases, oral and/or intravenous cyclophosphamide was combined with pulsed intravenous dexamethasone and was reported to be of benefit in otherwise extremely resistant BP. Treatment with oral cyclophosphamide 100 mg daily in a small series of 10 patients gave no steroid-sparing effect and an unacceptably high drug-related mortality and morbidity.[42] Cyclophosphamide should be considered only if other treatments have failed or are contraindicated (*Strength of recommendation D, Quality of evidence IV*).

Methotrexate

There are no controlled trials. In one small series methotrexate in low dosage (5–10 mg weekly) permit-

ted reduction of concomitant oral prednisolone. In a prospective open study of 11 patients with BP unresponsive to topical corticosteroids alone, methotrexate (dose range 5–12·5 mg weekly) as the only systemic treatment successfully controlled their disease for periods of 3 months to 2 years.[43] Methotrexate should be considered in patients with concomitant psoriasis and BP (*Strength of recommendation B, Quality of evidence IV*).

Cyclosporin

Experience with cyclosporin is limited to five individual case reports and a small series of seven patients. The evidence for benefit is conflicting, even with relatively high dosage, > 6 mg mg kg^{-1} daily, and responses mainly occurred in patients treated with concomitant oral corticosteroids[44] (*Strength of recommendation D, Quality of evidence IV*).

Mycophenolate mofetil

Mycophenolate mofetil is an inhibitor of purine synthesis in activated T and B cells and is a generally well-tolerated immunosuppressive agent used since 1997 in the prevention of renal graft rejection. It has been used successfully at doses of 0·5–1 g twice daily to control BP in six individual cases, in three cases as an adjunct to oral prednisolone. Further evidence is needed for its role in BP.

Intravenous immunoglobulin

The total published experience of intravenous immunoglobulin in BP amounts to five small series that suggest that it is of limited value. Used mainly at a dose of 0·4 mg kg^{-1} polyvalent immunoglobulin daily for 5 days, either as a sole treatment or with oral prednisolone, it produced some occasional dramatic but unfortunately very transient responses that were too short-lived to be useful[45,46] (*Strength of recommendation D, Quality of evidence III*).

Chlorambucil

In an open study of 26 patients with BP, treatment was started with prednisolone 40–60 mg daily and chlorambucil at approximately 0·1–0·15 mg kg^{-1} daily.[47] After 2 weeks the doses of both drugs were gradually reduced; the maintenance dose of chlorambucil was usually 2 mg daily. The mean duration of therapy and the mean total corticosteroid requirement were both lower than in other studies using corticosteroids plus azathioprine.

Chlorambucil should be considered as an alternative to other more established immunosuppressants if these have failed or are poorly tolerated or contraindicated. Careful monitoring is required for possible haematological toxicity (*Strength of recommendation B, Quality of evidence* III).

Plasmapheresis (plasma exchange)

There have been only two RCTs[10,11] (Table 1), several small series and a number of case reports (100–150 patients) of the use of plasmapheresis (plasma exchange) in the treatment of BP. The regimens used, the additional therapy, and the results have been very variable. There is no evidence to support the use of plasmapheresis in routine treatment of BP, although at low corticosteroid doses a steroid-sparing effect was seen (*Strength of recommendation D, Quality of evidence II-i*). There may be a limited role for plasmapheresis in resistant cases of BP where side-effects are a major issue or the disease is uncontrolled[48] (*Strength of recommendation B, Quality of evidence* III).

Follow-up

BP is a long-term disease, and ideally all patients should be followed until they are in complete remission and off all treatment. They should be regularly reviewed to ensure that they are not being continued on higher doses of topical or systemic treatment than are necessary to provide sufficient control of their disease. The occasional urticated lesion or blister is acceptable, and indicates that the patient is not being over-treated. We suggest attempted reduction of medication every 1–2 months in stable patients; this should be done on clinical rather than IF criteria.

Audit

There is no established optimum treatment for BP, and thus no gold standard against which to audit clinical practice.

Suggested audit points:

- Evidence of a clear management strategy
- Scrutiny of prednisolone dosage used

- Implementation of measures to minimize and reduce corticosteroid dosage
- Indications for use of azathioprine and other immunosuppressants
- Monitoring of drug therapy
  - Corticosteroid side-effects in relation to dose
  - Implementation of osteoporosis prophylaxis
  - TMPT screening prior to the use of azathioprine
  - Drug monitoring of dapsone, sulphonamide or immunosuppressant treatment.

Recommendations

BP is a common disease of the elderly. With our ageing population it will become increasingly frequent, and the age of the patients will add to the complexity of treatment. There is a clear need to determine how to stratify patients clinically, and to ascertain the optimum regimens for treating mild, moderate and severe BP.

- Systemic corticosteroids are the best established treatment. Recommended initial doses of prednisolone are 20 mg or 0.3 mg kg^{-1} daily in localized or mild disease, 40 mg or 0.6 mg kg^{-1} daily in moderate disease, and 50–70 mg or 0.75–1 mg kg^{-1} daily in severe disease. Measures to prevent osteoporosis must be implemented from the start of systemic corticosteroid therapy, whenever practicable.
- For localized BP, very potent topical corticosteroids are worth trying first.
- For mild to moderate disease tetracycline and nicotinamide should be considered.
- Immunosuppressants cannot be recommended routinely from the outset but should only be considered if the corticosteroid dose cannot be reduced to an acceptable level. Azathioprine is the best established; methotrexate may be considered in patients with additional psoriasis.
- Topical corticosteroids should be considered in any patient with BP; they may help to achieve control if this is only borderline using systemic agents. The aim of treatment is to suppress the clinical signs of BP sufficiently to make the disease tolerable to an individual patient. We recommend to aim for reduction, but not complete suppression, of blister formation, urticarial lesions and pruritus.

References

1 Bernard P, Vaillant L, Labeille B *et al.* Incidence and distribution of subepidermal autoimmune bullous skin diseases in three French regions. *Arch Dermatol* 1995; **131**: 48–52.

2 Zillikens D, Wever S, Roth A *et al.* Incidence of autoimmune subepidermal blistering dermatoses in a region of Central Germany. *Arch Dermatol* 1995; **131**: 957–8.

3 Venning VA, Wojnarowska F. The association of bullous pemphigoid and malignant disease: a case control study. *Br J Dermatol* 1990; **123**: 439–45.

4 Anstey A, Venning VA, Wojnarowska F *et al.* Determination of the optimum site for biopsy for direct immunofluorescence in bullous pemphigoid. *Clin Exp Dermatol* 1990; **15**: 438–41.

5 Lever WF. Pemphigus. *Medicine* 1953; **32**: 2–123.

6 Korman NJ. Bullous pemphigoid. The latest in diagnosis, prognosis and therapy. *Arch Dermatol* 1998; **134**: 1137–41.

7 Khumalo NP, Murrell DF, Wojnarowska F, Kirtschig G. A systematic review of treatments for bullous pemphigoid. *Arch Dermatol* 2002; **138**: 385–9.

8 Morel P, Guillaume J-C. Treatment of bullous pemphigoid with prednisolone only: 0.75 mg/kg/day versus 1.25 mg/kg/day. A multicenter randomized study. *Ann Dermatol Venereol* 1984; **111**: 925–8.

9 Burton JL, Harman RR, Peachey RD, Warin RP. Azathioprine plus prednisone in treatment of pemphigoid. *Br Med J* 1978; **ii**: 1190–1.

10 Roujeau JC, Guillaume J-C, Morel P *et al.* Plasma exchange in bullous pemphigoid. *Lancet* 1984; **ii**: 486–8.

11 Guillaume J-C, Vaillant L, Bernard P *et al.* Controlled trial of azathioprine and plasma exchange in addition to prednisolone in the treatment of bullous pemphigoid. *Arch Dermatol* 1993; **129**: 49–53.

12 Fivenson D, Breneman D, Rosen G *et al.* Nicotinamide and tetracycline therapy of bullous pemphigoid. *Arch Dermatol* 1994; **130**: 753–8.

13 Stevenson CJ. Treatment in bullous diseases with corticosteroid drugs and corticotrophin. *Br J Dermatol* 1960; **72**: 11–19.

14 Church R. Pemphigoid treated with corticosteroids. *Br J Dermatol* 1960; **72**: 434–41.

15 Downham TF, Chapel TA. Bullous pemphigoid. *Arch Dermatol* 1978; **114**: 1639–42.

16 Chosidow O, Saada V, Diquet B *et al.* Correlation between the pretreatment number of blisters and the time to control bullous pemphigoid with prednisone 1 mg/kg/day. *Br J Dermatol* 1992; **127**: 185–95.

17 Fine J-D. Management of acquired bullous skin diseases. *N Engl J Med* 1995; **333**: 1475–84.

18 Wojnarowska F, Eady RAJ, Burge SM. Bullous eruptions. In: *Textbook of Dermatology* (Champion RH, Burton JL, Burns DA, Breathnach SM, eds.), 6th edn. Oxford: Blackwell Science, 1998; 1817–98.

19 Venning VA, Wojnarowska F. Lack of predictive factors for the clinical course of bullous pemphigoid. *J Am Acad Dermatol* 1992; **26**: 585–9.

20 Person JR, Rogers RS, Perry HO. Localised pemphigoid. *Br J Dermatol* 1976; **95**: 531–3.

21 Siegel J, Eaglstein WH. High-dose methylprednisolone in the treatment of bullous pemphigoid. *Arch Dermatol* 1984; **120**: 1157–65.

22 Westerhof W. Treatment of bullous pemphigoid with topical clobetasol propionate. *J Am Acad Dermatol* 1989; **20**: 458–61.

23 Zimmermann R, Faure M, Claudy A. Prospective study of treatment of bullous pemphigoid by a class I topical corticosteroid. *Ann Dermatol Venereol* 1999; **126**: 13–16.

24 Muramatsu T, Iida T, Shirai T. Pemphigoid and pemphigus foliaceus successfully treated with topical corticosteroids. *J Dermatol* 1996; **23**: 683–8.

25 Spuls PI, Brakman M, Westerhof W, Bos JD. Treatment of generalized bullous pemphigoid with topical corticosteroids. *Acta Derm Venereol (Stockh)* 1995; **75**: 89 [Letter].

26 Paquet P, Richelle M, Lapiere CM. Bullous pemphigoid treated by topical corticosteroids. *Acta Derm Venereol (Stockh)* 1991; **71**: 534–5.

27 Loche F, Bazex J, Giard A *et al.* Efficacy and tolerability of topical corticosteroid treatment in the initial phase of bullous pemphigoid: an open study of 13 cases. *J Dermatol Treat* 1995; **6**: 69–72.

28 Joly P, Roujeau JC, Benichou J *et al.* A comparison of oral and topical corticosteroids in patients with bullous pemphigoid. *N Engl J Med* 2002; **346**: 321–7.

29 Fox BJ, Odom RB, Findlay RF. Erythromycin therapy in bullous pemphigoid: possible anti-inflammatory effects. *J Am Acad Dermatol* 1982; **7**: 504–10.

30 Altomare G, Capella GL, Fracchiolla C, Frigerio E. Treatment with erythromycin: a reappraisal. *Eur J Dermatol* 1999; **9**: 583–5.

31 Mensing H, Krauße S. Therapie des bullösen Pemphigoids mit Erythromycin. *Med Klin* 1990; **85**: 481–4.

32 Thomas I, Khorenian S, Arbesfeld DM. Treatment of generalized bullous pemphigoid with oral tetracycline. *J Am Acad Dermatol* 1993; **28**: 74–7.

33 Kawahara Y, Hashimoto T, Ohata Y, Nishikawa T. Eleven cases of bullous pemphigoid treated with a combination of minocycline and nicotinamide. *Eur J Dermatol* 1996; **6**: 427–9.

34 Kolbach DN, Remme JJ, Bos WH *et al.* Bullous pemphigoid successfully controlled by tetracycline and nicotinamide. *Br J Dermatol* 1995; **133**: 88–90.

35 Hornschuh B, Hamm H, Wever S *et al.* Treatment of 16 patients with bullous pemphigoid with oral tetracycline and niacinamide and topical clobetasol. *J Am Acad Dermatol* 1997; **36**: 101–3.

36 Depaire-Duclos F, Dandurand M, Basset-Seguin N *et al.* Treatment of bullous pemphigoid with tetracyclines and topical corticosteroids. *Eur J Dermatol* 1997; **7**: 570–3.

37 Phiamphonsongant T. Dapsone for the treatment of bullous pemphigoid. *Asian Pacific J Allergy Immunol* 1983; **1**: 19–21.

38 Venning VA, Millard PR, Wojnarowska F. Dapsone as first line therapy for bullous pemphigoid. *Br J Dermatol* 1989; **120**: 83–92.

39 Bouscarat F, Chosidow O, Picard-Dahan C *et al.* Treatment of bullous pemphigoid with dapsone: retrospective study of thirty-six cases. *J Am Acad Dermatol* 1996; **34**: 683–4.

40 Person J, Rogers R. Bullous pemphigoid responding to sulfapyridine and the sulfones. *Arch Dermatol* 1977; **113**: 610–15.

41 Jeffes EW, Ahmed AR. Adjuvant therapy of bullous pemphigoid with dapsone. *Clin Exp Dermatol* 1989; **14**: 132–6.

42 Itoh T, Hosokawa H, Shirai Y, Horio T. Successful treatment of bullous pemphigoid with pulsed intravenous cyclophosphamide. *Br J Dermatol* 1996; **134**: 931–3.

43 Heilborn JD, Stahle-Backdahl M, Albertioni F *et al.* Low-dose oral pulse methotrexate as monotherapy in elderly patients with bullous pemphigoid. *J Am Acad Dermatol* 1999; **40**: 741–9.

44 Barthelemy H, Thivolet J, Cambazard F *et al.* Cyclosporin in the treatment of bullous pemphigoid: preliminary study. *Ann Dermatol Venereol* 1986; **113**: 309–13.

45 Tappeiner G, Steiner A. High-dosage intravenous gamma globulin: therapeutic failure in pemphigus and pemphigoid. *J Am Acad Dermatol* 1989; **20**: 684–5.

46 Harman KE, Black MM. High-dose intravenous immune globulin for the treatment of autoimmune blistering diseases: an evaluation of its use in 14 cases. *Br J Dermatol* 1999; **140**: 865–74.

© 2002 British Association of Dermatologists

47 Milligan A, Hutchinson PE. The use of chlorambucil in the treatment of bullous pemphigoid. *J Am Acad Dermatol* 1990; **22**: 796–801.

48 Egan CA, Meadows KP, Zone JJ. Plasmapheresis as a steroid saving procedure in bullous pemphigoid. *Int J Dermatol* 2000; **39**: 230–5.

Appendix 1

Strength of recommendations

A There is good evidence to support the use of the procedure

B There is fair evidence to support the use of the procedure

C There is poor evidence to support the use of the procedure

D There is fair evidence to support the rejection of the use of the procedure

E There is good evidence to support the rejection of the use of the procedure.

Quality of evidence

I   Evidence obtained from at least one properly designed, randomized controlled trial

II-i   Evidence obtained from well-designed controlled trials without randomization

II-ii   Evidence obtained from well-designed cohort or case–control analytical studies, preferably from more than one centre or research group

II-iii Evidence obtained from multiple time series with or without the intervention. Dramatic results in uncontrolled experiments (such as the results of the introduction of penicillin treatment in the 1940s) could also be regarded as this type of evidence

III   Opinions of respected authorities based on clinical experience, descriptive studies or reports of expert committees

IV   Evidence inadequate due to problems of methodology (e.g. sample size, or length of comprehensiveness of follow-up or conflicts of evidence).

http://bad.org.uk/Portals/_Bad/Guidelines/Clinical
%20Guidelines/Bullous%20Pemphigoid.pdf

Comment

Further developments since the publication of 2002 guidelines [1] are the trend towards reducing the morbidity and mortality associated with prolonged high-dose prednisolone [2–5] with steroid sparing agents or topical corticosteroids. Joly *et al*'s study has demonstrated that topical corticosteroids can be successfully used to control bullous pemphigoid associated with a much-reduced morbidity [4]. An ongoing multicentre UK clinical trial is investigating the efficiency of tetracylines in the management of bullous pemphigoid [6].

REFERENCES

1 Wojnarowska F, Kirtschig G, Highet AS. Guidelines for the management of bullous pemphigoid. *Brit J Dermatol* 2002; 147: 214–21.
2 Kirtschig G, Middleton P, Hollis S, Wojnarowska F, Murrell DF. Interventions for bullous pemphigoid. *Cochrane Database Syst Rev* 2005; Issue 3: CD002292 (http://mrw.interscience.wiley.com/cochrane/clsysrev/articles/CD002292/frame.html).
3 Alexandroff AB, Harman KE. Blistering skin disorders: an evidence-based update. Conference report. *Br J Dermatol* 2009; 160: 502–4.
4 Joly P, Roujeau JC, Delaporte E, *et al*. A comparison of two regimens of topical corticosteroids in the treatment of patients with bullous pemphigoid: a multicenter randomized study. *J Invest Dermatol* 2009; 129: 1681–7.
5 Gürcan HM, Ahmed AR. Analysis of current data on the use of methotrexate in the treatment of pemphigus and pemphigoid. *Br J Dermatol* 2009; 161: 723–31.
6 http://www.ukdctn.org/ongoing/blister/Study_Synopsis.pdf

Additional professional resources

Chan L. Bullous pemphigoid. http://emedicine.medscape.com/article/1062391-overview.
http://www.dermnetnz.org/immune/pemphigoid.html
http://www.dermnetnz.org/immune/pemphigoid-gestationis.html

BAD patient information leaflet

http://www.bad.org.uk/site/852/default.aspx

Related to pemphigoid gestationis

http://www.bad.org.uk/site/853/default.aspx

Other patient resources

http://www.emedicine.com/derm/topic64.htm
http://www.medicinenet.com/bullous_pemphigoid/article.htm
http://www.dermnetnz.org/dna.bullous.pemphigoid/bulpem.html
http://www.patient.co.uk/pdf/pilsL387.pdf

Guidelines for the management of contact dermatitis: an update

J. Bourke, I. Coulson* and J. English†

Department of Dermatology, South Infirmary, Victoria Hospital, Cork, Ireland
*Department of Dermatology, Burnley General Hospital, Burnley, U.K.
†Department of Dermatology, Queen's Medical Centre, Nottingham University Hospital, Nottingham NG7 2UH, U.K.

Summary   These guidelines for management of contact dermatitis have been prepared for dermatologists on behalf of the British Association of Dermatologists. They present evidence-based guidance for investigation and treatment, with identification of the strength of evidence available at the time of preparation of the guidelines, ncluding details of relevant epidemiological aspects, diagnosis and investigation.

Disclaimer

These guidelines have been prepared for dermatologists on behalf of the British Association of Dermatologists and reflect the best data available at the time the report was prepared. Caution should be exercised in interpreting the data; the results of future studies may require alteration of the conclusions or recommendations in this report. It may be necessary or even desirable to depart from the guidelines in the interests of specific patients and special circumstances. Just as adherence to guidelines may not constitute defence against a claim of negligence, so deviation from them should not necessarily be deemed negligent.

Definition

The words 'eczema' and 'dermatitis' are often used synonymously to describe a polymorphic pattern of inflammation, which in the acute phase is characterized by erythema and vesiculation, and in the chronic phase by dryness, lichenification and fissuring. Contact dermatitis describes these patterns of reaction in response to external agents, which may be the result of the external agents acting either as irritants, where the T cell-mediated immune response is not involved, or as allergens, where cell-mediated immunity is involved.

Contact dermatitis may be classified into the following reaction types:

Subjective irritancy – idiosyncratic stinging and smarting reactions that occur within minutes of contact, usually on the face, in the absence of visible changes. Cosmetic or sunscreen constituents are common precipitants.

Acute irritant contact dermatitis – often the result of a single overwhelming exposure or a few brief exposures to strong irritants or caustic agents.

Chronic (cumulative) irritant contact dermatitis – this occurs following repetitive exposure to weaker irritants which may be either 'wet', such as detergents, organic solvents, soaps, weak acids and alkalis, or 'dry', such as low humidity air, heat, powders and dusts.

Allergic contact dermatitis – this involves sensitization of the immune system to a specific allergen or allergens with resulting dermatitis or exacerbation of pre-existing dermatitis.

Phototoxic, photoallergic and photoaggravated contact dermatitis – some allergens are also photoallergens. It is not always easy to distinguish between photoallergic and phototoxic reactions.

Systemic contact dermatitis – seen after the systemic administration of a substance, usually a drug, to which topical sensitization has previously occurred.

In practice, it is not uncommon for endogenous, irritant and allergic aetiologies to coexist in the development of certain eczemas, particularly hand and foot eczema. It is important to recognize and seek in the history, or by a home or workplace visit, any recreational and occupational factors in irritant and allergic dermatitis.

Other types of contact reactions are not discussed in these guidelines. Strength of recommendations and quality of evidence gradings are listed in Appendix 1.

Epidemiology

Properly designed and conducted studies to determine the prevalence of dermatitis in the general community are few but the point prevalence of dermatitis in the U.K. is estimated at about 20%, with atopic eczema forming the majority.[1] The best studies show a point prevalence of hand dermatitis in South Sweden of 2%[2] and the lifetime risk of developing hand eczema to be 20% in women.[3] Irritant contact dermatitis is more common than allergic dermatitis; allergic dermatitis usually carries a worse prognosis than irritant dermatitis unless the allergen is identified and avoided.

Contact dermatitis accounts for 4–7% of dermatological consultations. Chronicity is commonest in those allergic to nickel and chromate. Occupational dermatitis remains a burden for those affected. The most recent THOR/EPIDERM figures indicate that skin disease follows mental illness and musculoskeletal problems as a cause of occupational disease and accounts for approximately one in seven reported work-related cases in the U.K.[4] Occupational dermatitis makes up the bulk of occupational skin disease (approximately 70%) with a rate of 68 per million of the population presenting to dermatologists annually and 260 per million to occupational physicians who tend to see earlier and less severe skin disease.

The number of reports of allergic contact dermatitis in children is increasing.[5] The principle allergens which have been identified include nickel, topical antibiotics, preservative chemicals, fragrances and rubber accelerators. Children with eczematous eruptions should be patch tested, particularly those with hand and eyelid eczema[6] (*Quality of evidence II.ii*) (*Strength of recommendation A*).

Contact allergy to specific allergens has been estimated in the general population to be 4·5% for nickel,[7] and 1–3% of the population are allergic to ingredient(s) of a cosmetic.[8] The prevalence of allergy to the other common allergens in the general population is not known as almost all studies have patch tested selected groups rather than general populations.

Who should be investigated?

Many authors have identified the unreliability of clinical features alone in distinguishing allergic contact from irritant and endogenous eczema, particularly with hand and facial eczema.[9–12] Patch testing is therefore an essential investigation in patients with persistent eczematous eruptions when contact allergy is suspected or cannot be ruled out (*Quality of evidence II.ii*) (*Strength of recommendation A*). A prospective study[13] has confirmed the value of a specialist contact clinic in the diagnosis of contact dermatitis. It highlighted the importance of formal training in patch test reading and interpretation, testing with additional series and prick testing in the investigation of patients with contact dermatitis (*Quality of evidence II.i*) (*Strength of recommendation A*).

Referral rate

An approximate annual workload for a contact dermatitis investigation clinic has been suggested to be one individual investigated per 700 of the population served[14] (*Quality of evidence II.ii*) (*Strength of recommendation B*), i.e. 100 patients patch tested for every 70 000 of the catchment population per year. A positive linear relationship was found between the number of relevant allergic patch test reactions and the number of patients referred by individual consultants.

Diagnostic tests

Patch testing

The mainstay of diagnosis in allergic contact dermatitis is the patch test. This test has a sensitivity and specificity of between 70% and 80%[15] (*Quality of evidence II.ii*) (*Strength of recommendation A*).

Patch testing involves the reproduction under the patch tests of allergic contact dermatitis in an individual sensitized to a particular antigen(s). The standard method involves the application of antigen to the skin at standardized concentrations in an appropriate vehicle and under occlusion. The back is most commonly used principally for convenience because of the area available, although the limbs, in particular the outer upper arms, are also used. Various application systems are available of which the most commonly used are Finn chambers. With this system, the investigator adds the individual allergens to test discs that are loaded on to adhesive tape. Two preprepared series of patch tests are available – the TRUE (Pharmacia, Milton Keynes, U.K.) and the Epiquick (Hermal, Reinbek, Germany) tests. There are few comparative studies between the different systems. Preprepared tests are significantly more reliable than operator-prepared tests[16–20] (*Quality of evidence I*). There is also some evidence that larger chambers may give more reproducible tests,[21] but this may only apply to some allergens[22] (*Quality of evidence II.ii*), and can be used to obtain a more definite positive reaction when a smaller chamber has previously given a doubtful one. The International Contact Dermatitis Research Group has laid down the standardization of gradings, methods and nomenclature for patch testing.[23]

Timing of patch test readings

The optimum timing of the patch test readings is probably day 2 and day 4.[24] An additional reading at day 6 or 7 will pick up approximately 10% more positives that were negative at days 2 and 4[25] (*Quality of evidence II.ii*) (*Strength of recommendation A*). The commonest allergens that may become positive after day 4 are neomycin, tixocortol pivalate and nickel.

Relevance of positive reactions

An assessment should be made of the relevance of each positive reaction to the patient's presenting dermatitis. Unfortunately this is not always a simple task even with careful history taking and knowledge of the allergen's likely sources and the patient's occupation and/or hobbies. Textbooks on contact dermatitis are an invaluable resource in this regard (Appendix 2). A simple and pragmatic way of classifying clinical relevance of positive allergic patch test reactions is: (i) *current relevance* – the patient has been exposed to allergen during the current episode of dermatitis and improves when the exposure ceases; (ii) *past relevance* – past episode of dermatitis from exposure to allergen; (iii) *relevance not known* – not sure if exposure is current or old; (iv) *cross reaction* – the positive test is due to cross-reaction with another allergen; and (v) *exposed* – a history of exposure but not resulting in dermatitis from that exposure, or no history of exposure but a definite positive allergic patch test.

Patch test series

The usual approach to patch testing is to have a screening series, which will pick up approximately 80% of allergens.[26,27] Such series vary from country to country. There are two principal standard series, differing between the U.S.A. and Europe. Most dermatologists adapt these series by adding allergens that may be of local importance. The standard series should be revised on a regular basis. The North American Contact Dermatitis Group extended its standard series to a total of 49 allergens and the British Contact Dermatitis Society (BCDS) in 2001 expanded its series to include several common bases and preservatives (Appendix 3) and a number of other important allergens. There are six additions to the BCDS standard series. Following the emergence of new fragrance allergens, a new mix [Fragrance mix II: hydroxyisohexyl 3-cyclohexene carboxaldehyde (Lyral), citral, farnesol, citronellol, alpha-hexyl-cinnamic aldehyde] has been tested and validated as a useful screening tool for fragrance allergy.[28] The specific allergen Lyral is also tested separately because of the number of new cases of allergy reported.[29] Compositae mix (2·5% pet.) has

been recommended as it increases the rate of detecting Compositae allergy.[30] Disperse Blue mix, which contains the two commonest textile dye allergens Disperse Blue 106 and 124, has also been added to the standard series.[31] More recently, propolis and sodium metabisulphite have also been added to the standard series. Five supplemental series have also been recommended. These series are outlined in Appendix 3. Supplemental series should be used to complement the standard series for particular body sites or types of agents to which the patient is exposed (Appendixes 3 and 4). The patient's own cosmetics, toiletries and medicaments should be tested at non-irritant concentrations. This usually means 'as is' (undiluted product) for leave-on products and dilutions for wash-off products. Strong irritants such as powder detergents should not be patch tested. Occupational products should also be tested at nonirritant concentrations. The most useful reference source for documented test concentrations and vehicles of chemicals, groups of chemicals and products is that by De Groot.[32] Guidelines for testing patients' own materials can be found in the *Handbook of Occupational Dermatology*.[33] However, false positives and false negatives often occur when patch testing products brought by the patient.

Photopatch testing

Where photoallergic dermatitis is suspected, photopatch testing may be carried out.[34] Very briefly, the standard method of photopatch testing involves the application of the photoallergen series and any suspected materials in duplicate on either side of the upper back. One side is irradiated with 5 J cm^{-2} of ultraviolet (UV) A after an interval (1 or 2 days) and readings are taken in parallel after a further 2 days. The exact intervals for irradiation and the dose of UVA given vary from centre to centre. The U.K. multicentre study into photopatch testing has now been completed and published.[35] It is recommended that allergens be subjected to 5 J cm^{-2} UVA and a reading taken after 2 days. The incidence of photoallergy in suspected cases was low at under 5%; however, further readings at 3 and 4 days increased the detection rate. The issue of whether to irradiate the test site after 1 or 2 days of allergen application was addressed in a separate study, which found in favour of a 2-day interval[36] (*Quality of evidence II.ii*) (*Strength of recommendation A*).

Open patch testing

The open patch test is commonly used where potential irritants or sensitizers are being assessed. It is also useful in the investigation of contact urticaria and protein contact dermatitis. The open patch test is usually performed on the forearm but the upper outer arm or scapular areas may also be used. The site should be assessed at regular intervals for the first 30–60 min and a later reading should be carried out after 3–4 days. A repeated open application test, applying the suspect agent on to the forearm, is also useful in the assessment of cosmetics, where irritancy or combination effects may interfere with standard patch testing. This usually involves application of the product twice daily for up to a week, stopping if a reaction develops.

Preparation of the patient

A number of factors may alter the accuracy of patch testing. Principal among these are the characteristics of the individual allergens and the method of patch testing. Some allergens are more likely to cause irritant reactions than others. These reactions may be difficult to interpret and are easily misclassified as positive reactions. Nickel, cobalt, potassium dichromate and carba mix are the most notable offenders in the standard series. As indicated above, preprepared patch tests are better standardized in terms of the amount of allergen applied and are therefore more reproducible, but are prohibitively expensive in the U.K.

Patient characteristics are also important. It is essential that the skin on the back is free from dermatitis and that skin disease elsewhere is as well controlled as possible. This will help to avoid the 'angry back syndrome' with numerous false positives.[37] However, if a patient applies potent topical steroids to the back up to 2 days prior to the test being applied[38–40] (*Quality of evidence* I), or is taking oral corticosteroids or immunosuppressant drugs, then there is a significant risk of false negative results. It has been claimed that patch testing is reliable with doses of prednisolone up to 20 mg per day but that figure is based on poison ivy allergy, which causes strongly positive patch tests[41] (*Quality of evidence* II.iii). The effect of systemic steroids on weaker reactions has not been assessed but clinical experience would suggest that if the daily dose is no higher than 10 mg prednisolone, suppression of positive patch tests is unlikely. UV radiation may also interfere with patch test results[42] but the amount required to do so and the relevant interval between exposure and patch testing are poorly quantified (*Quality of evidence* II.iii).

Testing for immediate (type I) hypersensitivity

Although not strictly a part of assessment of contact dermatitis this is important particularly in the situation of hand dermatitis. Type I hypersensitivity to natural rubber latex (NRL) may complicate allergic, irritant or atopic hand dermatitis and may be seen in combination with delayed (type IV) hypersensitivity to NRL or rubber additives. The two skin tests in common use are the prick test and the use test. Prick testing involves an intradermal puncture through a drop of NRL extract. A positive reaction consists of an urticarial weal, which is usually apparent after 15 min, although it may take as long as 45 min to develop. A positive control test of histamine should be performed to check the patient does not give a false negative reaction from oral antihistamine ingestion. A negative control prick test with saline should also be performed to check if the patient is dermographic. The use test involves application of a glove that has been soaked for 20 min in water or saline. The prick test is generally favoured over the use test because of

reports of anaphylaxis following the latter[43] (*Quality of evidence* II.iii) (*Strength of recommendation* A). There are also occasional reports of anaphylaxis following prick testing with NRL extract.[44] With the advent of standardized commercially available NRL extracts this risk is probably greatly reduced. Some clinicians may prefer to perform a radioallergosorbent test (RAST) for NRL allergy, as they may not have adequate facilities or training to deal with anaphylaxis; however, the sensitivity and specificity may be less for RAST compared with prick testing. Skin prick and use tests are also useful when investigating protein contact dermatitis in occupations at risk such as chefs or veterinarians.

Intervention and treatment

Irritant contact dermatitis

The management of irritant contact dermatitis principally involves the protection of the skin from irritants. The most common irritants are soaps and detergents, although water itself is also an irritant. In occupational settings other irritants such as oils and coolants, alkalis, acids and solvents may be important. The principles of management involve avoidance, protection and substitution, as follows.

Avoidance

In general, this is self-evident. However, a visit to the workplace may be necessary to identify all potential skin hazards.

Protection

Most irritant contact dermatitis involves the hands. Gloves are therefore the mainstay of protection. For general purposes and household tasks, rubber or polyvinyl chloride household gloves, possibly with a cotton liner or worn over cotton gloves, should suffice. It is important to take off the gloves on a regular basis as sweating may aggravate existing dermatitis. There is also some evidence that occlusion by gloves may impair the stratum corneum barrier function[45] (*Quality of evidence* I). In an occupational setting, the type of glove used will depend upon the nature of the chemicals involved. Health and safety information for handling the chemical should stipulate which gloves ought to be used[46] (Appendix 5). Exposure time is an important factor in determining the most appropriate glove as so-called 'impervious' gloves have a finite permeation time for any particular substance; a glove may be protective for a few minutes but not for prolonged contact, e.g. NRL gloves and methacrylate bone cement.

Substitution

It may be possible to substitute nonirritating agents. The most common example of this is the use of a soap substitute. Correct recycling of oils in heavy industry and reduction of, or changing, the biocide additives may help.

Allergic contact dermatitis

Detection and avoidance of the allergen is often easier said than done. Again, a site visit may be necessary to identify the source of allergen contact and methods of avoidance. It may be necessary to contact manufacturers of products to determine if the allergen is present. It may also be necessary to contact a number of manufacturers to identify suitable substitutes.

Visiting the workplace

Visiting the workplace has an important place in the management of contact dermatitis. Apart from identifying potential allergens and irritants, it may be essential in the effective treatment and prevention of contact dermatitis (*Quality of evidence III*) (*Strength of recommendation B*). More information about the indications for visiting a patient's workplace and how to go about it are given elsewhere.[47]

Barrier creams and after-work creams?

Barrier creams by themselves are of questionable value in protecting against contact with irritants[48,49] (*Quality of evidence I*) (*Strength of recommendation E*). Their use should not be overpromoted as this may confer on workers a false sense of security and encourage them to be complacent in implementing the appropriate preventive measures.

After-work creams appear to confer some degree of protection against developing irritant contact dermatitis. There are controlled clinical trials showing benefit in the use of soap substitutes[50] and after-work creams[51] in reducing the incidence and prevalence of contact dermatitis (*Quality of evidence I*) (*Strength of recommendation A*). They should be encouraged and made readily available in the workplace.

Topical corticosteroids

Topical corticosteroids, soap substitutes and emollients are widely accepted as the treatment of established contact dermatitis. There is one study demonstrating a marginal benefit of the use of a combined topical corticosteroid/antibiotic combination[52] in infected or potentially infected eczema (*Quality of evidence IV*) (*Strength of recommendation C*). There is an open prospective randomized trial demonstrating the long-term intermittent use of mometasone furoate in chronic hand eczema[53] (*Quality of evidence I*) (*Strength of recommendation B*).

Topical tacrolimus has been shown to be effective in a nickel model of allergic contact dermatitis.[54]

Second-line treatments

Second-line treatments such as psoralen plus UVA, azathioprine and ciclosporin are used for steroid-resistant chronic hand dermatitis. There are several prospective clinical trials to support these treatments[55–57] (*Quality of evidence I*) (*Strength of recommendation A*). A randomized controlled trial of Grenz rays for chronic hand dermatitis showed a significantly better response with this therapy compared with use of topical corticosteroids[58] (*Quality of evidence I*) (*Strength of recommendation B*). Oral retinoids have been used in the treatment of chronic hand eczema with a recently published trial of alitretinoin showing promise[59] (*Quality of evidence I*) (*Strength of recommendation B*).

Nickel elimination diets

There is some evidence[60,61] to support the benefit of low nickel diets in some nickel-sensitive patients (*Quality of evidence IV*) (*Strength of recommendation C*).

Prognosis

Several studies have confirmed that the long-term prognosis for occupational contact dermatitis is often very poor. A Swedish study[62] demonstrated that only 25% of 555 patients investigated as having occupational contact dermatitis over a 10-year period had completely healed; one half still had periodic symptoms and one quarter permanent symptoms. Unfortunately, in 40% who changed their occupation, the overall prognosis was not improved. In a large follow-up study from Western Australia,[63] 55% of 949 patients still had dermatitis after 2 years from diagnosis (*Quality of evidence II.ii*). Prognosis for milder cases of contact dermatitis depends upon the ease of avoidance. If the patient can avoid the cause of the contact dermatitis then dermatitis will clear.

Summary of recommendations

1 Patients with persistent eczematous eruptions should be patch tested (*Quality of evidence II.ii*) (*Strength of recommendation A*).
2 A suggested annual workload for a patch test clinic serving an urban population of 70 000 is 100 patients patch tested (*Quality of evidence II.iii*) (*Strength of recommendation B*).
3 Patients should be patch tested to at least an extended standard series of allergens (*Quality of evidence II.ii*) (*Strength of recommendation A*).
4 An individual who has had training in the investigation of contact dermatitis prescribes appropriate patch tests and performs day 2 and day 4 readings in patients undergoing diagnostic patch testing (*Quality of evidence II.i*) (*Strength of recommendation A*).

Minimum standards (those marked * are potential audit points)

The BCDS recommends that certain minimum standards should apply to a contact dermatitis investigation unit. These include:
1 A named lead dermatologist for the unit who has received training for at least 6 months at a recognized contact dermatitis investigation unit or who can demonstrate comparable experience.*
2 That the contact dermatitis investigation unit conforms to best practice guidelines. The Unit and the staff should:

(i) Have a dedicated investigation clinic which should include an area for storage (refrigerator) and preparation of allergens.*

(ii) Record investigation results on an electronic database with a minimum data set:*

Site of onset of dermatitis and duration

Gender, occupational, atopy, hand dermatitis, leg dermatitis, face dermatitis and age index[64]

Details of occupation and leisure activities

Patch test results including type (allergic/irritant) and severity of reaction

Relevance of positive tests, occupational or otherwise

Final diagnosis

(iii) Participate in regular audit of data and 'benchmarks' results with nationally pooled data. This is evolving and will be reviewed periodically.

(iv) The lead dermatologist demonstrates regular attendance at CME-approved update meetings on contact dermatitis (at least every 2 years).*

(v) The unit should have up-to-date reference textbooks on contact dermatitis including occupational dermatitis and relevant journals.*

These minimum standards including the audit and benchmarking may be needed to demonstrate ongoing competency for the relicensing/revalidation of individuals working in and clinical leads for contact dermatitis.

References

1 Rea JN, Newhouse ML, Halil T. Skin diseases in Lambeth. A community study of prevalence and use of medical care. Br J Prev Soc Med 1976; **30**:107–14.

2 Agrup G. Hand eczema and other dermatoses in South Sweden. Acta Derm Venereol (Stockh) 1969; **49** (Suppl. 61):1–91.

3 Menné T, Buckmann E. Permanent disability from skin diseases. A study of 564 patients registered over a six-year period. Derm Beruf Umwelt 1979; **27**:37–42.

4 Turner S, Carder M, van Tongeren M et al. The incidence of occupational skin disease as reported to The Health and Occupation Reporting (THOR) network between 2002 and 2005. Br J Dermatol 2007; **157**:713–22.

5 Militello G, Jacob SE, Crawford GH. Allergic contact dermatitis in children. Curr Opin Pediatr 2006; **4**:385–90.

6 Beattie PE, Green C, Lowe G, Lewis-Jones MS. Which children should we patch test? Clin Exp Dermatol 2007; **32**:6–11.

7 Peltonen L. Nickel sensitivity in the general population. Contact Dermatitis 1979; **5**:27–32.

8 De Groot AC, Beverdam ET, Jong Ayong C et al. The role of contact allergy in the role of adverse effects caused by cosmetics and toiletries. Contact Dermatitis 1988; **19**:195–201.

9 Bettley FR. Hand eczema. Br Med J 1964; **ii**:151–5.

10 Agrup G, Dahlquist I, Fregert S, Rorsman H. Value of history and testing in suspected contact dermatitis. Arch Dermatol 1970; **101**:212–15.

11 Cronin E. Clinical prediction of patch test results. Trans St Johns Hosp Dermatol Soc 1972; **58**:153–62.

12 Podmore P, Burrows D, Bingham F. Prediction of patch test results. Contact Dermatitis 1984; **11**:283–4.

13 Goulden V, Wilkinson SM. Evaluation of a contact allergy clinic. Clin Exp Dermatol 2000; **25**:67–70.

14 Bhushan M, Beck MH. An audit to identify the optimum referral rate to a contact dermatitis investigation unit. Br J Dermatol 1999; **141**:570–2.

15 Nethercott J. Positive predictive accuracy of patch tests. Immunol Allergy Clin North Am 1989; **9**:549–53.

16 Lachapelle JM, Bruynzeel DP, Ducombs G et al. European multicenter study of the TRUE test. Contact Dermatitis 1988; **19**:91–7.

17 Fisher T, Maibach HI. Easier patch testing with the TRUE test. J Am Acad Dermatol 1989; **20**:447–53.

18 TRUE Test Study Group. Comparative studies with TRUE test and Finn chamber in eight Swedish hospitals. J Am Acad Dermatol 1989; **21**:486–9.

19 Wilkinson JD, Bruynzeel DD, Ducombs G et al. European multicenter study of TRUE test, Panel 2. Contact Dermatitis 1990; **22**:218–25.

20 Lachapelle JM, Antoine JL. Problems raised by the simultaneous reproducibility of positive allergic patch test reactions in man. J Am Acad Dermatol 1989; **21**:850–4.

21 Brasch J, Szliska C, Grabbe J. More positive patch test reactions with larger test chambers? Results from a study group of the German Contact Dermatitis Research Group (DKG). Contact Dermatitis 1997; **37**:118–20.

22 Gefeller O, Pfahlberg A, Geier J et al. The association between size of test chamber and patch test reaction: a statistical reanalysis. Contact Dermatitis 1999; **40**:14–18.

23 Wilkinson DS, Fregert S, Magnusson B et al. Terminology of contact dermatitis. Acta Derm Venereol (Stockh) 1970; **50**:287–92.

24 Shehade SA, Beck MH, Hillier VF. Epidemiological survey of standard series patch test results and observations on day 2 and day 4 readings. Contact Dermatitis 1991; **24**:119–22.

25 Jonker MJ, Bruynzeel DP. The outcome of an additional patch test reading on day 6 or 7. Contact Dermatitis 2000; **42**:330–5.

26 Sheretz EF, Swartz SM. Is the screening patch test tray still worth using? J Am Acad Dermatol 1993; **36**:1057–8.

27 Menné T, Dooms-Goosens A, Wahlberg JE et al. How large a proportion of contact sensitivities are diagnosed with the European standard series? Contact Dermatitis 1992; **26**:201–2.

28 Frosch PT, Pirker C, Rastogi SC et al. Patch testing with a new fragrance mix detects additional patients sensitive to perfumes and missed by the current fragrance mix. Contact Dermatitis 2005; **52**:207–15.

29 Baxter KF, Wilkinson SM, Kirk SJ. Hydroxymethyl pentylcyclohexenecarboxaldehyde (Lyral®) as a fragrance allergen in the UK. Contact Dermatitis 2003; **48**:117–18.

30 British Contact Dermatitis Group. Diluted Compositae mix versus sesquiterpene lactone mix as a screening agent for Compositae dermatitis: a multicentre study. Contact Dermatitis 2001; **45**:26–8.

31 IDVK and German Contact Dermatitis Research Group. Contact allergy to Disperse Blue 106 and Disperse Blue 124 in German and Austrian patients, 1995 to 1999. Contact Dermatitis 2001; **44**:173–7.

32 De Groot AC. Patch Testing. Test Concentrations and Vehicles for 3700 Chemicals, 2nd edn. Amsterdam: Elsevier, 1994.

33 Jolanki R, Estlander T, Alanko K, Kanerva L. Patch testing with a patient's own materials handled at work. In: Handbook of Occupational Dermatology (Kanerva L, Elsner P, Wahlberg JE, Maibach HI, eds). Berlin: Springer-Verlag, 2000; 375–83.

34 British Photodermatology Group. Workshop report: photopatch testing – methods and indications. Br J Dermatol 1997; **136**:371–6.

35 Bryden AM, Moseley H, Ibbotson SH et al. Photopatch testing of 1155 patients: results of the U.K. multicentre photopatch study group. Br J Dermatol 2006; **155**:737–47.

36 Batchelor RJ, Wilkinson SM. Photopatch testing – a retrospective review using the 1 day and 2 day irradiation protocols. Contact Dermatitis 2006; **54**:73–8.

37 Bruynzeel DP, Maibach HI. Excited skin syndrome (angry back). *Arch Dermatol* 1986; **122**:323–8.

38 Sukanto H, Nater JP, Bleumink E. Influence of topically applied corticosteroids on patch test reactions. *Contact Dermatitis* 1981; **7**:180–5.

39 Clark RA, Rietschel RL. 0·1% triamcinolone acetonide ointment and patch test responses. *Arch Dermatol* 1982; **118**:163–5.

40 Green C. The effect of topically applied corticosteroid on irritant and allergic patch test reactions. *Contact Dermatitis* 1996; **35**:331–3.

41 Condie MW, Adams RM. Influence of oral prednisolone on patch test reactions to rhus antigen. *Arch Dermatol* 1973; **107**:540–3.

42 Sjovall P, Christensen OB. Local and systemic effects of ultraviolet irradiation (UVB and UVA) on human allergic contact dermatitis. *Acta Derm Venereol (Stockh)* 1986; **66**:290–4.

43 Spaner D, Dolovich J, Tarlo S *et al.* Hypersensitivity to natural latex. *J Allergy Clin Immunol* 1989; **83**:1135–7.

44 Kelly KJ, Kurup V, Zacharisen M *et al.* Skin and serologic testing in the diagnosis of latex allergy. *J Allergy Clin Immunol* 1993; **91**:1140–5.

45 Ramsing DW, Agnew T. Effect of glove occlusion on human skin (II). Long-term experimental exposure. *Contact Dermatitis* 1996; **34**:258–62.

46 Mellstrom GA, Bowman A. Protective gloves. In: *Handbook of Occupational Dermatology* (Kanerva L, Elsner P, Wahlberg JE, Maibach HI, eds). Berlin: Springer-Verlag, 2000; 416–25.

47 English JSC. Occupational dermatoses. In: *Textbook of Dermatology* (Burns DA, Breathnach SM, Cox NH, Griffiths CEM, eds), 7th edn. Oxford: Blackwell Publishing, 2004; 21.8–21.9.

48 Goh CL, Gan SL. Efficacies of a barrier cream and an afterwork emollient cream against cutting fluid dermatitis in metalworkers: prospective study. *Contact Dermatitis* 1994; **31**:176–80.

49 Berndt U, Wigger-Alberti W, Gabard B, Elsner P. Efficacy of a barrier cream and its vehicle as protective measures against occupational irritant contact dermatitis. *Contact Dermatitis* 2000; **42**:77–80.

50 Lauharanta J, Ojajarvi J, Sarna S, Makela P. Prevention of dryness and eczema of the hands of hospital staff by emulsion cleansing instead of washing with soap. *J Hosp Infect* 1991; **17**:207–15.

51 Halkier-Sorensen L, Thestrup-Pedersen K. The efficacy of a moisturizer (Locobase) among cleaners and kitchen assistants during everyday exposure to water and detergents. *Contact Dermatitis* 1993; **29**:266–71.

52 Hjorth N, Schmidt H, Thomsen K. Fusidic acid plus betamethasone in infected or potentially infected eczema. *Pharmatherapeutica* 1985; **4**:126–31.

53 Veien NK, Olholm Larsen P, Thestrup-Pedersen K, Schou G. Long term, intermittent treatment of chronic hand eczema with mometasone furoate. *Br J Dermatol* 1999; **140**:882–6.

54 Belsito DV, Wilson DC, Warshaw E *et al.* A prospective randomized clinical trial of 0·1% tacrolimus ointment in a model of chronic allergic contact dermatitis. *J Am Acad Dermatol* 2006; **55**:40–6.

55 Rosen K, Mobacken H, Swanbeck G. Chronic eczematous dermatitis of the hands: a comparison of PUVA and UVB treatment. *Acta Derm Venereol (Stockh)* 1987; **67**:48–54.

56 Murphy GM, Maurice PD, Norris PG *et al.* Azathioprine treatment in chronic actinic dermatitis: a double-blind controlled trial with monitoring of exposure to ultraviolet radiation. *Br J Dermatol* 1989; **121**:639–46.

57 Granlund H, Erkko P, Eriksson E, Reitamo S. Comparison of the influence of cyclosporine and topical betamethasone-17,21-dipropionate treatment on quality of life in chronic hand eczema. *Acta Derm Venereol (Stockh)* 1997; **77**:54–8.

58 Lindelof B, Wrangsjo K, Liden S. A double-blind study of Grenz ray therapy in chronic eczema of the hands. *Br J Dermatol* 1987; **117**:77–80.

59 Ruzika T, Lynde CW, Jemec GBE *et al.* Efficacy and safety of oral alitretinoin (9-*cis* retinoic acid) in patients with severe chronic hand eczema refractory to topical corticosteroids: results of a randomized, double-blind, placebo-controlled, multicentre trial. *Br J Dermatol* 2008; **158**:808–17.

60 Veien NK, Hattel T, Laurberg G. Low nickel diet: an open, prospective trial. *J Am Acad Dermatol* 1993; **29**:1002–7.

61 Antico A, Soana R. Chronic allergic-like dermatopathies in nickel-sensitive patients. Results of dietary restrictions and challenge with nickel salts. *Allergy Asthma Proc* 1999; **20**:235–42.

62 Fregert S. Occupational dermatitis in a 10-year material. *Contact Dermatitis* 1975; **1**:96–107.

63 Wall LM, Gebauer KA. A follow up study of occupational skin disease in Western Australia. *Contact Dermatitis* 1991; **24**:241–3.

64 Smith HR, Wakelin SH, McFadden JP *et al.* A 15-year review of our MOAHLFA index. *Contact Dermatitis* 1999; **40**:227–8.

Appendix 1. Strength of recommendations and quality of evidence

Strength of recommendations

A There is good evidence to support the use of the procedure

B There is fair evidence to support the use of the procedure

C There is poor evidence to support the use of the procedure

D There is fair evidence to support the rejection of the use of the procedure

E There is good evidence to support the rejection of the use of the procedure

Quality of evidence

I Evidence obtained from at least one properly designed, randomized controlled trial

II.i Evidence obtained from well-designed controlled trials without randomization

II.ii Evidence obtained from well-designed cohort or case–control analytic studies, preferably from more than one centre or research group

II.iii Evidence obtained from multiple time series with or without the intervention. Dramatic results in uncontrolled experiments (such as the results of the introduction of penicillin treatment in the 1940s) could also be regarded as this type of evidence

III Opinions of respected authorities based on clinical experience, descriptive studies or reports of expert committees

IV Evidence inadequate owing to problems of methodology (e.g. sample size, or length of comprehensiveness of follow-up or conflicts in evidence)

Appendix 2. Recommended textbooks and journal on contact dermatitis

Adams RM, ed. *Occupational Skin Disease*, 3rd edn. Philadelphia: WB Saunders Co., 2000.

Burns DA, Breathnach SM, Cox NH, Griffiths CEM, eds. *Rook's Textbook of Dermatology*, 7th edn. Oxford: Blackwell Publishing, 2004.

Cronin E. *Contact Dermatitis*. London: Churchill Livingstone, 1980.

De Groot AC. *Patch Testing. Test Concentrations and Vehicles for 3700 Chemicals*, 2nd edn. Amsterdam: Elsevier, 1994.

Frosch P, Menné T, LePoittevin JP, eds. *Textbook of Contact Dermatitis*, 4th edn. Berlin: Springer-Verlag, 2006.

Kanerva L, Elsner P, Wahlberg JE, Maibach HI, eds. *Handbook of Occupational Dermatology*. Berlin: Springer-Verlag, 2000.

Rietschel RL, Fowler JF, eds. *Fisher's Contact Dermatitis*, 5th edn. Philadelphia: Lippincott Williams and Wilkins, 2001.

Contact Dermatitis. Copenhagen: Munksgaard.

Appendix 3. British Contact Dermatitis Society recommended standard series

Potassium dichromate	0·5%	pet.
Neomycin sulphate	20%	pet.
Thiuram mix	1%	pet.
p-Phenylenediamine	1%	pet.
Cobalt chloride	1%	pet.
Caine mix III	10%	pet.
Formaldehyde	1%	aq.
Colophony	20%	pet.
Quinoline mix	6%	pet.
Myroxylon pereirae (balsam of Peru)	25%	pet.
N-Isopropyl-N-phenyl-4-phenylenediamine	0·1%	pet.
Lanolin alcohol	30%	pet.
Mercapto mix	2%	pet.
Epoxy resin	1%	pet.
Parabens mix	16%	pet.
4-tert-Butylphenol formaldehyde resin	1%	pet.
Fragrance mix I	8%	pet.
Quaternium 15 (Dowicil 200)	1%	pet.
Nickel sulphate	5%	pet.
Cl- + Me-isothiazolinone	0·01%	aq.
Mercaptobenzothiazole	2%	pet.
Primin	0·01%	pet.
Sesquiterpene lactone mix	0·1%	pet.
p-Chloro-m-cresol	1%	pet.
2-Bromo-2-nitropropane-1,3-diol (Bronopol)	0·25%	pet.
Cetearyl alcohol	20%	pet.
Sodium fusidate	2%	pet.
Tixocortol-21-pivalate	1%	pet.
Budesonide	0·1%	pet.
Imidazolidinyl urea (Germal 115)	2%	pet.
Diazolidinyl urea (Germal 11)	2%	pet.
Methyldibromoglutaronitrile	0·3%	pet
Ethylenediamine dihydrochloride	1%	pet.
4-Chloro-3,5-xylenol (PCMX)	0·5%	pet.
Carba mix	3%	pet.
Fragrance mix II	14%	pet.
Disperse Blue mix 106/124	1%	pet.
Lyral	5%	pet.
Compositae mix (Chemo)	2·5%	pet.
Propolis	10%	pet.
Sodium metabisulphite	1%	pet.

Additional series

British Contact Dermatitis Society hairdressing series		
Diaminotoluene (toluene-2,5-diamine sulphate)	1%	pet.
Ammonium persulphate	2·5%	pet.
2-Nitro-p-phenylenediamine	1%	pet.
Glyceryl thioglycolate	1%	pet.
4-Aminophenol (p-aminophenol)	1%	pet.
3-Aminophenol (m-aminophenol)	1%	pet.
Hydroquinone	1%	pet.
Captan	0·5%	pet.
Ammonium thioglycolate (ammonium mercaptoacetate)	2·5%	aq.
Resorcinol	1%	pet.

British Contact Dermatitis Society footwear series		
Aminobenzene	0·25%	pet.
Diphenyl guanidine	1%	pet.
Direct Orange 34	5%	pet.
Urea formaldehyde resin	10%	pet.
Granuflex (gum rosin)	As is	
Disperse Orange 3	1%	pet.
Disperse Red 1	1%	pet.
Toluene sulf form resin	10%	pet.
Disperse Yellow 3	1%	pet.
Glutaraldehyde	0·2%	pet.
Octyl-isothiazolinone	0·1%	pet.
Diaminophenylmethane	0·5%	pet.
Acid Yellow 36	1%	pet.
Benzotriazole	1%	pet.
Diphenyl thiourea	1%	pet.
Hydroquinone	1%	pet.
Diethyl thiourea	1%	pet.
Dithiomorpholinone	1%	pet.
Basic Red 46	1%	pet.

British Contact Dermatitis Society steroid series		
Betamethasone-17-valerate	1%	pet.
Triamcinolone acetonide	1%	pet.
Alcomethasone dipropionate	1%	pet.
Clobetasol-17-propionate	1%	pet.
Dexamethasone phosphate	1%	pet.
Hydrocortisone-17-butyrate	1%	alc.
Prednisolone	1%	pet.

British Contact Dermatitis Society facial/cosmetic series

2,6-Di-tert-butyl-4-cresol (BHT)	2%	pet.
2-tert-Butyl-4-methoxyphenol (BHA)	2%	pet.
Toluenesulphonamide f resin	10%	pet.
Amerchol	50%	pet.
Cocamidopropyl betaine	1%	aq.
Sorbic acid	2%	pet.
tert-Butylhydroquinone	1%	pet.
Triclosan (Ingrasan DP 300)	2%	pet.
Propyl gallate	1%	pet.
Abitol	10%	pet.
Benzyl alcohol	1%	pet.
Methoxybenzophenone (Oxybenzone)	10%	Pet.
Triethanolamine	2%	pet.
DMDM hydantoin	2%	aq.
EDTA	1%	pet.
Propolis	10%	pet.
Tea tree oil	5%	pet.
Chloracetamide	0·2%	pet.
Iodopropynyl butylcarbamate	0·1%	pet.
Oleamidopropyl dimethylamine	0·1%	aq.
Sorbitan sesquioleate (Arlacel 83)	20%	pet.
Coconut diethanolamide	0·5%	pet.
Glyceryl monothioglycolate (GMTG)	1%	pet.
Methoxy-dibenzoylmethane (Parsol 1789)	10%	pet.

British Contact Dermatitis Society medicament series

Miconazole	1%	alc.
Bacitracin	5%	pet.
Chloramphenicol	5%	pet.
Clotrimazole	5%	pet.
Gentamicin sulphate	20%	pet.
Amerchol	50%	pet.
Benzalkonium chloride	0·1%	aq.
Econazole nitrate	1%	alc.
Chlorhexidine digluconate	0·5%	aq.
Polymyxin B	5%	pet.
Sodium metabisulphite Trolab	1%	pet.
Sorbic acid	2%	pet.
Coal tar (pix lithanthracis)	5%	pet.
Nystatin	2%	pet.
Propylene glycol	5%	pet.
Sorbitan sesquioleate (Arlacel 83)	20%	pet.
Triclosan (Ingrasan DP 300)	2%	pet.
2,6-Di-tert-butyl-4-cresol (BHT)	2%	pet.
2-tert-Butyl-4-methoxyphenol (BHA)	2%	pet.
Framycetin	10%	
Granuflex® dressing	As is	

Appendix 4. Commercially available additional patch test series

Trolab®	Chemotechnique Diagnostics
Antimicrobial, preservative and antioxidant	Bakery
	Corticosteroid
Cosmetics	Cosmetics
Dental materials	Dental screening
Hairdressing	Epoxy
Medicament (including corticosteroids, antibiotics, local anaesthetics and ophthalmics)	Fragrance
	Hairdressing
	Isocyanate
	Leg ulcer
	Medicament
Metal compounds	Adhesives, dental and other (meth) acrylate
Metalworking/technical oils	
Perfume and flavours	Nails – artificial (meth) acrylate
Photoallergens	Printing (meth) acrylate
Photographic chemicals	Oil and cooling fluid
Plant	Photographic chemicals
Plastics and glues	Plant
Rubber chemicals	Plastics and glues
Sunscreen agents	Rubber additives
Textile and leather dyes	Scandinavian photopatch test
Vehicles and emulsifiers	Shoe
Miscellaneous	Sunscreen
	Textile colours and finish
	Various allergens

Appendix 5. A guide to which gloves will give some degree of protection for specific types of hazard

Hazard	Type of glove
Microorganisms	NRL, thermoplastic elastomer
Disinfectants	NRL, PVC, PE, EMA
Pharmaceuticals	NRL (permeability time very short)
Composite materials	NRL (permeability time in minutes), 4H-glove
Solvents	PE, PVC, nitrile, NRL, neoprene, butyl rubber, Viton, 4H-glove
Corrosives	NRL, PE, PVC, neoprene, butyl rubber, Viton, 4H-glove
Detergents	NRL, EMA, PE, neoprene, PVC, nitrile (if addition of organic solvents)
Machining oils	NRL, PVC, nitrile, neoprene, 4H-glove

NRL, natural rubber latex; PVC, polyvinyl chloride; PE, polyethylene; EMA, ethylene methylmethacrylate.

http://www.bad.org.uk/Portals/_Bad/Guidelines/Clinical
%20Guidelines/Contact%20Dermatitis%20BJD
%20Guidelines%20May%202009.pdf

Comment

The main changes since the 2001 guidelines were published [1] place a greater emphasis on quality assurance through collecting a minimum data set and audit of patch test results recorded [2]. The British Contact Dermatitis Society has expanded the number of recommend patch test series, which now stands at the British Contact Dermatitis Society standard, facial and cosmetics, hairdressing, footwear, steroid and medicament series. There are two recent systematic reviews studying various aspects of occupational contact dermatitis [3, 4]. They have both highlighted a lack of good quality studies of prevention and management of occupational contact dermatitis.

REFERENCES

1 Bourke J, Coulson I, English J. Guidelines for the care of contact dermatitis. *Brit J Dermatol* 2001; 145: 877–85.

2 Bourke J, Coulson I, English J. Guidelines for the management of contact dermatitis: an update. *Brit J Dermatol* 2009; 160: 946–54.

3 NHS Plus, Royal College of Physicians, Faculty of Occupational Medicine. *Dermatitis: occupational aspects of management. A national guideline.* London: RCP, 2009 (http://www.rcplondon.ac.uk/pubs/contents/df3c4165-619f-4c2b-b371-06c3d31fe15c.pdf).

4 BOHRF guidelines, March 2010. http://www.bohrf.org.uk/projects/dermatitis.html.

Additional professional resources

Clinical Knowledge Summaries guidance 2008. http://www.cks.nhs.uk/dermatitis_contact#.

Saary J, Qureshi R, Palda V, *et al.* A systematic review of contact dermatitis treatment and prevention. *J Am Acad Dermatol* 2005; 53: 845–55.

Contact dermatitis: synopsis. World Allergy Organization review. http://www.worldallergy.org/professional/allergic_diseases_center/contactdermatitis/.

BAD patient information leaflet

http://www.bad.org.uk/site/804/Default.aspx

http://www.bad.org.uk/site/567/default.aspx (occupational dermatitis)

http://www.bcds.org.uk/downloads/patient/standard/index.html

Other patient resources

http://www.eczema.org

http://www.aad.org/pamphlets/eczema.html

http://www.dermnetnz.org

http://www.patient.co.uk/pdf/pilsL59.pdf (patch testing)

http://www.cks.nhs.uk/patient_information_leaflet/contact_dermatitis

http://www.nhs.uk/conditions/eczema-(contact-dermatitis)/Pages/Introduction.aspx (UK Department of Health Patient Information)

http://www.dermatology.org.uk/quality/info-sheets-dermatitis.html (Cardiff University, Wales, information sheets)

British Association of Dermatologists' guidelines for the management of lichen sclerosus 2010

S.M. Neill, F.M. Lewis,* F.M. Tatnall† and N.H. Cox‡

St John's Institute of Dermatology, St Thomas' Hospital, Westminster Bridge Road, London SE1 7EH, U.K.
*Heatherwood & Wexham Park Hospitals NHS Trust, Wexham Street, Slough SL2 4HL, U.K.
†Watford General Hospital, Vicarage Road, Watford WD18 0HB, U.K.
‡Cumberland Infirmary, Newtown Road, Carlisle CA2 7HY and University of Cumbria, Carlisle, U.K.

One of the aims of the British Association of Dermatologists (BAD) is to provide guidelines for the management of skin diseases using all available good-quality evidence-based data. The BAD guidelines writing and consultation process, and its revised formats, have been described elsewhere.[1-3]

These guidelines for the management of lichen sclerosus (LS) have been prepared for dermatologists on behalf of the BAD. They present evidence-based guidance for investigation and treatment, with identification of the strength of evidence available at the time of preparation of the guidelines.

Purpose and scope

The guidelines have been revised and updated in accordance with a predetermined scope, based on that used in the 2002 guidelines. Recommendations in these guidelines supersede those in the 2002 guidelines. The overall objective of the guidelines is to provide up-to-date recommendations for the management of LS in adults and children.

Stakeholder involvement

This guidance has been written by dermatologists and has been shown to a patient. The guidelines have also been seen by a urologist, gynaecologist and genitourinary physician, all of whom are involved in the management of patients with LS.

Methodology

These guidelines have been developed using the BAD's recommendations[3] and also with reference to the AGREE (Appraisal of Guidelines Research and Evaluation) instrument.[4] Medline and EMBASE databases were searched from 2002 to 2009 and full relevant papers obtained. The draft guidelines were made available for consultation and review by the BAD membership; the final document was peer reviewed by the Clinical Standards Unit of the BAD (made up of the Therapy & Guidelines and Audit & Clinical Standards Subcommittees) prior to publication.

There are few published randomized controlled trials to support the following guidelines for the management of LS; the recommendations made are those that are currently con-

© 2010 British Association of Dermatologists

sidered best practice but they will be modified at intervals in the light of new evidence. LS, although a dermatosis, occurs commonly at a genital site and consequently is not only managed by dermatologists; patients may be under the care of other specialist disciplines. There have been many long-standing difficulties in the appraisal and grading of the evidence for the treatment of LS. Historically, the nomenclature used to describe LS has been unclear. In addition, there may be difficulty in assessing the number of patients with active disease as, although asymptomatic, there is still ongoing activity as evidenced by scarring. There are also instances where the LS may be in remission but the patient still experiences symptoms due to a secondary sensory disorder, or additional irritant eczema.

Plans for revision

These guidelines will be revised as necessary to reflect changes in practice.

Limitations of the guidelines

These guidelines have been prepared for dermatologists on behalf of the BAD and reflect the best data available at the time the report was prepared. Caution should be exercised in interpreting the data; the results of future studies may require alteration of the conclusions or recommendations in this report. It may be necessary or even desirable to depart from the guidelines in the interests of specific patients and special circumstances. Just as adherence to guidelines may not constitute defence against a claim of negligence, so deviation from them should not necessarily be deemed negligent.

Definition

LS is an autoimmune, inflammatory dermatosis, characterized by a lymphocytic response that has a predilection for the genital skin in both sexes, and an association with several other autoimmune diseases.

The aetiology of LS is uncertain but there is mounting evidence to suggest that autoimmune mechanisms are involved in its pathogenesis;[5-7] there is an increased incidence of tissue-specific antibodies[8] and associations with other autoimmune diseases in patients with LS,[9,10] as well as positive associations with HLA class II antigens.[11-13] There is still controversy regarding the implication of Borrelia infection as an aetiological agent; although several studies have shown that this association does not occur in the U.S.A., some doubt still remains in Europe.[14,15] The presence of circulating extracellular matrix protein antibodies gives further support to an immune aetiopathology in female patients.[16] 'Balanitis xerotica obliterans' is now viewed as a synonymous term describing LS of the penis, and 'kraurosis vulvae' is now recognized as LS of the vulva. The term 'leucoplakia' (meaning white plaque) is not a diagnostic entity and is

descriptive only, as many conditions may present with white plaques. The term 'lichen sclerosus et atrophicus' has been abbreviated to 'lichen sclerosus' as some cases are associated with a hypertrophic, rather than atrophic, epithelium. There are instances when it can be difficult to differentiate between LS and lichen planus (LP) on the basis of the clinical and histological features; these cases appear to constitute an overlap syndrome, which is often associated with squamous cell hyperplasia and a poor response to ultrapotent topical corticosteroids.

In the main, these guidelines are for classical LS with typical clinical and histological features.

Incidence and patterns

LS is a relatively common dermatosis, although the true incidence is unknown, and probably underestimated, in part due to the distribution of patients among different clinical specialities and to the fact that it may be asymptomatic. Genital LS in female subjects has two peak ages of presentation – in the prepubertal and postmenopausal years.[17] Although childhood LS usually improves, there may be cases that persist into adulthood.[18] There is also a bimodal onset in male subjects, with age peaks in young boys and in adult men.[19]

Clinical features

Readers are referred to several reviews on the clinical, histological and pathogenetic aspects of LS[20-23] and to a historical review of the nomenclature and therapy.[24]

Female anogenital: adult

The typical lesions are porcelain-white papules and plaques, often associated with areas of ecchymosis. Follicular delling may be prominent, and occasionally hyperkeratosis is a prominent feature. The characteristic sites are the interlabial sulci, labia minora, clitoral hood, clitoris, perineal body and perineum. Genital mucosal involvement does not occur, the vagina and cervix always being spared (which is in contrast to LP), although there may be involvement at the mucocutaneous junctions (the vestibule), which may result in introital narrowing. Perianal lesions occur in women in 30% of cases. There may be extension to the buttocks and genitocrural folds. LS can Koebnerize and may first arise in an episiotomy scar.

Itch is the main symptom, but pain may be a consequence of erosions or fissures. However, LS may also be entirely asymptomatic and an incidental finding on examination. In those with itch, this is often worse at night and may be sufficiently severe to disturb sleep. Dyspareunia occurs in the presence of erosions, fissures or introital narrowing.

LS is a scarring process and may cause loss of the labia minora, sealing of the clitoral hood and burying of the clitoris. Severe introital stenosis may rarely occur, but is seen more frequently in the LS/LP overlap syndrome.

Female anogenital: children

The lesions are similar to those in adult women, but ecchymosis may be very striking and potentially mistaken as evidence of sexual abuse.[25] The confirmation of a diagnosis of LS does not, however, totally exclude coincident sexual abuse as some cases of LS may possibly be caused or aggravated by sexual abuse through Koebnerization.[26] Features that should arouse suspicion of this include LS arising in older prepubertal girls, poor response to treatment, the presence of associated sexually transmitted infection or other symptoms or signs of abuse.

Milia may also be present transiently in treated and untreated disease.

Perianal involvement is a frequent finding in young girls, who may present with constipation because of painful fissuring in this area.

Male genital: adult

The common sites of involvement of LS in adult men are the prepuce, coronal sulcus and glans penis, and more rarely lesions may be found on the shaft of the penis. The presenting complaint is usually tightening of the foreskin, which may lead to phimosis. This in turn results in erectile dysfunction and painful erections. One report documents that 30% of phimosis occurring in adults was due to LS,[27] although another study of 75 subjects with severe phimosis identified LS in only 11%.[28] Other presenting complaints are due to the appearance of lesions or changes in urinary stream, but itch is not a prominent symptom. Perianal disease is rarely, if ever, seen in male patients. The perimeatal area may be involved and postinflammatory scarring may lead to stenosis and obstruction. There may also be more proximal urethral involvement although this usually starts at the meatus.[23] These complications may require a multidisciplinary approach with input from both a dermatologist and urologist.

Male genital: children

The disease usually affects the prepuce and the most frequent presentation is phimosis. The reported incidence of LS in children with phimosis ranges from 14% to 100%.[29–31] Perianal involvement, as in adult men, is extremely rare. There is a report of a rare complication of renal failure following meatal obstruction.[32]

Extragenital: male, female and children

The classical sites for extragenital lesions are the upper trunk, axillae, buttocks and lateral thighs, and these are involved most frequently in adult women. Rarer sites include the mouth, face, scalp, hands, feet and nails. The typical lesions are porcelain-white plaques, which may have follicular dells and areas of ecchymosis, similar to the genital lesions. In extragenital sites, there may be difficulty in distinguishing the lesions from those of morphoea. The clinical types of extra-genital LS include an extensive bullous form,[33,34] as well as annular, Blaschkoid and keratotic variants.[35] Koebnerization is very common at extragenital sites, arising at pressure points, old surgical and radiotherapy scars and at sites of trauma.

Investigations

Biopsy

A confirmatory biopsy, although ideal, is not always practical, particularly in children. It is not always essential when the clinical features are typical. However, histological examination is advisable if there are atypical features or diagnostic uncertainty and is mandatory if there is any suspicion of neoplastic change. Patients under routine follow-up will need a biopsy if: (i) there is a suspicion of neoplastic change, i.e. a persistent area of hyperkeratosis, erosion or erythema, or new warty or papular lesions; (ii) the disease fails to respond to adequate treatment; (iii) there is extragenital LS, with features suggesting an overlap with morphoea; (iv) there are pigmented areas, in order to exclude an abnormal melanocytic proliferation; and (v) second-line therapy is to be used.

Immunology

An autoantibody screen to look for associated autoimmune disease is useful if there are clinical features to suggest an autoimmune disorder. In particular, thyroid disease is common in women with LS.[36]

Microbiology

Swabs are not required routinely but may be indicated in erosive disease to exclude herpes simplex or *Candida* as additional complicating problems.[37] Retesting for these infections may be necessary in disease that flares or fails to respond to treatment. If there is an abnormal vaginal discharge this will need appropriate investigation.

Complications

Malignancy

Squamous cell carcinoma (SCC) has been described predominantly in association with female genital LS and less commonly in penile LS. It is not associated with extragenital LS. Less commonly the malignancy is a verrucous carcinoma. Melanoma, basal cell carcinoma and Merkel cell carcinoma have all been reported rarely in patients with vulval LS but no studies suggest that there is an increased frequency of these tumours. There appear to be two pathogenetic mechanisms for vulval SCC: firstly, SCC in younger women is associated with the oncogenic human papillomavirus (HPV); and secondly, in older women, the association is with a chronic scarring dermatosis such as LS or LP with little, if any, evidence of a link with HPV.

Squamous cell carcinoma in female patients with genital lichen sclerosus

SCC arising within LS only occurs in anogenital disease. The risk is small, being < 5%.[17,23,38] However, histopathological examination of vulval SCCs indicates that about 60% occur on a background of LS.[39–41] LS may act as both an initiator and promoter of carcinogenesis by mechanisms that seem to be independent of HPV. Although there is little evidence for an important role for HPV in LS-associated SCC, there has been a suggestion that topical corticosteroid use may induce oncogenic HPV types. HPV may be found in vulval intraepithelial neoplasia (VIN) associated with LS.[42] SCC of the vulva should be managed by oncological gynaecologists experienced in this field as surgery has to be individualized according to the tumour size and location, particularly in early invasive disease.

Squamous cell carcinoma in men with genital lichen sclerosus

An association between LS and penile SCC has also been reported.[43–45] Although histological evidence of LS can be found in about 40% of penile carcinoma specimens, the actual risk of this complication in any individual patient with LS is uncertain. Published data suggest that the risk is about 5%, similar to the figure suggested for female patients.[43] In a 10-year multicentre cohort of 130 male patients with genital LS, histological changes of SCC were found in eight, verrucous carcinoma in two and erythroplasia of Queyrat (*in situ* SCC) in one.[46]

The role of HPV in penile LS-associated SCC has also been debated. Some studies using polymerase chain reaction have documented a negligible frequency of HPV in LS,[47,48] but other studies have suggested a frequency of up to 33%.[49,50] An additional feature that has been linked with penile LS-associated SCC is the occurrence of a prominent lichenoid infiltrate on long-standing, chronic LS, suggesting disease reactivation.[51]

Scarring

Introital narrowing

This is rare, but, if significant and causing dyspareunia or difficulty with micturition, surgery may need to be considered. Part of the posterior vaginal wall is used in the reconstruction to prevent further adhesions and stenosis due to Koebnerization.[52]

Pseudocyst of the clitoris

Occasionally, clitoral hood adhesions seal over the clitoris and keratinous debris builds up underneath forming a painful pseudocyst. This requires a subtotal or total circumcision.[53]

Preputial adhesions and phimosis

If subcoronal or transcoronal adhesions between the inner aspect of the prepuce and the glans persist despite adequate medical treatment, these will need to be treated surgically and a circumcision performed at the same time. Persistent phimosis will also require a circumcision. If the disease is still active at the time of surgery a topical steroid might be required to prevent Koebnerization and further scarring, particularly around the coronal sulcus.

Meatal stenosis

If this results in an impaired urinary stream, referral for urological assessment is advisable.

Sensory abnormalities: dysaesthesia

Vestibulodynia and vulvodynia

These conditions may occur after an inflammatory condition of the vulva or vestibule. Typically, the patient remains symptomatic despite objective clinical improvement or resolution of the skin lesions. Neuropathic pain does not respond to topical corticosteroids, and treatment must be directed to the eradication of the neuronal sensitization. Initially, 5% lidocaine ointment is recommended, with the addition of pain-modulating oral medication, such as a tricyclic antidepressant or gabapentin, in unresponsive cases.

Penile dysaesthesia

Men may develop a similar problem, with an abnormal burning sensation on the glans or around the urethral meatus. The management is as for female patients.

Psychosexual problems

Men and women who have any chronic genital disorder will often lose their interest in sexual activity, leading to problems with sexual dysfunction.[54,55] It is important to give the patient the opportunity to express their concerns about their sexual function, and to offer a referral to someone with the necessary expertise to address these problems. Women are more likely to bring up sexual matters if they have seen the doctor before and feel comfortable with the consultation. However, many patients are too embarrassed to bring up the topic of sexual function and it is important that the doctor asks a simple question about sexual activity and associated concerns. Sometimes it is the patient's partner who has a problem and does not wish to have physical contact for fear of hurting the partner or 'catching' the disease.

Management

Topical corticosteroids

Topical steroids have become the mainstay of medical treatment for LS.

Adult female anogenital lichen sclerosus

There are no randomized controlled trials providing evidence that a once- or twice-daily application of any one specific corticosteroid is the most effective, or documenting that one regimen is superior to another. However, the recommended and accepted first-line treatment is the very potent topical corticosteroid clobetasol propionate 0·05%[56–58] (*Strength of recommendation B; quality of evidence 2++*; see Appendix for definitions). The regimen recommended by the authors for a newly diagnosed case is clobetasol propionate 0·05% ointment applied once daily, at night, for 4 weeks, then on alternate nights for 4 weeks, and then twice weekly for a further 4 weeks, before review. The rationale for once-a-day application is based on pharmacodynamic studies showing that an ultrapotent steroid only needs to be applied once a day on extragenital skin.[59] If symptoms recur when the frequency of application is reduced, the patient is instructed to use the treatment more often until the symptoms resolve. They can then try to reduce the frequency again. A 30-g tube of clobetasol propionate 0·05% should last at least 12 weeks. If the treatment has been successful the hyperkeratosis, ecchymoses, fissuring and erosions should have resolved, but the atrophy, scarring and its associated pallor will persist. About 60% of patients experience complete remission of their symptoms.[60,61] Others will continue to have flares and remissions; they are advised to use clobetasol propionate 0·05% as required. Most patients with ongoing disease seem to require 30–60 g of clobetasol propionate 0·05% ointment annually. In our experience, the long-term use of clobetasol propionate in this way is safe and there has been no evidence of significant steroid damage or an increase in the incidence of SCC. There is one short-term study of up to 12 months showing the safety of continued use.[62]

One study using the less potent steroid mometasone furoate showed that this was also effective.[63]

A prospective open study of 34 postmenopausal women with vulval LS demonstrated that the use of an emollient, in addition to the topical steroid during the initial treatment phase, and then as maintenance therapy, is very beneficial.[64] No patients had worsening of scarring during follow-up. A soap substitute is also recommended.

An information sheet on LS, with the instructions for the use of the topical steroid, should be given to the patient.

Adult male genital lichen sclerosus

A retrospective study of 22 men treated with clobetasol propionate 0·05% documented this to be safe and effective, with significant improvement in discomfort and skin tightness, and also in urinary flow in the nine patients in whom this was affected.[65] The use of topical steroids in men may also reduce the need for circumcision[66] (*Strength of recommendation B; quality of evidence 2++*).

Child anogenital lichen sclerosus

There are no ongoing randomized controlled trials to base the recommendation of a potent topical corticosteroid as being the treatment of choice for childhood LS in either sex. In a series of 70 cases of childhood vulval LS, potent topical corticosteroids were effective treatment to alleviate symptoms, without significant side-effects.[67] Several smaller series support this conclusion.[68,69] A prospective study, completed by 111 boys with phimosis using betamethasone for 1 month, documented that 80% had normal retractability of the foreskin after this time, 10% proceeded to circumcision as treatment failures and 10% required ongoing topical treatment.[70] One placebo-controlled series using a medium potency steroid documented improvement in disease with little scarring.[71] Other studies have shown that preputial phimosis may resolve with the use of an ultrapotent or medium potency topical steroid, thus avoiding a need for circumcision.[72,73] Interestingly, in a series of 462 boys with phimosis, only 12 of whom had documented LS, 86% responded to twice-daily corticosteroid application for 6 weeks, but only nine of the patients with LS responded:[74] this suggests that phimosis due to causes other than LS may also respond to topical corticosteroids (*Strength of recommendation B; quality of evidence 2++*).

Extragenital LS

There are no randomized controlled trials on which to base recommendations but clobetasol propionate, with or without occlusion, is used once daily as and when required. In general, extragenital lesions are not as responsive as genital disease to topical corticosteroid therapy.

Testosterone and other hormonal treatments

Adult female anogenital lichen sclerosus

Although it has been extensively used in the past, there appears to be no evidence base for the use of topical testosterone.[58,75–77] There is a solitary report of the effective use of topical progesterone.[78]

Although LS predominantly affects the genital region in female patients, suggesting a hormonal influence, neither pregnancy nor hormone replacement therapy seems to have any effect on the condition.

Male genital lichen sclerosus

Similarly, testosterone is no longer used.

Child anogenital lichen sclerosus

There is no supportive evidence for the use of topical oestrogens or testosterone in children.

Surgery, cryotherapy, photodynamic therapy, phototherapy, laser

Adult female anogenital lichen sclerosus

There is no indication for removal of vulval tissue in the management of uncomplicated LS, and surgery should be used exclusively for malignancy and postinflammatory sequelae.

In one small study of 12 patients with vulval LS and severe intractable itch, 75% obtained symptom relief with cryotherapy, 50% for 3 years[79] (*Strength of recommendation D; quality of evidence 3*).

In an open study of photodynamic therapy (PDT) for vulval LS (topical 5-aminolaevulinic acid, argon laser light, one to three treatments), 10 of 12 patients derived significant improvement[80] (*Strength of recommendation D; quality of evidence 3*). Another study demonstrated good symptomatic benefit in six of 10 patients treated with aminolaevulinic acid PDT using a bioadhesive patch.[81]

A single study of ultraviolet (UV) A1 in seven women with vulval LS that had not been controlled by topical steroids[82] reported initial improvement in five patients, although two relapsed and the others required ongoing treatment with topical steroids (*Strength of recommendation D; quality of evidence 3*).

Laser treatment, in a small study of 10 patients, was helpful symptomatically but did not stop the disease recurring. It was ineffective in one patient with urethral LS[83] (*Strength of recommendation D; quality of evidence 3*).

There is a solitary report of the beneficial use of focused ultrasound in 17 out of 31 cases of untreated LS using frequencies of 5–8 MHz[84] (*Strength of recommendation D; quality of evidence 3*).

Male genital lichen sclerosus

Although the first-line treatment for male patients with LS is a potent topical corticosteroid, it is not always successful when scarring has led to structural changes. The role of surgery for penile LS with symptoms due to persistent phimosis or meatal stenosis is supported with large studies documenting satisfactory results. In a multicentre series of 215 men with penile LS, and mean follow-up of almost 5 years, circumcision (indicated in 34 cases) was successful in 100%, meatotomy (n = 15) in 80%, circumcision and meatotomy (n = 8) in 100%, and various forms of urethroplasty (n = 111) in 73–91%.[85] LS is rare in the circumcised male, but circumcision does not always ensure protection against further flares of the disease. One series showed that 50% of men requiring circumcision continued to have lesions of LS,[19] and that the LS may Koebnerize in the circumcision scar. Koebnerization may be the explanation for the recurrence of urethral stricture, which is seen more frequently after surgery in patients with LS. This complication appears to be most common in those having a one-stage repair rather than stricture excision with a two-stage repair[86] (*Strength of recommendation D; quality of evidence 3*).

Laser treatment has been used to treat meatal stenosis,[83,87] but this is not standard practice. One study of 50 men with LS showed good long-term results after CO_2 laser treatment 13–19 years earlier, 80% having no evidence of LS[88] (*Strength of recommendation D; quality of evidence 3*). First-line treatment is urethral dilatation or formal meatoplasty. A topical steroid may be required at the same time as surgery.

Child anogenital lichen sclerosus

Surgical treatment of childhood phimosis by circumcision has demonstrated the presence of LS in a high proportion of cases. It is now being recognized that a trial of a topical steroid should be tried prior to circumcision in all cases of phimosis independent of aetiology and that circumcision should be reserved for treatment failures[70] (*Strength of recommendation D; quality of evidence 3*).

Extragenital LS

Shave (tangential) excision has been used,[89] and CO_2 laser has been reported to produce improvement in symptoms and appearance of lesions.

Various forms of phototherapy have been used for extragenital LS, including narrowband UVB, psoralen-UVA (PUVA) (alone or with topical tacrolimus) and UVA1. The latter appears to be the most successful in reducing clinical sclerosis as well as symptoms.[90–94] All of these treatments have only been reported as individual cases or small case series. One study compared the use of methyl aminolaevulinic acid pulsed dye laser (PDL)-mediated PDT vs. PDL alone on two areas of extragenital LS in one patient. The site treated with the PDT-PDL showed a slightly better response than the PDL alone[95] (*Strength of recommendation D; quality of evidence 3*).

Other treatments

Topical calcineurin inhibitors

The use of topical tacrolimus and pimecrolimus has been studied in women with vulval LS, after initial anecdotal reports and small series suggested benefit.[96–99] A study of 84 patients (49 women, 32 men and three girls) has supported the efficacy of tacrolimus.[100] A small study on the use of pimecrolimus in four prepubertal girls also noted an improvement in symptoms.[101] However, stinging on application was often reported. Furthermore, the long-term safety profile of these drugs is not established and there are concerns about an increased risk of neoplasia with their use in a disease with a premalignant potential.[102–104] There are case reports of SCC developing in patients who have been using these treatments[105,106] and longer-term studies are therefore of particular importance in LS. It is therefore recommended that the calcineurin inhibitors should not be used as first-line treatment (*Strength of recommendation D; quality of evidence 3*).

Ciclosporin, methotrexate and other immunosuppressive agents

A pilot trial of topical ciclosporin failed to have any beneficial clinical or histological effect in five cases of vulval LS.[107] However, oral ciclosporin was reported as effective in reducing symptoms and erosions in a series of five patients with refractory LS.[108]

Methotrexate has been used with success in an individual case of extragenital disease,[109] and hydroxycarbamide may also be an option for resistant LS[110] (*Strength of recommendation D; quality of evidence 3*).

There is a single study of the use of pulsed steroid and methotrexate which showed an improvement over 6 months[111] (*Strength of recommendation D; quality of evidence 3*).

Retinoids

Both topical and systemic retinoids have been used to treat LS.[112–114] There is no evidence that these are particularly effective in uncomplicated LS. However there is some evidence that they may have a role in hyperkeratotic and hypertrophic disease that does not respond to an ultrapotent steroid.

Potassium *para*-aminobenzoate

One report of five patients with LS at various sites, and resistant to numerous other therapies, documented good improvement with potassium *para*-aminobenzoate in all five (at quite wide dose ranges from 4 to 24 g daily, in divided doses)[115] (*Strength of recommendation D; quality of evidence 3*).

Others

There are reports of benefits from calcitriol, antimalarials, stanozolol, antipruritic and antihistamine agents, such as oxatomide, and various antibiotics (for which the main rationale is the uncertain link with *Borrelia* infection). These and others are summarized in reviews listed previously, but must all be viewed as less well-proven or anecdotal.[20–24]

Treatment failure

If treatment with topical corticosteroids appears to fail to bring LS under control then it is important to consider the following:

- Is noncompliance an issue? Sometimes patients may be alarmed at the contents of the package information insert warning against the use of topical corticosteroids in the anogenital area. Elderly patients disabled with poor eyesight and limited mobility may not be able to apply the medication appropriately.
- Has the correct diagnosis been made or is there an additional superimposed problem such as the development of a contact allergy to the medication, urinary incontinence, herpes simplex infection, intraepithelial neoplasia, malignancy, psoriasis or mucous membrane pemphigoid?
- Is there a secondary sensory problem? Has the LS been successfully treated, but the patient remains symptomatic because a

---

secondary sensory problem (vulvodynia) has developed, or are there problems with intercourse which the individual feels too embarrassed to reveal?
- Is there a mechanical problem due to scarring, such as severe phimosis or meatal stenosis in males, in which case surgery may be indicated?

Follow-up

The risk of malignancy in uncomplicated genital LS that has been diagnosed and treated appropriately is very small. If malignancy occurs it tends to develop rapidly.

The authors suggest two follow-up visits after the initial consultation: one at 3 months to assess response to treatment and to ensure that the patient is using the topical corticosteroid appropriately and judiciously, and a second final assessment 6 months later to ensure that the patient is confident in treating their problem and to take the opportunity to discuss any residual problems that the patient might have before discharge back to the care of their primary physician. If patients continue to use a topical steroid it is suggested that they see their primary care physician once a year. Written instruction should be given to the patient at the time of their discharge from the clinic warning them that any persistent area of well-defined erythema, ulceration or new growth must be reported to their family practitioner straight away, who will then make an urgent referral back to an appropriate specialist. However, as over half of women discharged from U.K. vulval clinics are not subsequently followed up in primary care appropriately,[116] it is important that instructions for self-monitoring are fully understood.

Long-term follow-up in a secondary care specialist clinic is appropriate for patients with genital LS associated with troublesome symptoms, localized skin thickening, previous cancer or VIN, or pathological uncertainty about VIN.[117] The same advice is suggested for male patients with this problem. Biopsies of persistent ulcers, erosions, hyperkeratosis and fixed erythematous areas are advised to exclude intraepithelial neoplasia or invasive SCC. These patients usually have LS with a histological pattern that has features of both LS and LP with squamous cell hyperplasia. Clinically these patients seem to have an overlap syndrome and their disease runs a relentless course despite trials of various therapies, and a small percentage do go on to develop one or more SCCs.

Recommendations and conclusions

1 An ultrapotent topical corticosteroid is the first-line treatment for LS in either sex or age group, at any site, but there are no randomized controlled trials comparing steroid potency, frequency of application and duration of treatment.
2 Asymptomatic patients with evidence of clinically active LS (ecchymosis, hyperkeratosis and progressing atrophy) should be treated.

---

3 Anogenital LS is associated with SCC but the development of this complication is rare in clinical practice, < 5%. It is not yet known whether treatment lessens the long-term risk of malignant change.

4 Long-term follow-up in a specialized clinic is unnecessary for uncomplicated disease that is well-controlled clinically using small amounts of a topical corticosteroid, i.e. < 60 g in 12 months.

5 Secondary care follow-up should be reserved for patients with complicated LS that is unresponsive to treatment and those patients who have persistent disease with a history of a previous SCC.

6 A dermatology opinion should be sought in any patient with atypical or poorly controlled LS.

7 Surgical intervention is only indicated for the complications of scarring, premalignant change or an invasive SCC, in female patients. It may be useful in male patients with severe irreversible phimosis.

8 If psychosexual issues arise, these should be addressed and, if appropriate, referral made to a practitioner experienced in this field.

Audit points

1 Has a biopsy been performed in patients with clinically active LS that has not responded to treatment?

2 Are follow-up arrangements in place for patients with ongoing symptomatic disease?

3 Are patients with genital LS aware of the need to report any suspicious lesions within the affected skin?

4 Has a topical steroid of adequate potency and duration been used prior to circumcision in males with symptomatic LS?

5 Is histology always reported on male circumcision specimens?

Acknowledgement

The authors would like to acknowledge the considerable contribution made by the late Neil Cox to the preparation of both the original guidelines and this latest revision. Neil's dedication to dermatology, teaching and the care of his patients cannot be overemphasized. He was a very generous collaborator and his passing is a great loss to us all.

References

1 Griffiths CEM. The British Association of Dermatologists guidelines for the management of skin disease. Br J Dermatol 1999; 141:396–7.

2 Cox NH, Williams HC. The British Association of Dermatologists Therapeutic Guidelines: can we AGREE? Br J Dermatol 2003; 148:621–5.

3 Bell HK, Ormerod AD. Writing a British Association of Dermatologists clinical guideline: an update on the process and guidance for authors. Br J Dermatol 2009; 160:725–8.

4 Appraisal of Guidelines Research and Evaluation. AGREE Instrument 2004. Available at: http://www.agreecollaboration.org/instrument/ (last accessed 3 August 2010).

5 Dickie RJ, Horne CHW, Sutherland HW. Direct evidence of localised immunological damage in lichen sclerosus et atrophicus. J Clin Pathol 1982; 35:1395–9.

6 Carli P, Cattaneo A, Pimpenelli N et al. Immunohistochemical evidence of skin immune system involvement in vulvar lichen sclerosus et atrophicus. Dermatologica 1991; 182:18–22.

7 Farrell AM, Marren P, Dean D, Wojnarowska F. Lichen sclerosus: evidence that immunological changes occur at all levels of the skin. Br J Dermatol 1999; 140:1087–92.

8 Cooper SM, Ali I, Baldo M, Wojnarowska F. The association of lichen sclerosus and erosive lichen planus of the vulva with autoimmune disease: a case–control study. Arch Dermatol 2008; 144:1432–5.

9 Harrington CI, Dunsmore IR. An investigation into the incidence of autoimmune disorders in patients with lichen sclerosus et atrophicus. Br J Dermatol 1981; 104:563–6.

10 Meyrick Thomas RH, Ridley CM, Black MM. The association of lichen sclerosus atrophicus and autoimmune related disease in males. Br J Dermatol 1983; 109:661–4.

11 Marren P, Charnock FM, Bunce M et al. The associations between lichen sclerosus and antigens of the HLA system. Br J Dermatol 1995; 132:197–203.

12 Azurdia RM, Luzzi GA, Byren L et al. Lichen sclerosus in adult men: a study of HLA associations and susceptibility to autoimmune disease. Br J Dermatol 1999; 140:79–83.

13 Powell J, Wojnarowska F, Winsey S et al. Lichen sclerosus premenarche: autoimmunity and immunogenetics. Br J Dermatol 2000; 142:481–4.

14 De Vito JR, Merogi AJ, Vo T et al. Role of Borrelia burgdorferi in the pathogenesis of morphoea/scleroderma and lichen sclerosus et atrophicus: a PCR study of thirty-five cases. J Cutan Pathol 1996; 23:350–8.

15 Fujiwara H, Fujiwara K, Hashimoto K et al. Detection of Borrelia burgdorferi DNA (B. garinii or B. afzelii) in morphoea and lichen sclerosus et atrophicus tissue of German and Japanese but not of US patients. Arch Dermatol 1997; 133:41–4.

16 Chan I, Oyama N, Neill SM et al. Characterization of IgG autoantibodies to extracellular matrix protein 1 in lichen sclerosus. Clin Exp Dermatol 2004; 29:499–504.

17 Wallace HJ. Lichen sclerosus et atrophicus. Trans St Johns Hosp Dermatol Soc 1971; 57:9–30.

18 Powell J, Wojnarowska F. Childhood vulvar lichen sclerosus: the course after puberty. J Reprod Med 2002; 47:706–9.

19 Lipscombe TK, Wayte J, Wojnarowska F et al. A study of clinical and aetiological factors and possible associations of lichen sclerosus in males. Australas J Dermatol 1997; 38:132–6.

20 Meffert JJ, Davis BM, Grimwood RE. Lichen sclerosus. J Am Acad Dermatol 1995; 32:393–412.

21 Powell JJ, Wojnarowska F. Lichen sclerosus. Lancet 1999; 353:1777–83.

22 Smith YR, Haefner HK. Vulvar lichen sclerosus: pathophysiology and treatment. Am J Clin Dermatol 2004; 5:105–25.

23 Pugliese JM, Morey AF, Peterson AC. Lichen sclerosus: review of the literature and current recommendations for management. J Urol 2007; 178:2268–76.

24 Neill SM, Lewis FM, eds. Ridley's The Vulva. London: Wiley-Blackwell, 2009; 115–23.

25 Handfield-Jones SE, Hinde FR, Kennedy CTC. Lichen sclerosus et atrophicus in children misdiagnosed as sexual abuse. BMJ 1987; 294:1404–5.

26 Warrington S, San Lazaro C. Lichen sclerosus and sexual abuse. Arch Dis Child 1996; 75:512–16.

27 Aynaud O, Piron D, Casanova JM. Incidence of preputial lichen sclerosus in adults: histologic study of circumcision specimens. J Am Acad Dermatol 1999; 41:923–6.

28 Liatsikos EN, Perimenis P, Dandinis K et al. Lichen sclerosus et atrophicus. Findings after complete circumcision. Scand J Urol Nephrol 1997; **31**:453–6.

29 Chalmers RJ, Burton PA, Bennett RF et al. Lichen sclerosus et atrophicus. A common and distinctive cause of phimosis in boys. Arch Dermatol 1984; **120**:1025–7.

30 Meuli M, Briner J, Hanimann B. Lichen sclerosus et atrophicus causing phimosis in boys: a prospective study with 5-year follow up after complete circumcision. J Urol 1994; **152**:987–9.

31 Kiss A, Király L, Kutasy B, Merksz M. High incidence of balanitis xerotica obliterans in boys with phimosis: prospective 10-year study. Pediatr Dermatol 2005; **22**:305–8.

32 Christman MS, Chen JT, Holmes NM. Obstructive complications of lichen sclerosus. J Pediatr Urol 2009; **5**:165–9.

33 Madan V, Cox NH. Extensive bullous lichen sclerosus with scarring alopecia. Clin Exp Dermatol 2009; **34**:360–2.

34 Ballister I, Bañuls J, Pérez-Crespo M, Lucas A. Extragenital bullous lichen sclerosus atrophicus. Dermatol Online J 2009; **15**:6.

35 Criado PR, Lima FH, Miguel DS et al. Lichen sclerosus – a keratotic variant. J Eur Acad Dermatol Venereol 2002; **16**:504–5.

36 Birenbaum DZ, Young RC. High prevalence of thyroid disease in patients with lichen sclerosus. J Reprod Med 2007; **32**:28–30.

37 Yesudian PD, Mendelssohn S, O'Mahoney C. Herpes simplex superinfection simulating erosive lichen sclerosus. Br J Dermatol 2006; **155** (Suppl. 1):28 (abstr.)

38 Hart WR, Norris HJ, Helwig EB. Relation of lichen sclerosus et atrophicus of the vulva to development of carcinoma. Obstet Gynecol 1975; **45**:369–77.

39 Leibowitch M, Neill S, Pelisse M, Moyal-Baracco M. The epithelial changes associated with squamous cell carcinoma of the vulva: a review of the clinical, histological and viral findings in 78 women. Br J Obstet Gynaecol 1990; **97**:1135–9.

40 Walkden V, Chia Y, Wojnarowska F. The association of squamous cell carcinoma and lichen sclerosus; implications for follow up. J Obstet Gynaecol 1997; **17**:551–3.

41 Vilmer C, Cavalier-Balloy B, Nogues C et al. Analysis of alterations adjacent to invasive vulvar cancer and their relationship with the associated carcinoma: a study of 67 cases. Eur J Gynaecol Oncol 1998; **19**:25–31.

42 van Seters M, ten Kate FJ, van Beurden M et al. In the absence of (early) invasive carcinoma, vulvar intraepithelial neoplasia associated with lichen sclerosus is mainly of undifferentiated type: new insights in histology and aetiology. J Clin Pathol 2007; **60**:504–9.

43 Nasca MR, Innocenzi D, Micali G. Penile cancer among patients with genital lichen sclerosus. J Am Acad Dermatol 1999; **41**:911–14.

44 Depasquale I, Park AJ, Bracka A. The treatment of balanitis xerotica obliterans. BJU Int 2000; **86**:459–65.

45 Powell J, Robson A, Cranston D et al. High incidence of lichen sclerosus in patients with squamous cell carcinoma of the penis. Br J Dermatol 2001; **145**:85–9.

46 Barbagli G, Palminteri E, Mirri F et al. Penile carcinoma in patients with genital lichen sclerosus: a multicenter survey. J Urol 2006; **175**:1359–63.

47 Cupp MR, Malek RS, Goellner JR et al. The detection of human papillomavirus deoxyribonucleic acid in intraepithelial, in situ, verrucous and invasive carcinoma of the penis. J Urol 1995; **154**:1024–9.

48 Lau PW, Cook N, Andrews H et al. Detection of human papillomavirus types in balanitis xerotica obliterans and other penile conditions. Genitourin Med 1995; **71**:228–30.

49 Nasca MR, Innocenzi D, Micali G. Association of penile lichen sclerosus and oncogenic human papillomavirus. Int J Dermatol 2006; **45**:681–3.

50 Prowse DM, Ktori EN, Chandrasekaran D et al. Human papillomavirus-associated increase in p16INK4A expression in penile lichen sclerosus and squamous cell carcinoma. Br J Dermatol 2008; **158**:261–5.

51 Innocenzi D, Nasca MR, Skroza N et al. Penile lichen sclerosus: correlation between histopathologic features and risk of cancer. Acta Dermatovenerol Croat 2006; **14**:225–9.

52 Paniel BJ, Berville-Levy S, Moyal-Baracco M. La vulvopérinéoplastie. J Gynécol Obstét Biol Reprod 1984; **31**:91–9.

53 Paniel BJ, Rouzier R. Surgical procedures in benign disease. In: Ridley's The Vulva (Neill SM, Lewis FM, eds). London: Wiley-Blackwell, 2009; 236.

54 Dalziel K. Effect of lichen sclerosus on sexual function and parturition. J Reprod Med 1995; **40**:351–4.

55 Marin MG, King R, Dennerstein GJ, Sfameni S. Dyspareunia and vulval disease. J Reprod Med 1998; **43**:952–8.

56 Dalziel K, Millard PR, Wojnarowska F. The treatment of vulvar lichen sclerosus with a very potent topical corticosteroid (clobetasol propionate 0.05%) cream. Br J Dermatol 1991; **124**:461–4.

57 Lorenz B, Kaufman RH, Kutzner SK. Lichen sclerosus. Therapy with clobetasol propionate. J Reprod Med 1998; **43**:790–4.

58 Ayhan A, Guven S, Guvendag Guven ES et al. Topical testosterone versus clobetasol for vulvar lichen sclerosus. Int J Gynaecol Obstet 2007; **96**:117–21.

59 Lagos BR, Maibach HI. Frequency of application of topical corticosteroids: an overview. Br J Dermatol 1998; **139**:763–6.

60 Renaud-Vilmer C, Cavalier-Balloy B, Porcher R, Dubertret L. Vulvar lichen sclerosus. Arch Dermatol 2004; **140**:709–12.

61 Cooper SM, Gao XH, Powell J, Wojnarowska F. Does treatment of vulvar lichen sclerosus influence its prognosis? Arch Dermatol 2004; **140**:702–6.

62 Diakomanolis ES, Haidopoulos D, Syndos M et al. Vulvar lichen sclerosus in postmenopausal women: a comparative study for treating advanced disease with clobetasol propionate 0.05%. Eur J Gynaecol Oncol 2002; **23**:519–22.

63 Cattaneo A, de Magnis A, Botti E et al. Topical mometasone furoate for vulvar lichen sclerosus. J Reprod Med 2003; **48**:444–8.

64 Simonart T, Lahaye M, Simonart JM. Vulvar lichen sclerosus: effect of maintenance treatment with a moisturizer on the course of the disease. Menopause 2008; **15**:74–7.

65 Dahlman-Ghozlan K, von Hedblad MA, Krogh G. Penile lichen sclerosus treated with clobetasol dipropionate 0.05% cream: a retrospective clinical and histopathological study. J Am Acad Dermatol 1999; **40**:451–7.

66 Riddell L, Edwards A, Sherrard J. Clinical features of lichen sclerosus in men attending a department of genitourinary medicine. Sex Transm Infect 2000; **76**:311–13.

67 Powell J, Wojnarowska F. Childhood vulvar lichen sclerosus: an increasingly common problem. J Am Acad Dermatol 2001; **44**:803–6.

68 Fischer G, Rogers M. Treatment of childhood vulval lichen sclerosus with potent topical corticosteroid. Pediatr Dermatol 1997; **14**:235–8.

69 Garzon MC, Paller AS. Ultrapotent topical corticosteroid treatment of childhood lichen sclerosus. Arch Dermatol 1999; **135**:525–8.

70 Yang SSD, Tsai YC, Wu CC et al. Highly potent and moderately potent topical steroids are effective in treating phimosis: a prospective randomized study. J Urol 2005; **173**:1361–3.

71 Kiss A, Csontai A, Nyirady P et al. The response of balanitis xerotica obliterans to local steroid application compared with placebo in children. J Urol 2001; **165**:219–20.

72 Jørgensen ET, Svensson A. The treatment of phimosis in boys, with a potent topical steroid (clobetasol propionate 0.05%) cream. Acta Derm Venereol (Stockh) 1993; **73**:55–4.

73 Lindhagen T. Topical clobetasol propionate compared with placebo in the treatment of unretractable foreskin. Eur J Surg 1996; **162**:969–72.

74 Ghysel C, Vander Eeckt K, Bogaert GA. Long-term efficiency of skin stretching and a topical corticoid cream application for unretractable foreskin and phimosis in prepubertal boys. *Urol Int* 2009; **82**:81–8.

75 Sideri M, Origoni M, Spinaci L, Ferrari A. Topical testosterone in the treatment of vulvar lichen sclerosus. *Int J Gynaecol Obstet* 1994; **46**:53–6.

76 Cattaneo A, Carli P, De Marco A et al. Testosterone maintenance therapy. Effects on vulval lichen sclerosus treated with clobetasol propionate. *J Reprod Med* 1996; **41**:99–102.

77 Bornstein J, Heifetz S, Kellner Y et al. Clobetasol dipropionate 0.05% versus testosterone 2% topical application for severe vulvar lichen sclerosus. *Am J Obstet Gynecol* 1998; **178**:80–4.

78 Jasionowski EA, Jasionowski PA. Further observations of the effect of topical progesterone on vulvar disease. *Am J Obstet Gynecol* 1979; **134**:565–7.

79 August PJ, Milward TM. Cryosurgery in the treatment of lichen sclerosus et atrophicus of the vulva. *Br J Dermatol* 1980; **103**:667–70.

80 Hillemans P, Untch M, Prove F et al. Photodynamic therapy of vulvar lichen sclerosus with 5-aminolevulinic acid. *Obstet Gynecol* 1999; **93**:71–4.

81 Zawislak AA, McCluggage WG, Donnelly RF et al. Response of vulval lichen sclerosus and squamous hyperplasia to photodynamic treatment using sustained topical delivery of aminolevulinic acid from a novel bioadhesive patch system. *Photodermatol Photoimmunol Photomed* 2009; **25**:111–13.

82 Beattie PE, Dawe RS, Ferguson J, Ibbotson SH. UVA1 phototherapy for genital lichen sclerosus. *Clin Exp Dermatol* 2006; **31**:343–7.

83 Kartamaa M, Reitamo S. Treatment of lichen sclerosus with carbon dioxide laser vaporization. *Br J Dermatol* 1997; **136**:356–9.

84 Li C, Bian D, Chen W et al. Focussed ultrasound therapy of vulvar dystrophies: a feasibility study. *Obstet Gynecol* 2004; **104**:915–21.

85 Kulkarni S, Barbagli G, Kirpekar D et al. Lichen sclerosus of the male genitalia and urethra: surgical options and results in a multi-center international experience with 215 patients. *Eur Urol* 2009; **55**:945–54.

86 Levine LA, Strom KH, Lux MM. Buccal mucosa graft urethroplasty for anterior urethral stricture repair: evaluation of the impact of stricture location and lichen sclerosus on surgical outcome. *J Urol* 2007; **178**:2011–15.

87 Hrebinko RL. Circumferential laser vaporization for severe meatal stenosis secondary to balanitis xerotica obliterans. *J Urol* 1996; **156**:1735–6.

88 Windahl T. Is carbon dioxide laser treatment of lichen sclerosus effective in the long run? *Scand J Urol Nephrol* 2006; **40**:208–11.

89 Klein LE, Cohen SR, Weinstein M. Bullous lichen sclerosus et atrophicus: treatment by tangential excision. *J Am Acad Dermatol* 1984; **10**:346–50.

90 Breuckmann F, Gambichler T, Altmeyer P, Kreuter A. UVA/UVA1 phototherapy and PUVA photochemotherapy in connective tissue diseases and related disorders: a research based review. *BMC Dermatol* 2004; **4**:11.

91 Colbert RL, Chiang MP, Carlin CS, Fleming M. Progressive extra-genital lichen sclerosus successfully treated with narrowband UV-B phototherapy. *Arch Dermatol* 2007; **143**:19–20.

92 Valdivielso-Ramos M, Bueno C, Hernanz JM. Significant improvement in extensive lichen sclerosus with tacrolimus ointment and PUVA. *Am J Clin Dermatol* 2008; **9**:175–9.

93 Kroft EB, Berkhof NJ, van de Kerkhof PC et al. Ultraviolet A phototherapy for sclerotic skin diseases: a systematic review. *J Am Acad Dermatol* 2008; **59**:1017–30.

94 Rombold S, Lobisch K, Katzer K et al. Efficacy of UVA1 phototherapy in 230 patients with various skin diseases. *Photodermatol Photoimmunol Photomed* 2008; **24**:19–23.

95 Passeron T, Lacour JP, Ortonne JP. Comparative treatment of extra-genital lichen sclerosus with methyl amino laevulinic acid pulsed dye laser mediated photodynamic therapy or pulsed dye laser alone. *Dermatol Surg* 2009; **35**:878–80.

96 Goldstein AT, Marinoff SC, Christopher K. Pimecrolimus for the treatment of vulvar lichen sclerosus: a report of 4 cases. *J Reprod Med* 2004; **49**:778–80.

97 Luesley DM, Downey GP. Topical tacrolimus in the management of lichen sclerosus. *Br J Obstet Gynaecol* 2006; **113**:823–4.

98 Nissi R, Eriksen H, Risteli J, Niemimaa M. Pimecrolimus cream 1% in the management of lichen sclerosus. *Gynecol Obstet Invest* 2007; **127**:808–16.

99 Virgili A, Lauriola MM, Mantovani L, Corrazza M. Vulvar lichen sclerosus: 11 women treated with tacrolimus 0.1% ointment. *Acta Derm Venereol* 2007; **87**:69–72.

100 Hengge UR, Krause W, Hofmann H et al. Multicentre, phase II trial on the safety of topical tacrolimus ointment for the treatment of lichen sclerosus. *Br J Dermatol* 2006; **155**:1021–8.

101 Boms S, Gambichler T, Frietag M et al. Pimecrolimus 1% cream for anogenital lichen sclerosus in childhood. *BMC Dermatol* 2004; **4**:14.

102 Bunker CB, Neill SM, Staughton RCD. Topical tacrolimus, genital lichen sclerosus and risk of squamous cell carcinoma. *Arch Dermatol* 2004; **140**:1169.

103 Ormerod AD. Topical tacrolimus and pimecrolimus and the risk of cancer: how much cause for concern? *Br J Dermatol* 2005; **153**:701–5.

104 Becker JC, Houben R, Vetter CS, Brocker EB. The carcinogenic potential of tacrolimus ointment beyond immune suppression: a hypothesis creating case report. *BMC Cancer* 2006; **6**:7.

105 Edey K, Bisson D, Kennedy C. Topical tacrolimus in the management of lichen sclerosus. *Br J Obstet Gynaecol* 2006; **113**:1482.

106 Fischer G, Bradford J. Topical immunosuppressants, genital lichen sclerosus and the risk of squamous cell carcinoma: a case report. *J Reprod Med* 2007; **52**:329–31.

107 Carli P, Cattaneo A, Taddei G, Gianotti B. Topical cyclosporine in the treatment of vulvar lichen sclerosus: clinical histologic and immunohistochemical findings. *Arch Dermatol* 1992; **128**:1279–80.

108 Bulbul Baskan E, Turan H, Tunali S et al. Open-label trial of cyclosporine for vulvar lichen sclerosus. *J Am Acad Dermatol* 2007; **57**:276–8.

109 Nayeemuddin F, Yates VM. Lichen sclerosus et atrophicus responding to methotrexate. *Clin Exp Dermatol* 2008; **33**:651–2.

110 Tomson N, Sterling JC. Hydroxycarbamide: a treatment for lichen sclerosus? *Br J Dermatol* 2007; **157**:622.

111 Kreuter A, Tigges C, Gaifullina R et al. Pulsed high-dose corticosteroids combined with low-dose methotrexate treatment in patients with refractory generalized extragenital lichen sclerosus. *Arch Dermatol* 2009; **145**:1303–8.

112 Mork N-J, Jensen P, Hoel PS. Vulval lichen sclerosus treated with etretinate (Tigason). *Acta Derm Venereol (Stockh)* 1986; **66**:363–5.

113 Bousema MT, Romppanen U, Geiger J-M et al. Acitretin in the treatment of lichen sclerosus et atrophicus of the vulva: a double blind placebo controlled study. *J Am Acad Dermatol* 1994; **30**:225–31.

114 Virgili A, Corazza M, Bianchi A et al. Open study of topical 0.025% tretinoin in the treatment of vulval lichen sclerosus. One year of therapy. *J Reprod Med* 1995; **40**:614–18.

115 Penneys NS. Treatment of lichen sclerosus with potassium para-aminobenzoate. *J Am Acad Dermatol* 1984; **10**:1039–42.

116 Balasubramaniam P, Lewis FM. Long-term follow-up of patients with lichen sclerosus: does it really happen? *J Obstet Gynaecol* 2007; **27**:282.

117 Jones RW, Curry J, Neill S, MacLean AB. Guidelines for the follow-up of women with vulvar lichen sclerosus in specialist clinics. *Am J Obstet Gynecol* 2008; **198**:496.e1–3.

Appendix 1: Recommendation and evidence gradings

Level of evidence

Level of evidence	Type of evidence
1++	High-quality meta-analyses, systematic reviews of RCTs, or RCTs with a very low risk of bias
1+	Well-conducted meta-analyses, systematic reviews of RCTs, or RCTs with a low risk of bias
1−	Meta-analyses, systematic reviews of RCTs, or RCTs with a high risk of bias[a]
2++	High-quality systematic reviews of case–control or cohort studies. High-quality case–control or cohort studies with a very low risk of confounding, bias or chance and a high probability that the relationship is causal
2+	Well-conducted case–control or cohort studies with a low risk of confounding, bias or chance and a moderate probability that the relationship is causal
2−	Case–control or cohort studies with a high risk of confounding, bias or chance and a significant risk that the relationship is not causal[a]
3	Nonanalytical studies (e.g. case reports, case series)
4	Expert opinion, formal consensus

[a]Studies with a level of evidence '−' should not be used as a basis for making a recommendation. RCT, randomized controlled trial.

Strength of recommendation

Class	Evidence
A	• At least one meta-analysis, systematic review, or RCT rated as 1++, and directly applicable to the target population, **or** • A systematic review of RCTs or a body of evidence consisting principally of studies rated as 1+, directly applicable to the target population and demonstrating overall consistency of results • Evidence drawn from a NICE technology appraisal
B	• A body of evidence including studies rated as 2++, directly applicable to the target population and demonstrating overall consistency of results, **or** • Extrapolated evidence from studies rated as 1++ or 1+
C	• A body of evidence including studies rated as 2+, directly applicable to the target population and demonstrating overall consistency of results, **or** • Extrapolated evidence from studies rated as 2++
D	• Evidence level 3 or 4, **or** • Extrapolated evidence from studies rated as 2+, **or** • Formal consensus
D (GPP)	• A good practice point (GPP) is a recommendation for best practice based on the experience of the guideline development group

RCT, randomized controlled trial; NICE, National Institute for Health and Clinical Excellence.

http://bad.org.uk/Portals/_Bad/Guidelines/Clinical
%20Guidelines/Lichen%20Sclerosus.pdf

Comment

The mainstay of treatment for lichen sclerosus (LS) remains ultra-potent topical corticosteroids [1]. Since the 2002 guidelines [2], there is weak evidence for the use of various other treatments such as photodynamic therapy, ultraviolet light (UVA1) and laser radiation [1]. Topical tacrolimus has been recommended as a second-line therapy [1] because of its unknown potential as a co-carcinogen. Long-term studies looking at the safety of ultra-potent topical corticosteroid use in LS are needed.

REFERENCES

1 Neill SM, Lewis FM, Tatnall FM, Cox NH. Guidelines for the management of lichen sclerosus. *Brit J Dermatol* 2010; 163: 672–82.
2 Neill SM, Tatnall FM, Cox NH. Guidelines for the management of lichen sclerosus. *Brit J Dermatol* 2002; 147: 640–49.

Additional professional resources

http://bad.org.uk/Portals/_Bad/Guidelines/Clinical
%20Guidelines/Lichen%20Sclerosus.pdf
http://www.bashh.org/documents/113/113.pdf   (British Association for Sexual Health and HIV)

BAD patient information leaflet

http://www.bad.org.uk/site/838/Default.aspx

Related to vulval skin care
http://www.bad.org.uk/site/1237/Default.aspx
http://www.dermnetnz.org/immune/lichen-sclerosus.html

Other patient resources

http://www.lichensclerosus.org
http://www.patient.co.uk/pdf/pilsL409.pdf
http://www.emedicine.com/derm/topic234.htm
http://www.dermnetnz.org/dna.ls/ls.html

Guidelines for the management of pemphigus vulgaris

K.E.HARMAN, S.ALBERT AND M.M.BLACK

St John's Institute of Dermatology, St Thomas' Hospital, London, SE1 7EH U.K.

Accepted for publication 15 May 2003

Summary   These guidelines for management of pemphigus vulgaris have been prepared for dermatologists on behalf of the British Association of Dermatologists. They present evidence-based guidance for treatment, with identification of the strength of evidence available at the time of preparation of the guidelines, and a brief overview of epidemiological aspects, diagnosis and investigation.

Key words: guidelines, immunosuppression, management, pemphigus vulgaris, therapy, treatment

Disclaimer

These guidelines have been prepared for dermatologists on behalf of the British Association of Dermatologists and reflect the best data available at the time the report was prepared. Caution should be exercised in interpreting the data; the results of future studies may require alteration of the conclusions or recommendations in this report. It may be necessary or even desirable to depart from the guidelines in the interests of patients and special circumstances. Just as adherence to guidelines may not constitute a defence against a claim of negligence, so deviation from them should not necessarily be deemed negligent.

Introduction

Pemphigus vulgaris (PV) is an acquired autoimmune disease in which IgG antibodies target desmosomal proteins to produce intraepithelial, mucocutaneous blistering. Desmoglein (Dsg) 3 is the major antigen but 50–60% of patients have additional antibodies to

Correspondence: Dr K.E.Harman.
Dept. of Dermatology, Leicester Royal
Infirmary, Leicester, LE1 5WW, U.K.
E-mail: karenharman@doctors.org.uk

These guidelines were commissioned by the British Association of Dermatologists Therapy Guidelines and Audit subcommittee. Members of the committee are N.H.Cox (Chairman), A.S.Highet, D.Mehta, R.H.Meyrick Thomas, A.D.Ormerod, J.K.Schofield, C.H.Smith and J.C.Sterling.

Dsg1, the antigen in pemphigus foliaceus (PF).[1-3] The underlying antibody profile is a major determinant of the clinical phenotype of PV.[3-5]

The mortality of PV was 75% on average before the introduction of corticosteroids (CS) in the early 1950s.[6] This figure may be an underestimate due to lack of diagnostic criteria, inclusion of all subtypes of pemphigus and inclusion of other blistering disorders, such as bullous pemphigoid, which have a better prognosis. However, not all cases of PV have such a dismal prognosis. Studies differentiating according to clinical phenotype have shown a lower mortality in patients with predominantly mucosal PV (1–17%) compared with those with mucocutaneous PV (34–42%).[7,8]

Clinical presentation

The diagnosis of PV should be suspected in any patient with mucocutaneous erosions or blisters. The oral mucosa is the first site of involvement in the majority of cases and PV may remain confined to the mucosal surfaces or extend to involve the skin (average lag period 4 months). A minority will present with cutaneous erosions but oral erosions occur in (almost) all cases. PV presents across a wide age range with peak frequency in the third to sixth decades.

Laboratory diagnosis

A skin or mucosal biopsy should be taken for histology and direct immunofluorescence (DIF), the latter requiring perilesional, intact skin or clinically uninvolved skin.[9] Suprabasal acantholysis and blister formation is highly suggestive of PV but the diagnosis should be confirmed by the characteristic deposition of IgG in the intercellular spaces of the epidermis. Indirect immuno-fluorescence (IIF) is less sensitive than DIF[10–12] but may be helpful if a biopsy is difficult, e.g. children and uncooperative adults. Enzyme-linked immunosorbent assays (ELISA) are now available for direct measurement of Dsg1 and Dsg3 antibodies in serum. They offer advantages over IIF and may supersede this technique.[13,14] Five millilitres of blood is sufficient for IIF and ELISA.

In patients with oral pemphigus, an intraoral biopsy is the optimum but IIF or DIF on a skin biopsy may suffice. One study showed that the sensitivity of DIF was 71% in oral biopsies compared with 61% in normal skin taken from 28 patients with oral PV.[15] Another study reported that the sensitivity of DIF was 89% in oral biopsies compared with 85% for IIF.[16]

Baseline investigations

The following investigations are suggested prior to commencing treatment: biopsy (or IIF) as above, full blood count and differential, urea and electrolytes, liver function tests, glucose, antinuclear antibody (differential of pemphigus erythematosus), thiopurine methyl-transferase (TPMT) levels (if azathioprine is to be used), chest X-ray, urinalysis and blood pressure. Current guidelines on osteoporosis should be followed, so a bone density scan early in the course of treatment may be recommended.

Evaluating therapies in pemphigus vulgaris

In general, the quality of published data concerning the therapy of PV is poor. There are few controlled trials, partly reflecting the rarity of PV. The majority of data is confined to case reports and small case series with short follow-up periods in which PV cases of variable severity are included, often with other subtypes of pemphigus. Drugs are often used in combination, particularly adjuvant drugs given concurrently with steroids, and dosing schedules vary widely. Controls are often indirect, involving comparisons of remission and mortality rates with historical controls or comparison of maintenance steroid doses before and after the addition of a given therapy. Therefore, in most studies, it is difficult to judge the effect of individual drugs and make firm treatment recommendations. In these guidelines, we have listed the highest ranking level of evidence and

given an overall recommendation for each therapy. A summary of treatment options is given in Table 1.

General principles of management

The initial aim of treatment is to induce disease remission. This should be followed by a period of maintenance treatment using the minimum drug doses required for disease control in order to minimize their side-effects. Occasional blisters are acceptable and indicate that the patient is not being overtreated. The ultimate aim of management should be treatment withdrawal and a recent study reported complete remission rates of 38%, 50% and 75% achieved 3, 5 and 10 years from diagnosis.[17]

Most patients are treated with systemic corticosteroids (CS), which are effective. Adjuvant drugs are commonly used in combination with the aims of increasing efficacy and of having a steroid-sparing action, thereby allowing reduced maintenance CS doses and reduced CS side-effects. Although mortality and complete remission rates have improved since the introduction of adjuvant drugs, this is in comparison with historical controls; a more recent study of PV patients treated with CS alone demonstrated outcomes comparable with studies using adjuvants.[18] There are no prospective, controlled studies that conclusively demonstrate the benefits of adjuvant drugs in PV. Therefore, some respected authorities do not use adjuvant drugs unless there are contraindications or side-effects of CS, or if tapering the CS dose is associated with repeated relapses.[6] However, most centres do use adjuvant drugs as standard practice. In general, adjuvant drugs are slower in onset than CS and are therefore rarely used alone to induce remission in PV.

Oral corticosteroids

Systemic CS are the best established therapy for the management of PV (*Strength of recommendation A, Quality of evidence II-iii*; see Appendix 1). Their introduction in the early 1950s resulted in a dramatic fall in mortality to an average of 30%[6] with complete remission rates of 13–20%.[6,19] Outcomes have continued to improve and in a recent study, the mortality was zero and the complete remission rate was 29% in 17 patients treated with steroids alone and followed for 4–6 years.[18]

Clinical improvement may be seen within days of starting CS. On average, cessation of blistering takes 2–3 weeks[20–22] and full healing may take 6–8 weeks.[23]

Table 1. Summary of treatment options

Drug	Strength of recommendation; Quality of evidence	Evidence and indication(s)	Principal side-effects	Advantages	Disadvantages
Oral steroids	A; II-iii	The cornerstone of therapy; effective; optimum dosing schedule not known	Diabetes; osteoporosis; adrenal suppression; peptic ulceration; weight gain; increased susceptibility to infection; mood changes; proximal myopathy; Cushing's syndrome; cataracts	Effective; rapid onset; oral administration; inexpensive	Side-effect profile
Pulsed i.v. steroids	C; IV	Few studies;[27,28] aims are theoretical. *Consider for remission induction in severe or recalcitrant disease, particularly if unresponsive to high oral doses*	Mood changes; flushing	Rapid onset; inexpensive	i.v. administration
Adjuvant drugs		Generally slower in onset than steroids, so rarely used alone to induce remission. *Commonly used in conjunction with CS for their steroid-sparing actions; may be used alone to maintain remission after CS withdrawal*			
Azathioprine	B; II-iii	Reports show steroid-sparing action;[29–33] complete remission rates 28–45%;[6,19,31] mortality rates 1·4–7%;[7,19,31] consider measuring TPMT activity for dose.[35–37] *Commonly used in combination with oral CS for steroid-sparing effect; monotherapy possible for mild disease.*	Myelosuppression and nausea (related to TPMT activity); hepatotoxicity and hypersensitivity reactions (unrelated to TPMT activity); increased susceptibility to infection	Oral administration; inexpensive	Slow onset; side-effect profile
Oral cyclophosphamide	B; III	Five small studies.[39–43] *Could be considered as an alternative to azathioprine if secondary infertility is not a concern*	Neutropenia; alopecia; GI disturbances; raised transaminases; thrombocytopenia; secondary infertility	Inexpensive; oral administration	Potential risk of haemorrhagic cystitis and carcinoma of bladder
Pulsed cyclophosphamide and dexamethasone or methylprednisolone	B; II-iii	Large series of 300 patients.[45] *Consider for severe or recalcitrant PV; repeated courses; may not be practical*	Alopecia, infections; amenorrhoea; ovarian/testicular failure; haemorrhagic cystitis; acne; hiccup	Possibly fewer steroid side-effects than conventional CS therapy;	i.v. administration; labour-intensive
Mycophenolate mofetil	B; III	Several reports;[38,49,50] largest series 12 patients;[49] two reports of monotherapy.[51,52] *Could be considered for recalcitrant cases or if azathioprine/ cyclophosphamide unsuitable; may supersede azathioprine as adjuvant of choice in future*	GI disturbances; lymphopenia; anaemia; thrombocytopenia; increased risk of opportunistic infections	Well tolerated and relatively less toxic compared with other immunosuppressive agents	Expensive

Table 1. Continued

Drug	Strength of recommendation; Quality of evidence	Evidence and indication(s)	Principal side-effects	Advantages	Disadvantages
Gold	B/C; III	Several series;[53–56] complete remission rates 15–44% but side-effects requiring drug withdrawal in 17–35%;[55,56] ineffective in up to 28% of cases. *Reports of use as monotherapy;[53,54] more commonly used as an adjuvant, enabling steroid dose reduction; an alternative to more established adjuvant drugs[56]*	Rashes; nephrotic syndrome; myelosuppression; hypersensitivity syndromes	Inexpensive	Intramuscular administration; slow onset
Methotrexate	C; III	Early reports of high mortality;[57–60] more recent small studies show benefit[61]	Myelosuppression; hepatotoxicity; pneumonitis	Oral administration; inexpensive	Slow onset
Ciclosporin	C; I	A few small case series suggest a steroid-sparing effect[22,62,63] but a randomized controlled trial showed no additional benefit and more side-effects compared with methylprednisolone alone;[18] therefore cannot be recommended as an adjuvant drug in PV	Hypertension; renal impairment; GI disturbances; hypertrichosis; hypertrophic gingivitis		Side-effects; expensive
Tetracyclines and nicotinamide	C; IV	Some reports of benefit with nicotinamide and tetracycline[64,65] or nicotinamide, tetracycline and prednisolone[64] or tetracycline/minocycline and prednisolone.[66–68] *Tetracycline/nicotinamide could be considered as an adjuvant in milder PV*	Flushing and headaches due to vasodilation with nicotinamide; GI upset (tetracyclines); hyperpigmentation, particularly at sites of blistering (minocycline); discoloration of teeth (avoid tetracyclines in children and pregnant/lactating females)	Inexpensive	Lots of tablets
Dapsone/ sulphonamides	C; IV	Very few reports and small numbers but may have a steroid-sparing action[69–71]	Haemolysis; methaemoglobinaemia; hypersensitivity reactions	Inexpensive	Minimal data
Chlorambucil	C; IV	One case series only, suggesting steroid-sparing effect[72]	Myelosuppression	Oral administration; inexpensive	Minimal data
IVIG	B; III	Reports of 48 patients treated;[73–83] most beneficial when used as adjuvant when improvement may be rapid but transient unless repeated.[75,81,82] *Possible adjuvant maintenance agent for recalcitrant PV failed on other regimens; could be considered in severe cases to induce remission while slower-acting drugs take effect*	During infusion, chills, tachycardia, hypertension, muscle pains, pyrexia, nausea and headache are common, self-limited and respond to slowing the infusion; anaphylaxis is rare	Rapid action reported in some cases	i.v. administration; expensive; labour-intensive; theoretical risk of blood-borne virus infections

Table 1. Continued

Drug	Strength of recommendation; Quality of evidence	Evidence and indication(s)	Principal side-effects	Advantages	Disadvantages
Plasma exchange	C; I	One randomized study showed no benefit over and above steroids;[84] some case reports suggest steroid-sparing effect/clinical benefit.[85–96] *Not recommended as routine; may be considered for difficult cases if combined with steroids and immunosuppressants*	Septicaemia; fluid and electrolyte imbalance	Direct and immediate removal of IgG and therefore removal of PV antibodies	Central venous access; specialist equipment; trained staff; limited availability; labour-intensive; expensive rebound production of PV antibodies after PE
Extracorporeal photopheresis	B; III	Nine patients with recalcitrant PV improved allowing reduced steroid/immunosuppressive doses.[101–104] *Could be considered in recalcitrant disease where conventional treatment has failed*	Symptoms of hypovolaemia during procedure	Can be performed via peripheral venous access	Specialist equipment; trained staff; labour-intensive; expensive; limited availability; limited data; UV protective sunglasses on the day of treatment; venous access can be a problem

CS, corticosteroids; GI, gastrointestinal; i.v. intravenous; IVIG, intravenous immunoglobulin; PE, plasma exchange, UV, ultraviolet; PV, pemphigus vulgaris; TPMT, thiopurine methyltransferase.

IIF titres fall with CS treatment but lag behind clinical improvement.[24]

The optimum CS dosing schedule is not known and dosing schedules are largely empirical and based on practical experience. Early studies advocated high doses, e.g. initial doses of 120–180 mg prednisolone daily.[23] However, CS side-effects were common and dose related[25,26] and one study estimated that up to 77% of deaths were CS related.[25] Therefore, a more moderate approach to CS therapy has been advocated. However, only one controlled trial has compared dosing schedules; initial therapy with low-dose prednisolone (45–60 mg day^{-1}) was compared with high-dose prednisolone (120–180 mg day^{-1}) in patients with severe pemphigus (19 with PV, three with PF) affecting more than 50% of their body surface. There was no significant difference in the duration to achieve remission and in relapse rates at 5 years, and there were no deaths.[21]

A tailored dosing schedule has been advocated according to disease severity[6,23] and a modified regimen is suggested here. Patients with mild disease are treated with initial prednisolone doses of 40–60 mg day^{-1} and in more severe cases, 60–100 mg day^{-1}. If there is no response within 5–7 days, the dose should be increased in 50–100% increments until there is disease control, i.e. no new lesions and healing of existing ones. If doses above 100 mg day^{-1} are required, pulsed intravenous CS could be considered.

Once remission is induced and maintained with healing of the majority of lesions, the dose of CS can be cautiously tapered. A 50% reduction every 2 weeks has been suggested.[6] In our own practice, we initially reduce by 5–10 mg of prednisolone weekly and more slowly below 20 mg prednisolone daily.

It is strongly recommended that guidelines for the prevention of CS-induced osteoporosis are followed.

Pulsed intravenous corticosteroids

This refers to the intermittent administration of high doses of intravenous CS, usually methylprednisolone (250–1000 mg) or equivalent doses of dexamethasone given on one to five consecutive days. The theoretical aims of pulsing are to achieve more rapid and effective disease control compared with conventional oral dosing, thus allowing a reduction in long-term maintenance CS doses and CS side-effects. This has yet to be demonstrated conclusively. One small retrospective study concluded that pulsed intravenous methylprednisolone (one course of 250–1000 mg day^{-1} for 2–5 days in eight cases, two courses in one case) resulted in increased complete remission rates (44% vs. 0%) and lower mean maintenance oral CS doses in nine patients with recalcitrant PV compared with six controls.[27] One report records disease control in 7–10 days in five of nine patients given pulsed methylprednisolone.[28]

Pulsed CS could be considered in severe or recalcitrant PV to induce remission, particularly if there has been no response to high oral doses (*Strength of recommendation C, Quality of evidence IV*).

Adjuvant drugs

Azathioprine

Azathioprine is a commonly prescribed adjuvant drug in PV and small case series report a steroid-sparing effect.[29–33] The complete remission rates of 28–45%[6,19,31] and mortality rates of 1·4–7%[6,7,19,31] exceed those seen in historical controls treated with CS alone.

In three cases, azathioprine was successfully used as a monotherapy to induce and maintain clinical remission with a fall in antibody titre.[30,34] However, there is a latent period of at least 6 weeks before the effects of azathioprine are seen[29–31,34] and its use as monotherapy to induce remission should be reserved for mild cases only.

Azathioprine doses of 1–3 mg kg^{-1} have been used in previous studies but ideally should be titrated according to the individual activity of TPMT. Azathioprine is best avoided in patients with very low TPMT levels (1 : 200–300 of the general population[35]), and should be used at reduced doses, e.g. 0·5 mg kg^{-1}, in those with low levels ($\approx$ 10%[35]). Patients with high levels ($\approx$ 10%[35]) are at risk of undertreatment using standard doses.[36,37] The dose should be titrated upwards according to clinical response and side-effects, and doses up to 3·5–4 mg kg^{-1} may be required.[38]

Azathioprine is a well-established choice as an adjuvant drug for the management of pemphigus (*Strength of recommendation B, Quality of evidence II-iii*).

Oral cyclophosphamide

Several authors have reported the steroid-sparing effects of cyclophosphamide at doses of 50–200 mg day^{-1} in case series of up to six patients.[39–43] In some cases, prolonged remission with cessation of all therapy was possible.[40] In a randomized study, the efficacy of

prednisolone (40 mg day^{-1}) alone was compared with prednisolone/cyclophosphamide (100 mg) and prednisolone/ciclosporin (5 mg kg^{-1}) in 28 patients with oral pemphigus.[15] There was no significant difference in the duration to achieve remission or in relapse rates between the three groups. However, cyclophosphamide and ciclosporin were given for a brief period of only 2–3 months.[15]

Oral cyclophosphamide could be considered as an alternative to azathioprine (*Strength of recommendation B, Quality of evidence III*).

Pulsed intravenous cyclophosphamide with dexamethasone or methylprednisolone

This refers to the intermittent administration of high doses of intravenous CS and cyclophosphamide, usually three daily doses of dexamethasone (100 mg) or methylprednisolone (500–1000 mg) and a single dose of cyclophosphamide (500 mg) given monthly. Pasricha and Ramji first described this therapy for PV.[44] Doses and frequency are arbitrary.

A large case series of 300 Indian patients with pemphigus (255 with PV) treated with dexamethasone–cyclophosphamide pulse (DCP) therapy at 4-weekly intervals has been reported.[45] Low-dose daily oral cyclophosphamide (50 mg) was administered between pulses. Pulsing continued until clinical remission and was followed by a consolidation phase of a further six DCP courses. Oral cyclophosphamide was then continued alone and if there were no relapses after 1 year all treatment was withdrawn. The number of DCPs required to induce clinical remission was variable, with 49% requiring six pulses or fewer but 11% needing more than 2 years of pulsing. Overall, 190 patients (63%) achieved complete remission, 123 (41%) for more than 2 years and 48 (16%) for more than 5 years. The overall mortality rate was 4%. The authors report relative freedom from steroid side-effects but 62% of menstruating females (18 of 29) developed amenorrhoea and azoospermia was also noted. Haemorrhagic cystitis occurred in 0·6%[46] and pituitary–adrenal suppression in 55% of patients (17 of 33).[47]

Another study of 50 Indian patients (45 PV) reported DCP therapy to be effective in most and ineffective in 12%. The mortality was 6% compared with an estimated 25–30% mortality in historical cohorts on conventional CS therapy at the same institute.[48]

Pulsed CS cyclophosphamide therapy could be considered in severe or recalcitrant cases of PV.

However, it may not be practical to administer repeated courses (*Strength of recommendation B, Quality of evidence II-iii*).

Mycophenolate mofetil

Mycophenolate mofetil (MMF) is a relatively new agent in PV therapy. Total daily doses of 2–2·5 g are typically given in two divided doses with prednisolone.[38,49,50] In a series of 12 patients who had relapsed on CS/azathioprine, 11 improved on MMF (2 g day^{-1}) and prednisolone (2 mg kg^{-1}), allowing a reduction in the prednisolone dose to 5 mg day^{-1} or less during the follow-up of 1 year. The patients responded rapidly, with a fall in IIF titres, and were free of lesions within 8 weeks of initiating MMF.[49] However, based on nine patients, Nousari and Anhalt commented that higher doses of MMF (2·5–3 g day^{-1}) were often required to induce remission in PV and at least 8 weeks' treatment was necessary before clinical and immunological improvement was observed.[38]

MMF given as monotherapy has been reported to be beneficial in two cases.[51,52]

On the basis of current evidence, MMF could be considered in recalcitrant cases or when azathioprine and cyclophosphamide cannot be used (*Strength of recommendation B, Quality of evidence III*). However, as experience increases, it may supersede other agents as the adjuvant drug of choice in view of its efficacy and more favourable side-effect profile.

Gold

Most studies have used intramuscular gold, initially at a dose of 50 mg week^{-1} if test doses were tolerated. It was used successfully as monotherapy in five patients,[53,54] with an associated fall in IIF titre.[53] However, it has more commonly been used as an adjuvant drug and steroid-sparing effects are reported. The two largest reported case series are of 18 and 26 patients.[55,56] Complete remission occurred in 15–44% and there were no deaths. The average dose of prednisolone was reduced from 55 mg pregold to 9 mg at the end of the study.[56] However, gold was considered ineffective in 15–28% and side-effects necessitated stopping the drug in 17–35% of patients.

Gold could be considered as an alternative to more established adjuvant drugs if they cannot be used (*Strength of recommendation B/C, Quality of evidence III*).

Methotrexate

High mortality and morbidity rates were attributed to methotrexate in studies from the late 1960s and early 1970s[57–60] and for this reason it has not been a commonly used adjuvant drug for PV. For example, three of four patients cited in one report died, but high doses of methotrexate had been used (125–420 mg week^{-1}) in combination with 40–240 mg of prednisolone daily.[59] However, a recent study of nine patients with recalcitrant PV on CS reports favourable outcomes and few side-effects in response to the addition of a mean dose of 12 mg of methotrexate weekly. CS were completely withdrawn within 6 months in six patients (67%) compared with an estimated 5–7% of similar patients treated previously at the same centre with CS alone.[61]

Methotrexate could be considered as an adjuvant drug if more established drugs cannot be used (*Strength of recommendation C, Quality of evidence III*).

Ciclosporin

Initial small case series reported that ciclosporin was a useful adjuvant with steroid-sparing effects in PV.[22,62,63] However, a single randomized, prospective, controlled trial of 33 patients comparing oral methylprednisolone 1 mg kg^{-1} alone vs. methylprednisolone with ciclosporin 5 mg kg^{-1} found no statistically significant difference in outcome measures such as time to healing, complete remission rate and cumulative CS dose.[18] More side-effects were encountered in the ciclosporin group during a mean follow-up period of 5 years.[18] There were no deaths and 10 patients (five from each group) were in complete remission, off all therapy, while the others were taking an average of prednisone 2·5 mg day^{-1}.[18]

On the basis of current evidence, ciclosporin cannot be recommended as an adjuvant drug in PV (*Strength of recommendation C, Quality of evidence I*).

Tetracyclines/nicotinamide

Variable combinations of tetracyclines with or without nicotinamide have been described in PV. Sixteen patients were given nicotinamide 1·5 g and tetracycline 2 g daily. In 12, no systemic steroids were given and of these only three cleared and three improved.[64,65] Of the four patients given additional prednisolone, there was clearance in one, partial improvement in two and no response in another.[64]

Thirteen new patients with PV were given tetracycline 2 g daily in combination with oral prednisolone. They had a faster response rate and reduced prednisolone requirement compared with seven historical CS-treated controls.[66]

Two studies using minocycline 50–200 mg day^{-1} as an adjuvant drug reported improvement and a steroid-sparing effect in seven of 13 patients.[67,68]

Tetracyclines with or without nicotinamide could be considered as adjuvant treatment, perhaps in milder cases of PV (*Strength of recommendation C, Quality of evidence IV*).

Dapsone/sulphonamides

Dapsone was reported to be beneficial as an adjuvant drug in four cases of PV.[69–71] However, in two of these cases, it was started either with or shortly after prednisolone and in two cases, it was started after the long-standing prednisolone was increased to high doses. Therefore, it is difficult to be certain if dapsone had a significant role and there is little evidence to recommend the use of dapsone in PV (*Strength of recommendation C, Quality of evidence IV*).

Chlorambucil

Seven patients with PV who had failed to respond to other steroid/immunosuppressive combinations were given oral chlorambucil 4 mg day^{-1} titrated upwards according to clinical response. There was improvement or remission in five patients and a steroid-sparing effect was reported. A fall in IIF titres was reported in three of four cases.[72] Chlorambucil could be considered as an adjuvant drug if more established options cannot be used but there are limited data to support its use (*Strength of recommendation C, Quality of evidence IV*).

Intravenous immunoglobulin

Several reports describe a total of 48 patients with PV who have been treated with intravenous immunoglobulin (IVIG).[73–83] Doses of 1·2–2 g kg^{-1} divided over 3–5 days were infused every 2–4 weeks for 1–34 cycles. It was beneficial and steroid-sparing in 44 cases,[74–79,81–83] with falls in IIF titres.[77,79,81–83] Clinical improvement was rapid in some cases[75,81,83] but may be transient unless repeated courses of IVIG are given.[75,81,82] In all cases where beneficial, IVIG was initially given as an adjuvant therapy. Of the four

treatment failures, three were given one course of IVIG as monotherapy.[73]

The largest series is of 21 patients with recalcitrant PV who were given 2 g kg^{-1} of IVIG divided over 3 days monthly. Improvement was noted after 4·5 months on average. A mean of 18 cycles was given (range 14–34). It was possible to withdraw all other therapies including CS, then reduce the frequency and finally stop IVIG infusions. All patients have been in complete remission for an average of 20 months (range 13–73).[82]

Repeated courses of IVIG could be considered as an adjuvant, maintenance agent in patients with recalcitrant disease who have failed more conventional therapies. In view of reports of a rapid action in some cases, it could be used to help induce remission in patients with severe PV while slower-acting drugs take effect (*Strength of recommendation B, Quality of evidence III*).

Plasma exchange

One randomized study of patients with newly diagnosed pemphigus treated with oral CS with (n 19) or without (n 15) additional plasma exchanges (PEs, 10 over 4 weeks) failed to demonstrate any additional clinical benefit of PE. Cumulative steroid doses and changes in IIF titre in the two groups were similar. Furthermore, there were four deaths from sepsis in the PE group.[84] This is in contrast to case reports and small case series which have reported clinical benefit, short-term falls in IIF titres and a steroid-sparing effect of PE.[85–96] In general, these were 'problem' patients with either steroid side-effects, poorly controlled disease on conventional therapy or life-threatening disease. In most cases, PEs were combined with both CS and immunosuppressive drugs and it is thought that the latter is necessary for clinical effect in order to prevent the rebound production of autoantibodies stimulated by PE.[85,88,93,94,97–100]

PE cannot be recommended as a routine treatment option in newly presenting patients with PV. However, it could be considered in difficult cases if combined with CS and immunosuppressant drugs (*Strength of recommendation C, Quality of evidence I*).

Extracorporeal photopheresis

Nine patients with recalcitrant PV were treated with extracorporeal photopheresis (ECP), 2-day cycles given every 2–4 weeks for a minimum of two cycles. In all cases, there was clinical improvement and it was possible to taper the concurrent doses of prednisolone and immunosuppressant drugs.[101–104] Two reports documented a fall in IIF titre[101,103] while another showed no change.[102]

ECP could be considered in recalcitrant cases of PV where there has been failure to improve with more conventional therapy (*Strength of recommendation B, Quality of evidence III*).

Topical therapy

PV is largely managed with systemic therapy but adjuvant topical therapy may be of additional benefit, although there are no controlled studies to confirm this. Rarely, patients with mild disease, particularly if confined to the mucosal surfaces, can be managed on topical therapy alone. Huilgol and Black have reviewed topical therapy for pemphigus and pemphigoid in detail.[105,106]

For oral pemphigus, measures such as soft diets and soft toothbrushes help minimize local trauma. Topical analgesics or anaesthetics, for example benzydamine hydrochloride 0·15% (Difflam Oral Rinse®), are useful in alleviating oral pain, particularly prior to eating or toothbrushing. Oral hygiene is crucial otherwise PV may be complicated by dental decay; toothbrushing should be encouraged and antiseptic mouthwashes may be used, such as chlorhexidine gluconate 0·2% (Corsodyl®), hexetidine 0·1% (Oraldene®), or 1 : 4 hydrogen peroxide solutions. Patients are susceptible to oral candidiasis, which should be treated. Topical CS therapy may help reduce the requirement for systemic agents.[105,106] For multiple oral erosions, mouthwashes are most practical, for example, soluble betamethasone sodium phosphate 0·5 mg tablet dissolved in 10 mL water may be used up to four times daily, holding the solution in the mouth for about 5 min. Isolated oral erosions could be treated with application of triamcinolone acetonide 0·1% in adhesive paste (Adcortyl in Orabase®), 2·5 mg hydrocortisone lozenges or sprayed directly with an asthma aerosol inhaler, for example beclomethasone dipropionate 50–200 µg or budesonide 50–200 µg. Topical ciclosporin (100 mg mL^{-1}) in oral pemphigus has been described and may be of some benefit but is expensive.[107,108]

Follow-up

Once remission is induced, there should follow a period of maintenance treatment using the minimum drug doses required for disease control and during which occasional blisters are acceptable. Drug doses should be slowly reduced and patients should remain under follow-up while they remain on therapy. Ultimately, treatment may be withdrawn if there has been prolonged clinical remission. This decision should largely be clinical but the chances of relapse are reduced if immunofluorescence studies are negative, e.g. the risk of relapse is 13–27% if DIF is negative, 44–100% if DIF is positive, 24% if IIF is negative, and 57% if IIF is positive.[109,110] However, DIF can occasionally remain positive in patients who are in remission and off all treatment.[11]

Suggested audit topics

- Measurement of baseline parameters prior to starting treatment
- Appropriate investigations to establish diagnosis
- Evidence of appropriate drug monitoring
- Adherence to guidelines for prophylaxis and management of steroid-induced osteoporosis.

References

1 Amagai M, Hashimoto T, Shimizu N, Nishikawa T. Absorption of pathogenic autoantibodies by the extracellular domain of pemphigus vulgaris antigen (Dsg3) produced by baculovirus. *J Clin Invest* 1994; **94**: 59–67.

2 Emery DJ, Diaz LA, Fairley JA *et al.* Pemphigus foliaceus and pemphigus vulgaris autoantibodies react with the extracellular domain of desmoglein-1. *J Invest Dermatol* 1995; **104**: 323–8.

3 Harman KE, Gratian MJ, Bhogal BS *et al.* A study of desmoglein 1 autoantibodies in pemphigus vulgaris: racial differences in frequency and the association with a more severe phenotype. *Br J Dermatol* 2000; **143**: 343–8.

4 Ding X, Aoki V, Mascaro JM Jr *et al.* Mucosal and mucocutaneous (generalized) pemphigus vulgaris show distinct autantibody profiles. *J Invest Dermatol* 1997; **109**: 592–6.

5 Amagai M, Tsunoda K, Zillikens D *et al.* The clinical phenotype of pemphigus is defined by the anti-desmoglein autoantibody profile. *J Am Acad Dermatol* 1999; **40**: 167–70.

6 Bystryn JC, Steinman NM. The adjuvant therapy of pemphigus. An update. *Arch Dermatol* 1996; **132**: 203–12.

7 Wolf R, Landau M, Tur E, Brenner S. Early treatment of pemphigus does not improve the prognosis. A review of 53 patients. *J Eur Acad Dermatol Venereol* 1995; **4**: 131–6.

8 Mourellou O, Chaidemenos GC, Koussidou TH, Kapetis E. The treatment of pemphigus vulgaris. Experience with 48 patients seen over an 11-year period. *Br J Dermatol* 1995; **133**: 83–7.

9 Bhogal BS, Black MM. Diagnosis, diagnostic and research techniques. In: *Management of Blistering Diseases* (Wojnarowska F, Briggaman RA, eds). London: Chapman & Hall, 1990; 15–34.

10 Bhogal BS, Wojnarowska F, Black MM *et al.* The distribution of immunoglobulins and the C3 component of complement in multiple biopsies from the uninvolved and perilesional skin in pemphigus. *Clin Exp Dermatol* 1986; **11**: 49–53.

11 Judd KP, Lever WF. Correlation of antibodies in skin and serum with disease severity in pemphigus. *Arch Dermatol* 1979; **115**: 428–32.

12 Lever WF. Pemphigus and pemphigoid. A review of the advances made since 1964. *J Am Acad Dermatol* 1979; **1**: 2–31.

13 Amagai M, Komai A, Hashimoto T *et al.* Usefulness of enzyme-linked immunosorbent assay using recombinant desmogleins 1 and 3 for serodiagnosis of pemphigus. *Br J Dermatol* 1999; **140**: 351–7.

14 Harman KE, Gratian MJ, Seed PT *et al.* Diagnosis of pemphigus by ELISA: a critical evaluation of two ELISAs for the detection of antibodies to the major pemphigus antigens, desmoglein 1 and 3. *Clin Exp Dermatol* 1999; **25**: 236–40.

15 Chryssomallis F, Ioannides D, Teknetzis A *et al.* Treatment for oral pemphigus. *Int J Dermatol* 1994; **33**: 803–7.

16 Scully C, Paes de Almeida O, Porter SR, Gilkes JJH. Pemphigus vulgaris: the manifestations and long-term management of 55 patients with oral lesions. *Br J Dermatol* 1999; **140**: 84–9.

17 Herbst A, Bystryn JC. Patterns of remission in pemphigus vulgaris. *J Am Acad Dermatol* 2000; **42**: 422–7.

18 Ioannides D, Chrysomallis F, Bystryn JC. Ineffectiveness of cyclosporin as an adjuvant to corticosteroids in the treatment of pemphigus. *Arch Dermatol* 2000; **136**: 868–72.

19 Carson PJ, Hameed A, Ahmed AR. Influence of treatment on the clinical course of pemphigus vulgaris. *J Am Acad Dermatol* 1996; **34**: 645–52.

20 Lever WF, Schaumburg-Lever G. Treatment of pemphigus vulgaris. Results obtained in 84 patients between 1961 and 1982. *Arch Dermatol* 1984; **120**: 44–7.

21 Ratnam KV, Phay KL, Tan CK. Pemphigus therapy with oral prednisolone regimens. *Int J Dermatol* 1990; **29**: 363–7.

22 Lapidoth M, David M, Ben-Amitai D *et al.* The efficacy of combined treatment with prednisolone and cyclosporin in patients with pemphigus: preliminary study. *J Am Acad Dermatol* 1994; **30**: 752–7.

23 Lever WF, White H. Treatment of pemphigus with corticosteroids. Results obtained in 46 patients over a period of 11 years. *Arch Dermatol* 1963; **87**: 12–25.

24 Katz SI, Halprin KM, Inderbitzin TM. The use of human skin for the detection of anti-epithelial autoantibodies. *J Invest Dermatol* 1969; **53**: 390–9.

25 Rosenberg FR, Sanders S, Nelson CT. Pemphigus. A 20-year review of 107 patients treated with corticosteroids. *Arch Dermatol* 1976; **112**: 962–70.

26 Hirone T. Pemphigus: a survey of 85 patients between 1970 and 1974. *J Dermatol* 1978; **5**: 43–7.

27 Werth VP. Treatment of pemphigus vulgaris with brief, high-dose intravenous glucocorticoids. *Arch Dermatol* 1996; **132**: 1435–9.

28 Chryssomallis F, Dimitriades A, Chaidemenos GC *et al.* Steroid-pulse therapy in pemphigus vulgaris long term follow-up. *Int J Dermatol* 1995; **34**: 438–42.

29 Wolff K, Schreiner E. Immunosuppressive Therapie bei Pemphigus vulgaris. *Arch Klin Exp Dermatol* 1969; **235**: 63–77.

30 van Dijk TJA, van Velde JL. Treatment of pemphigus and pemphigoid with azathioprine. *Dermatologica* 1973; **147**: 179–85.

31 Aberer W, Wolff-Schreiner EC, Stingl G, Wolff K. Azathioprine in the treatment of pemphigus vulgaris. *J Am Acad Dermatol* 1987; **16**: 527–33.

32 Krakowski A, Covo J, Rozanski Z. Pemphigus vulgaris. *Arch Dermatol* 1969; **100**: 117.

33 Burton JL, Greaves MW, Marks J, Dawber RPR. Azathioprine in pemphigus vulgaris. *Br Med J* 1970; **3**: 84–6.

34 Roenigk HH, Deodhar S. Pemphigus treatment with azathioprine. *Arch Dermatol* 1973; **107**: 353–7.

35 Holme SA, Duley J, Anstey AV. Thiopurine methyltransferase screening prior to azathioprine treatment in the United Kingdom. *Br J Dermatol* 2001; **145** (Suppl. 59): 12(Abstr.)

36 Snow JL, Gibson LE. The role of genetic variation in thiopurine methyltransferase activity and the efficacy and/or side effects of azathioprine therapy in dermatologic patients. *Arch Dermatol* 1995; **131**: 193–7.

37 Anstey A. Azathioprine in dermatology: a review in the light of advances in understanding methylation pharmacogenetics. *J R Soc Med* 1995; **88**: 155–60.

38 Nousari HC, Anhalt GJ. The role of mycophenolate mofetil in the management of pemphigus. *J Am Acad Dermatol* 1999; **135**: 853–4.

39 Krain LS, Landau JW, Newcomer VD. Cyclophosphamide in the treatment of pemphigus vulgaris and bullous pemphigoid. *Arch Dermatol* 1972; **106**: 657–61.

40 Fellner MJ, Katz JM, McCabe JB. Successful treatment of cyclophosphamide and prednisolone for initial treatment of pemphigus vulgaris. *Arch Dermatol* 1978; **114**: 889–94.

41 Pasricha JS, Sood VD, Minocha Y. Treatment of pemphigus with cyclophosphamide. *Br J Dermatol* 1975; **93**: 573–6.

42 Piamphongsant T. Treatment of pemphigus with corticosteroids and cyclophosphamide. *J Dermatol* 1979; **6**: 359–63.

43 Ahmed AR, Hombal S. Use of cyclophosphamide in azathioprine failures in pemphigus. *J Am Acad Dermatol* 1987; **17**: 437–42.

44 Pasricha JS, Ramji G. Pulse therapy with dexamethasone–cyclophosphamide in pemphigus. *Indian J Dermatol Venereol Leprol* 1984; **50**: 199–203.

45 Pasricha JS, Khaitan BK, Raman RS, Chandra M. Dexamethasone–cyclophosphamide pulse therapy for pemphigus. *Int J Dermatol* 1995; **34**: 875–82.

46 Pasricha JS, Khaitan BK. Curative treatment for pemphigus. *Arch Dermatol* 1996; **132**: 1518–19.

47 Kumrah L, Ramam M, Shah P *et al.* Pituitary–adrenal function following dexamethosone–cyclophosphamide pulse therapy for pemphigus. *Br J Dermatol* 2001; **145**: 944–8.

48 Kaur S, Kanwar AJ. Dexamethasone–cyclophosphamide pulse therapy in pemphigus. *Int J Dermatol* 1990; **29**: 371–4.

49 Enk AH, Knop J. Mycophenolate mofetil is effective in the treatment of pemphigus vulgaris. *Arch Dermatol* 1999; **135**: 54–6.

50 Nousari HC, Sragovich A, Kimyai-Asadi A *et al.* Mycophenolate mofetil in autoimmune and inflammatory skin disorders. *J Am Acad Dermatol* 1999; **40**: 265–8.

51 Bredlich RO, Grundmann-Kollmann M, Behrens S *et al.* Mycophenolate mofetil monotherapy for pemphigus vulgaris. *Br J Dermatol* 1999; **141**: 934 (Letter).

52 Grundmann-Kollmann M, Kaskel P, Leiter U *et al.* Treatment of pemphigus vulgaris and bullous pemphigoid with mycophenolate mofetil monotherapy. *Arch Dermatol* 1999; **135**: 724–5.

53 Penneys NS, Eaglstein WH, Indgin S, Frost P. Gold sodium thiomalate treatment of pemphigus. *Arch Dermatol* 1973; **108**: 56–60.

54 Sutej PG, Jorizzo JL, White W. Intramuscular gold therapy for young patients with pemphigus vulgaris: a prospective, open, clinical study utilising a dermatologist/rheumatologist team approach. *J Eur Acad Dermatol Venereol* 1995; **5**: 222–8.

55 Penneys NS, Eaglstein WH, Frost P. Management of pemphigus with gold compounds. A long-term follow-up report. *Arch Dermatol* 1976; **112**: 185–7.

56 Pandya AG, Dyke C. Treatment of pemphigus with gold. *Arch Dermatol* 1998; **134**: 1104–7.

57 Lever WF, Goldberg HS. Treatment of pemphigus vulgaris with methotrexate. *Arch Dermatol* 1969; **100**: 70–8.

58 Jablonska S, Chorzelski T, Blaszczyk M. Immunosuppressants in the treatment of pemphigus. *Br J Dermatol* 1970; **83**: 315–23.

59 Ryan JG. Pemphigus. A 20-year survey of experience with 70 cases. *Arch Dermatol* 1971; **104**: 14–20.

60 Lever WF. Methotrexate and prednisone in pemphigus vulgaris. Therapeutic results obtained in 36 patients between 1961 and 1970. *Arch Dermatol* 1972; **106**: 491–7.

61 Smith TJ, Bystryn JC. Methotrexate as an adjuvant treatment for pemphigus vulgaris. *Arch Dermatol* 1999; **135**: 1275–6.

62 Barthelemy H, Frappaz A, Cambazard F *et al.* Treatment of nine cases of pemphigus vulgaris with cyclosporin. *J Am Acad Dermatol* 1988; **18**: 1262–6.

63 Alijotas J, Pedragosa R, Bosch J, Vilardell M. Prolonged remission after cyclosporin therapy in pemphigus vulgaris: report of two young siblings. *J Am Acad Dermatol* 1990; **23**: 701–3.

64 Chaffins ML, Collison D, Fivenson DP. Treatment of pemphigus and linear IgA dermatosis with nicotinamide and tetracycline: a review of 13 cases. *J Am Acad Dermatol* 1993; **28**: 998–1000.

65 Alpsoy E, Yilmaz E, Basaran E *et al.* Is the combination of tetracycline and nicotinamide therapy alone effective in pemphigus? *Arch Dermatol* 1995; **131**: 1339–40.

66 Calebotta A, Saenz AM, Gonzalez F *et al.* Pemphigus vulgaris: benefits of tetracycline as adjuvant therapy in a series of thirteen patients. *Int J Dermatol* 1999; **38**: 217–21.

67 Gaspar ZS, Walkden V, Wojnarowska F. Minocycline is a useful adjuvant therapy for pemphigus. *Australas J Dermatol* 1996; **37**: 93–5.

68 Ozog DM, Gogstetter DS, Scott G, Gaspari AA. Minocycline-induced hyperpigmentation in patients with pemphigus and pemphigoid. *Arch Dermatol* 2000; **136**: 1133–8.

69 Piamphongsant T. Pemphigus controlled by dapsone. *Br J Dermatol* 1976; **94**: 681–6.

70 Haim S, Friedman-Birnbaum R. Dapsone in the treatment of pemphigus vulgaris. *Dermatologica* 1978; **156**: 120–3.

71 Bjarnason B, Skoglund C, Flosadottir E. Childhood pemphigus vulgaris treated with dapsone: a case report. *Pediatr Dermatol* 1998; **15**: 381–3.

72 Shah N, Green AR, Elgart GW, Kerdel F. The use of chlorambucil with prednisolone in the treatment of pemphigus. *J Am Acad Dermatol* 2000; **42**: 85–8.

73 Tappeiner G, Steiner A. High-dosage intravenous gamma globulin: therapeutic failure in pemphigus and pemphigoid. *J Am Acad Dermatol* 1989; **20**: 684–5.

74 Humbert P, Derancourt C, Aubin F, Agache P. Effects of intravenous gamma-globulin in pemphigus. *J Am Acad Dermatol* 1990; **22**: 326.

75 Messer G, Sizmann N, Feucht H, Meurer M. High-dose intravenous immunoglobulins for immediate control of severe pemphigus vulgaris. *Br J Dermatol* 1995; **133**: 1010–18.

76 Beckers RCY, Brand A, Vermeer BJ, Boom BW. Adjuvant high-dose intravenous gammaglobulin in the treatment of pemphigus and bullous pemphigoid: experience in six patients. *Br J Dermatol* 1995; **133**: 289–93.

77 Bewley AP, Keefe M. Successful treatment of pemphigus vulgaris by pulsed intravenous immunoglobulin therapy. *Br J Dermatol* 1996; **135**: 128–9.

78 Wever S, Zillikens D, Brocker EB. Successful treatment of refractory mucosal lesions of pemphigus vulgaris using intra-venous gammaglobulin as adjuvant therapy. *Br J Dermatol* 1996; **135**: 862–3.

79 Colonna L, Cianchini G, Frezzolini A. Intravenous immuno-globulins for pemphigus vulgaris: adjuvant or first choice therapy. *Br J Dermatol* 1998; **138**: 1102–3.

80 Jolles S, Hughes J, Rustin M. Therapeutic failure of high-dose intravenous immunoglobulin in pemphigus vulgaris. *J Am Acad Dermatol* 1999; **40**: 499–500.

81 Harman KE, Black MM. High-dose intravenous immune globulin for the treatment of autoimmune blistering diseases: an evaluation of its use in 14 cases. *Br J Dermatol* 1999; **140**: 865–74.

82 Ahmed AR. Intravenous immunoglobulin therapy in the treatment of patients with pemphigus vulgaris unresponsive to conventional immunosuppressive treatment. *J Am Acad Dermatol* 2001; **45**: 679–90.

83 Bystryn JC, Jiao D, Natow S. Treatment of pemphigus with intravenous immunoglobulin. *J Am Acad Dermatol* 2002; **47**: 358–63.

84 Guillaume JC, Roujeau JC, Morel P *et al.* Controlled study of plasma exchange in pemphigus. *Arch Dermatol* 1988; **124**: 1659–63.

85 Ruocco V, Rossi A, Argenziano G *et al.* Pathogenicity of the intercellular antibodies of pemphigus and their periodic removal from the circulation by plasmapheresis. *Br J Dermatol* 1978; **98**: 237–41.

86 Cotterill JA, Barker DJ, Millard LG, Robinson EA. Plasma exchange in the treatment of pemphigus vulgaris. *Br J Dermatol* 1978; **98**: 243.

87 Meurer M, Braun-Falco O. Plasma exchange in the treatment of pemphigus vulgaris. *Br J Dermatol* 1979; **100**: 231–2.

88 Auerbach R, Bystryn JC. Plasmapheresis and immunosuppressive therapy. Effect on levels of intercellular antibodies in pemphigus vulgaris. *Arch Dermatol* 1979; **115**: 728–30.

89 Swanson DL, Dahl MV. Pemphigus vulgaris and plasma exchange: clinical and serologic studies. *J Am Acad Dermatol* 1981; **4**: 325–8.

90 Roujeau JC, Kalis B, Lauret P *et al.* Plasma exchange in corticosteroid-resistant pemphigus. *Br J Dermatol* 1982; **106**: 103–4.

91 Roujeau JC, Andre C, Joneau Fabre M *et al.* Plasma exchange in pemphigus. Uncontrolled study of ten patients. *Arch Dermatol* 1983; **119**: 215–21.

92 Ruocco V, Astarita C, Pisani M. Plasmapheresis as an alternative or adjunctive therapy in problem cases of pemphigus. *Dermatologica* 1984; **168**: 219–23.

93 Euler HN, Loeffler H, Christophers E. Synchronisation of plasmapheresis and pulse cyclophosphamide therapy in pemphigus vulgaris. *Arch Dermatol* 1987; **123**: 1205–10.

94 Tan-Lim R, Bystryn JC. Effect of plasmapheresis therapy on circulating levels of pemphigus antibodies. *J Am Acad Dermatol* 1990; **22**: 35–40.

95 Sondergaard K, Carstens J, Jorgensen J, Zachariae H. The steroid-sparing effect of long-term plasmapheresis in pemphigus. *Acta Derm Venereol* (Stockh)1995; **75**: 150–2.

96 Turner MS, Sutton D, Sauder DN. The use of plasmapheresis and immunosuppression in the treatment of pemphigus vulgaris. *J Am Acad Dermatol* 2000; **43**: 1058–64.

97 Bystryn JC. Plasmapheresis therapy of pemphigus. *Arch Dermatol* 1988; **124**: 1702–4.

98 Blaszczyk M, Chorzelski TP, Jablonska S *et al.* Indications for future studies on the treatment of pemphigus with plasmapheresis. *Arch Dermatol* 1989; **125**: 843–4 (Letter).

99 Roujeau JC. Plasmapheresis therapy of pemphigus and bullous pemphigoid. *Semin Dermatol* 1988; **7**: 195–200.

100 Ruocco V. Plasmapheresis and pulse cyclophosphamide therapy in pemphigus vulgaris: a novelty or reappraisal? *Arch Dermatol* 1988; **124**: 1716–18.

101 Rook AH, Jegasothy BV, Heald P *et al.* Extracorporeal photo-chemotherapy for drug-resistant pemphigus vulgaris. *Ann Intern Med* 1990; **112**: 303–5.

102 Liang G, Nahass G, Kerdel FA. Pemphigus vulgaris treated with photopheresis. *J Am Acad Dermatol* 1992; **26**: 779–80.

103 Gollnick HPM, Owsianowski M, Taube KM, Orfanos CE. Unresponsive severe generalised pemphigus vulgaris successfully controlled by extracorporeal photopheresis. *J Am Acad Dermatol* 1993; **28**: 122–4.

104 Wollina U, Lange D, Looks A. Short-time extracorporeal photochemotherapy in the treatment of drug-resistant autoimmune bullous diseases. *Dermatology* 1999; **198**: 140–4.

105 Huilgol SC, Black MM. Management of the immunobullous disorders. II. Pemphigus. *Clin Exp Dermatol* 1995; **20**: 283–93.

106 Huilgol SC, Black MM. Management of the immunobullous disorders. I. Pemphigoid. *Clin Exp Dermatol* 1995; **20**: 189–201.

107 Eisen D, Ellis CN. Topical cyclosporin for oral mucosal disorders. *J Am Acad Dermatol* 1990; **23**: 1259–64.

108 Goopta C, Staughton RCD. Use of topical cyclosporin in oral pemphigus. *J Am Acad Dermatol* 1998; **38**: 860–1.

109 David M, Weissman-Katzenelson V, Ben-Chetrit A *et al.* The usefulness of immunofluorescent tests in pemphigus patients in clinical remission. *Br J Dermatol* 1989; **120**: 391–5.

110 Ratnam KV, Pang BK. Pemphigus in remission: value of negative direct immunofluorescence in management. *J Am Acad Dermatol* 1994; **30**: 547–50.

111 Griffiths CEM.. The British Association of Dermatologists guidelines for the management of skin disease. *Br J Dermatol* 1999; **141**: 396–7.

112 Cox NH. Williams HC. The British Association of Dermatologists therapeutic guidelines: can we AGREE? *Br J Dermatol* 2003; **148**: 621–5.

Appendix 1

The consultation process and background details for the British Association of Dermatalogists guidelines have been published elsewhere[111,112]

Strength of recommendations

A There is good evidence to support the use of the procedure.

B There is fair evidence to support the use of the procedure.

C There is poor evidence to support the use of the procedure.

D There is fair evidence to support the rejection of the use of the procedure.

E There is good evidence to support the rejection of the use of the procedure.

Quality of evidence

I Evidence obtained from at least one properly designed, randomized controlled trial.

II–i Evidence obtained from well–designed controlled trials without randomization.

II–ii Evidence obtained from well–designed cohort or case–control analytical studies, preferably from more than one centre or research group.

II–iii Evidence obtained from multiple time series with or without the intervention. Dramatic results in uncontrolled experiments (such as the introduction of penicillin treatment in the 1940s) could also be regarded as this type of evidence.

III Opinions of respected authorities based on clinical experience, descriptive studies or reports of expert committees.

IV Evidence inadequate owing to problems of methodology (e.g. sample size, of length or comprehensiveness of follow–up or conflicts of evidence).

http://bad.org.uk/Portals/_Bad/Guidelines/Clinical
%20Guidelines/Pemphigus%20Vulgaris.pdf

Comment

Since the 2003 guidelines [1] the Cochrane systematic
review [2] has confirmed that the best therapeutic regimen for treating pemphigus vulgaris and foliaceous is
still not determined. High-dose corticosteroids are the
mainstay therapy apart from the use of various steroid-
sparing agents such as mycophenolate mofetil, intravenous immunoglobulin (IVIg) [3] (low-dose regime)
[4] and methotrexate [5]. The role of rituximab has still
not been adequately studied [4]. Further research into
the diagnosis and optimum management of the different
subtypes of pemphigus vulgaris is warranted.

REFERENCES

1 Harman KE, Albert S, Black MM. Guidelines for the management of pemphigus vulgaris. *Brit J Dermatol* 2003; 149:
926–37.
2 Martin LK, Agero AL, Werth V, Villanueva E, Segall J, Murrell
DF. Interventions for pemphigus vulgaris and pemphigus
foliaceus. *Cochrane Database Syst Rev* 2009; Issue 1: CD006263
(http://mrw.interscience.wiley.com/cochrane/clsysrev/articles/
CD006263/frame.html).
3 Arnold DF, Burton J, Shine B, *et al.* An 'n-of-1' placebo-
controlled crossover trial of intravenous immunoglobulin as
adjuvant therapy in refractory pemphigus vulgaris. *Brit J Dermatol* 2009; 160: 1098–102.
4 Alexandroff AB, Harman KE. Blistering skin disorders: an
evidence-based update. Conference report. *Br J Dermatol*
2009; 160: 502–4.
5 Gürcan HM, Ahmed AR. Analysis of current data on the use of
methotrexate in the treatment of pemphigus and pemphigoid.
Br J Dermatol 2009; 161: 723–31.

Additional professional resources

http://www.dermnetnz.org/immune/pemphigus-
vulgaris.html
http://www.dermnetnz.org/immune/pemphigus-
foliaceus.html
http://www.dermnetnz.org/immune/pemphigoid-
gestationis.html

BAD patient information leaflet

http://www.bad.org.uk/site/854/default.aspx

Other patient resources

http://www.pemphigus.org/
http://www.dermnetnz.org/dna.pemphigus/pgus.html
http://www.nhs.uk/conditions/pemphigus-vulgaris/
Pages/Definition.aspx
http://www.patient.co.uk/pdf/pilsL386.pdf

Guidelines for evaluation and management of urticaria in adults and children

C.E.H. Grattan and F. Humphreys* on behalf of the British Association of Dermatologists Therapy Guidelines and Audit Subcommittee

Department of Dermatology, Norfolk and Norwich University Hospital, Norwich NR4 7UY, and St John's Institute of Dermatology, St Thomas' Hospital, London SE1 7EH, U.K.

*Department of Dermatology, Warwick Hospital, Warwick CV34 5BW, U.K.

Summary

Appropriate management of urticaria depends on the correct evaluation of clinical patterns and causes where these can be identified. Guidance for treatment is presented, based on the strength of evidence available at the time of preparation. As many of the recommendations relate to the off-licence use of drugs, it is particularly important that clinicians should be familiar with dosing and side-effects of treatment in the context of managing urticaria.

Disclaimer

These guidelines have been prepared for dermatologists on behalf of the British Association of Dermatologists and reflect the best data available at the time the report was prepared. Caution should be exercised in interpreting the data; the results of future studies may require alterations of the conclusions or recommendations in this report. It may be necessary or even desirable to depart from the guidelines in the interests of specific patients and special circumstances. Just as adherence to the guidelines may not constitute defence against a claim of negligence, so deviation from them should not necessarily be deemed negligent.

Definition

The term urticaria is widely used to describe an eruption of weals. It is now also increasingly being used to define a disease characterized by short-lived itchy weals, angio-oedema or both together. Most patients with urticaria do not have systemic reactions, but allergic and some physical urticarias may occasionally progress to anaphylaxis. Conversely, urticaria is often a feature of anaphylactic and anaphylactoid reactions.

Clinical classification

For clinical purposes it is often more helpful to classify urticaria by presentation than by aetiology, which is often difficult to establish. A classification based on clinical features may be used to guide appropriate investigation and management. It is usually possible to distinguish clearly recognizable patterns of urticaria on the clinical presentation, supported, where appropriate, by challenge tests and skin biopsy (Table 1). The presentation of urticaria in childhood is similar to that in adults. Clinical and aetiological classifications should be complementary rather than exclusive: for example, chronic ordinary urticaria (COU) is most appropriate when the aetiology remains uncertain. Where there is evidence of histamine-releasing autoantibodies the patient has autoimmune COU (syn. chronic autoimmune urticaria) but where there is no evidence of functional autoantibodies the patient has idiopathic COU (syn. chronic idiopathic urticaria).

Ordinary urticaria is the commonest pattern, presenting with spontaneous weals anywhere on the body with or without angio-oedema. Although the underlying tendency to urticaria is spontaneous it is often possible to identify aggravating factors, such as heat or pressure from clothing, that appear

Table 1 Clinical classification of the urticarias

Ordinary urticaria
  Acute (up to 6 weeks of continuous activity)
  Chronic (6 weeks or more of continuous activity)
  Episodic (acute intermittent or recurrent activity)
Physical urticarias (reproducibly induced by the same
  physical stimulus)
  Mechanical
    Delayed pressure urticaria
    Symptomatic dermographism
    Vibratory angio-oedema
  Thermal
    Cholinergic urticaria
    Cold contact urticaria
    Localized heat urticaria
  Other
    Aquagenic urticaria
    Solar urticaria
    Exercise-induced anaphylaxis
Angio-oedema without weals
  Idiopathic
  Drug-induced
  C1 esterase inhibitor deficiency
Contact urticaria (contact with allergens or chemicals)
Urticarial vasculitis (defined by vasculitis on skin biopsy)
Autoinflammatory syndromes
  Hereditary
    Cryopyrin-associated periodic syndromes (*CIAS1* mutations)
  Acquired
    Schnitzler syndrome
---

to encourage urticarial lesions. It may follow an acute, episodic (syn. intermittent) or chronic course. Weals occur
continuously every day or almost daily while the disease is
active.

Physical urticarias are triggered reproducibly by one or more
physical stimuli. Swellings are induced rather than spontaneous. Defining the stimulus provides an opportunity to minimize or prevent urticaria through lifestyle changes. The
most readily identifiable triggers are mechanical or thermal.
Some authorities distinguish cholinergic urticaria from the
physical urticarias because it is primarily induced by the
stimulus for sweating rather than overheating *per se* (even
though the usual reason for sweating is a raised core
temperature).

Angio-oedema without weals should be distinguished from angio-
oedema occurring with weals as it may be caused by angiotensin-converting enzyme (ACE) inhibitors or be a presentation of C1 esterase inhibitor (C1 inh) deficiency. Patients with
C1 inh deficiency may present with abdominal pain without
obvious angio-oedema. Angio-oedema without weals may also
be idiopathic.

Contact urticaria occurs only when the eliciting substance is
absorbed percutaneously or through mucous membranes. It is
never spontaneous. Percutaneous or mucosal absorption of an
allergen may result in a localized or a systemic reaction. The

latter may occasionally progress to anaphylaxis in a highly
sensitized individual (e.g. latex allergy).

Urticarial vasculitis presents with urticaria clinically but small
vessel vasculitis histologically. Other features of this systemic
disease may include joint and renal involvement.

Autoinflammatory syndromes presenting with urticaria typically
develop spontaneous weals, pyrexia and malaise, with other
features that define the disease phenotype (such as renal amyloidosis and sensorineural deafness in Muckle–Wells syndrome). The inherited patterns usually present in early
childhood.

The duration of individual weals can be very helpful in distinguishing between these clinical patterns: weals typically last
from 2 to 24 h in ordinary urticaria and up to 2 h in contact
urticaria. The weals of physical urticaria are gone within
an hour except those in delayed pressure urticaria, which take
2–6 h to develop and up to 48 h to fade. The weals of urticarial vasculitis usually persist for days. Angio-oedema may
last up to 3 days without treatment.

Aetiology

Despite thorough evaluation many cases remain unexplained
('idiopathic') but it may be possible to assign a specific aetiology to individual cases of urticaria (Table 2).

Immunological urticaria

At least 30% of patients with COU have histamine-releasing
autoantibodies. These degranulate mast cells and basophils
in vitro by activating high-affinity IgE receptors directly or IgE
bound to them.[1] Patients with evidence of functional autoantibodies are increasingly being regarded as having an autoimmune subset of urticaria. Cross-linking of specific IgE on
cutaneous mast cells by allergens can cause contact urticaria,
anaphylaxis and some cases of acute or episodic ordinary urticaria, but experience shows that allergy is not the cause
of chronic continuous disease in adults. Urticarial vasculitis
and acute urticarial reactions to drugs or blood products
(serum sickness) are thought to result from the lodging of
immune complexes in small blood vessels. The angio-oedema
of C1 inh deficiency is mediated by kinins resulting from

Table 2 Aetiologies of urticaria

Idiopathic
Immunological
  Autoimmune (autoantibodies against FcεRI or IgE)
  Allergic (IgE-mediated type I hypersensitivity reactions)
  Immune complex (urticarial vasculitis)
  Complement-dependent (C1 esterase inhibitor deficiency)
Nonimmunological
  Direct mast cell-releasing agents (e.g. opiates)
  Aspirin, nonsteroidal anti-inflammatories and dietary
    pseudoallergens
  Angiotensin-converting enzyme inhibitors
---

complement activation and bradykinin formation rather than histamine.

Nonimmunological urticaria

Degranulation of mast cells and basophils can occur independently of IgE receptor activation after exposure to certain drugs (e.g. codeine) and other agents (e.g. radiocontrast media). The mechanism by which aspirin, nonsteroidal anti-inflammatory drugs (NSAIDs) and dietary pseudoallergens (such as salicylates, azo dyes and food preservatives) cause or aggravate urticaria remains uncertain but probably involves leukotriene formation as well as histamine release. Angio-oedema due to ACE inhibitors is believed to result from inhibition of kinin breakdown by ACE.

Associations

Thyroid autoimmunity in COU (14%) is more prevalent than in population controls (6%)[2] (*Quality of evidence* II-ii; see Appendix 1). A significantly higher prevalence of coeliac disease in children and adolescents with severe chronic urticaria than in case-matched controls has been reported.[3] Associations between chronic urticaria and occult infection (e.g. dental abscess[4] and gastrointestinal candidiasis[5]) have been proposed but there is little evidence to support them (*Quality of evidence* III). A meta-analysis of therapeutic trials for *Helicobacter pylori* found that resolution of chronic urticaria was more likely when antibiotic therapy was successful than when it was not (*Quality of evidence* I, *Strength of recommendation* B).[6] There is no statistical association between malignancy and urticaria[7] (*Quality of evidence* II-ii) although individual case reports have been published.

Appropriate investigations

The diagnosis of urticaria is primarily clinical.[8] Any investigations should be guided by the history and should not be performed in all patients. Relevant clinical and laboratory tests for the different clinical patterns of urticaria are summarized in Table 3.

Acute or episodic ordinary urticaria

No investigations are required except where suggested by the history. IgE-mediated reactions to environmental allergens (such as latex, nuts or fish) as a cause of acute allergic or contact urticaria can be confirmed by skin-prick testing (where there are facilities) and CAP fluoroimmunoassay (previously radioallergosorbent tests, RAST) on blood. Results of both have to be interpreted in the clinical context. Single-blind oral challenge with food additives or aspirin may be appropriate in the evaluation of episodic urticaria in the appropriate clinical setting in centres where challenge capsules are available.

Chronic ordinary urticaria

No investigations are required for the majority of patients with mild disease responding to H1 antihistamines. A useful screening profile for nonresponders with more severe disease could include a full blood count and white cell differential (for instance, to detect the eosinophilia of bowel helminth infections or the leucopenia of systemic lupus erythematosus), and erythrocyte sedimentation rate (usually normal in COU but may be raised in urticarial vasculitis and always raised in autoinflammatory syndromes). Thyroid autoantibodies and thyroid function tests should be performed, especially if an autoimmune aetiology of urticaria is likely. There is currently no routine laboratory test for histamine-releasing autoantibodies but intradermal injection of autologous serum (the autologous serum skin test, ASST) offers a reasonably sensitive and specific screening test[9] in centres with experience of doing it. The basophil histamine release assay remains the gold standard investigation for functional autoantibodies in centres where it is available.

Table 3 Relevant investigations

	FBC	ESR	TA/TFT	IgE	C4	Skin biopsy	Physical challenge
Ordinary urticaria							
Acute/episodic	–	–	–	(+)	–	–	–
Chronic	(+)	(+)	(+)	–	–	–	–
Physical urticaria	–	–	–	–	–	–	+
Angio-oedema without weals	–	–	–	–	+	–	–
Contact urticaria	–	–	–	(+)	–	–	–
Urticarial vasculitis	+	+	–	–	+	+	–
Autoinflammatory syndrome	+	+	–	–	–	–	–

FBC, full blood count; ESR, erythrocyte sedimentation rate; TA, thyroid autoantibodies; TFT, thyroid function tests; IgE, specific IgE (CAP) or skin prick tests; C4, component of complement as a marker for C1 esterase inhibitor deficiency in hypocomplementaemic urticarial vasculitis; (+), discretionary investigations.

Physical urticarias

Physical urticarias may occur alone or coexist with ordinary urticaria. International standards for the diagnosis of physical urticarias and definitions of challenge testing have been proposed.[10]

Angio-oedema without weals

Serum C4 should be used as an initial screening test for hereditary and acquired C1 inh deficiency. A low C4 level between and during attacks (< 30% mean normal) has a very high sensitivity but low specificity for C1 inh deficiency.[11] If low, C1 inh deficiency can be confirmed by quantitative and functional C1 inh assays. Immunochemical and functional C1 inh are both low in type I hereditary angio-oedema (HAE) whereas only functional activity is low in type II HAE. C1q is also reduced in acquired C1 inh deficiency.

Urticarial vasculitis

Lesional skin biopsy is essential to confirm the presence of small-vessel vasculitis histologically (leucocytoclasia, endothelial cell damage, perivascular fibrin deposition and red cell extravasation are key changes although there is no single defining feature). Patients with urticarial vasculitis need a full vasculitis screen, including serum complement assays for C3 and C4 to distinguish normocomplementaemic from hypocomplementaemic disease, which carries a worse prognosis.

Interventions

General measures

Nonspecific aggravating factors, such as overheating, stress, alcohol and drugs with the potential to worsen urticaria (e.g. aspirin and codeine) should be minimized. The risk of cross-reactions between aspirin and NSAIDs is difficult to quantify but may relate to potency of cyclooxygenase inhibition and dose. NSAIDs should be avoided in aspirin-sensitive patients with urticaria. ACE inhibitors should be avoided in patients with angio-oedema without weals and used with caution in urticaria if angio-oedema is also present. Oestrogens should be avoided in HAE. Cooling antipruritic lotions, such as calamine or 1% menthol in aqueous cream, can be soothing (*Quality of evidence III, Strength of recommendation A*). Clearly written information sheets, such as the British Association of Dermatologists' publication on urticaria and angio-oedema, can be very helpful to patients. It is important to explain to the patient that a cause of the condition is unlikely to be found but the prognosis for eventual recovery from ordinary, physical and vasculitic urticarias is excellent. Some physical urticarias may be especially persistent.

Pharmacological agents

Antihistamines

The efficacy and safety of antihistamines in urticaria is undisputed although not all patients respond and some, very occasionally, become worse. The outcome of randomized controlled studies of nonsedating H1 antihistamines has been summarized.[12] Seven nonsedating H1 antihistamines are currently licensed for urticaria in the U.K. Cetirizine, desloratadine, fexofenadine, levocetirizine, loratadine and mizolastine are taken once daily. Acrivastine is taken three times a day in view of its short half-life (T½). It is now available in the U.K. only in a nonprescription presentation. Cetirizine (the active metabolite of hydroxyzine) may be sedating, especially at higher doses. Mizolastine is contraindicated in clinically significant cardiac disease and when there is prolongation of the Q-T interval. It should not be taken concurrently with drugs that inhibit hepatic metabolism via cytochrome P450 (including macrolide antibiotics and imidazole antifungals) and with drugs that have potential arrythmic properties (including tricyclic antidepressants, such as doxepin). Cetirizine has the shortest time to attain maximum concentration, which may be an advantage where rapid availability is clinically important. Desloratadine has the longest elimination T½ at 27 h and should therefore be discontinued 6 days before skin prick testing.

All patients should be offered the choice of at least two nonsedating H1 antihistamines because responses and tolerance vary between individuals (*Strength of recommendation A*). It has become common practice to increase the dose above the manufacturer's licensed recommendation for patients who do not respond when the potential benefits are considered to outweigh any risks (*Quality of evidence III, Strength of recommendation C*). 'Antiallergic' effects on mast-cell mediator release of possible clinical importance have been shown with cetirizine[13] and loratadine,[14] especially at higher doses. Adjustments to the timing of medication can be helpful to ensure that the highest drug levels are obtained when urticaria is anticipated. The use of sedating antihistamines as monotherapy is now less common because of concerns about reduced concentration and performance but they can be effective and well tolerated by some individuals. Doxepin has useful antihistaminic properties but has sedating and anticholinergic side-effects. Addition of a sedating antihistamine at night [e.g. chlorphenamine (chlorpheniramine) 4–12 mg, hydroxyzine 10–50 mg] to a nonsedating antihistamine by day may help patients sleep better although it probably has little additional clinical effect on urticaria if the H1 receptor is already saturated. The off-licence addition of an H2 antihistamine, on the other hand, may sometimes give better control of urticaria than an H1 antihistamine taken alone (*Quality of evidence II, Strength of recommendation C*)[15,16] although, in practice, it may be more helpful for dyspepsia that may accompany severe urticaria.

Renal impairment. Acrivastine should be avoided in moderate renal impairment (creatinine clearance 10–20 mL min^{-1}) and the dose of cetirizine, levocetirizine and hydroxyzine should be halved. Cetirizine, levocetirizine and alimemazine (trimeprazine) should be avoided in severe renal impairment (creatinine clearance < 10 mL min^{-1}). Loratadine and desloratadine should be used with caution in severe renal impairment.

Hepatic impairment. Mizolastine is contraindicated by significant hepatic impairment. Alimemazine should be avoided in hepatic impairment because it is hepatotoxic and may precipitate coma in severe liver disease. Chlorphenamine and hydroxyzine should also be avoided in severe liver disease because their sedating effect is inappropriate.

Antihistamines in pregnancy. It is best to avoid all antihistamines in pregnancy, especially during the first trimester, although none has been shown to be teratogenic in humans. Hydroxyzine is the only antihistamine to be specifically contraindicated during the early stages of pregnancy in its current U.K. manufacturer's Summary of Product Characteristics. Avoidance or caution is recommended for the others, particularly in the first trimester and during lactation. Chlorphenamine is often chosen by clinicians in the U.K. when antihistamine therapy is necessary because of its long safety record. Loratadine and cetirizine are classified as U.S. Food and Drug Administration Pregnancy Category B drugs, implying there is no evidence of harm to the fetus during pregnancy, although well-controlled studies in humans are not available to exclude harmful effects.

Antihistamines in childhood. None of the currently licensed antihistamines is contraindicated in children 12 years and older. As dosing and age restrictions for individual products vary in younger children, it is recommended that the relevant Data Sheets are consulted before prescribing.

Antileukotrienes

Antileukotrienes may be taken in addition to an H1 antihistamine for poorly controlled urticaria but there is little evidence that they are useful as monotherapy. They appear more likely to benefit aspirin-sensitive and ASST-positive COU than other patterns of urticaria[17] but a good response is unpredictable. Montelukast is usually chosen.

Corticosteroids

Oral corticosteroids may shorten the duration of acute urticaria (e.g. prednisolone 50 mg daily for 3 days in adults[18]) although lower doses are often effective. Parenteral hydrocortisone is often given as an adjunct for severe laryngeal oedema and anaphylaxis although its action is delayed. Short tapering courses of oral steroids over 3–4 weeks may be necessary for urticarial vasculitis and severe delayed pressure urticaria (*Quality of evidence III*) but long-term oral corticosteroids should not be used in chronic urticaria (*Strength of recommendation A*) except in very selected cases under regular specialist supervision.

Epinephrine (syn. adrenaline)

Intramuscular epinephrine can be life saving in anaphylaxis and in severe laryngeal angio-oedema but should be used with caution in hypertension and ischaemic heart disease. Dosing is weight dependent. The British National Formulary recommends 0·5 mL of 1 : 1000 (500 µg) epinephrine by intramuscular injection for adults and adolescents older than 12 years. Fixed-dose epinephrine pens delivering 300 µg for adults or 150 µg in children between 15 and 30 kg may be carried by patients for emergency self-administration if the history indicates that the individual is at risk of further life-threatening attacks. If after the first dose of epinephrine there is no significant relief of symptoms, a further dose should be given. Epinephrine is not considered helpful for angio-oedema caused by C1 inh deficiency (*Quality of evidence III*). There is currently no licensed epinephrine aerosol inhaler available in the U.K., although Primatene® Mist (Wyeth, Madison, NJ, U.S.A.) is available as a named patient import from the U.S.A. where it is licensed for asthma. It should be sprayed directly on to the affected area of the mouth rather than inhaled or used sublingually with the intention of achieving systemic absorption.

Immunomodulating therapies

Ciclosporin has been the best studied immunsuppressive drug for COU to date. It was effective in about two thirds of patients with severe autoimmune urticaria unresponsive to antihistamines at 4 mg kg^{-1} daily[19] for up to 2 months (*Quality of evidence I, Strength of recommendation A*) but only 25% of the responders remained clear or much improved 4–5 months later. In a recent large multicentre study, there were fewer therapeutic failures when ciclosporin was taken for 16 weeks than 8 weeks.[20] Optimal patient selection, dose and duration of treatment still need to be defined. Some patients with chronic urticaria without evidence of functional autoantibodies (with a negative ASST) also respond, although this is not well documented in the literature and a beneficial outcome from immunosuppressive treatment is less predictable. Similar overall responses have been seen in open studies of tacrolimus[21] and mycophenolate mofetil.[22] Plasmapheresis[23] and intravenous immunoglobulins[24] may also be effective in severe autoimmune chronic urticaria (*Quality of evidence II-ii*) but are expensive and not widely available. There have been anecdotal reports of success with methotrexate[25] and cyclophosphamide.[26,27] Resolution of cold urticaria has been noted in a patient treated with omalizumab for asthma,[28] improvement of delayed pressure urticaria occurred during treatment of psoriasis with etanercept[29] but no improvement was seen in a patient with severe corticosteroid-dependent COU given rituximab.[30]

Other interventions

Although some food additives and natural salicylates may aggravate aspirin-sensitive chronic urticaria[31] the value of avoidance is controversial. In one prospective open study of inpatients with chronic urticaria, 73% of 64 improved within 2 weeks of a strict pseudoallergen diet but confirmed exacerbations on provocation testing with individual pseudoallergens were demonstrated in only 19% of them[32] (*Quality of evidence III, Strength of recommendation B*). Oral sodium cromoglycate is not absorbed from the gastrointestinal tract and is not effective for urticaria. Nifedipine has been shown to reduce pruritus and wealing in idiopathic COU[33] (*Quality of evidence II-i, Strength of recommendation C*), but the benefit in clinical practice is usually disappointing. Thyroxine treatment of euthyroid patients with idiopathic COU and with evidence of thyroid autoimmunity may occasionally result in improvement of urticaria[34] (*Quality of evidence III, Strength of recommendation C*). Although the published evidence for using sulfasalazine or dapsone in delayed pressure urticaria is anecdotal, they may be successful in otherwise corticosteroid-dependent cases. Sulfasalazine has also been reported to benefit idiopathic COU in a retrospective review[35] (*Quality of evidence III, Strength of recommendation C*) but there is a risk of aggravating urticaria in aspirin-sensitive patients. Some patients with idiopathic COU have responded to warfarin[36] (*Quality of evidence III, Strength of recommendation C*). Idiopathic angio-oedema without weals may respond to tranexamic acid[37] (*Quality of evidence II-ii, Strength of recommendation B*). A double-blind randomized placebo-controlled study appeared to show a benefit from stanozolol with cetirizine over placebo with cetirizine[38] (*Quality of evidence II-i, Strength of recommendation C*). Hydoxychloroquine improved the quality of life scores but did not reduce the requirement for other medication in patients with idiopathic COU.[39] Psoralen photochemotherapy,[40] ultraviolet B phototherapy[41] and relaxation therapies[42] for chronic urticaria have yielded inconsistent results (*Quality of evidence VI, Strength of recommendation D*) although narrow-band ultraviolet B phototherapy may be more promising.[43] Using a very potent topical steroid in a foam vehicle on the most affected area has been reported for delayed pressure urticaria,[44] and some immediate benefit was noted at the site of application of a potent topical steroid under occlusion for 2 weeks in patients with idiopathic COU,[45] but the routine use of topical steroids is not recommended.

Treatment of C1 esterase inhibitor deficiency

The management of C1 inh has been comprehensively reviewed[11] (Table 4). Maintenance therapy is only necessary for patients with symptomatic recurring angio-oedema or related abdominal pain. Anabolic steroids are the treatment of choice for most adults (*Quality of evidence III, Strength of recommendation B*) but should be avoided in children if possible. Virilizing side-effects may occur even at the low doses needed for long-term maintenance. Regular monitoring for hepatic inflammation and hepatocellular adenomas is essential. Tranexamic acid may be used for maintenance but is contraindicated in patients with a history of thrombosis. Regular eye examinations and liver function tests are recommended by the manufacturer in the long-term treatment of HAE. Prophylaxis before planned surgery or dental procedures includes taking tranexamic acid 2 days before and afterwards or increasing the dose of established maintenance therapies with tranexamic acid or anabolic steroids. C1 inh concentrate should be given for emergency treatment of serious angio-oedema attacks or as prophylaxis before surgery, especially when intubation or dental extractions are necessary. Fresh frozen plasma may be used as a substitute in an emergency if C1 inh is not available.

Prognosis

A comprehensive survey published in 1969 before the advent of nonsedating antihistamines showed that 50% of patients with chronic urticaria attending a hospital clinic with weals alone were clear by 6 months. By contrast, over 50% of patients with weals and angio-oedema still had active disease after 5 years[46] and therefore had a poorer outlook. A retrospective survey in 1998 did not address prognosis directly but found that 44% of hospitalized patients with urticaria reported a good response to antihistamines.[47] It is possible that the more potent antihistamines now available result in better disease control although the prognosis for complete recovery has probably not changed over 40 years.

Key points

1 Urticaria can usually be classified on the clinical presentation without extensive investigation. The weals of physical urticaria usually last less than 1 h (except delayed pressure urticaria) whereas those of ordinary urticaria typically last from 2 to 24 h. Urticarial vasculitis should be sought by skin biopsy if weals last longer.

Table 4 Summary of treatments for C1 esterase inhibitor deficiency

Drug	Maintenance	Short-term prophylaxis	Emergency
Stanozolol[a]	2 mg alternate days to 10 mg daily	10 mg, 48 h before and after procedure	–
Danazol[b]	200 mg Mon–Fri to 400 mg daily	600 mg, 48 h before and after procedure	–
Tranexamic acid	0·5–3·0 g daily	$\leq 4\cdot5$ g, 48 h before and after procedure	–
C1 esterase inhibitor concentrate	–	1000 U, 1 h before procedure	500–1500 U
Fresh frozen plasma	–	–	3 units

[a]No longer available in the U.K. but obtainable through IDIS World Medicines (Weybridge, U.K.). [b]Not licensed for hereditary angio-oedema in the U.K. Dose ranges given are for adults only.

2 Urticaria often remains idiopathic after allergic, infectious, physical and drug-related causes have been excluded as far as possible. At least 30% of patients with the ordinary presentation of chronic urticaria appear to have an autoimmune aetiology. The ASST is a reasonably sensitive and specific marker for histamine-releasing autoantibodies in this group.

3 Advice on general measures and information can be helpful for most patients with urticaria, especially if an avoidable physical or dietary trigger can be identified. Over 40% of hospitalized patients with urticaria show a good response to antihistamines, which are the mainstay of therapy.

4 It has become common practice to increase the dose of second-generation H1 antihistamines above the manufacturer's licensed recommendation for patients when the potential benefits are considered to outweigh any risks.

5 Combinations of nonsedating H1 antihistamines with other agents, such as H2 antihistamines, sedating antihistamines at night or the addition of antileukotrienes, can be useful for resistant cases.

6 Oral corticosteroids should be restricted to short courses for severe acute urticaria or angio-oedema affecting the mouth, although more prolonged treatment may be necessary for delayed pressure urticaria or urticarial vasculitis.

7 Immunomodulating therapies for chronic autoimmune urticaria should be restricted to patients with disabling disease who have not responded to optimal conventional treatments.

Audit points

1 The use of investigations above the minimum standard for the different clinical presentations of urticaria.

2 Use of antihistamines above the manufacturers' recommended dose.

References

1 Niimi N, Francis DM, Kermani F et al. Dermal mast cell activation by autoantibodies against the high affinity IgE receptor in chronic urticaria. J Invest Dermatol 1996; **106**:1001–6.

2 Leznoff A, Sussman GL. Syndrome of idiopathic chronic urticaria and angioedema with thyroid autoimmunity: a study in 90 patients. J Allergy Clin Immunol 1989; **84**:66–71.

3 Caminiti L, Passalacqua G, Magazzu G et al. Chronic urticaria and associated coeliac disease in children: a case–control study. Pediatr Allergy Immunol 2005; **16**:428–32.

4 Resch CA, Evans RR. Chronic urticaria and dental infection. Cleve Clin Q 1958; **25**:147–50.

5 James J, Warin RP. An assessment of the role of Candida albicans and food yeasts in chronic urticaria. Br J Dermatol 1971; **84**:227–37.

6 Federman DG, Kirsner RS, Moriarty JP, Concato J. The effect of antibiotic therapy for patients infected with Helicobacter pylori who have chronic urticaria. J Am Acad Dermatol 2003; **49**:861–4.

7 Lindelöf B, Sigurgeirsson B, Wahlgren CF, Eklund G. Chronic urticaria and cancer: an epidemiological study study of 1155 patients. Br J Dermatol 1990; **123**:453–6.

8 Kozel MM, Mekkes JR, Bossuyt PMM, Bos JD. The effectiveness of a history-based diagnostic approach in chronic urticaria and angioedema. Arch Dermatol 1998; **134**:1575–80.

9 Sabroe RA, Grattan CEH, Francis DM et al. The autologous serum skin test: a screening test for autoantibodies in chronic idiopathic urticaria. Br J Dermatol 1999; **140**:446–53.

10 Kobza Black A, Lawlor F, Greaves MW. Consensus meeting on the definition of physical urticarias and urticarial vasculitis. Clin Exp Dermatol 1996; **21**:424–6.

11 Gompels MM, Lock RJ, Abinun M et al. C1 inhibitor deficiency: consensus document. Clin Exp Immunol 2005; **139**:379–94.

12 Wedi B, Kapp A. Chronic urticaria: assessment of current treatment. Exp Rev Clin Immunol 2005; **1**:459–73.

13 Spencer CM, Faulds D, Peters DH. Cetirizine. A reappraisal of its pharmacological properties and therapeutic use in selected allergic disorders. Drug 1993; **46**:1055–80.

14 Bousquet J, Czarlewski W, Danzig MR. Antiallergic properties of loratadine: a review. Adv Ther 1995; **12**:283–98.

15 Bleehen SS, Thomas SE, Greaves MW. Cimetidine and chlorpheniramine in the treatment of chronic idiopathic urticaria: a multi-centre randomized double-blind study. Br J Dermatol 1987; **117**:81–8.

16 Paul E, Bödeker RH. Treatment of chronic urticaria with terfenadine and ranitidine: a randomized double-blind study in 45 patients. Eur J Clin Pharmacol 1986; **31**:277–80.

17 Di Lorenzo G, Pacor ML, Mansuetto P et al. Is there a role for antileukotrienes in the management of urticaria? Clin Exp Dermatol 2006; **31**:327–34.

18 Zuberbier T, Ifflländer J, Semler C, Henz BM. Acute urticaria: clinical aspects and therapeutic responsiveness. Acta Derm Venereol (Stockh) 1996; **76**:295–8.

19 Grattan CEH, O'Donnell BF, Francis DM et al. Randomized double-blind study of cyclosporin in chronic 'idiopathic' urticaria. Br J Dermatol 2000; **143**:365–72.

20 Vena GA, Cassano N, Colombo D et al. Cyclosporine in chronic idiopathic urticaria: a double-blind, randomised, placebo controlled trial. J Am Acad Dermatol 2006; **55**:705–9.

21 Kessel A, Bamberger E, Toubi E. Tacrolimus in the treatment of severe chronic idiopathic urticaria: an open-label prospective study. J Am Acad Dermatol 2005; **52**:145–8.

22 Shahar E, Bergman R, Guttman-Yassky E, Pollack S. Treatment of severe chronic idiopathic urticaria with oral mycophenolate mofetil in patients not responding to antihistamines and/or corticosteroids. Int J Dermatol 2006; **45**:1224–7.

23 Grattan CEH, Francis DM, Slater NGP et al. Plasmapheresis for severe, unremitting, chronic urticaria. Lancet 1992; **339**:1078–80.

24 O'Donnell BF, Barr RM, Kobza Black A et al. Intravenous immunoglobulin in autoimmune chronic urticaria. Br J Dermatol 1998; **138**:101–6.

25 Gach JE, Sabroe RA, Greaves MW, Kobza Black A. Methotrexate-responsive chronic idiopathic urticaria: a report of two cases. Br J Dermatol 2001; **145**:340–3.

26 Bernstein JA, Garramone SM, Lower EG. Successful treatment of autoimmune chronic idiopathic urticaria with intravenous cyclophosphamide. Ann Allergy Asthma Immunol 2002; **89**:212–14.

27 Asero R. Oral cyclophosphamide in a case of cyclosporin and steroid-resistant chronic urticaria showing autoreactivity on autologous serum skin testing. Clin Exp Dermatol 2005; **30**:578–602.

28 Boyce JA. Successful treatment of cold-induced urticaria/anaphylaxis with anti-IgE. J Allergy Clin Immunol 2006; **117**:1415–18.

29 Magerl M, Philipp S, Manasterski M et al. Successful treatment of delayed pressure urticaria with anti-TNF-α. J Allergy Clin Immunol 2007; **119**:752–4.

30 Mallipeddi R, Grattan CEH. Lack of response of severe steroid-dependent chronic urticaria to rituximab. Clin Exp Dermatol 2007; **32**:333–4.

31 Doeglas HMG. Reactions to aspirin and food additives in patients with chronic urticaria, including the physical urticarias. Br J Dermatol 1975; **93**:135–43.

32 Zuberbier T, Chantraine-Hess S, Harmann K, Czarnetski BM. Pseudoallergen-free diet in the treatment of chronic urticaria. A prospective study. Acta Derm Venereol (Stockh) 1995; **75**:484–7.

33 Bressler RB, Sowell K, Huston DP. Therapy of chronic idiopathic urticaria with nifedipine: demonstration of beneficial effect in a double-blinded, placebo controlled, crossover trial. J Allergy Clin Immunol 1989; **83**:756–63.

34 Rumbyrt JS, Katz JL, Schocket AL. Resolution of chronic urticaria in patients with thyroid autoimmunity. J Allergy Clin Immunol 1995; **96**:901–5.

35 McGirt LY, Vasagar K, Gober LM et al. Successful treatment of recalcitrant chronic idiopathic urticaria with sulfasalazine. Arch Dermatol 2006; **142**:1337–42.

36 Parslew R, Pryce D, Ashworth J, Friedmann PS. Warfarin treatment of chronic idiopathic urticaria and angio-oedema. Clin Exp Allergy 2000; **30**:1161–5.

37 Munch EP, Weeke B. Non-hereditary angioedema treated with tranexamic acid. Allergy 1985; **40**:92–7.

38 Parsad D, Pandhi R, Juneja A. Stanozolol in chronic urticaria: a double-blind, placebo-controlled trial. J Dermatol 2001; **28**:299–302.

39 Reeves GEM, Boyle MJ, Bonfield J et al. Impact of hydoxychloroquine on chronic urticaria: chronic autoimmune urticaria study and evaluation. Int J Med 2004; **34**:182–6.

40 Olafsson JH, Larkö O, Roupe G et al. Treatment of chronic urticaria with angio-oedema with PUVA or UVA plus placebo: a double-blind study. Arch Dermatol Res 1986; **278**:228–31.

41 Hannuksela M, Kokkonen E-L. Ultraviolet light therapy in chronic urticaria. Acta Derm Venereol (Stockh) 1985; **65**:449–50.

42 Shertzer CL, Lookingbill DP. Effects of relaxation therapy and hypnotizability in chronic urticaria. Arch Dermatol 1987; **123**:913–16.

43 Berroeta L, Clark C, Ibbotson SH et al. Narrow-band (TL-01) ultraviolet B phototherapy for chronic urticaria. Clin Exp Dermatol 2004; **29**:91–9.

44 Vena GA, Cassano N, D'Argento V, Milani M. Clobetasol propionate 0.05% in a novel foam formulation is safe and effective in the short-term treatment of patients with delayed pressure urticaria: a randomized double-blinded placebo-controlled trial. Br J Dermatol 2006; **154**:353–6.

45 Ellingsen AR, Thestrup-Pedersen K. Treatment of chronic idiopathic urticaria with topical steroids. Acta Derm Venereol (Stockh) 1996; **76**:43–4.

46 Champion RH, Roberts SOB, Carpenter RG, Roger JH. Urticaria and angio-oedema: a review of 554 patients. Br J Dermatol 1969; **81**:588–97.

47 Humphreys F, Hunter JAA. The characteristics of urticaria in 390 patients. Br J Dermatol 1998; **138**:635–8.

Appendix 1

Strength of recommendations and quality of evidence

Strength of recommendations

A   There is good evidence to support the use of the procedure

B   There is fair evidence to support the use of the procedure

C   There is poor evidence to support the use of the procedure

D   There is fair evidence to support the rejection of the use of the procedure

E   There is good evidence to support the rejection of the use of the procedure

Quality of evidence

I   Evidence obtained from at least one properly designed, randomized controlled trial

II-i   Evidence obtained from well-designed controlled trials without randomization

II-ii   Evidence obtained from well-designed cohort or case–control analytical studies, preferably from more than one centre or research group

II-iii   Evidence obtained from multiple time series with or without the intervention. Dramatic results in uncontrolled experiments (such as the results of the introduction of penicillin treatment in the 1940s) could also be regarded as this type of evidence

III   Opinions of respected authorities based on clinical experience, descriptive studies or reports of expert committees

IV   Evidence inadequate owing to problems of methodology (e.g. sample size, or length or comprehensiveness of follow-up or conflicts in evidence)

http://bad.org.uk/Portals/_Bad/Guidelines/Clinical
%20Guidelines/Urticaria%20and%20Angiodema%20
(2007).pdf

Comment

Differences between the BAD guidelines [1] and the
British Society for Allergy and Clinical Immunology's
guidelines [2] are remarkably few. They both highlight the
need for high-quality clinical trials in chronic urticaria
to clarify which antihistamines should be used in what
dose and for how long, and what treatment(s) should be
used when chronic urticaria does not respond to standard
therapy. A survey of Spanish dermatologists and allergists has shown that allergists were more likely to follow
the published guidelines [3] compared with dermatologists. Whether this is applicable to other countries with
different healthcare systems is not possible to say but perhaps highlights the need to advertise more to specialists
the publication of guidelines and to undertake local and
national audits. A recent study has highlighted the efficacy
of methotrexate in severe, antihistamine un-responsive
urticaria [4].

REFERENCES

1 Grattan CEH, Humphreys F. Guidelines for the evaluation
and management of urticaria in adults and children. *Brit J
Dermatol* 2007; 157: 1116–23.
2 Powell RJ, Du Toit GL, Siddique N, *et al.* BSACI guidelines
for the management of chronic urticaria and angio-oedema.
http://www3.interscience.wiley.com/journal/117999818/home
Clin Exp Allergy 2007; 37: 631–50.
3 Ferrer M, Jáuregui I, Bartra J, *et al.* Chronic urticaria: do
urticaria nonexperts implement treatment guidelines? A survey of adherence to published guidelines by nonexperts. *Brit J
Dermatol* 2009; 160: 823–7.
4 Perez A, Woods A, Grattan CE. Methotrexate: a useful steroid-
sparing agent in recalcitrant chronic urticaria. *Brit J Dermatol*
2010; 162: 191–4.

Additional professional resources

Angio-oedema and anaphylaxis. Clinical Knowledge Summaries 2007. http://www.cks.nhs.uk/patient_
information_leaflet/angioedema.
Urticaria and angioedema: synopsis (World Allergy
Organization review). http://www.worldallergy.org/
professional/allergic_diseases_center/urticaria/
urticariasynopsis.php
NHS Plus, Royal College of Physicians, Faculty of Occupational Medicine. *Latex allergy: occupational aspects of
management. A national guideline.* London: RCP, 2008
(http://www.rcplondon.ac.uk/pubs/contents/f0ba0178-
f790-48e8-a764-b319357f974a.pdf).
Patient Safety Information: protecting people with allergy
associated with latex. National Patient Safety Agency.
http://www.nrls.npsa.nhs.uk/resources/?entryid45
=59791.

BAD patient information leaflet

http://www.bad.org.uk/site/740/default.aspx

Related to urticaria pigmentosa
http://www.bad.org.uk/site/797/Default.aspx

Other patient resources

http://www.dermnet.org.nz/dna.urticaria/urt.html
http://www.allergyuk.org
http://www.cks.nhs.uk/patient_information_leaflet/
angioedema
Allergy and allergy tests: a guide for patients and relatives (Royal College of Pathologists 2005). http://www.
rcpath.org/resources/pdf/allergy_doc.pdf

VITILIGO

Guideline for the diagnosis and management of vitiligo

D.J. Gawkrodger, A.D. Ormerod, L. Shaw, I. Mauri-Sole, M.E. Whitton,*† M.J. Watts, A.V. Anstey, J. Ingham‡ and K. Young‡

British Association of Dermatologists, 4 Fitzroy Square, London W1T 5HQ, U.K.

*Vitiligo Society, 125 Kennington Road, London SE11 6SF, U.K.

†Cochrane Skin Group, Centre of Evidence Based Dermatology, King's Meadow Campus, University of Nottingham NG7 2NR, U.K.

‡Royal College of Physicians, St Andrew's Place, Regent's Park, London NW1 4LE, U.K.

Summary

This detailed and user-friendly guideline for the diagnosis and management of vitiligo in children and adults aims to give high quality clinical advice, based on the best available evidence and expert consensus, taking into account patient choice and clinical expertise.

The guideline was devised by a structured process and is intended for use by dermatologists and as a resource for interested parties including patients. Recommendations and levels of evidence have been graded according to the method developed by the Scottish Inter-Collegiate Guidelines Network. Where evidence was lacking, research recommendations were made.

The types of vitiligo, process of diagnosis in primary and secondary care, and investigation of vitiligo were assessed. Treatments considered include offering no treatment other than camouflage cosmetics and sunscreens, the use of topical potent or highly potent corticosteroids, of vitamin D analogues, and of topical calcineurin inhibitors, and depigmentation with p-(benzyloxy)phenol. The use of systemic treatment, e.g. corticosteroids, ciclosporin and other immunosuppressive agents was analyzed.

Phototherapy was considered, including narrowband ultraviolet B (UVB), psoralen with ultraviolet A (UVA), and khellin with UVA or UVB, along with combinations of topical preparations and various forms of UV. Surgical treatments that were assessed include full-thickness and split skin grafting, mini (punch) grafts, autologous epidermal cell suspensions, and autologous skin equivalents. The effectiveness of cognitive therapy and psychological treatments was considered. Therapeutic algorithms using grades of recommendation and levels of evidence have been produced for children and for adults with vitiligo.

Key recommendations

Grades of recommendation/levels of evidence are given (see Tables 1 and 2).

Therapeutic algorithm in children

1. Diagnosis

Where vitiligo is classical, the diagnosis is straightforward and can be made in primary care (D/4) but atypical presentations may require expert assessment by a dermatologist (D/4).

2. No treatment option

In children with skin types I and II, in the consultation it is appropriate to consider, after discussion, whether the initial approach may be to use no active treatment other than use of camouflage cosmetics and sunscreens (D/4).

3. Topical treatment

• Treatment with a potent or very potent topical steroid should be considered for a trial period of no more than 2 months. Skin atrophy has been a common side-effect (B/1+).

Table 1 Levels of evidence (from Scottish Inter-Collegiate Guidelines Network)

	Levels of evidence
1++	High-quality meta-analyses, systematic reviews of RCTs, or RCTs with a very low risk of bias
1+	Well-conducted meta-analyses, systematic reviews of RCTs, or RCTs with a low risk of bias
1−	Meta-analyses, systematic reviews of RCTs, or RCTs with a high risk of bias
2++	High-quality systematic reviews of case–control or cohort studies
	High-quality case–control or cohort studies with a very low risk of confounding, bias, or chance and a high probability that the relationship is causal
2+	Well-conducted case–control or cohort studies with a low risk of confounding, bias, or chance and a moderate probability that the relationship is causal
2−	Case–control or cohort studies with a high risk of confounding, bias, or chance and a significant risk that the relationship is not causal
3	Nonanalytical studies, e.g. case reports, case series
4	Expert opinion

RCT, randomized controlled trial.

Table 2 Grades of recommendation (from Scottish Inter-Collegiate Guidelines Network)

	Grades of recommendation
A	At least one meta-analysis, systematic review, or RCT rated as 1++, and directly applicable to the target population; or
	A systematic review of RCTs or a body of evidence consisting principally of studies rated as 1+, directly applicable to the target population, and demonstrating overall consistency of results
B	A body of evidence including studies rated as 2++, directly applicable to the target population, and demonstrating overall consistency of results; or Extrapolated evidence from studies rated as 1++ or 1+
C	A body of evidence including studies rated as 2+, directly applicable to the target population and demonstrating overall consistency of results; or Extrapolated evidence from studies rated as 2++
D	Evidence level 3 or 4; or Extrapolated evidence from studies rated as 2+

RCT, randomized controlled trial.

• Topical pimecrolimus or tacrolimus should be considered as alternatives to the use of a highly potent topical steroid in view of their better short-term safety profile (B/1+).

4. Phototherapy

Narrowband (NB) ultraviolet (UV) B phototherapy should be considered only in children who cannot be adequately managed with more conservative treatments (D/4), who have widespread vitiligo, or have localized vitiligo associated with a significant impact on patient's quality of life (QoL). Ideally, this treatment should be reserved for patients with darker skin types and monitored with serial photographs every 2–3 months (D/3). NB-UVB should be used in preference to PUVA in view of evidence of greater efficacy, safety and lack of clinical trials of PUVA in children (A/1+).

5. Systemic and surgical treatments

The use of oral dexamethasone to arrest progression of vitiligo cannot be recommended due to an unacceptable risk of side-effects (B/2++). There are no studies of surgical treatments in children.

6. Psychological treatments

Clinicians should make an assessment of the psychological and QoL effects of vitiligo on children (C/2++). Psychological interventions should be offered as a way of improving coping mechanisms (D/4). Parents of children with vitiligo should be offered psychological counselling.

Therapeutic algorithm in adults

1. Diagnosis

Where vitiligo is classical, the diagnosis is straightforward and can be made in primary care (D/4) but atypical presentations may require expert assessment by a dermatologist (D/4). A blood-test to check thyroid function should be considered in view of the high prevalence of autoimmune thyroid disease in patients with vitiligo (D/3).

2. No treatment option

In adults with skin types I and II, in the consultation it is appropriate to consider, after discussion, whether the initial approach may be to use no active treatment other than use of camouflage cosmetics and sunscreens (D/4).

3. Topical treatment

• In adults with recent onset of vitiligo, treatment with a potent or very potent topical steroid should be considered for a trial period of no more than 2 months. Skin atrophy has been a common side-effect (B/1+).
• Topical pimecrolimus should be considered as an alternative to a topical steroid, based on one study. The side-effect profile of topical pimecrolimus is better than that of a highly potent topical steroid (C/2+).
• Depigmentation with p-(benzyloxy)phenol (monobenzyl ether of hydroquinone) should be reserved for adults severely affected by vitiligo (e.g. more than 50% depigmentation or extensive depigmentation on the face or hands) who cannot

or choose not to seek repigmention and who can accept permanently not tanning (D/4).

4. Phototherapy

NB-UVB phototherapy (or PUVA) should be considered for treatment of vitiligo only in adults who cannot be adequately managed with more conservative treatments (D/4), who have widespread vitiligo, or have localized vitiligo with a significant impact on QoL. Ideally, this treatment should be reserved for patients with darker skin types and monitored with serial photographs every 2–3 months (D/3). NB-UVB should be used in preference to oral PUVA in view of evidence of greater efficacy (A/1+).

5. Systemic therapy

The use of oral dexamethasone to arrest progression of vitiligo cannot be recommended due to an unacceptable risk of side-effects (B/2++).

6. Surgical treatments

- Surgical treatments are reserved for cosmetically sensitive sites where there have been no new lesions, no Koebner phenomenon and no extension of the lesion in the previous 12 months (A/1++).
- Split-skin grafting gives better cosmetic and repigmentation results than minigraft procedures and utilizes surgical facilities that are relatively freely available (A/1+). Minigraft is not recommended due to a high incidence of side-effects and poor cosmetic results (A/1+). Other surgical treatments are generally not available.

7. Psychological treatments

Clinicians should make an assessment of the psychological and QoL effects of vitiligo on patients (C/2++). Psychological interventions should be offered as a way of improving coping mechanisms in adults with vitiligo (D/4).

Introduction

Vitiligo is a disease process that results in depigmented areas in the skin. It usually begins after birth and, although it can develop in childhood, the average age at onset is about 20 years.[1] Most commonly, vitiligo produces symmetrical depigmented areas of skin that otherwise appears normal. A less common type is the segmental form in which asymmetrical, one-sided depigmentation develops.

An important aspect of vitiligo is the psychological effect of the disease. Vitiligo is often immediately visible to others and those with the condition may suffer social and emotional consequences including low self-esteem, social anxiety, depression, stigmatization and, in extreme cases, rejection by those

around them.[2] In people with a pale white skin colour, vitiligo may cause little concern.

There is increasing evidence to support the view that vitiligo is an autoimmune disease and that it shows a familial trait in about 18% of cases.[3] The diagnosis of vitiligo is in many cases regarded as being straightforward, although this is not always the case. However, the treatment of vitiligo is acknowledged as being difficult. Hence, an evidence-based review of the management of the disease is timely.

Method of guideline development

The development of this guideline was a combined effort involving the Therapy Guidelines and Audit Subcommittee of the British Association of Dermatologists, the Clinical Standards Department of the Royal College of Physicians of London, The Cochrane Skin Group, and the Vitiligo Society. The Guideline Development Group (GDG) included one trainee dermatologist who is also a paediatrician (L.S.), one general practitioner with an interest in dermatology (I.M.-S.), one nurse (M.J.W.), one patient representative of the Vitiligo Society who is also a member of The Cochrane Skin Group (M.E.W.), and three dermatologists (A.V.A., A.D.O. and D.J.G.). Technical and methodological support was provided by the Royal College of Physicians Clinical Standards Department (J.I., K.Y. and Karen Reid), and administrative support by the British Association of Dermatologists. The Cochrane Skin Group has already published a systematic review of interventions for vitiligo.[4]

Aims

The objective of the process was to produce a detailed and user-friendly guideline giving the best available clinical advice for the management of vitiligo, based on the best available evidence and expert consensus, taking into account patient choice and clinical expertise. The guideline is intended for use by dermatologists (with an abbreviated version available for other healthcare professionals) and as a resource for interested parties including patients.

Scope

Diagnosis and management for adults and children with any type of vitiligo were considered. Other depigmenting diseases were considered in the differential diagnosis but their further management was not included.

Audience

The audience for this guideline is healthcare professionals, including doctors, nurses, psychologists, and indeed patients themselves and their carers. Commissioning organizations and health service providers may also find the guideline helpful.

Process

Nine meetings were held over a period of 12 months. A systematic approach was taken to the development of the guideline, using the method developed by the Scottish Inter-Collegiate Guidelines Network (SIGN; http://www.sign.ac.uk/methodology/index.html). In the initial meetings, the questions to be answered were formulated. Subsequently, literature searches were performed to obtain the evidence, which was subsequently appraised. This appraisal was performed in a standardized way according to the method described by SIGN (see Tables 1 and 2).

Tables showing the results were produced and are available on the website (http://www.bad.org.uk). The evidence was discussed at meetings of the group where the level of the evidence and the grade of the recommendations were agreed. Where no evidence was available, consensus statements were drawn up. Lastly, the entire guideline was agreed by the GDG.

Funding, declaration of interests and review

The expenses for the meetings of the GDG were underwritten by the British Association of Dermatologists. The Royal College of Physicians of London bore the costs of the work done by the members from the Clinical Standards Department. The members of the Group were not paid for their work.

The guideline will be reviewed in 5 years time.

What symptoms and signs are suggestive of vitiligo?

Introduction

Vitiligo vulgaris/nonsegmental vitiligo is an acquired chronic depigmentation disorder characterized by white patches. These are often symmetrical and usually increase in size with time. This corresponds with a substantial loss of functioning epidermal and, sometimes, hair follicle melanocytes. Segmental vitiligo is a variant of vitiligo confined to one unilateral segment. One unique segment is involved in most patients but two or more segments on the same or opposite sides may be involved or depigmentation may follow a dermatome distribution or Blaschko's lines. Depigmenting or hypopigmenting skin diseases that are considered in the differential diagnosis of vitiligo are listed in Table 3.

In symmetrical vitiligo, the commonest sites to be affected are the fingers and wrists, the axillae and groins and the body orifices such as the mouth, eyes and genitalia. As the pigment cells are destroyed, sometimes a 'trichrome' appearance of a white centre with an intermediate, pale area around it is found. In vitiligo skin there is no surface change and usually no redness. Very occasionally, inflammation is seen at the advancing edge of a vitiligo macule. Vitiligo can affect melanocytes in the hair roots, resulting in white eyelashes and white hair within the pale skin patches. Depigmentation can

Table 3 Differential diagnosis of vitiligo

Halo naevus
Hypopigmented naevus
Idiopathic guttate hypomelanosis
Leprosy
Lichen sclerosus (for genital vitiligo)
Melanoma-associated leucoderma
Melasma
Mycosis fungoides-associated depigmentation
Naevus anaemicus
Naevus of Ito
Piebaldism
Pityriasis alba
Pityriasis versicolor
Postinflammatory depigmentation, e.g. scleroderma, psoriasis, atopic eczema
Post-traumatic depigmentation
Topical or drug-induced depigmentation
Tuberous sclerosis

affect mucosal areas such as in the mouth. This can be prominent in darkly pigmented people.

The three main diseases that can be mistaken for vitiligo are tinea (pityriasis) versicolor, piebaldism and guttate hypomelanosis. Tinea versicolor is a superficial yeast infection that can cause loss of pigment in darker skinned individuals. It presents as pale macules typically on the upper trunk and chest, with a fine dry surface scale. Piebaldism is an autosomal dominant disease in which there is absence of melanocytes from the affected areas of the skin. It usually presents at birth with depigmented areas that are usually near the mid-line on the front, including a forelock of white hair. In idiopathic guttate hypomelanosis, multiple small, white macules are noted, mostly on the trunk or on sun-exposed parts of the limbs. When vitiligo affects only the genital areas, it can be difficult to exclude lichen sclerosus, which sometimes can coexist with vitiligo.

Patients with vitiligo often develop autoimmune thyroid disease or other autoimmune diseases and a history of autoimmune disease in a family member is obtained in 32% of patients.[3] In one series of 41 adults, a history of autoimmune thyroid disease was found in 14 (34%), suggesting that screening for abnormal thyroid function or the presence of autoantibodies to thyroid antigens may be helpful in the management of adults with vitiligo.[3]

As part of the initial assessment, the patient's skin type should be noted. The definitions are shown in Table 4.

Methods

Evidence for this question came from consensus within the GDG.

Evidence statements

General evidence on the diagnosis of vitiligo was considered and a consensus view was made by the group. This specific

Table 4 Skin types (from http://www.dermnetnz.org)

Skin type	Typical features	Tanning ability
I	Pale white skin, blue/ hazel eyes, blond/ red hair	Always burns, does not tan
II	Fair skin, blue eyes	Burns easily, tans poorly
III	Darker white skin	Tans after initial burn
IV	Light brown skin	Burns minimally, tans easily
V	Brown skin	Rarely burns, tans darkly easily
VI	Dark brown or black skin	Never burns, always tans darkly

question has been addressed recently by Taieb and Picardo,[5] who undertook an assessment and evaluation of vitiligo, including a definition of the disease, in a consensus group (level of evidence 4).

Evidence to recommendations

The group found that, in many cases, the diagnosis of vitiligo is straightforward but some cases present a difficult diagnostic challenge.

Recommendations

1. Where vitiligo is classical, as in the symmetrical types, the diagnosis is straightforward and can be made with confidence in primary care.

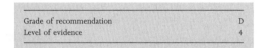

Grade of recommendation	D
Level of evidence	4

2. In patients with an atypical presentation, diagnosis is more difficult and referral for expert assessment by a dermatologist is recommended.

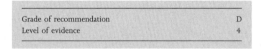

Grade of recommendation	D
Level of evidence	4

3. In adults with vitiligo, a blood test to check thyroid function should be considered in view of the high prevalence of autoimmune thyroid disease in patients with vitiligo.

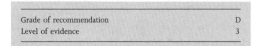

Grade of recommendation	D
Level of evidence	3

What is the accuracy of Wood's light compared with naked eye examination in the diagnosis of vitiligo?

Introduction

Wood's light is a hand-held ultraviolet (UV) irradiation device that emits UVA. It has been used to identify areas of depigmentation that may not be visible to the naked eye, especially in pale skin.

Methods

The GDG considered the limited evidence, consisting of two observational studies, and consensus statements regarding Wood's light.

Evidence statements

Wood's light delineates areas of pigment loss. Actively depigmenting areas may appear larger under UV illumination than with visible light, whereas areas showing repigmentation can appear larger or smaller with UV than with visible light. Thus combined assessment of a selected area in natural and Wood's light is useful.[5] Photography using a UV camera is also reported as useful in documenting pigmentary disorders.[6] Although Wood's light has not been scientifically evaluated, it has potential as a tool for objective assessment of vitiligo in research and clinical trials.

Evidence to recommendations

Wood's light can give the dermatologist additional information about the extent and activity of patches of vitiligo. Experience is needed in the use of the machine and evaluation of the results (level of evidence 4).

Recommendation

1. Wood's light may be of use in the diagnosis of vitiligo and in the demonstration of the extent and activity of the disease in subjects with skin types I and II. Wood's light can be of use in monitoring response to therapy.

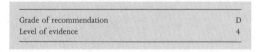

Grade of recommendation	D
Level of evidence	4

What is the natural history of vitiligo?

Introduction

Despite being a common condition that may cause severe and long-lasting disability, the epidemiology of vitiligo has not been established with clarity.

Methods

No studies on the natural history of vitiligo were identified by the search of the literature. Evidence and recommendations are based on consensus views.

Evidence statements

The natural history for the condition remains unclear, as no long-term follow-up study has been performed. This is relevant to the large number of therapeutic studies that have been carried out on vitiligo, as few have attempted to assess the longevity of any therapeutic response. There is no convincing evidence to suggest that any treatment has an effect on the natural history of vitiligo.

Textbooks of dermatology usually fail to comment on the natural history of vitiligo. Although some patients have been reported to undergo spontaneous repigmentation, this is probably uncommon. More typically, vitiligo is a chronic persistent disorder that progresses in a step-wise fashion with long periods when the disease is relatively inactive or static interspersed with shorter periods when areas of pigment loss extend. The genetic basis for vitiligo postulates a contribution from multiple recessive alleles at unlinked autosomal loci.[7]

The most detailed attempt at an epidemiological study was performed on the island of Bornholm in 1970–71.[8] This involved a single attempt to establish the prevalence of vitiligo in a population of sufficient size (47 033) to eliminate (or minimize) bias. Age-specific rates were established and showed that vitiligo is rare in the 0–9-year age group, with prevalence rising steadily thereafter to a peak at 60–70 years. Although this does not prove the natural history, it provides indirect evidence consistent with the notion that vitiligo is a life-long condition, with new cases in each age-band joining others who previously developed the condition. This study did not attempt a cross-sectional sample, which might have diagnosed more patients including those who were unaware of the study, or who had mild disease unapparent to them or who chose not to come forward.

A study from South Korea reported progressive disease in > 90% of a series of 318 patients with vitiligo.[9] This was a selected group and the methods used to assess disease progression were crude (patient recall on questionnaire). Nevertheless, it suggested that progression rather than spontaneous resolution is the norm. Finally, an epidemiological study from South America used a case–control design, identifying significant differences in age at presentation between unilateral (younger) and generalized vitiligo,[10] but no differences for rate of disease progression between the two groups (level of evidence 4).

Evidence to recommendations

No study has specifically determined the natural history of vitiligo. Indirect evidence and clinical experience of the GDG suggest that, in most cases, vitiligo is a chronic and persistent disorder characterized by periods of disease activity and often long periods of relative inactivity or stasis. Response to treatment should be considered in the light of this, recognizing that spontaneous repigmentation may occur, albeit uncommonly.

Recommendation

1. The response to treatment of vitiligo should be considered in the context of the natural history, recognizing that spontaneous repigmentation may occur but is uncommon.

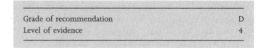

Grade of recommendation	D
Level of evidence	4

Research recommendation

1. A longitudinal epidemiological study is needed to define the natural history of vitiligo. This should use photographs combined with computerized image analysis, to quantify how the vitiligo changes with time.

What is the quality of life in patients with vitiligo compared with other skin diseases?

Introduction

Vitiligo can be a psychologically devastating disease which has a significant impact on quality of life (QoL) and self-esteem.[4,11] It may cause social isolation and significant depression,[12,13] create difficulties in sexual relationships, and affect perceived suitability for marriage.[14,15]

Some assessment of the impact of vitiligo on the patient's QoL should be made at the initial consultation, along with an assessment of the disease extent. The assessment of 'quality of life' is likely to be done differently by different clinicians and patients, unless standardized. Vitiligo differs from other diseases as it has no physical symptoms to speak of – its main impact is psychological.

QoL indices are important outcome measures in studies of vitiligo because there may be discrepancy between a researcher's definition of successful outcome and the patient's. For example, a study may show a statistical significance using an outcome measure of > 50% repigmentation when only 10% of patients with vitiligo consider this a successful result.[16] Hence, there is discrepancy between doctor and patient assessment of disease severity which may reflect the fact that psychological factors are important in overall morbidity.[17]

Methods

Several large studies have recorded a dermatology QoL index score (Dermatology Life Quality Index, DLQI) for vitiligo.[2,14,15,18–25] The scores range widely (3·5–15). This probably reflects the disease severity in the patient group examined, i.e. varying between primary care and tertiary centres. Few studies directly compare QoL scores in vitiligo with other skin diseases. Two studies compared vitiligo and psoriasis using the DLQI.[15,26] Both had patient populations that were not well matched. Two other studies used Skindex and the World Health Organization's GHQ12 scoring system.[27,28]

Evidence statements

One study comparing QoL in vitiligo and psoriasis showed a higher DLQI for psoriasis than vitiligo (mean 6·26 and 4·95, respectively).[26] The scoring pattern was different, with vitiligo scoring lower on the symptoms and treatment subscales and higher on the social, clothing and leisure subscales. This suggests that QoL scales with a weighting on the effect of symptoms and treatment effects underestimate the effect of vitiligo on QoL. DLQI might not be the most appropriate tool for assessing QoL in vitiligo as it may inevitably give a rather low score (level of evidence 2+).

In a study using Skindex and the GHQ12 score vitiligo scored higher than psoriasis on the social functioning subscale and emotions subscale but much lower on the symptoms subscale (level of evidence 2+).[27] The GHQ questionnaire reveals that QoL is more affected by vitiligo than by psoriasis (level of evidence 3).[28]

Race, colour and culture all influence how vitiligo affects QoL. DLQI is higher in studies looking at more racially pigmented groups. Loss of pigmentation may be seen as a threat to racial identity.[29] There may be cultural perceptions that wrongdoing in a previous life causes vitiligo. This stigma may itself affect QoL. There may be lay confusion with leprosy. Vitiligo causes unique psychosocial problems in some parts of the world (level of evidence 3).[30]

Gender also influences the way vitiligo affects QoL. Women are more severely affected, being more likely to be depressed about their appearance and more likely to internalize stigmatization and attribute an internal cause (level of evidence 3).[20] Women with vitiligo scored as highly on the DLQI as did women with psoriasis, whereas men with vitiligo scored significantly lower than men with psoriasis (level of evidence 2+).[26]

Psychological effects are prominent when visible body areas, e.g. the hands and face, are affected (level of evidence 3).[20] Studies of treatments for vitiligo should employ measures of QoL to assess the end result of any treatment, i.e. patient satisfaction with their response to therapy (consensus view of the GDG).

Evidence to recommendations

Vitiligo has an impact on a patient's QoL comparable with that of psoriasis. The DLQI may not be the best tool for measuring QoL in vitiligo, because vitiligo has no physical symptoms and is often not treated. Vitiligo has more impact on QoL in women, in those with racially pigmented skin, and in a cultural setting where there is attribution of blame for disfigurement.

Recommendations

1. Clinicians should make an assessment of the psychological and QoL effects of vitiligo on patients.

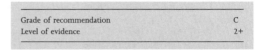

Grade of recommendation	C
Level of evidence	2+

2. In therapeutic trials relating to vitiligo, researchers should make the patient's improvement in QoL the most important outcome measure.

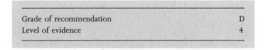

Grade of recommendation	D
Level of evidence	4

Research recommendation

1. More research is needed on appropriate QoL assessments for vitiligo and they should always be used as outcome measures.

In all patients with vitiligo, what is the accuracy of a scoring index in showing the outcome of common treatments compared with simple photography?

Introduction

A problem when assessing efficacy of treatment for vitiligo is to quantify the response with an objective, valid and reproducible scoring system. The most important aspect of therapeutic response is how the patient feels about their vitiligo after the treatment (see above). Another, which may well include how a patient feels, is the degree of repigmentation that has occurred. When patients are asked 'what degree of repigmentation do you want?' the answer is 'complete'. However, 100% repigmentation is very rarely achievable and something less has usually to be accepted. Assessment of repigmentation in vitiligo studies usually involves the use of photography or sometimes, the 'rule of nines'. Both methods have serious drawbacks. Inevitably, photography is a two-dimensional medium. The rule of nines is an estimate of surface area. A better method is needed that takes into account more than just the surface area.

Methods

Only three papers were identified, two clinical trials and one observational study.

Evidence statements

The vitiligo area-scoring index (VASI), based on the PASI score for psoriasis,[31] is a quantitative tool that can be used to evaluate the extent of vitiligo based on a composite estimate of the overall area of depigmented patches at baseline and the degree of macular repigmentation within these patches. The VASI correlated well with physician and patient global assessments ($P = 0.05$ and $P = 0.001$, respectively). A problem with VASI is that it takes into account only the area of vitiligo, and not other factors.

The Vitiligo European Task Force (VETF) assessed vitiligo and treatment outcomes using a system that combines analysis of extent, stage of disease and disease progression.[5] Extent is evaluated by the rule of nines; staging is based on cutaneous and hair pigmentation, and assessment of spreading is based on Wood's light examination. For extent, the investigators' correlations were very close (92% of evaluations were within 1% of the mean value). There were no patients with skin type VI in the study (20% of patients were skin type IV or V, which may not be representative for the U.K.). In addition, the measurements were not always consistent and no κ value was given for interobserver variability for extent of disease.

The use of digitized photographs subjected to morphometric computer analysis to delineate the degree of repigmentation has been described.[32] This method seemed to be workable and compared well with physicians' visual evaluations.

Evidence to recommendations

The response to treatments for vitiligo have typically been analysed using nominal binary scales in which the proportion of treated patients who achieve a specified degree of repigmentation is compared using nonparametric analysis based on physicians' assessment. The VETF tool adds two parameters, namely severity (staging) and progression (spreading). The VETF tool may give a more accurate assessment of vitiligo in research studies and seems to be the current gold standard but is impractical for routine clinic use. Digital photography with morphometric evaluation may be helpful in clinical trials.

Recommendations

1. The VASI and VETF tools offer a more accurate measure of disease extent than simple clinical photography alone (even when combined with computerized morphometry) and should be used in a research setting. Additionally, the VETF assesses severity and spreading.

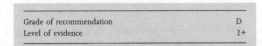

Grade of recommendation	D
Level of evidence	2+

2. For routine clinical use, serial photographs should be used to monitor response to treatment in vitiligo.

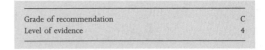

Grade of recommendation	C
Level of evidence	4

Research recommendation

1. Further research is needed to establish a simple, meaningful and reproducible method to monitor treatment response of vitiligo in the clinic and in clinical trials.

In all patients with vitiligo, what is the efficacy of applying betamethasone, clobetasol, fluocinolone, fluticasone or mometasone vs. placebo or other active treatment in terms of condition progression, area reduction and quality of life score?

Introduction

In the management of vitiligo, the physician typically makes an initial assessment of the patient and discusses the disease and treatment options. In many instances, the first-line therapy involves topical medicaments. In most cases, patients are offered advice about use of sunscreens and cosmetic camouflage including fake tanning products. There is evidence from one study that use of cosmetic camouflage can produce an improvement in QoL (DLQI 7.3 to 5.9).[15] With regard to topical therapy that might influence the state of the disease, the use of topical steroids is the usual first-line treatment.

Methods

Seven papers met the criteria for inclusion, underlining the paucity of good quality clinical studies of topical treatments in vitiligo. Only studies in which there were 20 or more evaluations were included. In all trials, only patients with generalized (symmetrical) types of vitiligo were included. In some studies, the researchers had excluded patients with vitiligo on the hands, presumably as they assumed the lesions would not respond to treatment. A left-vs.-right treatment methodology has been used in some studies and this presents potential problems. Studies on children have been separated from those on adults.

Evidence statements

The studies of Clayton[33] and Kandil,[34] although easily criticized, show that the use of a highly potent (clobetasol) or potent (betamethasone) topical steroid can repigment vitiligo but only in a small proportion of cases. Clayton found 15–25% repigmentation in 10 of 23 subjects (ages not stated) and > 75% in two of 23 (the other 11 showed no response), while Kandil found 90–100% repigmentation in six of 23 subjects (ages not given for all but one was aged 12 years) and 25–90% in three (with six showing 'beginning' repigmentation).[33,34] Clayton found that all steroid users had skin atrophy with clobetasol, a highly potent topical steroid (used for 8 weeks), while Kandil noted hypertrichosis in two subjects and acne in three subjects, related to 4 months use of the potent topical steroid, betamethasone.[33,34]

Westerhof and colleagues,[35] in probably the best controlled study to date of a topical treatment, compared topical fluticasone alone or combined with UVA in 135 adults. They found that the potent topical steroid fluticasone used alone for 9 months induced mean repigmentation of only 9% (compared with UVA alone of 8%) whereas the combination of fluticasone and UVA induced mean repigmentation of 31%: no steroid atrophy was noted in steroid users.

Comparison of a potent or highly potent topical steroid with another topical agent has been made but the studies are not robust. In a left-vs.-right comparison over an 8-week period in 10 adults, topical pimecrolimus was found to give 50–100% repigmentation in eight of 10 patients compared with an equivalent degree of repigmentation in seven of 10 patients treated with clobetasol.[36] A study of topical betamethasone vs. calcipotriol vs. a combination of the two over 5–10 weeks in 15, 16 and 18 adults, respectively, showed > 50% repigmentation in two, one and four, respectively, each out of 15 evaluable cases, with a conclusion that the results favoured the combination of topical betamethasone and calcipotriol.[37]

In children, Khalid *et al.* noted that topical use of the highly potent steroid clobetasol induced better repigmentation than PUVA-sol alone, finding > 50% repigmentation in 15 of 22 (vs. four of 23 for PUVA-sol) following use for 6 months, but six steroid users developed skin atrophy.[38] Another study in 20 children (aged less than 18 years of age) over an 8-week period compared topical clobetasol and tacrolimus and described '41%' repigmentation for clobetasol vs. '49%' repigmentation for tacrolimus.[32]

Evidence to recommendations

There is evidence that very potent or potent topical corticosteroids can repigment vitiligo in adults but the studies that support this statement have often been poorly conducted and side-effects are common if treatment lasts for more than a few weeks. For generalized symmetrical types of vitiligo, topical clobetasol used over 2–6 months repigments vitiligo to some degree. There is weak evidence for clinically meaningful repigmentation with topical betamethasone, used over a period of 4 months, and for topical fluticasone used over 9 months. There are significant potential side-effects, mainly of skin atrophy and hypertrichosis, especially for clobetasol and betamethasone, less so with fluticasone. For generalized symmetrical types of vitiligo, the combination of topical betamethasone with calcipotriol was better than betamethasone alone over a 5–10-week period. The combination of topical fluticasone with UVA used over 9 months was much more effective than fluticasone used alone. In children, topical clobetasol induced repigmentation but skin atrophy was a side-effect.

Recommendations

1. In children, and adults with recent onset of vitiligo, treatment with a potent or very potent topical steroid should be considered for a trial period of no more than 2 months. Although benefits have been observed, skin atrophy has been a common side-effect.

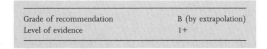

| Grade of recommendation | B (by extrapolation) |
| Level of evidence | 1+ |

2. In patients with skin types I and II, in the consultation it is appropriate to consider, after discussion with the patient, whether the initial approach may be to use no active treatment other than consideration of the use of camouflage cosmetics including fake tanning products and the use of sunscreens.

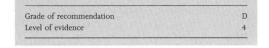

| Grade of recommendation | D |
| Level of evidence | 4 |

In all patients with vitiligo, what is the efficacy of applying calcipotriol or tacalcitol vs. placebo or an active treatment in terms of condition progression, area reduction and quality of life score?

Introduction

The vitamin D analogues, calcipotriol and tacalcitol, may have a place in the treatment of vitiligo.

Methods

Nine papers met the criteria for inclusion as used for topical corticosteroids. In all trials but one (Chiaverini *et al.*,[39] in which localized forms of vitiligo were included), only patients with generalized (symmetrical) types of vitiligo were studied.

Evidence statements

The best study of calcipotriol is the randomized open left-vs.-right study of Chiaverini *et al.*,[39] in which the effect over a 3–6-month period of the once daily application of calcipotriol is compared in symmetrical target lesions in 24 patients (15 females, nine males; age range 5–59 years) with localized and generalized vitiligo. No repigmentation was noted in 21 of 23 patients after 3–6 months. One patient had 5% repigmentation with calcipotriol; two had repigmentation with and without calcipotriol (P > 0·5). An unpublished clinical trial of the efficacy of topical calcipotriol vs. vehicle for vitiligo showed no beneficial effect for the calcipotriol over the vehicle placebo (A. Bibby, LEO Pharma A/S, personal communication, 2008).

A study of topical betamethasone vs. calcipotriol vs. a combination of the two over 5–10 weeks in 15, 16 and 18 adults, respectively, showed > 50% repigmentation in two, one and four each out of 15 evaluable cases.[37] The conclusion was that the results favoured the combination of topical betamethasone and calcipotriol over betamethasone alone. However, the numbers here are too small for a definitive conclusion and there has been no other study of this sort. An open study of twice daily topical calcipotriol (with PUVA in four patients) in 26 patients (16 females, 10 males; age range 5–61 years; 22 Asians) for 3–9 months showed that 17 of 22 receiving monotherapy with calcipotriol had 30–100% repigmentation which was > 50% in 12.[40]

There have been studies of the effect of combining topical calcipotriol with phototherapy (see below).[19,41–44]

Evidence to recommendations

For generalized symmetrical or localized types of vitiligo, topical calcipotriol by itself has no effect in vitiligo and is not recommended. For generalized symmetrical types of vitiligo, the addition of topical calcipotriol to narrowband (NB) UVB does not add any benefit and is not recommended. The use of topical calcipotriol with PUVA may produce earlier repigmentation but it is not clear whether the final degree of repigmentation is enhanced. There is insufficient evidence to make a comment about the use of tacalcitol.

Recommendation

1. The use of topical calcipotriol as a monotherapy is not recommended.

Grade of recommendation	B
Level of evidence	2++

In all patients with vitiligo, what is the efficacy of applying tacrolimus or pimecrolimus vs. placebo or an active treatment in terms of condition progression, area reduction and quality of life score?

Introduction

The calcineurin inhibitors have found use in a variety of inflammatory skin diseases and have been tried in vitiligo.

Methods

Four papers met the criteria for inclusion as used for topical corticosteroids. Studies on children will be considered separately from those on adults.

Evidence statements

Coskun and colleagues,[36] in a left-vs.-right comparison over an 8-week period in 10 adults, compared topical pimecrolimus with topical clobetasol. They found topical pimecrolimus resulted in 50–100% repigmentation in eight of 10 patients, most noticeable for lesions on the trunk or extremities, compared with an equivalent degree of repigmentation in seven of 10 patients treated with clobetasol. No skin atrophy was noted but burning was a side-effect with pimecrolimus. The number of subjects in this study is small, making a reliable conclusion difficult.

In an open proof-of-concept study of 26 children aged over 6 years and adults with generalized symmetrical forms of vitiligo, treated for head and neck lesions with topical 1% pimecrolimus twice daily, total repigmentation of a target lesion was found in 50% of patients after 6 months of therapy.[45]

Twenty children treated over 8 weeks with either topical clobetasol or tacrolimus were shown to have repigmentation that amounted to 41% with clobetasol and 49% with tacrolimus.[32] Lesions on the face and thorax responded better than those on the abdomen or legs: lesions on hands did not respond. Skin atrophy was noted in five of the 20 treated with the steroid, while two of 20 who received tacrolimus noted burning.

Comparisons have been made of topical tacrolimus alone with tacrolimus and Excimer UV radiation. In one study of 14 patients aged over 12 years, 23 vitiligo lesions received a combination of tacrolimus ointment twice daily and Excimer UV twice weekly for 12 weeks and were compared with 20 lesions that received Excimer UV alone for 12 weeks.[46] For the combination of topical tacrolimus and Excimer UV, 16 of 23 had 75% or more repigmentation compared with four of 20 lesions treated using the Excimer alone (P < 0·001). In UV-exposed areas, i.e. face, neck, trunk or limbs, 75% or more repigmentation was seen in 10 of 13 using the combination treatment compared with none of 13 lesions that received the Excimer alone (P < 0·001). Side-effects included stinging in the tacrolimus group, moderate erythema at least once in all patients, and bullous lesions in four of 43 lesions. Another study that included only 20 lesions in eight adults, comparing Excimer plus topical tacrolimus vs. Excimer plus placebo, found repigmentation to be more in the tacrolimus/ Excimer group.[47]

Further studies on the efficacy of topical calcineurin inhibitors are required. The long-term side-effects of the calcineurin inhibitor drugs are unknown and this should be borne in mind if prolonged treatment (e.g. longer than 12 months) is proposed.

Evidence to recommendations

In adults with generalized symmetrical types of vitiligo, in a small study, topical pimecrolimus for 8 weeks induced 50–100% repigmentation (a similar degree to that seen with topical clobetasol) for lesions on the trunk or extremities. Stinging was a side-effect. In children with generalized symmetrical vitiligo, topical tacrolimus used over an 8-week period induced nearly 50% repigmentation of vitiligo lesions (a similar degree to that seen with topical clobetasol) for lesions on the face or thorax but not the hands. Stinging was a side-effect. The combination of topical tacrolimus with Excimer UV radiation appeared to enhance the degree of repigmentation over that for Excimer alone, for UV-sensitive sites but not for areas over bony prominences.

Recommendations

1. In adults with symmetrical types of vitiligo, topical pimecrolimus should be considered as an alternative to the use of a topical steroid, based on evidence from one study. The side-effect profile of topical pimecrolimus is better than that of a highly potent topical steroid.

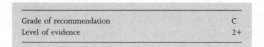

Grade of recommendation	C
Level of evidence	2+

2. In children with vitiligo, topical pimecrolimus or tacrolimus should be considered as alternatives to the use of a highly potent topical steroid in view of their better short-term safety profile.

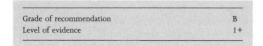

Grade of recommendation	B
Level of evidence	1+

Research recommendation

1. Further research is needed to clarify the roles of tacrolimus and pimecrolimus in adults and children with vitiligo. A head-to-head study of tacrolimus vs. pimecrolimus is suggested.

In all patients with vitiligo, what is the efficacy of applying *p*-(benzyloxy)phenol (monobenzyl ether of hydroquinone) vs. placebo or an active treatment in terms of reducing areas of pigmentation?

Introduction

The use of medicaments to induce complete depigmentation may be considered in patients with vitiligo under certain situations.

Methods

There were no randomized controlled trials (RCTs). Case studies or consensus reports were considered.

Evidence statements

Several products, some of which are marketed as cosmetics, have been used to reduce pigmentation of the skin. In certain countries such products are legally available over the counter; in others the products are available but not legally. These products may contain mercuric iodide (as in a germicidal soap), antiseptics containing phenolic derivatives and hydroquinone or related chemicals. In vitiligo, depigmentation may be considered as a therapeutic option when the patient has a naturally dark skin and has very obvious vitiligo extensively affecting cosmetically sensitive areas such as the face and backs of the hands. To induce depigmentation, the main method used has been the application of p-(benzyloxy)phenol (monobenzyl ether of hydroquinone, MBEH). There have been concerns about whether p-(benzyloxy)phenol is carcinogenic and it was banned from use in cosmetics in the EU in 2001. More recently, one study has examined the effect of topical 4-methoxyphenol (4MP) as a depigmenting agent.

Only two clinical trials that examine treatments aimed at depigmenting the normally pigmented skin in vitiligo were found. Both met the criteria for inclusion although one had only 13 subjects and the other 18. In both trials, it appears that only patients with generalized (symmetrical) types of vitiligo were included.

In the clinical trial described by Njoo et al.,[48] topical 4MP and the Q-switched ruby laser (QSRL) were used as the depigmenting agents. Topical 4MP produced total depigmentation in 11 of 16 subjects (69%; 95% confidence interval, CI 41–90%) with the onset of depigmentation within 4–12 months. Of the 11, four had a recurrence of pigment after 2–36 months. Side-effects of 4MP included mild burning or itching. Four of the five nonresponders to 4MP did depigment when treated using the QSRL. In the group treated using the QSRL, total depigmentation was found in nine of the 13 treated (69%; 95% CI 39–91%) with an onset within 7–14 days. Four had recurrence of pigment after 2–18 months. There were no side-effects in the QSRL group.

In an open study of p-(benzyloxy)phenol (MBEH),[49] 18 patients 'severely' affected by vitiligo (type of vitiligo not stated) were treated with the topical application of 20% MBEH. Eight achieved complete depigmentation after 10 months and three had 'dramatic' depigmentation, but in three there was no effect at all (after 4 months use).

Four papers on the management of vitiligo discuss the consensus view of the place of depigmentation treatment.[50–53] Expert consensus opinion concludes that patients with a dark skin type selected for depigmentation treatments must understand the cultural effects the depigmentation may have. It is usual to consider for depigmentation only subjects in whom the area of skin involved by vitiligo is extensive, usually taken to mean more than 50% of the skin surface area.[54] If there is extensive involvement of the cosmetically sensitive areas of the face and hands, and covering cosmetics are ineffective, depigmentation can be considered although it is usual to treat only the exposed sites.

Hydroquinones and related chemicals may cause side-effects. Irritation and occasionally contact dermatitis are recognized, as is the infrequent occurrence of ochronosis.[55] This had led to the banning of hydroquinones from over-the-counter products in Europe. Of more concern is the possibility of carcinogenesis from hydroquinones.[56] However, this is still a matter for debate.[55]

Evidence to recommendations

In patients with extensive generalized forms of vitiligo, the topical use of MBEH and 4MP or the use of the QSRL are effective in inducing depigmentation. MBEH and 4MP can take a long time to have an effect, with onset of depigmentation often delayed until after 4 months, and may be associated with local irritation and sometimes recurrence of pigmentation. With the QSRL, onset of the effect is much quicker and there are apparently fewer side-effects. This treatment may be preferred. However, there are few papers on this treatment and it is unwise to make a major recommendation based on one report.

Expert consensus recommends that patient selection is important in depigmentation treatment. It is vital that patients with a dark skin type understand the cultural implications. In general, depigmentation is undertaken only when the patient has more than 50% pigment loss in their skin due to vitiligo, or when the depigmentation is extensive in the cosmetically sensitive areas of the hands and face, when depigmentation of the exposed areas can be considered. This treatment is not recommended for children.

Recommendation

1. Depigmentation with p-(benzyloxy)phenol (MBEH) or 4MP should be reserved for adults severely affected by vitiligo (e.g. who have more than 50% depigmentation or who have extensive depigmentation on the face or hands) who cannot or choose not to seek repigmentation and who can accept the permanence of never tanning.

Grade of recommendation	D
Level of evidence	4

In all patients with vitiligo, what is the efficacy of a course of narrowband UVB including high-intensity light sources compared with placebo in terms of condition progression, area reduction and quality of life score?

Introduction

Phototherapy with UVB has been used in the treatment of vitiligo for many years. Phototherapy with broadband UVB appeared less effective than PUVA and was less frequently used. In the early 1990s, NB-UVB became widely available in Europe due to its widespread use in psoriasis. NB-UVB appeared to be more effective for treating vitiligo than the broadband UVB that it replaced. It is only recently that the efficacy of NB-UVB in the treatment of vitiligo has been assessed objectively in clinical trials. By convention, NB-UVB is usually given three times each week. An arbitrary limit of 200 NB-UVB treatments for vitiligo has been suggested, although in practice most patients have fewer.[57]

NB-UVB has the advantage for patients of being more acceptable than PUVA because they do not need to take oral medication before exposure to radiation or to wear protective sunglasses. Both PUVA and NB-UVB require a great degree of commitment by the patient. This should be explained at the time of consultation.

Methods

Nine studies identified using a computer-assisted search are included in the evidence table.

Evidence statements

Nine studies were assessed, two of which[31,57] follow the study design of an RCT. The study by Hamzavi and Shapiro[31] is of limited importance due to the small patient numbers, and the fact that most of the patients were white. This study did, however, establish that NB-UVB is an effective treatment for vitiligo compared with no treatment (P < 0·001). It also highlighted the differential response within patients according to body site.

The most important study, by Yones et al.,[57] was the first double-blind, randomized trial of oral PUVA vs. NB-UVB therapy in vitiligo. It demonstrated therapeutic efficacy for both treatment modalities. However, NB-UVB was more effective, easier to administer and produced a better colour match. Vitiligo relapse was reported following both treatments in some patients by 12 months post-therapy.

Three of the remaining seven studies included 50 or more patients, but all three were methodologically weak. The largest, by Menchini et al.,[58] was an open study of 734 patients treated with a filtered xenon arc lamp which was claimed to deliver UVB. There were no controls and no attempt to analyse responses statistically. None the less, the authors claimed that this treatment was 'highly effective with no side-effects'. The second largest study, by Westerhof and Nieuweboer-Krobotova,[59] included 175 patients. Response was compared with baseline and no attempt was made to analyse results statistically. The authors concluded that TL-01 phototherapy was as efficient as topical PUVA in inducing repigmentation in vitiligo, but with fewer side-effects. The third largest report, an open study of NB-UVB in the treatment of 51 children with vitiligo, concluded that this was a safe and effective treatment.[22]

The final four reports are small open studies which are not objective or controlled. Three describe responses to the

Excimer laser.[60–62] Each study reports a positive response (i.e. repigmentation) but no data are presented on the amount of repigmentation, or cosmetic acceptability or permanence. A small study that made a good attempt to assess the responses objectively concluded that NB-UVB was effective at treating vitiligo while broadband UVB was not.[19]

Evidence to recommendations

There is good evidence that some patients with vitiligo respond well to phototherapy with NB-UVB. A single randomized double-blind trial comparing oral PUVA with NB-UVB has convincingly demonstrated the superiority of NB-UVB over PUVA. Twelve-month follow-up showed that some patients relapsed and ended up with worse vitiligo than they had before PUVA (28%) or NB-UVB (12%) started. However, maintenance of > 75% repigmentation of surface area was seen in 24% in the PUVA group and 36% in the NB-UVB group.

Recommendations

1. NB-UVB phototherapy should be considered for treatment of vitiligo only in children or adults who cannot be adequately managed with more conservative treatments.

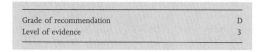

| Grade of recommendation | D |
| Level of evidence | 4 |

2. A trial of NB-UVB therapy should be considered for children or adults with widespread vitiligo, or localized vitiligo associated with a significant impact on patient's QoL. Ideally, this treatment should be reserved for patients with darker skin types.

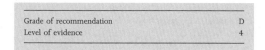

| Grade of recommendation | D |
| Level of evidence | 3 |

3. Before starting treatment, children, their parents and carers, and adults should be made aware that there is no evidence that NB-UVB phototherapy alters the natural history of vitiligo. They should also be made aware that not all patients respond to this treatment, and that some body sites, such as the hands and feet, respond poorly in all patients. They should also be informed of the limit to the number of treatments due to possible side-effects.

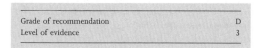

| Grade of recommendation | D |
| Level of evidence | 3 |

4. If phototherapy is to be used for treating nonsegmental vitiligo, NB-UVB should be used in preference to oral PUVA.

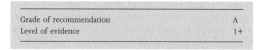

| Grade of recommendation | A |
| Level of evidence | 1+ |

5. Evidence is lacking to define an upper limit for the number of treatments with NB-UVB for patients with vitiligo. Taking into account the published data for patients with psoriasis (see below) and in view of the greater susceptibility of vitiliginous skin to sunburn and possible photodamage (due to absence of melanin), it is advised that safety limits for NB-UVB for the treatment of vitiligo are more stringent than those applied to psoriasis, with an arbitrary limit of 200 treatments for skin types I–III. This could be higher for skin types IV–VI at the discretion of the clinician and with the consent of the patient.

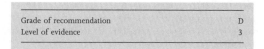

| Grade of recommendation | D |
| Level of evidence | 3 |

6. It is recommended that physicians prescribing NB-UVB for vitiligo monitor response closely with the assistance of serial clinical photographs (every 2–3 months), more easily to identify patients who fail to respond adequately or in whom the disease progresses during treatment.

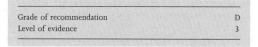

| Grade of recommendation | D |
| Level of evidence | 3 |

In all patients with vitiligo, what is the efficacy of a course of PUVA or PUVA-sol compared with placebo in terms of condition progression, area reduction and quality of life score?

Introduction

Psoralen derived from plants applied to the skin followed by exposure to sunlight has been used as treatment for vitiligo since biblical times. El Mofty in 1948 first published on this treatment in a contemporary journal.[63] Since then, there have been many publications on the efficacy of PUVA in vitiligo.

Methods

Fifteen papers were identified by the computer-assisted search strategy, but only five of these were relevant to the question.

Evidence statements

Two studies used an RCT study design.[57,64] The study by Pathak had a poor assessment method and lacked statistical analysis but included 366 patients and a placebo group.[64] This study confirmed that PUVA is an effective treatment for vitiligo compared with placebo, yet failed to address the issue of disease progression and impact on QoL. Yones *et al.* compared the efficacy of NB-UVB with oral PUVA in nonsegmental vitiligo in a well-conducted study that showed that both treatments were effective.[57] However, PUVA was less effective at inducing repigmentation and the colour match of the repigmented skin was not as good as for NB-UVB. At 12 months follow-up > 25% of PUVA-treated patients had vitiligo that was worse than at baseline. However, a similar proportion of patients had maintained more than 75% improvement in body surface area repigmented at 12 months.

Khalid *et al.* reported on 50 children less than 12 years old with vitiligo, using photographs to compare PUVA-sol with topical clobetasone.[38] They reported a good response to PUVA-sol but used no formal statistical analysis. In a study of 89 patients with vitiligo, Sehgal found three different psoralen products to be efficacious in inducing repigmentation compared with baseline but used no control group and no statistical analysis.[65]

Two studies have compared efficacy of PUVA compared with NB-UVB. Westerhof and Nieuweboer-Krobotova compared PUVA and NB-UVB in 28 patients with vitiligo, reporting 46% repigmentation for the PUVA group.[59] Another (open) study of NB-UVB and PUVA using systemic trimethylpsoralen showed a better response to NB-UVB in 50 subjects.[66]

Evidence to recommendations

Both PUVA and PUVA-sol are efficacious in the treatment of some patients with vitiligo. However, most studies fail adequately to address the degree of this response, its durability or its effect on QoL. PUVA has now been demonstrated to be less effective than NB-UVB in the treatment of vitiligo, and sustained improvement at 12 months following treatment end is seen in < 25% of patients. No study has looked at long-term dangers of PUVA in vitiligo.

Recommendations

1. PUVA therapy should be considered for treatment of vitiligo only in adults who cannot be adequately managed with more conservative treatments. PUVA is not recommended in children.

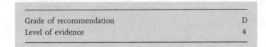

Grade of recommendation — D
Level of evidence — 4

2. If phototherapy is to be used for treating nonsegmental vitiligo, NB-UVB should usually be used in preference to oral PUVA.

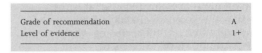

Grade of recommendation — A
Level of evidence — 1+

3. A trial of PUVA therapy should be considered only for adults with widespread vitiligo, or localized vitiligo associated with a significant impact on patient's QoL. Ideally, this treatment should be reserved for patients with darker skin types.

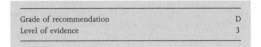

Grade of recommendation — D
Level of evidence — 3

4. Before starting PUVA treatment patients should be made aware that there is no evidence that this treatment alters the natural history of vitiligo. They should also be made aware that not all patients respond, and that some body sites, such as the hands and feet, respond poorly in all patients. They should also be informed of the limit to the number of treatments due to possible side-effects.

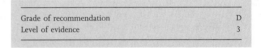

Grade of recommendation — D
Level of evidence — 3

5. Evidence is lacking to define an upper limit for the number of treatments with PUVA for patients with vitiligo. Taking into account the published data for patients with psoriasis (see below) and in view of the greater susceptibility of vitiligo skin to psoralen-induced burning and possible photodamage (due to absence of melanin), it is advised that safety limits for PUVA in the treatment of vitiligo are more stringent than those for psoriasis, with an arbitrary limit of 150 treatments for patients with skin types I–III. This could be higher for skin types IV–VI at the discretion of the clinician and with the consent of the patient.

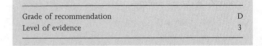

Grade of recommendation — D
Level of evidence — 3

6. It is recommended that physicians prescribing PUVA for vitiligo monitor response closely using serial clinical photographs (every 2–3 months) to identify patients who fail to respond adequately or in whom the disease progresses during treatment.

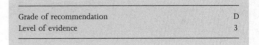

Grade of recommendation — D
Level of evidence — 3

In all patients with vitiligo, what is the efficacy of a course of khellin with sunlight UVA or UVB compared with PUVA or PUVA-sol in terms of progression, area reduction and quality of life score?

Introduction

Khellin is a naturally occurring furochromone which is a structural isomer of methoxsalen. In combination with UVA or sunlight khellin is reported to induce repigmentation of vitiliginous skin. The exact mechanism of action of khellin plus UVA in vitiligo is unknown.

Methods

Five papers were identified by the computer-assisted search strategy and all five are relevant to the question. However, none of these papers adhered strictly to an RCT design.

Evidence statements

In a study comparing khellin or placebo both with natural sunlight, 12 of 30 in the khellin group showed > 50% repigmentation compared with none in the control group.[67] A left-vs.-right study of 72 patients compared khellin with UVA vs. UVA alone and concluded that repigmentation was due to the UVA, not the khellin.[68] A left-vs.-right study compared khellin plus sunlight with vehicle plus sunlight in 41 patients and found no difference between the khellin and placebo groups.[69] However, in a later study the same authors compared a khellin gel and UVA with UVA alone, finding that both groups responded but khellin plus UVA was superior to UVA alone (P < 0·01).[70] A study with 33 patients compared topical khellin plus UVA with PUVA, concluding that khellin plus UVA may induce repigmentation comparable with that induced by systemic PUVA, but required a longer duration.[71]

Evidence to recommendations

Despite apparent initial promise, research in this area is inconclusive and at times contradictory.

Recommendation

1. There is currently insufficient evidence to recommend khellin with UV in the treatment of vitiligo.

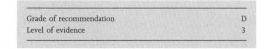

| Grade of recommendation | D |
| Level of evidence | 3 |

Late complications of PUVA or narrowband UVB therapy in patients with vitiligo: are patients who have received large doses of PUVA (more than 150 treatment sessions) or narrowband UVB (more than 150 treatment sessions) at increased risk of developing premalignant or malignant skin changes?

Introduction

It is not uncommon for patients with vitiligo to be given large numbers of PUVA or UVB treatments, occasionally over a relatively short period. As the areas of vitiligo have no melanin they are particularly susceptible to the damaging effects of UVB (or PUVA) and may therefore be more susceptible to developing premalignant or malignant changes.

Methods

There is only one study on vitiligo in which the issue of chronic cutaneous damage with long-term PUVA is specifically assessed.[72]

Evidence statements

Harrist et al. followed up annually with a skin examination 596 patients with vitiligo treated with PUVA (230 for up to 55 months) but did not include a control group.[72] No skin cancers were observed, but vitiligo and perilesional skin showed dermal changes of chronic photodamage.

There is a paucity of studies of skin cancer in vitiligo, but there are retrospective reports from centres that have treated patients with vitiligo with phototherapies over long periods of time. Wildfang et al. reported no actinic keratoses, lentigines or skin cancer in a retrospective study on 59 patients with vitiligo treated with PUVA.[73] Chuan et al. reported no actinic keratoses or skin cancer in 21 patients with vitiligo treated with PUVA followed for up to 7 years.[74] Westerhof and Schallreuter reported no skin cancer in > 2500 patients (but not in a study).[75] Halder et al. in a study of 326 patients with vitiligo treated with PUVA with 4 years of follow up reported no actinic keratoses, cutaneous carcinomas or lentigines, but acknowledged that the follow-up period was almost certainly too short to detect an increase in skin cancer.[76]

Reports of skin cancer in patients with vitiligo treated with PUVA are limited. Buckley and Rogers describe a patient who developed multiple invasive squamous cell carcinomas in areas of vitiligo which had failed to repigment despite a prolonged continuous course of PUVA.[77] A similar patient had multiple squamous cell carcinomas in situ in vitiligo areas following PUVA therapy over a 9-year period.[78] Multiple bizarre-looking lentigines were reported in a patient with vitiligo following years of topical and systemic PUVA, but with no malignancy and benign histology.[79] Park et al. reported a patient with vitiligo who developed a squamous cell carcinoma in an area of vitiligo following long-term PUVA.[80]

Evidence to recommendations

The risk of skin cancer in patients with vitiligo treated with PUVA is currently unclear. There is no long-term follow-up study of the type carried out by Stern and Lange which established the clear cancer risk for PUVA in patients with psoriasis.[81] Despite some authors' claims that high doses of PUVA in vitiligo are safe, it is counterintuitive to believe that patients with vitiligo are at a lower risk of skin cancer with PUVA than patients who have psoriasis. Indeed, the absence of functional melanocytes could put patients with vitiligo at a greater risk. In the absence of persuasive evidence to the contrary, it is logical to recommend more stringent limits on PUVA for vitiligo than apply for psoriasis.

Recommendations

1. In view of uncertainty regarding the cancer risk, clinicians prescribing NB-UVB or PUVA should be cautious in prescribing these treatments in vitiligo. A clear explanation of the risks and benefits of treatment must be given *before* treatment, with a Patient Information Leaflet written in lay terms.

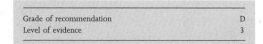

Grade of recommendation	D
Level of evidence	3

2. Patients treated with PUVA or UVB should have their treatment closely supervised by a consultant dermatologist and the treatment regimen for patients with skin types I–III should not exceed 200 treatments for NB-UVB and 150 treatments for PUVA. This recommendation is based on published evidence for patients with psoriasis. Evidence is lacking to define an upper limit for patients with skin types IV–VI for NB-UVB or PUVA.

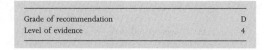

Grade of recommendation	D
Level of evidence	4

3. In most patients, NB-UVB should be used in preference to PUVA.

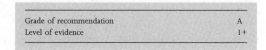

Grade of recommendation	A
Level of evidence	1+

Research recommendation

1. In view of the possible long-term risk of skin cancer with extended courses of NB-UVB or PUVA in patients with vitiligo, further research to define this potential risk is recommended.

In all patients with vitiligo, what is the efficacy of a course of narrowband UVB with a vitamin D analogue compared with narrowband UVB with placebo in terms of condition progression, area reduction and quality of life score?

Introduction

The use of combination treatments has been commonplace in the treatment of vitiligo.

Methods

Authors have attempted to assess whether the combination of a topical vitamin D analogue with NB-UVB is more effective than NB-UVB alone.

Evidence statements

For calcipotriol, there are two studies with directly contradictory results. In a small single-blinded RCT with 20 patients, there was no additional benefit from adding calcipotriol to NB-UVB when compared with UVB alone.[82] In contrast, a slightly larger open study with 24 patients showed that the combination of calcipotriol with NB-UVB was more effective than UVB alone.[83] In a similar randomized but open-label study with 32 patients, the combination of tacalcitol with NB-UVB was more effective at inducing repigmentation in vitiligo than UVB alone.[84] Another open, bilateral comparison study with 20 subjects compared NB-UVB with NB-UVB and calcipotriene; results suggested a better response to the combination but the results were inconclusive.[85]

Two studies attempted to assess the response of vitiligo to the Excimer laser with and without topical tacrolimus. A double-blind study in eight patients whose vitiligo was treated with the Excimer laser with tacrolimus ointment 0·1% or placebo showed better results for the tacrolimus-treated group.[47] This study failed to include a tacrolimus-only limb or a Excimer laser-only limb so the results are hard to interpret. A second study compared Excimer monotherapy with Excimer and tacrolimus ointment and reported a superior response to the combination but also failed to include a tacrolimus-only limb or an ointment placebo with the Excimer.[46]

A combination study of 27 patients found no benefit of combining NB-UVB with vitamin B_{12} and folate vs. NB-UVB as monotherapy.[86] In addition, mention is made of the treatment of vitiligo using topical application of pseudocatalase and calcium in combination with UVB therapy or Dead Sea climatotherapy reported by Schallreuter et al.[87,88] In an open study of 33 patients, complete repigmentation on the face and hands was reported in 90% of the group starting within 2–4 months.[87] This treatment cannot be considered further as it was not a controlled study and the work has not been reproduced.

Evidence to recommendations

There is no convincing evidence to suggest that topical vitamin D analogues in combination with NB-UVB phototherapy
are superior to NB-UVB alone.

Recommendation

1. Topical vitamin D analogues in combination with NB-UVB
therapy should not be used in the treatment of vitiligo.

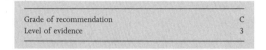

| Grade of recommendation | C |
| Level of evidence | 3 |

In all patients with vitiligo, what is the efficacy of a course of PUVA with a vitamin D analogue compared with PUVA with placebo in terms of condition progression, area reduction and quality of life score?

Introduction

The use of combination therapies has been common in the
treatment of vitiligo.

Methods

Studies were identified which have attempted to assess
whether PUVA or PUVA-sol in combination with a vitamin
D analogue was more effective than PUVA or PUVA-sol
alone.

Evidence statements

Five studies were identified – two used an RCT design. A
study of 27 patients treated with PUVA monotherapy or
PUVA with calcipotriol showed an earlier and better overall
response for the combination than for PUVA
monotherapy.[41] These findings were similar to the second
RCT of 19 patients in which the combination of PUVA
with calcipotriol was more effective and faster than PUVA
alone.[43] In contrast, another study showed no improvement
for the combination of PUVA with calcipotriol compared
with PUVA alone.[42] Other open studies report the
combination of calcipotriol with PUVA to be more effective than PUVA alone, especially at initiating repigmentation.[40,44]

Evidence to recommendations

Five small studies fail to provide convincing evidence for an
additional therapeutic effect for PUVA combined with a vitamin D analogue compared with PUVA monotherapy.

Recommendation

1. Topical vitamin D analogues in combination with PUVA
therapy should not be used in the treatment of vitiligo.

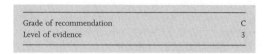

| Grade of recommendation | C |
| Level of evidence | 3 |

In all patients with vitiligo, what is the efficacy of systemic (i.e. orally and parenterally administered) treatments, including corticosteroids, ciclosporin and other immunosuppressive agents, in terms of condition progression, area reduction and quality of life score?

Introduction

There is evidence that in many cases autoimmune mechanisms
are involved in causing vitiligo. It is not surprising that systemic immunosuppressive treatments have been used in
patients with vitiligo.

Methods

There is only one satisfactory RCT of any systemic treatment
for vitiligo, a double-blind placebo-controlled trial of *Gingko
biloba* extract. This product is said to have antioxidant and
immunomodulatory properties. The study looked at cessation
of progression in spreading generalized and focal types of vitiligo and at repigmentation.[89]

Evidence statements

Numerous open studies lacking any comparator arm have suggested a beneficial effect for systemic treatments, often of oral
corticosteroids, on patients (often with Asian skin types) with
usually generalized (symmetrical) forms of vitiligo.[90–96] These
have been excluded from consideration here. The paper of
Pasricha and Khera has been excluded as the effects of treatment are unclear – the trial design is suboptimal.[97] The study
of Orecchia *et al.* regarding the use of phenylalanine was
excluded as it had fewer than 20 subjects in comparator
groups.[98]

Some other studies, usually also lacking a comparator, were
of mixed treatment modalities, e.g. including some sort of
phototherapy, and are excluded from consideration here
although they may be considered elsewhere.[99–107]

A double-blind placebo-controlled trial looked at the effect
of *G. biloba* extract for 6 months, in adults with spreading generalized and focal types of vitiligo, and also on repigmentation, in 47 subjects divided into two groups.[89] The authors
showed that the *G. biloba* extract induced cessation of activity
of the vitiligo in all subjects with acrofacial type (placebo

induced cessation in one of six), in a third of those with symmetrical type called here 'vulgaris' (placebo one of six) and in a quarter with focal type (placebo seven of 10).[89] The G. *biloba* extract was associated with some degree of repigmentation in four of nine with focal, two of nine with vulgaris and four of seven with acrofacial type, whereas only two subjects with focal type who had placebo experienced any repigmentation. The conclusion seems to be that G. *biloba* extract can arrest active vitiligo of the acrofacial type. This is the only study on G. *biloba* extract, and it is therefore unwise to place too much reliance on this result without confirmation of a beneficial effect.

Azathioprine has not been tried as a monotherapy in vitiligo but, at a dose of 0·75 mg kg^{-1} daily, has been combined with PUVA in adults with symmetrical types of vitiligo.[101] Earlier (after five treatments compared with six) and a greater degree of repigmentation (58% compared with 25%) was noted in the group that received azathioprine and PUVA (compared with PUVA alone), without any serious side-effects. No recommendation can be made based on this single study.

A well-conducted but open study of 25 European adults with active generalized types of vitiligo (and four with stable disease) examined the effect of oral dexamethasone 10 mg twice a week for 24 weeks, evaluating pigment change using photographs.[108] The authors showed that disease progression was arrested in 22 of the 25 subjects with active vitiligo, after a mean treatment of 18 ± 5 weeks. 'Marked' repigmentation (51–75%) occurred in two subjects (7%) and 'moderate' or 'slight' repigmentation (26–50%; < 25%) was noted in three (10%), with no response being found in 21 (72%). Side-effects were common, being seen in 20 of 29 subjects, and included weight gain, acne, menstrual irregularity and hypertrichosis.

One study of intralesional triamcinolone in 35 patients with one (12 subjects) or more (23 subjects) areas of vitiligo is worthy of mention.[109] The 25 patients were randomly allocated to receive weekly injections of triamcinolone (0·1 mL of 10 mg mL^{-1} strength) for 8 weeks, vs. 10 who received distilled water. Seventeen of the treatment group (69%) vs. six in the control group (60%) had a 'fair-to-excellent' response, indicating that the intralesional triamcinolone was no better than placebo.

Evidence to recommendations

In adult patients with active generalized (symmetrical) types of vitiligo, oral dexamethasone 10 mg twice weekly can arrest the progression of the disease after a mean of 18 weeks, but there is poor objective evidence for repigmentation and side-effects are common. The use of oral G. *biloba* extract in active generalized vitiligo cannot be recommended unless further studies confirm the effect of the one reported study.

There is no convincing evidence at present that any systemic treatment (apart from PUVA) has a role in the treatment of vitiligo.

Recommendation

1. The use of oral dexamethasone to arrest progression of vitiligo cannot be recommended due to an unacceptable risk of side-effects.

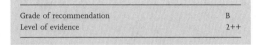

Grade of recommendation	B
Level of evidence	2++

In patients with vitiligo what is the efficacy of a skin graft and of various forms of placebo in terms of condition progression, area reduction and quality of life score? This may include punch grafts, full-thickness skin graft, split-thickness skin graft, autologous epidermal cell suspension, and autologous skin equivalent (commercial skin equivalent)

Introduction

Surgical interventions are based on the idea of transplanting functional melanocytes to the depigmented area. To be successful this requires preparation of the affected area with debridement, laser peeling of the skin, suction blisters or removal of punch biopsies. There are several methods of varied sophistication for harvesting melanocytes, the simplest being by punch biopsy. These techniques require a donor site, which may be scarred and in which vitiligo may be induced by the Koebner phenomenon.

Methods

It is difficult to design RCTs for treatments that use skin grafts. Many papers refer to methodology or small patient series. Case series, cohorts or randomized clinical trials of 20 or more patients were included. A systematic review has looked at a set of 39 nonrandomized studies carried out prior to 1998, so only papers that followed were selected. Eleven papers were identified, of which five were RCTs, five case series and one a systematic review.

Evidence statements

Njoo *et al.* performed a systematic review that evaluated 39 studies assessing split-thickness graft, minigraft using punch biopsies, epidermal suction blisters as preparation and donor and transplantation of noncultured cell suspension or cultured melanocytes.[110] The highest mean success rates (87%) were achieved with split-skin grafting (95% CI 82–91%) and epidermal blister grafting (87%; 95% CI 83–90%). The mean success rate of five culturing techniques varied from 13% to 53%. However, in four of the five culturing methods, fewer than 20 patients were studied and there was insufficient evidence. Minigrafting had the highest rates of adverse effects, with poor colour match in < 10%, cobblestone appearance in 27%, milia in 13%, partial take in 11% and thick margins in 5%. Split-skin grafting and epidermal blister grafting were recommended as the most effective and safest techniques. Barman et al. studied 50 patients in an RCT comparing punch graft followed by PUVA with punch graft followed by topical fluocinolone acetonide and found spread of pigment similar in each group, both of which had significant side-effects as above.[111] Khandpur et al., in an RCT of 64 patients, compared minipunch grafting with split-skin grafting: 15 of 34 (44%) punch grafts had excellent (> 75%) repigmentation, compared with 25 of 30 (83%) of the split-skin grafts.[112] Cosmetic results were better with split-skin grafts.

Ozdemir and colleagues, in an unblended RCT, studied 20 patients comparing, within patients, suction blister alone with suction blister grafting, suction and a split-skin graft or area of thin split-skin graft.[113] Using suction blisters, repigmentation was 25–65% as compared with 90% with split-skin graft.[114] Gupta and Kumar, in a retrospective series of 143 patients, evaluated suction blister transfer supplemented by PUVA.[114] The success rate was 50% and was higher in segmental or focal disease and in patients under 20 years. The results were not affected by site. Kim and Kang reported a case series of 40 patients using suction blister transfer who were followed up for 3 months–2·5 years.[115] Of these, 71–73% had complete repigmentation but relapse was more common in patients with progressive disease (40%) than in those with stable vitiligo (10%).

Van Geel and colleagues, in a high-quality RCT that included 28 patients, looked at autologous cell suspension applied to laser-debrided skin followed by NB-UVB or PUVA, compared with a placebo application to another area, and analysed images of the outcome.[116] Pigmentation was seen only in sites receiving cell suspension and progressed from 55% to 77%, showing > 70% repigmentation between 3 and 12 months. Pianigiani et al. reported a case series of 93 patients treated with laser abrasion and grafting of cultured epidermal cells and NB-UVB and followed for 18 months.[117] Complete repigmentation was seen in 60% and partial (> 50%) in 30%. Relapses were not seen at 18 months. Pandya and colleagues studied 27 patients in a case series allocated to dermabrasion and application of cultured melanocytes or dermabrasion with application of autologous disaggregated epidermal cell suspension.[118] Excellent responses of > 90% repigmentation were seen in 50% and 52%, respectively, with no scarring. There were more good responses in the noncultured group.

Chen et al., in a case series of 120 patients treated with laser abrasion followed by application of cultured epidermal cells, observed > 90% repigmentation in 84%, 90–100% coverage in localized disease, 54% in stable generalized vitiligo, and only 14% in active generalized vitiligo.[119] Guerra et al. reported 32 patients treated with programmed diathermy (TIMED surgery) to prepared sites followed by the application of autologous cultured epidermal cells, and found 88–96% repigmentation, with less successful repigmentation on the

extremities (8%) and in a periorificial distribution (35%).[120] Guerra et al. also evaluated the use of skin preparation using erbium-YAG laser followed by application of cultured epidermal cells in 21 patients with vitiligo.[121] Repigmentation was noted in 76%. The same authors treated six patients with piebaldism using this technique, with good results.[122]

Evidence to recommendations

Surgical techniques were among the most effective interventions in the systematic review and have been assessed in RCTs. They are limited by their invasive nature and often studies applied only to a target area which may not equate to any perceived benefit for the patient, unless the area is particularly disfiguring, e.g. lips or eyelids. There was some evidence for successful treatment of such difficult sites, but results are less good in the extremities and around orifices. The least scarring is seen with the method using laser-abraded skin preparation and application of cell suspensions. This requires special facilities. A 'lab in a box' kit for producing cell suspensions has been produced recently (Recell®; Clinical Cell Culture Europe Ltd, Cambridge, U.K.) but has not been evaluated in any meaningful studies. Surgical treatment gives a high rate of successful repigmentation that appears to be durable in patients with stable inactive vitiligo. Patient selection is important.

Recommendations

1. Surgical treatments in vitiligo should be used only for cosmetically sensitive sites where there have been no new lesions, no Koebner phenomenon and no extension of the lesion in the previous 12 months.

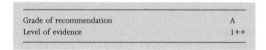

Grade of recommendation	A
Level of evidence	1++

2. Split-skin grafting is the best option when a surgical treatment is required.

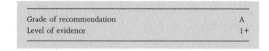

Grade of recommendation	A
Level of evidence	1+

3. Minigraft is not recommended due to a high incidence of side-effects and poor cosmetic results including cobblestone appearance and polka dot appearance.

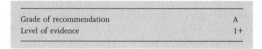

Grade of recommendation	A
Level of evidence	1+

4. Autologous epidermal suspension applied to laser-abraded lesions followed by NB-UVB or PUVA therapy is the optimal

surgical transplantation procedure but does require special facilities.

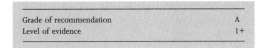

| Grade of recommendation | A |
| Level of evidence | 1+ |

5. Expanding the autologous cells in tissue culture prior to grafting is feasible and treats larger areas successfully, without the need for additional phototherapy. However, the culturing introduces growth factors leading to uncertain risks and cultures can fail, reducing the value of the procedure.

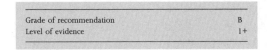

| Grade of recommendation | D |
| Level of evidence | 3 |

6. Transfer of suction blisters is an alternative transplantation method, which shows evidence of benefit over placebo but gives less good coverage than split-skin grafting or laser and cell suspension.

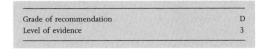

| Grade of recommendation | B |
| Level of evidence | 1+ |

In all patients with vitiligo, what is the efficacy of cognitive therapy vs. psychological support or no treatment in terms of condition progression, area reduction and quality of life score?

Introduction

Cognitive behavioural techniques (CBT) may help patients to cope with skin diseases. There is some suggestion that QoL and coping mechanisms improve over time in vitiligo.[123] Cognitive strategies rather than avoidance or concealment may be associated with better coping.[124] This suggests that cognitive behavioural strategies are potentially helpful (level of evidence 3).

Methods

Two papers were identified which addressed the question.[2,125] The first study was small, with only seven patients in each treatment arm.[2] The intervention was not purely CBT but involved training in practical coping strategies with general psychological support. This intervention cannot be blinded and this introduces potential bias. The second study was an RCT of 45 patients randomized into three arms: one received group CBT, one group received person-centred therapy and the other group were controls.[125] Whereas the first study used

individual therapy the second one used group therapy which did not allow for the individual assessment of participants. This study did not show that group CBT was effective in improving the condition or improving QoL score.

Evidence statements

The first study compared before, after, and a nontreatment arm.[2] The CBT intervention arm showed a sustained improvement in QoL, self-esteem and body image. The effects reported were statistically and clinically significant with patients 'coming into the normal range'. Given the methodological limitations it did not offer sound evidence of the benefit of CBT but it did offer some support for the intervention used. Patients' own cognitive strategies may help coping over time. CBT may offer benefit to patients with vitiligo. Only one study has looked at this directly and it was small in size.[2] Parents of children affected by vitiligo are often very concerned.

Evidence to recommendations

Despite the small evidence base on CBT the GDG feels that psychological support and strategies to cope with the psychological effects of disfigurement are an important part of the treatment of vitiligo. This is reflected in the views expressed by the members of the Vitiligo Society. The value of the support given by patient organizations should not be underestimated. Patients should be given information about the Vitiligo Society as part of the management of the disorder. Parents of children with vitiligo may require psychological counselling.

Recommendation

1. Psychological interventions should be offered as a way of improving coping mechanisms in patients with vitiligo. Parents of affected children should be offered psychological counselling.

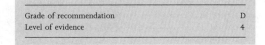

| Grade of recommendation | D |
| Level of evidence | 4 |

Footnote: The organization 'Changing Faces' (The Squire Centre, 33–37 University Street, London WC1E 6JN, U.K.: http://www.changingfaces.org.uk) can give practical help and support to patients and their families. They advise that adjustment is not related to extent of disfigurement but is helped by quality social support, realistic information about treatment options and effective coping strategies, especially on how to manage social anxiety.

Research recommendations

During the development of this guideline it was apparent that more research effort needs to be put into the scientific investigation of the causes of vitiligo. Anyone reading the guideline will be struck by the paucity of effective treatments available and the lack of treatments specifically introduced for vitiligo itself. Almost all treatments have been borrowed from therapies whose prime target is another disease. Not even the greater understanding of the science underlying vitiligo, e.g. evidence of autoimmune disease or of oxidative stress in melanocytes, has resulted yet in a treatment specifically tailored towards vitiligo. The interrogation of the available studies and clinical trials did throw up some questions pertinent to the currently available treatments and research recommendations based on these are detailed below.

1. A longitudinal epidemiological study is needed to define the natural history of vitiligo. This should use photographs combined with computerized image analysis, to quantify how the vitiligo changes with time.

2. More research is needed on more appropriate QoL tools in vitiligo and they should always be used as outcome measures on studies in vitiligo.

3. Further research is needed to establish simple, meaningful and reproducible methods of monitoring accurately the response of vitiligo to treatment both in the clinic and in clinical trials.

4. Further research is needed to clarify the roles of tacrolimus and pimecrolimus in adults and children with vitiligo. A head-to-head study of tacrolimus vs. pimecrolimus is suggested.

5. In view of the possible long-term risk of skin cancer with extended courses of NB-UVB or PUVA in patients with vitiligo, further research to define this potential risk is recommended.

Final recommendations

The recommendations have been distilled and set into the form of algorithms for use by dermatologists and other physicians for the treatment of children and adults with vitiligo. The level of the recommendation and the level of the evidence are shown in parentheses. It is anticipated that phototherapy and surgical treatments will be available only to dermatologists (and their associates) but other approaches, e.g. topical treatments [with the exception of the use of p-(benzyloxy)phenol] and psychological support, may be widely available.

Assessment, prognosis and social impact in children and adults

1. Diagnosis of vitiligo

Where vitiligo is classical, as in the symmetrical types, the diagnosis is straightforward and can be made with confidence in primary care (D/4). In patients with an atypical presentation, diagnosis is more difficult and referral for expert assessment by a dermatologist is recommended (D/4). Assessment of skin type is useful in the initial examination, together with photographs to record the extent of the disease. Wood's light

may be of benefit in the diagnosis of vitiligo and in the demonstration of the extent and activity of the disease in subjects with skin types I and II. Wood's light can be of use in monitoring response to therapy (D/4). A blood test to check thyroid function should be considered in view of the high prevalence of autoimmune thyroid disease in adults with vitiligo (D/3).

2. Natural history

A longitudinal epidemiological study is needed to define the natural history of vitiligo with time. This should use photographs combined with computerized image analysis, to quantify how the vitiligo changes with time (D/4). The response of vitiligo to treatment should be considered in the context of the natural history, recognizing that spontaneous repigmentation may occur but is uncommon (D/4).

3. Psychological impact

Clinicians should make an assessment of the psychological and QoL effects of vitiligo on patients (C/2++). In therapeutic trials relating to vitiligo, researchers should make the patient's improvement in QoL the most important outcome measure (D/4).

4. Assessment tools

In a research setting, the VASI and VETF assessment tools offer a more accurate measurement of disease extent than simple clinical photography alone (even when combined with computerized morphometry). The VETF gives further assessment of severity and spreading (D/2+). In clinical practice, serial photographs should be used to record progress (C/4).

Therapeutic algorithm in children

1. No treatment option

In children with skin types I and II, in the consultation it is appropriate to consider, after discussion with the patient, whether the initial approach may be to use no active treatment other than consideration of the use of camouflage cosmetics and sunscreens (D/4).

2. Topical treatment

• In all children with vitiligo who are under 18 years, treatment with a potent or very potent topical steroid should be considered for a trial period of no more than 2 months. Although benefits have been observed, skin atrophy has been a common side-effect (B/1+).

• In children with vitiligo, topical pimecrolimus or tacrolimus should be considered as alternatives to the use of a highly potent topical steroid in view of their better short-term safety profile (B/1+).

3. Phototherapy

• NB-UVB phototherapy should be considered for treatment of vitiligo only in children who cannot be adequately managed with more conservative treatments (D/4), who have widespread vitiligo, or have localized vitiligo associated with a significant impact on patient's QoL. Ideally, this treatment should be reserved for patients with darker skin types and monitored with serial photographs every 2–3 months (D/3).

• If phototherapy is to be used for treating nonsegmental vitiligo, NB-UVB should be used in preference to PUVA in view of evidence of greater efficacy, safety and lack of clinical trials of PUVA in children (A/1+).

• Taking into account the published data for patients with psoriasis and in view of the greater susceptibility of vitiligo skin to sunburn and photodamage due to absence of melanin, it is advised that safety limits for the treatment of vitiligo are more stringent than those applied to psoriasis, with an arbitrary limit for NB-UVB of 200 treatments for skin types I–III. Evidence is lacking to define an upper limit for skin types IV–VI (D/3).

4. Systemic therapy

The use of oral dexamethasone to arrest progression of vitiligo cannot be recommended due to an unacceptable risk of side-effects (B/2++).

5. Surgical treatment

There are no studies of surgical treatment in children and it is not recommended.

6. Psychological treatments

Psychological interventions should be offered as a way of improving coping mechanisms in children with vitiligo (D/4). Parents of children with vitiligo should be offered psychological counselling.

Therapeutic algorithm in adults

1. No treatment option

In adults with skin types I and II, in the consultation it is appropriate to consider, after discussion with the patient, whether the initial approach may be to use no active treatment other than consideration of the use of camouflage cosmetics and sunscreens (D/4).

2. Topical treatment

• In adults with recent onset of vitiligo, treatment with a potent or very potent topical steroid should be considered for a trial period of no more than 2 months. Although benefits have been observed, skin atrophy has been a common side-effect (B/1+).

• In adults with symmetrical types of vitiligo, topical pimecrolimus should be considered as an alternative to the use of a topical steroid, based on one study. The side-effect profile of topical pimecrolimus is better than that of a highly potent topical steroid (C/2+).

• Depigmentation with p-(benzyloxy)phenol (MBEH) should be reserved for patients severely affected by vitiligo (e.g. who have more than 50% depigmentation or who have extensive depigmentation on the face or hands) who cannot or choose not to seek repigmention and who can accept the permanence of never tanning (D/4).

3. Phototherapy

• NB-UVB phototherapy (or PUVA) should be considered for treatment of vitiligo only in patients who cannot be adequately managed with more conservative treatments (D/4), who have widespread vitiligo, or have localized vitiligo associated with a significant impact on patient's QoL. Ideally, this treatment should be reserved for patients with darker skin types and monitored with serial photographs every 2–3 months (D/3).

• If phototherapy is to be used for treating nonsegmental vitiligo, NB-UVB should be used in preference to oral PUVA in view of evidence of greater efficacy (A/1+).

• Taking into account the data published for patients with psoriasis and in view of the greater susceptibility of vitiliginous skin to sunburn and photodamage due to absence of melanin, it is advised that safety limits for the treatment of vitiligo are more stringent than those applied to psoriasis, with an arbitrary limit of 200 treatments with NB-UVB for patients with skin types I–III, and 150 treatments with PUVA for patients with skin types I–III. Evidence is lacking to define an upper limit for the number of treatments with NB-UVB or PUVA for patients with skin types IV–VI (D/3).

4. Systemic therapy

The use of oral dexamethasone to arrest progression of vitiligo cannot be recommended due to an unacceptable risk of side-effects (B/2++).

5. Surgical treatments

• Surgical treatments are best reserved for cosmetically sensitive sites in patients in whom there have been no new lesions, no Koebner phenomenon and no extension of the lesion in the previous 12 months (A/1++).

• Split-skin grafting gives better cosmetic and repigmentation results than minigraft procedures and utilizes surgical facilities that are relatively freely available (A/1+). Minigraft is not recommended due to a high incidence of side-effects and poor cosmetic results (A/1+).

• Autologous epidermal suspension applied to laser-abraded lesions followed by NB-UVB or PUVA therapy is the optimal surgical transplantation procedure but requires special facilities (A/1+). Expanding the autologous cells in tissue culture prior to grafting is feasible and can treat larger areas successfully, without the need for additional phototherapy (D/3).

• Transfer of suction blisters is an alternative transplantation method, which shows evidence of benefit over placebo but gives less good coverage than split-skin grafting or laser and cell suspension (B/1+).

6. Psychological treatments

Psychological interventions should be offered as a way of improving coping mechanisms in patients with vitiligo (D/4).

References

1 Nordlund JJ, Majumder PP. Recent investigations on vitiligo vulgaris. *Dermatol Clin* 1997; **15**:69–78.

2 Papadopoulos L, Bor R, Legg C. Coping with the disfiguring effects of vitiligo: a preliminary investigation into the effects of cognitive-behavioural therapy. *Br J Med Psychol* 1999; **72**:385–96.

3 Mason CP, Gawkrodger DJ. Vitiligo presentation in adults. *Clin Exp Dermatol* 2005; **30**:344–5.

4 Whitton ME, Ashcroft DM, Barrett CW, Gonzalez U. Interventions for vitiligo. *Cochrane Database Syst Rev* 2006; **1**:CD003263.

5 Taieb A, Picardo M. The definition and assessment of vitiligo: a consensus report of the Vitiligo European Task Force. *Pigment Cell Res* 2007; **20**:27–35.

6 Fulton JE Jr. Utilizing the ultraviolet (UV detect) camera to enhance the appearance of photodamage and other skin conditions. *Dermatol Surg* 1997; **23**:163–9.

7 Nath SK, Majumder PP, Nordlund JJ. Genetic epidemiology of vitiligo: multilocus recessivity cross-validated. *Am J Hum Genet* 1994; **55**:981–90.

8 Howitz J, Schwartz M, Thomsen K. Prevalence of vitiligo. *Arch Dermatol* 1977; **113**:47–52.

9 Chun WH, Hann S-H. The progression of nonsegmental vitiligo: clinical analysis of 318 patients. *Int J Dermatol* 1997; **36**:908–10.

10 Barona MI, Arrunategui A, Falabella R, Alzatwe A. An epidemiologic case–control study in a population with vitiligo. *J Am Acad Dermatol* 1995; **33**:621–5.

11 Firooz A, Bouzari N, Fallah N et al. What patients with vitiligo believe about their condition. *Int J Dermatol* 2004; **43**:811–14.

12 McMichael AJ, Shaw K, Cayce K et al. Facial blemishes and QoL. *J Cosmet Dermatol* 2004; **17**:107–13.

13 Mattoo SK, Handa S, Kaur L et al. Psychiatric morbidity in vitiligo: prevalence and correlates in India. *J Eur Acad Dermatol Venereol* 2002; **16**:573–8.

14 Parsad D, Pandhi R, Dogra S et al. DLQI score in vitiligo and its impact on treatment outcome. *Br J Dermatol* 2003; **148**:373–4.

15 Ongenae K, Dierckxsens L, Brochez L et al. Quality of life and stigmatization profile in a cohort of vitiligo patients and effect of the use of camouflage. *Dermatology* 2005; **210**:279–85.

16 van Geel NAC, Ongenae K, Vander Haeghen YMSJ, Naeyaert JM. Autologous transplantation techniques for vitiligo: how to evaluate treatment outcome. *Eur J Dermatol* 2004; **14**:46–51.

17 Porter JP, Beuf AH, Nordlund JJ, Lerner AB. Personal responses of patients to vitiligo: the importance of the patient–physician interaction. *Arch Dermatol* 1978; **114**:1384–5.

18 Agarwal S, Ramam M, Sharma VK et al. A randomized placebo-controlled double-blind study of levamisole in the treatment of limited and slowly spreading vitiligo. *Br J Dermatol* 2005; **153**:163–6.

19 Hartmann A, Lurz C, Hamm H et al. Narrow-band UVB 311 nm vs. broad-band UVB therapy in combination with topical calcipotriol vs. placebo in vitiligo. *Int J Dermatol* 2005; **44**:736–42.

20 Ongenae K, van Geel N, De Schepper S, Naeyaert JM. Effect of vitiligo on self-reported health-related quality of life. *Br J Dermatol* 2005; **152**:1165–72.

21 Aghaei S, Sodaifi M, Jafari P et al. DLQI scores in vitiligo: reliability and validity of the Persian version. *BMC Dermatol* 2004; **4**:8.

22 Njoo MD, Boss JD, Westerhof W. Treatment of generalised vitiligo in children with narrow-band (TL-01) UVB radiation therapy. *J Am Acad Dermatol* 2000; **42**:245–53.

23 Kent GG, Al'Abadie MSK. Psychologic effects of vitiligo: a critical incident analysis. *J Am Acad Dermatol* 1996; **35**:895–8.

24 Kent GG, Al'Abadie MSK. Factors affecting responses on DLQI items amongst vitiligo sufferers. *Clin Exp Dermatol* 1996; **21**:330–3.

25 Kent GG. Correlates of perceived stigma in vitiligo. *Psychol Health* 1999; **14**:241–51.

26 Stangier U, Gieler U, Ehlers A. Measuring adjustment to chronic skin disorders: validation of a self-report measure. *Psychol Assess* 2003; **15**:532–49.

27 Sampogna F, Picardi A, Chren M-M et al. Association between poorer QoL and psychiatric morbidity in patients with different dermatological conditions. *Psychosom Med* 2004; **66**:620–4.

28 Sharma N, Koranne RV, Singh RK. Psychiatric morbidity in psoriasis and vitiligo: a comparative study. *J Dermatol* 2001; **28**:419–23.

29 Porter JR, Beuf AH. Racial variation in reaction to physical stigma: a study of degree of disturbance by vitiligo among black and white patients. *J Health Soc Behav* 1991; **32**:192–204.

30 Papadopoulos L, Bor R, Walker C et al. Different shades of meaning: illness beliefs among vitiligo sufferers. *Psychology* 2002; **7**:425–33.

31 Hamzavi I, Shapiro J. Parametric modelling of narrow band UV-B phototherapy for vitiligo using a novel quantitative tool. *Arch Dermatol* 2004; **140**:677–83.

32 Lepe V, Moncada B, Castanedo-Cazares JP et al. A double-blind randomized trial of 0·1% tacrolimus vs. 0·05% clobetasol for the treatment of childhood vitiligo. *Arch Dermatol* 2003; **139**:581–5.

33 Clayton R. A double-blind trial of 0·05% clobetasol propionate in the treatment of vitiligo. *Br J Dermatol* 1977; **96**:71–3.

34 Kandil E. Treatment of vitiligo with 0·1 per cent betamethasone 17-valerate in isopropyl alcohol – a double-blind trial. *Br J Dermatol* 1974; **91**:457–60.

35 Westerhof W, Nieuweboer-Krobotova L, Mulder PGH, Glazenburg EJ. Left–right comparison study of the combination of fluticasone propionate and UV-A vs. either fluticasone propionate or UV-A alone for the long-term treatment of vitiligo. *Arch Dermatol* 1999; **135**:1061–6.

36 Coskun B, Saral Y, Turgut D. Topical 0·05% clobetasol propionate versus 1% pimecrolimus ointment in vitiligo. *Eur J Dermatol* 2005; **15**:88–91.

37 Kumaran MS, Kaur I, Kumar B. Effect of topical calcipotriol, betamethasone dipropionate and their combination in the treatment of localized vitiligo. *J Eur Acad Dermatol Venereol* 2006; **20**:269–73.

38 Khalid M, Mujtaba G, Haroon TS. Comparison of 0·05% clobetasol propionate cream and topical Puvasol in childhood vitiligo. *Int J Dermatol* 1995; **34**:203–5.

39 Chiaverini C, Passeron T, Ortonne JP. Treatment of vitiligo by topical calcipotriol. *J Eur Acad Dermatol Venereol* 2002; **16**:137–8.

40 Ameen M, Exarchou V, Chu AC. Topical calcipotriol as monotherapy and in combination with psoralen plus ultraviolet A in the treatment of vitiligo. Br J Dermatol 2001; **145**:476–9.

41 Ermis O, Alpsoy E, Cetin L, Yilmaz E. Is the efficacy of psoralen plus ultraviolet-A therapy for vitiligo enhanced by concurrent topical calcipotriol? A placebo-controlled double-blind study. Br J Dermatol 2001; **145**:472–5.

42 Baysal V, Yildirim M, Erel A, Kesici D. Is the combination of calcipotriol and PUVA effective in vitiligo? J Eur Acad Dermatol Venereol 2003; **17**:299–302.

43 Parsad D, Saini R, Verma N. Combination of PUVAsol and topical calcipotriol in vitiligo. Dermatology 1998; **197**:167–70.

44 Cherif F, Azaiz MI, Ben Hamida A et al. Calcipotriol and PUVA as treatment for vitiligo. Dermatol Online J 2003; **9**:4.

45 Boone B, Ongenae K, van Geel N et al. Topical pimecrolimus in the treatment of vitiligo. Eur J Dermatol 2007; **17**:55–61.

46 Passeron T, Ostovari N, Zakaria W et al. Topical tacrolimus and the 308-nm excimer laser: a synergistic combination for the treatment of vitiligo. Arch Dermatol 2004; **140**:1065–9.

47 Kawalek AZ, Spencer JM, Phelps RG. Combined excimer laser and topical tacrolimus for the treatment of vitiligo: a pilot study. Dermatol Surg 2004; **30**:130–5.

48 Njoo MD, Vodegel RM, Westerhof W. Depigmentation therapy in vitiligo universalis with topical 4-methoxyphenol and the Q-switched ruby laser. J Am Acad Dermatol 2000; **42**:760–9.

49 Mosher DB, Parrish JA, Fitzpatrick TB. Monobenzylether of hydroquinone. A retrospective study of treatment of 18 vitiligo patients and a review of the literature. Br J Dermatol 1977; **97**:669–79.

50 Shaffrali F, Gawkrodger D. Management of vitiligo. Clin Exp Dermatol 2000; **25**:575–9.

51 Bolognia JL, Lapia K, Somma S. Depigmentation therapy. Dermatol Ther 2001; **14**:29–34.

52 Le Poole C, Boissy RE. Vitiligo. Semin Cutan Med Surg 1997; **16**:3–14.

53 Kenney JA Jr, Grimes PE. How we treat vitiligo. Cutis 1983; **32**:347–8.

54 Antoniou C, Katsambas A. Guidelines for the treatment of vitiligo. Drugs 1992; **43**:490–8.

55 Nordlund JJ, Grimes PE, Ortonne JP. The safety of hydroquinone. J Eur Acad Dermatol Venereol 2006; **20**:781–7.

56 Kooyers TJ, Westerhof W. Toxicology and health risks of hydroquinone in skin lightening formulations. J Eur Acad Dermatol Venereol 2006; **20**:777–80.

57 Yones SS, Palmer RA, Garibaldinos TM, Hawk JLM. Randomised double-blind trial of treatment of vitiligo. Efficacy of psoralen-UVA vs. narrowband-UVB therapy. Arch Dermatol 2007; **143**:578–84.

58 Menchini G, Tsoureli-Nikita E, Hercogova J. Narrow-band UV-B micro-phototherapy: a new treatment for vitiligo. J Eur Acad Dermatol Venereol 2003; **17**:171–7.

59 Westerhof W, Nieuweboer-Krobotova L. Treatment of vitiligo with UV-B radiation vs. topical psoralen plus UVA. Arch Dermatol 1997; **133**:1525–8.

60 Spencer JM, Nossa R, Ajmeri J. Treatment of vitiligo with the 308-nm excimer laser: a pilot study. J Am Acad Dermatol 2002; **46**:727–31.

61 Hofer A, Hassan AS, Legat FJ et al. The efficacy of excimer laser (308 nm) for vitiligo at different body sites. J Eur Acad Dermatol Venereol 2006; **20**:558–64.

62 Hong SB, Park HH, Lee MH. Short-term effects of 308-nm xenon-chloride excimer laser and narrow-band ultraviolet B in the treatment of vitiligo: a comparative study. J Korean Med Sci 2005; **20**:273–8.

63 El Mofty AM. A preliminary clinical report on the treatment of leucoderma with Ammi majus Linn. J Egypt Med Assoc 1948; **31**:651–65.

64 Pathak MA. Mechanisms of psoralen photosensitization reactions. Natl Cancer Inst Monogr 1984; **66**:41–6.

65 Sehgal VN. A comparative clinical evaluation of trimethylpsoralen, psoralen and 8-methoxypsoralen in treating vitiligo. Int J Dermatol 1975; **14**:205–8.

66 Bhatnagar A, Kanwar AJ, Parsad D. Comparison of systemic PUVA and NB-UVB in the treatment of vitiligo: an open prospective study. J Eur Acad Dermatol Venereol 2007; **21**:638–42.

67 Abdel-Fattah A, Aboul-Enein MN, Wassel GM, El-Menshawi BS. An approach to treatment of vitiligo by khellin. Dermatologica 1982; **165**:136–40.

68 Procaccini EM, Riccio G, Montfrecola G. Ineffectiveness of topical khellin in photochemotherapy of vitiligo. J Dermatolog Treat 1995; **6**:117–20.

69 Orecchia G, Perfetti L. Photochemotherapy with topical khellin and sunlight in vitiligo. Dermatology 1992; **184**:120–3.

70 Orecchia G, Sangalli ME, Gazzaniga A, Giordano F. Topical photochemotherapy of vitiligo with new khellin formulation: preliminary clinical results. J Dermatolog Treat 1998; **9**:65–9.

71 Valkova S, Trashlieva M, Christova P. Treatment of vitiligo with local khellin and UVA: comparison with systemic PUVA. Clin Exp Dermatol 2004; **29**:180–4.

72 Harrist TJ, Pathak MA, Mosher DB, Fitzpatrick TB. Chronic cutaneous effects of long-term psoralen and ultraviolet radiation therapy in patients with vitiligo. Natl Cancer Inst Monogr 1984; **66**:191–6.

73 Wildfang IL, Jacobsen FK, Thestrup-Pedersen K. PUVA treatment of vitiligo. A retrospective study of 59 patients. Acta Derm Venereol (Stockh) 1992; **72**:305–6.

74 Chuan MT, Tsai YJ, Wu MC. Effectiveness of psoralen photochemotherapy for vitiligo. J Formos Med Assoc 1999; **98**:335–40.

75 Westerhof W, Schallreuter KU. PUVA for vitiligo and skin cancer. Clin Exp Dermatol 1996; **22**:54.

76 Halder RM, Battle EF, Smith EM. Cutaneous malignancies in patients treated with psoralen photochemotherapy (PUVA) for vitiligo. Arch Dermatol 1995; **131**:734–5.

77 Buckley DA, Rogers S. Multiple keratoses and squamous carcinoma after PUVA treatment of vitiligo. Clin Exp Dermatol 1996; **21**:43–5.

78 Takeda H, Mitsuhashi Y, Kondo S. Multiple squamous cell carcinomas in situ in vitiligo lesions after long-term PUVA therapy. J Am Acad Dermatol 1998; **38**:268–70.

79 Abdel Naser MB, Wollina U, El Okby M, El Shiemy S. Psoralen plus ultraviolet-A irradiation-induced lentigines arising in vitiligo: involvement of vitiliginous and normal appearing skin. Clin Exp Dermatol 2004; **29**:380–2.

80 Park HS, Lee YS, Chun DK. Squamous cell carcinoma in vitiligo lesion after long-term PUVA therapy. J Eur Acad Dermatol Venereol 2003; **17**:578–80.

81 Stern RS, Lange R. Non-melanoma skin cancer occurring in patients treated with PUVA five to ten years after first treatment. J Invest Dermatol 1988; **91**:120–4.

82 Ada S, Sahin S, Boztepe G et al. No additional effect of topical calcipotriol on narrow-band UVB phototherapy in patients with generalised vitiligo. Photodermatol Photoimmunol Photomed 2005; **21**:79–83.

83 Goktas EO, Aydin F, Senturk N et al. Combination of narrow-band UVB and topical calcipotriol for the treatment of vitiligo. J Eur Acad Dermatol Venereol 2006; **20**:553–7.

84 Leone G, Pacifico P, Lacovelli P et al. Tacalcitol and narrow-band phototherapy in patients with vitiligo. *Clin Exp Dermatol* 2006; **31**:200–5.

85 Kullavanijaya P, Lim HW. Topical calcipotriene and narrowband ultraviolet B in the treatment of vitiligo. *Photodermatol Photoimmunol Photomed* 2004; **20**:248–51.

86 Tjioe M, Gerritsen MJ, Juhlin L, van de Kerkhof PC Treatment of vitiligo vulgaris with narrow band UVB (311 nm) for one year and the effect of addition of folic acid and vitamin B12. *Acta Derm Venereol (Stockh)* 2002; **82**: 369–72. Erratum in: *Acta Derm Venereol (Stockh)* 2002; **82**: 485.

87 Schallreuter KU, Wood JM, Lemke KR, Levenig C. Treatment of vitiligo with a topical application of pseudocatalase and calcium in combination with short-term UVB exposure: a case study on 33 patients. *Dermatology* 1995; **190**:223–9.

88 Schallreuter KU, Moore J, Behrens-Williams S et al. Rapid initiation of repigmentation in vitiligo with Dead Sea climatotherapy in combination with pseudocatalase (PC-KUS). *Int J Dermatol* 2002; **41**:482–7.

89 Parsad D, Pandhi R, Juneja A. Effectiveness of oral *Ginkgo biloba* in treating limited, slowly spreading vitiligo. *Clin Exp Dermatol* 2003; **28**:285–7.

90 Banerjee K, Barbhuiya J, Ghosh A et al. The efficacy of low-dose oral corticosteroids in the treatment of vitiligo patient. *Indian J Dermatol Venereol Leprol* 2003; **69**:135–7.

91 Seiter S, Ugurel S, Tilgen W, Reinhold U. Use of high-dose methylprednisolone pulse therapy in patients with progressive and stable vitiligo. *Int J Dermatol* 2000; **39**:624–7.

92 Kim SM, Lee HS, Hann SK. The efficacy of low-dose oral corticosteroids in the treatment of vitiligo patients. *Int J Dermatol* 1999; **38**:546–50.

93 Pasricha JS, Khaitan BK. Oral mini-pulse therapy with betamethasone in vitiligo patients having extensive or fast-spreading disease. *Int J Dermatol* 1993; **32**:753–7.

94 Schulpis CH, Antoniou C, Michas T, Strarigos J. Phenylalanine plus ultraviolet light: preliminary report of a promising treatment for childhood vitiligo. *Pediatr Dermatol* 1989; **6**:332–5.

95 Hernandez Perez E. Vitiligo treated with ACTH. *Int J Dermatol* 1979; **18**:578–9.

96 Imamura S, Tagami H. Treatment of vitiligo with oral corticosteroids. *Dermatologica* 1976; **153**:179–85.

97 Pasricha JS, Khera V. Effect of prolonged treatment with levamisole on vitiligo with limited and slow-spreading disease. *Int J Dermatol* 1994; **33**:584–7.

98 Orecchia G, Perfetti L, Borghini F, Malagoli P. Phenylalanine in the treatment of vitiligo. *Ann Ital Dermatol Clin Sper* 1992; **46**:143–6.

99 Don P, Iuga A, Dacko A, Hardick K. Treatment of vitiligo with broadband ultraviolet B and vitamins. *Int J Dermatol* 2006; **45**:63–5.

100 Mulekar SV. Stable vitiligo treated by a combination of low-dose oral pulse betamethasone and autologous, noncultured melanocyte-keratinocyte cell transplantation. *Dermatol Surg* 2006; **32**:536–41.

101 Radmanesh M, Saedi K. The efficacy of combined PUVA and low-dose azathioprine for early and enhanced repigmentation in vitiligo patients. *J Dermatolog Treat* 2006; **17**:151–3.

102 Handa S, Pandhi R, Kaur I. Vitiligo: a retrospective comparative analysis of treatment modalities in 500 patients. *J Dermatol* 2001; **28**:461–6.

103 Juhlin L, Olsson MJ. Improvement of vitiligo after oral treatment with vitamin B12 and folic acid and the importance of sun exposure. *Acta Derm Venereol (Stockh)* 1997; **77**:460–2.

104 Al Khawajah MM. The failure of L-phenylalanine and UVA in the treatment of vitiligo. *J Dermatolog Treat* 1996; **7**:181–2.

105 Salafia A. Vitiligo. Successful treatment with dapsone. *Chron Dermatol* 1995; **5**:171–88.

106 Patel IK, Vora NS, Dave JN et al. Comparative study of various drug regimens in vitiligo. *Indian J Dermatol Venereol Leprol* 1993; **59**:247–50.

107 Farah FS, Kurban AK, Charglassian HT. The treatment of vitiligo with psoralens and triamcinolone by mouth. *Br J Dermatol* 1967; **79**:89–91.

108 Radakovic-Fijan S, Fürnsinn-Friedl AM, Hönigsmann H, Tanew A. Oral dexamethasone pulse treatment for vitiligo. *J Am Acad Dermatol* 2001; **44**:814–17.

109 Vasistha LK, Singh G. Vitiligo and intralesional steroids. *Indian J Med Res* 1979; **69**:308–11.

110 Njoo MD, Westerhoff W, Bos JD, Bossuyt PM. A systematic review of autologous transplantation methods in vitiligo. *Arch Dermatol* 1998; **134**:1543–9.

111 Barman KD, Khaitan BK, Verma K. A comparative study of punch grafting followed by topical corticosteroid versus punch grafting followed by PUVA therapy in stable vitiligo. *Dermatol Surg* 2004; **30**:49–53.

112 Khandpur S, Sharma VK, Manchandra Y. Comparison of mini-punch grafting versus split skin grafting in chronic stable vitiligo. *Dermatol Surg* 2005; **31**:436–41.

113 Ozdemir M, Cetinkale O, Wolf R et al. Comparison of two surgical approaches for treating vitiligo – a preliminary study. *Int J Dermatol* 2002; **41**:135–8.

114 Gupta S, Kumar B. Epidermal grafting in vitiligo: influence of age, site of lesion and type of disease on outcome. *J Am Acad Dermatol* 2003; **49**:99–104.

115 Kim HY, Kang KY. Epidermal grafts for the treatment of stable and progressive vitiligo. *J Am Acad Dermatol* 1999; **40**:412–17.

116 van Geel NA, Ongenae K, De Mil M et al. Double-blind placebo-controlled study of autologous transplanted epidermal cell suspensions for repigmenting vitiligo. *Arch Dermatol* 2004; **140**:1203–8.

117 Pianigiani E, Risulo M, Andreassi A et al. Autologous epidermal cultures and narrow-band ultraviolet B in the treatment of vitiligo. *Dermatol Surg* 2005; **31**:155–9.

118 Pandya V, Parma KS, Shah BJ, Bilimoria FE. A study of autologous melanocyte transfer in treatment of chronic stable vitiligo. *Indian J Dermatol Venereol Leprol* 2005; **71**:393–7.

119 Chen YF, Yang PY, Hu DN et al. Treatment of vitiligo by transplantation of cultured pure melanocyte suspension – analysis of 120 cases. *J Am Acad Dermatol* 2004; **51**:68–74.

120 Guerra L, Cappirro S, Melchi F et al. Treatment of stable vitiligo by TimedSurgery and transplantation of cultured epidermal grafts. *Arch Dermatol* 2000; **136**:1380–9.

121 Guerra L, Primavera G, Raskovic D et al. Erbium YAG laser and cultured epidermis in the surgical therapy of stable vitiligo. *Arch Dermatol* 2003; **139**:1303–10.

122 Guerra L, Primavera G, Raskovic D et al. Permanent repigmentation of piebaldism by erbium YAG laser and autologous cultured epidermis. *Br J Dermatol* 2004; **150**:715–21.

123 Papadopoulos L, Bor R, Legg C. Psychological factors in cutaneous disease; an overview of research. *Psychol Health Med* 1999; **4**:107–26.

124 Thomson AR, Kent G, Smith JA. Living with vitiligo: dealing with difference. *Br J Health Psychol* 2002; **7**:213–25.

125 Papadopoulos L, Walker C, Anrhis L. Living with vitiligo: a controlled investigation into the effects of group cognitive-behavioural and person-centred therapies. *Dermatol Psychosom* 2004; **5**:172–7.

Appendix 1. Contents

Key recommendations:
The main points of note.

Introduction: D.J. Gawkrodger
Includes method of guideline development, aims, scope, audience, process, funding, declaration of interests and review.

Symptoms and signs: A.D. Ormerod
What symptoms and signs are suggestive of vitiligo?

Wood's light: A.D. Ormerod
What is the accuracy of Wood's light compared with naked eye examination in the diagnosis of vitiligo?

Natural history: A.V. Anstey
What is the natural history of vitiligo?

Quality of life: L. Shaw, I. Mauri-Sole
What is the quality of life in patients with vitiligo compared with other skin diseases?

Scoring indices: M.J. Watts, M.E. Whitton
In all patients with vitiligo, what is the accuracy of a scoring index in showing the outcome of common treatments compared with simple photography?

Topical treatments: D.J. Gawkrodger
Includes: In all patients with vitiligo, what is the efficacy of applying betamethasone, clobetasol, fluocinolone, fluticasone or mometasone vs. placebo or other active treatment in terms of condition progression, area reduction and quality of life score?
In all patients with vitiligo, what is the efficacy of applying calcipotriol or tacalcitol vs. placebo or an active treatment in terms of condition progression, area reduction and quality of life score?
In all patients with vitiligo, what is the efficacy of applying tacrolimus or pimecrolimus vs. placebo or an active treatment in terms of condition progression, area reduction and quality of life score?
In all patients with vitiligo, what is the efficacy of applying p-(benzyloxy)phenol (monobenzyl ether of hydroquinone) vs. placebo or an active treatment in terms of reducing areas of pigmentation?

Phototherapy: A.V. Anstey
Includes: In all patients with vitiligo, what is the efficacy of a course of narrowband UVB including high-intensity light sources compared with placebo in terms of condition progression, area reduction and quality of life score?

In all patients with vitiligo, what is the efficacy of a course of PUVA or PUVA-sol compared with placebo in terms of condition progression, area reduction and quality of life score?
In all patients with vitiligo, what is the efficacy of a course of khellin with sunlight UVA or UVB compared with PUVA or PUVA-sol in terms of progression, area reduction and quality of life score?
Late complications of PUVA or narrowband UVB therapy in patients with vitiligo: are patients who have received large doses of PUVA (more than 150 treatment sessions) or narrowband UVB (more than 150 treatment sessions) at increased risk of developing premalignant or malignant skin changes?

Combination phototherapy: A.V. Anstey
Includes: In all patients with vitiligo, what is the efficacy of a course of narrowband UVB with a vitamin D analogue compared with narrowband UVB with placebo in terms of condition progression, area reduction and quality of life score?
In all patients with vitiligo, what is the efficacy of a course of PUVA with a vitamin D analogue compared with PUVA with placebo in terms of condition progression, area reduction and quality of life score?

Systemic therapies: D.J. Gawkrodger
In all patients with vitiligo, what is the efficacy of systemic (i.e. orally and parenterally administered) treatments, including corticosteroids, ciclosporin and other immunosuppressive agents, in terms of condition progression, area reduction and quality of life score?

Surgical treatments: A.D. Ormerod
In patients with vitiligo what is the efficacy of a skin graft and of various forms of placebo in terms of condition progression, area reduction and quality of life score? This may include punch grafts, full-thickness skin graft, split-thickness skin graft, autologous epidermal cell suspension, and autologous skin equivalent (commercial skin equivalent).

Psychological treatments: L. Shaw, I. Mauri-Sole
In all patients with vitiligo, what is the efficacy of cognitive therapy vs. psychological support or no treatment in terms of condition progression, area reduction and quality of life score?

Research recommendations:
Areas for future research to improve treatment of vitiligo are suggested.

Final recommendations:
An approach to the overall management of vitiligo is outlined based on the evidence evaluated in this guideline.

Guideline for the diagnosis and management of vitiligo:
http://bad.org.uk/Portals/_Bad/Guidelines/Clinical
%20Guidelines/Vitiligo%202008.pdf

Comment

This very thorough multidisciplinary produced guideline
[1] has explored the diagnosis and management of vitiligo.
Unfortunately, it has unearthed a paucity of effective treatments for vitiligo. The authors recommend research into
the causes, epidemiology and natural history of vitiligo
as well as developing specific treatments for vitiligo. They
also stated that the total safe dosage of radiation of UVB
and PUVA in the treatment of vitiligo has yet to be determined. A recently published study [2] has examined the
efficacy and safety of topical PGE2 in localised stable
vitiligo and concludes that it is a promising therapy. A
recently published updated Cochrane review has confirmed Gawkrodger *et al*'s guideline findings [3].

REFERENCES

1 Gawkrodger DJ, Omerod AD, Shaw L, *et al*. Guideline for the
   diagnosis and management of vitiligo. *Brit J Dermatol* 2008;
   159: 1051–76.
2 Kapoor R, Phiske MM, Jerajani HR. Evaluation of safety and
   efficacy of topical prostaglandin E2 in treatment of vitiligo.
   Brit J Dermatol 2009; 160: 861–3.
3 Whitton ME, Pinart M, Batchelor J, *et al*. Interventions for
   vitiligo. *Cochrane Database Syst Rev* 2010; Issue 1: CD003263
   (http://www.library.nhs.uk/skin/ViewResource.aspx?resID=
   237714&tabID=289&catID=8431).

Additional professional resources

http://www.dermnet.org.nz/colour/vitiligo.html
http://www.cks.nhs.uk/patient_information_leaflet/
   vitiligo

BAD patient information leaflet

http://www.bad.org.uk/site/885/Default.aspx

Other patient resources

http://www.vitiligosociety.org.uk
http://www.nvfi.org
http://www.aad.org/dermaz/Default.aspx

2 Infections

The British Association of Dermatologists (BAD) have produced guidelines on three areas of cutaneous infection: viral warts, onychomycosis and tinea capitis. In all three areas, more research is needed into more effective treatments, but none the less useful information is provided by each guideline to highlight the utility of various interventions. Guidance for other cutaneous infections is available from the Clinical Knowledge Summaries.

http://www.cks.nhs.uk/boils_and_paronychia
http://www.cks.nhs.uk/candida_skin
http://www.cks.nhs.uk/cellulitis_acute#-336656
http://www.cks.nhs.uk/chickenpox
http://www.cks.nhs.uk/fungal_skin_infection_body_and_groin
http://www.cks.nhs.uk/fungal_skin_infection_foot
http://www.cks.nhs.uk/head_lice
http://www.cks.nhs.uk/impetigo
http://www.cks.nhs.uk/lyme_disease
http://www.cks.nhs.uk/molluscum_contagiosum
http://www.cks.nhs.uk/pubic_lice
http://www.cks.nhs.uk/scabies

British Association of Dermatologists' Management Guidelines, 1st edition. Edited by Neil Cox and John English.
© 2011 British Association of Dermatologists.

Guidelines for the management of cutaneous warts

J.C.STERLING,* S.HANDFIELD-JONES,† P.M.HUDSON‡

*Department of Dermatology, Addenbrooke's Hospital. Cambridge, U.K.
†West Suffolk Hospital, Bury St Edmunds, U.K.
‡Peterborough District Hospital, Peterborough, U.K.

Accepted for publication DD MONTH 2000

Summary

These guidelines for the management of cutaneous warts have been prepared for dermatologists on behalf of the British Association of Dermatologists. They present evidence-based guidance for treatment, with identification of the strength of evidence available at the time of preparation of the guidelines, and a brief overview of epidemiological aspects, diagnosis and investigation.

Disclaimer

These guidelines have been prepared for dermatologists on behalf of the British Association of Dermatologists and reflect the best data available at the time the report was prepared. Caution should be exercised in interpreting the data; the results of future studies may require alteration of the conclusions or recommendations in this report. It may be necessary or even desirable to depart from the guidelines in the interests of specific patients and special circumstances. Just as adherence to guidelines may not constitute defence against a claim of negligence, so deviation from them should not necessarily be deemed negligent.

Definition

Warts are caused by infection of the epidermis with human papillomavirus (HPV). HPVs are divided into separate genotypes on the basis of their DNA sequence. Different HPV types may preferentially infect either cornified stratified squamous epithelium of skin or uncornified mucous membranes. The appearance of the lesion is influenced not only by viral type but also by environmental and host factors.

These guidelines omit detail regarding therapy for anogenital warts. Patients with such warts are best seen and investigated by genito-urinary physicians to exclude the possibility of other sexually transmitted

Correspondence: Dr Jane C. Sterling, Department of Dermatology, Box 46, Addenbrooke's Hospital, Hills Road, Cambridge, CB2 2QQ, U.K.
E-mail: jcs12@mole.bio.cam.ac.uk

Guidelines prepared for the British Association of Dermatologists Therapy Guidelines and Audit subcommittee. Members of the committee are N.H. Cox (Chairman), A. Anstey, C. Bunker, M.Goodfield, A. Highet, D. Mehta, R. Meyrick Thomas, J. Schofield.

disease. Children with ano-genital warts, particularly over the age of 3 years, may need paediatric assessment if sexual abuse is considered a possibility.

Epidemiology and prevalence

Most people will experience infection with HPV at some time in their life. The prevalence of viral warts in children and adolescents in the United Kingdom has been recorded at between 3·9% and 4·9%.[1] Other surveys in the northern hemisphere quote prevalence rates of between 3% and 20% in children and teenagers[2–4] and 3·5% in adults aged 25–34 years.[5,6]

There are marked regional differences in wart prevalence, rates being higher in the north than in the south of the U.K. Visible warts were twice as common in white Europeans compared to other ethnic groups in the National Child Development Study of 1958.[7] This study also suggests that in 90% of children, warts at the age of 11 years had cleared by the age of 16 years. Other studies have suggested spontaneous clearance rates of 23% at two months, 30% at 3 months and 65–78% at 2 years.[2,3,8–10]

Most large studies have found no evidence of a sex difference in wart prevalence.[1] Population studies suggest that there is no increased risk of viral warts in children with atopic eczema.[11]

Common forms of warts and their HPV type are described in Table 1.

Other warty conditions

Epidermodysplasia verruciformis

Epidermodysplasia verruciformis (EV) is an inherited disorder in which there is a mild defect of cell-mediated

Table 1. Morphology of warts

Clinical type	Appearance	HPV type
Common warts	Firm, rough keratotic papules and nodules on any skin surface. May be single or grouped papules.	1,2,4,57
Plane warts (flat warts)	2–4 mm in diameter, slightly elevated. Most commonly flat topped papules with minimal scaling.	3,10
Intermediate warts	Features of common and plane warts.	2,3,10,28
Myrmecia	Deep burrowing wart.	1
Plantar warts	May start as sago grain-like papules which develop a more typical keratotic surface with a collar of thickened keratin.	1,2,4,57
Mosaic warts	Occur when palmar or plantar warts coalesce into large plaques.	2
(Ano) Genital warts (Condyloma acuminata or venereal warts)	Epidermal and dermal nodules and papules in the perineum and on the genitalia. Their occurrence in children especially under the age of 3 is not always a sign of sexual abuse; vertical transmission is possible.	6,11
Oral warts	Small white or pink elevated papules on the oral mucosa. (HPV 16 has been detected in 80% of cases of oral leukoplakia.)	6,11,32

immunity and widespread and persistent infection with HPV. The lesions vary considerably and may be flat, wart-like lesions, often pigmented, red or atrophic macules or branny pityriasis versicolor-like plaques. The flat, wart-like lesions are frequently localized to the extremities and the face and thicker plaques may resemble seborrhoeic keratoses. The lesions are found to harbour a large variety of HPV types including those causing plane warts, but also several which do not cause disease in normal individuals. There is a risk of development of squamous cell carcinoma on sun-exposed skin.

Bowenoid papulosis

Also known as vulval, penile and anal intraepithelial neoplasia (VIN, PIN, AIN), Bowenoid papulosis presents as small papules, usually multiple, sometimes pigmented, on the cutaneous and mucosal surfaces of the ano-genital regions in both sexes. It usually affects young adults but no age is exempt and there is a strong association with HPV 16 infection.

Focal epithelial hyperplasia

Also known as Heck's disease, this is a rare benign, familial disorder with no sex predisposition. It is characterized by multiple soft circumscribed sessile nodular elevations of the oral mucosa. The disease is seen most commonly in native Americans and in Inuits in Greenland but has been reported rarely from many other countries. HPV 13 and HPV 32 appear to be the causal agents in patients with a genetic predisposition.

Epithelioma cuniculatum and verrucous carcinoma

Epithelioma cuniculatum is a squamous cell carcinoma that appears as a soft bulbous mass with a squashy consistency on the sole of the foot. Multiple sinuses open onto the surface and when pressed, the lesion may appear like a giant plantar wart, but is distinguished by its relentless growth and local invasion. Verrucous carcinoma may develop in the oral cavity and on the genital mucosa and appear as cauliflower-like lesions. The bland histology contrasts with its aggressive behaviour.

Diagnosis

Diagnosis of warts is usually based on clinical examination but can be suggested by the histological appearances of acanthotic epidermis with papillomatosis, hyperkeratosis and parakeratosis, with elongated rete ridges often curving towards the centre of the wart. Dermal capillary vessels may be prominent and thrombosed. There may be large keratinocytes with eccentric pyknotic nuclei surrounded by a perinuclear halo (koilocytes are characteristic of HPV-associated papillomas). HPV infected cells may have small eosinophilic granules and diffuse clumps of basophilic keratohyaline granules. These are not HPV particles. Flat warts have less acanthosis and hyperkeratosis and do not have parakeratosis or papillomatosis.

HPV typing is limited to a few laboratories but may be useful in some cases of genital warts in children with suspected sexual abuse. Knowledge of the HPV genotype in benign warts does not influence choice of therapy.

Table 2. Summary of treatments for warts

Strength of evidence	Treatment	Suggested method of use
A, I	Cryotherapy	15–20 s single or double freeze of warts, every 3–4 weeks
B, I	Photodynamic therapy	3 treatments: 20% topical amino-laesulinic acid + irradiation
B, II ii	Salicylic acid (SA)	Daily application of 15–20% SA in suitable base. 25–50% SA may be used cautiously on plantar warts. 2–5% SA cream may be used for plane face warts.
	Bleomycin	Single intralesional delivery
	Retinoids	Topical: 0·05% tretinoin cream daily Systemic: 1 mg/kg/day acitretin for 3 months
C, II ii	Formaldehyde	Daily application of 0·7% gel or 3% solution as short soak for mosaic plantar warts
C, III	Thermocautery	Single surgical removal of wart; risk of scarring
	Glutaraldehyde	Daily application of 10–20% in suitable base.
C, IV	Chemical cautery	Twice weekly application
	CO_2 laser	Single treatment
	Pulsed dye laser	Single treatment
	Topical sensitization	Sensitization with 2% diphencyprone, then weekly application of appropriate dilution of the allergen.
D, I	Cimetidine, oral	Up to 40 mg/kg/day for 3 months
	Homeopathy	
Insufficient evidence	Podophyllin	
	Folk remedies	
	Hypnosis	
	Heat treatment	
	Interferon	
	Imiquimod	

Differential diagnosis

Plantar warts must be distinguished from callosities which are ill-defined areas of waxy, yellowish thickening, which on paring reveal no capillaries. Corns occur on pressure points and are usually smaller and painful with a central plug. Plane warts must be distinguished from lichen planus which will normally show a violaceous discoloration and Wickham's striae. The lesions of lichen planus are usually pruritic and often accompanied by characteristic mucosal lesions. Epidermal naevi may resemble clusters of filiform and digitate warts. The individual lesions of molluscum contagiosum are white umbilicated papules sometimes showing a central depression.

Transmission of warts

Warts are spread by contact, either directly from person to person, or indirectly via fomites left on surfaces. Infection via the environment is more likely to occur if the skin is macerated and in contact with roughened surfaces, the conditions which are common in swimming pools and communal washing areas.[12]

Warts and malignancy

Benign warts in immunocompetent individuals almost never undergo malignant transformation. There are a small number of reports of lesions that have initially appeared as warts and later become invasive squamous cell carcinomas. Periungual warts in combination with genital HPV disease warrant particular attention.

Warty lesions are especially common in immunosuppressed and transplant patients – approximately 50% of renal transplant patients develop warts within 5 years of transplantation.[13] Sun exposure increases the incidence of warty lesions and also acts as a cocarcinogen. Dysplastic change is quite common and there is frequently poor correlation between clinical and histological appearances. The lesions may appear typical of virus warts, solar or Bowenoid keratoses or keratoacanthomata or occasionally frank squamous carcinomata. Numerous HPV types have been found in benign and malignant squamous lesions in immunocompromised patients and the precise role they play in initiation and progression of malignancy is yet to be elucidated.

Table 3. Treatments for consideration according to site of warts

Face	Hands	Feet	Body
Consider no treatment	Consider no treatment	Consider no treatment	Consider no treatment
Plane warts	(1)	(1)	**Single**
Salicylic acid (cream)	Salicylic acid paint	Salicylic acid paint	Curettage + cautery
Cryotherapy	Glutaraldehyde	Glutaraldehyde	Cryotherapy
Curettage + light cautery	Formaldehyde	Formaldehyde	
Filiform warts	(2)	(2)	**Multiple**
Cryotherapy	Cryotherapy	Cryotherapy	Cryotherapy
Curettage + light cautery	Curettage + cautery	Silver nitrate	Curettage + cautery
	Silver nitrate		Retinoid, systemic
	(3)	(3)	
	PDT	PDT	
	Bleomycin	Bleomycin	
	CO_2 laser	CO_2 laser	
	Pulsed dye laser	Pulsed dye laser	
	Retinoid, systemic	Retinoid, systemic	
	Topical immunotherapy	Topical immunotherapy	

Published evidence is inadequate to permit development of clear rules for treating particular types of warts in specific sites in individuals of various ages. The above-mentioned therapies could all be considered alone, sequentially or in combination. Treatment in groups (1) or (2) could be performed by general practitioner but those in group (3) are more specialized.

Treatment

There is no single treatment that is 100% effective and different types of treatment may be combined. Research into efficacy of treatment must take into account the possibility of spontaneous regression. It is a valid management option to leave warts untreated if this is acceptable to patients but plantar warts can be painful and hand warts sufficiently unsightly to affect school attendance or cause occupational difficulty. Warts in adults, in those with a long duration of infection and in immunosuppressed patients are less likely to resolve spontaneously and are more recalcitrant to treatment.[14–16]

Different types of warts and those at different sites may need differing treatments.[17] Genital warts are not dealt with in depth in these guidelines. Facial warts should not be treated with wart paints because of the risk of severe irritation and possible scarring. Plane warts Koebnerize readily and any destructive technique may exacerbate the problem. The majority of warts can be treated in general practice and increasingly, wart clinics are run by nursing staff. A summary of treatments is given in Tables 2 and 3.

The ideal aims of treatment of warts are: (i) to remove the wart with no recurrence; (ii) to produce no scars; and (iii) to induce life-long immunity. Certain general principles in the treatment of warts should be observed:

1 Not all warts need to be treated

2 Indications for treatment are: pain; interference with function; cosmetic embarrassment; and risk of malignancy

3 No treatment has a very high success rate (average 60–70% clearance in 3 months)

4 An immune response is usually essential for clearance. Immunocompromised individuals may never show wart clearance.

5 Highest clearance rates for various treatments are usually in younger individuals who have a short duration of infection.

Destructive treatments

Salicylic acid (Strength of evidence [Appendix]: B, IIii).
Salicylic acid is a keratolytic that acts by slowly destroying the virus-infected epidermis. The resulting mild irritation may stimulate an immune response. Salicylic acid alone has been shown to produce clearance in 67% of patients with hand warts and 84% in those with plantar warts in 12 weeks.[14]

There are many commercially available preparations but there is limited information to enable comparison to be made between products:

1 Salicylic acid 11–17% in collodion and collodion-like gels ± lactic acid, copper.

2 Salicylic acid 26% in polyacrylic base – designed to be self-occlusive.

3 Salicylic acid 25% with podophyllin in ointment base – for use on plantar warts.

4 Salicylic acid 50% ointment for use on plantar warts.

Before application of wart paints, excess keratin should be pared away or filed with sandpaper or emery board and the area softened by soaking in warm water. Collodion-based products form a film that should be peeled off before re-application. Occlusion has been shown to improve clearance rates of plantar warts.[18]

Comparisons between salicylic acid-containing paints, and monotherapy with glutaraldehyde, fluorouracil, podophyllin, benzalklonium or liquid nitrogen cryotherapy, failed to find any preparation more effective than salicylic acid.[14]

Cryotherapy (Strength of evidence: A, I). Liquid nitrogen (LN_2, $-196\,°C$) is the most commonly used agent. Carbon dioxide slush ($-79\,°C$) is now less commonly used. Dimethyl ether/propane mixtures ($-57\,°C$) are used because of their convenience but efficacy in inducing tissue temperatures adequate for cell necrosis appears low.[19] Cryotherapy may have an effect on wart clearance either by simple necrotic destruction of HPV-infected keratinocytes, or possibly by inducing local inflammation conducive to the development of an effective cell-mediated response.

Techniques differ between practitioners with variations in freeze times, mode of application and intervals between treatment. Many practitioners use a spray, but cotton wool-tipped sticks are still widely used and can be preferable when treating children or for warts near the eyes. It is common practice to freeze until a halo of frozen tissue appears around the wart and then time for 5–30 s depending on site and size of wart. When reapplying LN_2 with a cotton stick it is important to be aware that HPV and other viruses such as HIV can survive in stored liquid nitrogen.

Destruction of warts by freezing every three weeks can give a clearance rate of 69% of patients with hand warts in 12 weeks.[14] This study used liquid nitrogen applied with a cotton bud until a frozen halo appeared round the wart (5–30 s). Clearance rates are increased when cryotherapy is combined with salicylic acid paints although this did not reach significance.[14]

Two freeze–thaw cycles have been shown to improve clearance in plantar warts but not in hand warts.[20] The ideal interval between freeze treatments is unclear – Bunney's study showed that intervals above 3 weeks reduced cure rates at 12 weeks,[14] others have shown that clearance was dependent on the number of treatments so that weekly treatments resulted in more rapid clearance.[21]

Patients should be warned that cryotherapy is painful and blistering may occur. Caution must be used when freezing warts over tendons and in patients with poor circulation. Hypo- and hyper-pigmentation can occur, particularly in black skin. Onychodystrophy can follow treatment of periungual warts.

Thermocautery/curettage and cautery (Strength of evidence: C, III). Surgical removal of warts is widely practised, particularly by curettage or blunt dissection, followed by cautery. It may be particularly useful for filiform warts on the face and limbs. In open studies, a patient success rate of 65–85% is reported.[22,23] Scarring is usual after these procedures and recurrence occurs in up to 30%. The development of scarring is a relative contraindication to this form of surgery on the sole.

Chemical cautery: silver nitrate stick (Strength of evidence: C, IV). Chemical cautery with repeated daily use of silver nitrate stick can induce adequate destruction to effect wart clearance, but occasionally pigmented scars may develop. In a placebo-controlled study of 70 patients, three applications of silver nitrate over nine days resulted in clearance of all warts in 43% and improvement in warts in 26% one month after treatment compared to 11% and 14%, respectively, in the placebo group.[24]

Carbon dioxide laser (Strength of evidence: C, IV). The destruction produced by the CO_2 laser has been used to treat viral warts. Periungual and subungual lesions, which can be difficult to eradicate by other methods, may be particularly appropriate for this treatment. A cure rate of individual warts of 64–71% at 12 months is reported in two case series[25,26] but postoperative pain and scarring may occur.

Pulsed dye laser (Strength of evidence: C, IV). The use of the pulsed dye laser depends upon the energy absorption within the capillary loops of the wart and hence localized tissue necrosis. Uncontrolled studies have suggested a wart clearance rate of 70–90%[27,28] and a patient clearance rate of 48%.[29] Pain and scarring are less than with the CO_2 laser.

Photodynamic therapy (Strength of evidence: B, I). This treatment depends upon the uptake by abnormal cells of a chemical, usually amino-laevulinic acid (ALA), involved in the porphyrin pathway and subsequent photo-oxidation invoked by irradiation using laser or non-laser light of affected tissue. Comparison of response in 45 patients who received 3 treatments of 589–700 nm laser light after application of either 20% ALA or placebo cream showed that the active treatment produced a significant improvement in clearance or reduction of wart size after 4 months with ALA and irradiation.[30]

Virucidal Methods

Formaldehyde (Strength of evidence: C, IIii). Formaldehyde is virucidal and is available commercially as a 0·7% gel or a 3% solution. As a soak it may hasten clearance of viral warts when combined with regular paring. Two hundred children with plantar warts were treated for 6–8 weeks with 3% formaldehyde solution and this produced clearance in 80% of warts.[22] A controlled study comparing formaldehyde soaks with both water soaks and with saccharose by mouth showed no difference in wart clearance rates between the three groups.[31]

Glutaraldehyde (Strength of evidence: C, III). Glutaraldehyde is available as a 10% solution or gel and like formaldehyde it hardens the skin and makes paring easier. An uncontrolled trial with a 20% solution applied once daily cleared warts in 72% of 25 patients in three months.[32] It has the disadvantage of staining the skin brown and there has been a report of cutaneous necrosis following the application of 20% glutaraldehyde.[33]

Antimitotic therapy

Podophyllin/Podophyllotoxin. Podophyllotoxin, the active ingredient within the cruder mixture of podophyllin, acts as an antimitotic by binding to the spindle during mitosis. Cellular division is blocked. The agent is used extensively in the treatment of anogenital warts, but penetration of a thick stratum corneum is poor and podophyllin is much less effective in the treatment of skin warts. Applied under occlusion after paring of the wart (see Keratolytics section), the treatment may be effective[34] but there is risk of intense inflammation, sterile pustule formation and secondary infection.

Bleomycin (Strength of evidence: B, IIii). Intralesional application of the cytotoxic agent bleomycin[35] has been used to treat warts that have failed to respond to other modalities of treatment. Studies have used concentrations of bleomycin of 250–1000 U/mL (old units 0·25–1 U/mL) with no obvious benefits for the higher

concentrations.[36] Response rates of between 31% and 100% are reported.

Pain both on application and afterwards is the main limiting factor. The resultant necrosis can cause scarring, pigmentary change and nail damage. Injected or topical local anaesthesia is often needed. Bleomycin may be injected with a normal syringe but studies have also looked at using modified tattooing apparatus, dermal multipuncture injection or simply applying a drop of bleomycin and pricking the wart repeatedly with a Monolet™ needle. The latter uncontrolled study of 62 patients treated monthly gave a success rate of 92% of treated individuals after an average of four months.[37] Bleomycin should not be used in pregnant women since significant absorption of bleomycin has been reported following intralesional injection.[36]

Retinoids (Strength of evidence B, IIii). Retinoids disrupt epidermal growth and differentiation thereby reducing the bulk of the wart. A randomized controlled trial of 25 children treated with 0·05% tretinoin cream showed clearance rates of 85% of the children compared with 32% in 25 controls.[38] There are a number of case reports and a limited number of trials showing the effect of systemic retinoids in the treatment of warts.[39,40] Sixteen of 20 children with extensive warts given etretinate for a period not exceeding 3 months at a dosage of 1 mg/kg per day showed complete regression of the disease without relapse.[41] In 4 patients the lesions recurred following partial regression.

Immune stimulation

Topical sensitization (Strength of evidence: C, IV). The induction of delayed hypersensitivity has been used as a treatment of warts. Dinitrochlorobenzene[42] and squaric acid dibutylester[43] have been used but most studies have looked at the effect of diphencyprone. Two large open studies of diphencyprone have shown encouraging results. In one, diphencyprone was applied weekly for 8 weeks in 134 patients and gave a response rate of 60% (complete clearance 44% of individuals at 4 months).[44] In another retrospective study, of 48 patients treated on average every 3 weeks, 88% of patients were clear of warts within 14 weeks.[45] Drawbacks of this treatment are that some patients cannot be sensitized whilst others get troublesome eczematous reactions.

Cimetidine (Strength of evidence: D, I). Cimetidine has weak, undefined immunomodulatory effects and its use to treat warts has been advocated. Several open trials suggested efficacy, but a controlled trial showed no advantage over placebo.[9]

Other treatments

Many other treatments have been used to treat warts, although few have received adequate assessment.

Folk remedies[45,46] are still practised but remain unevaluated.

Homoeopathy (Strength of evidence: D, I), using a variety of remedies including calcium, sodium and sulphur has shown no benefit over placebo.[8]

Hypnosis has been evaluated in a double-blind, placebo-controlled trial of 40 individuals treated over 6 weeks. The hypnosis-treated group lost more warts than individuals treated either with topical salicylic acid or with placebo.[47]

Local heat treatment has been tested in 13 patients. Of 29 treated warts, 86% cleared while 41% of placebo-treated warts regressed.[48]

Intralesional interferon has shown some effect in cutaneous warts in a limited number of open trials.[49]

Topical imiquimod applied in a 5% cream for 9–11 weeks has been used in a small number of patients, including immunosuppressed individuals, with encouraging results.[50,51]

Irradiation, once used quite frequently, now has no place in the management of this benign condition.

Potential audit points

1 Liquid nitrogen cryotherapy – is the treatment regimen used in accordance with recommended frequency, duration, etc., and what is the clearance rate?

2 Topical salicylic acid – is the treatment used in a regimen most likely to produce an effect and what is the clearance rate?

Appendix 1

Strength of recommendations

A There is good evidence to support the use of the procedure

B There is fair evidence to support the use of the procedure

C There is poor evidence to support the use of the procedure

D There is fair evidence to support the rejection of the use of the procedure

E There is good evidence to support the rejection of the use of the prodedure

Appendix 2

Quality of evidence

I Evidence obtained from at least one properly designed, randomized trial

II-i Evidence obtained from well designed control trials without randomization

II-ii Evidence obtained from well designed cohort or case control analytic studies, preferably from more than one centre or research group.

II-iii Evidence obtained from multiple time series with or without the intervention. Dramatic results in uncontrolled experiments (such as the results of the introduction of penicillin treatment in the 1940s) could also be regarded as this type of evidence.

III Opinions of respected authorities based on clinical experience, descriptive studies or reports of expert committees.

IV Evidence inadequate due to problems of methodology (e.g. sample size, or length of comprehensiveness of follow-up or conflicts of evidence).

References

1 Williams HC, Potter A, Strachan D. The descriptive epidemiology of warts in British schoolchildren. *Br J Dermatol* 1993; **128**: 504–11.

2 Van der Werf E, Lent T. Een onderzoek naar het vóókomen en het verloop van wratten bij schoolkindren. *Ned Tijdschr Geneeskd* 1959; **103**: 1204–8.

3 Larsson PA, Lidén S. Prevalence of skin diseases among adolescents 12–16 years of age. *Acta Dermatovener* 1980; **60**: 415–23.

4 East Anglian Branch of the School Medical Officers of Health. The incidence of warts and plantar warts amongst schoolchildren in East Anglia. *Med Officer* 1955; **94**: 55–9.

5 Rea JN, Newhouse ML, Halil T. Skin disease in Lambeth: a community study of prevalence and use of medical care. *Br J Prev Soc Med* 1976; **30**: 107–14.

6 Barr A, Coles RB. Warts on the hands. A statistical survey. *Trans St John's Hosp Derm Soc* 1969; **55**: 69–73.

7 Shepherd PM. *The National Child Development Study: An introduction to the Origins of the Study and the Methods of Data Collection* London: NCDS User Support Group, City University, 1985.

8 Kaintz JT, Kozel G, Haidvogl M, Smolle J. Homoeopathic versus placebo therapy of children with warts on the hands: a randomized, double-blind clinical trial. *Dermatology* 1996; **193**: 318–20.

9 Yilmaz E, Alpsoy E, Basaran E. Cimetidine therapy for warts: a

placebo-controlled, double-blind study. *J Am Acad Dermatol* 1995; **34**: 1005–7.

10 Massing AM, Epstein WL. Natural history of warts. *Arch Dermatol* 1963; **87**: 306–10.

11 Williams HC, Pottier A, Strachan D. Are viral warts seen more commonly in children with eczema? *Arch Dermatol* 1993; **129**: 717–21.

12 Johnson LW. Communal showers and the risk of plantar warts. *J Fam Pract* 1995; **40**: 136–8.

13 Rudlinger R, Smith IW, Bunney MH *et al.* Human papilloma virus infections in a group of renal transplant recipients. *Br J Dermatol* 1986; **115**: 681–92.

14 Bunney MH, Nolan M, Williams D. An assessment of methods of treating viral warts by comparative treatment trials based on a standard design. *Br J Dermatol* 1976; **94**: 667–9.

15 Larsen PØ, Laurberg G. Cryotherapy of viral warts. *J Derm Treatment* 1996; **7**: 29–31.

16 Berth-Jones J, Hutchinson PE. Modern treatment of warts: cure rates at 3 and 6 months. *Br J Dermatol* 1992; **127**: 262–5.

17 Anonymous. Tackling warts on the hands and feet. *Drug Ther Bull* 1998; **36**: 22–4.

18 Veien NK, Madsen SM, Avrach W *et al.* The treatment of plantar warts with a keratolytic agent and occlusion. *J Dermatol Treat* 1991; **2**: 59–61.

19 Gaspar ZS, Dawber RP. An organic refrigerant for cryosurgery: fact or fiction? *Aust J Dermatol* 1997; **38**: 71–2.

20 Berth-Jones J, Bourke J, Eglitis *et al.* Value of a second freeze–thaw cycle in cryotherapy of common warts. *Br J Dermatol* 1994; **131**: 883–6.

21 Bourke J, Berth-Jones J, Hutchinson PE. Cryotherapy of common viral warts at intervals of 1, 2 and 3 weeks. *Br J Dermatol* 1995; **132**: 433–6.

22 Vickers CFH. Treatment of plantar warts in children. *Br Med J* 1961; **ii**: 743–5.

23 Pringle WM, Helms DC. Treatment of plantar warts by blunt dissection. *Arch Dermatol* 1973; **8**: 79–82.

24 Yazar S, Basaran E. Efficacy of silver nitrate pencils in the treatment of common warts. *J Dermatol* 1994; **21**: 329–33.

25 Street ML, Rœnigk RK. Recalcitrant periungual verrucae: the role of carbon dioxide laser vaporization. *J Am Acad Dermatol* 1990; **23**: 115–20.

26 Sloan K, Haberman H, Lynde CW. Carbon dioxide laser treatment of resistant verrucae vulgaris: retrospective analysis. *J Cutan Med Surg* 1998; **2**: 142–5.

27 Jain A, Storwick GS. Effectiveness of the 585 nm flashlamp-pulsed dye laser (PTDL) for treatment of plantar verrucae. *Lasers Surg Med* 1997; **21**: 500–5.

28 Kenton-Smith J, Tan ST. Pulsed dye laser therapy for viral warts. *Br J Plastic Surg* 1999; **52**: 554–8.

29 Ross BS, Levine VJ, Nehal K *et al.* Pulsed dye laser treatment of warts: an update. *Derm Surg* 1999; **25**: 377–80.

30 Stender I-M, Na R, Fogh H *et al.* Photodynamic therapy with 5-aminolaevulinic acid or placebo for recalcitrant foot and hand warts: randomised double-blind trial. *Lancet* 2000; **355**: 963–6.

31 Anderson I, Shirreffs E. The treatment of plantar warts. *Br J Dermatol* 1963; **75**: 29–32.

32 Hirose R, Hori M, Shukuwa T *et al.* Topical treatment of resistant warts with glutaraldehyde. *J Dermatol* 1994; **21**: 248–53.

33 Prigent F, Iborra C, Meslay C. Glutaraldehyde-induced cutaneous necrosis after topical treatment of a wart. *Ann Dermatol Venereol* 1996; **123**: 644–6.

34 Duthie DA, McCallum D. Treatment of plantar warts with elastoplast and podophyllin. *Br Med J* 1951; **2**: 216–18.

35 James MP, Collier PM, Aherna W. Histologic, pharmacologic and immunocytochemical effects of injection of bleomycin into viral warts. *J Am Acad Dermatol* 1993; **28**: 933–7.

36 Hayes ME, O'Keefe EJ. Reduced dose of bleomycin in the treatment of recalcitrant warts. *J Am Acad Dermatol* 1986; **15**: 1002–6.

37 Munn SE, Higgins E, Marshall M, Clement M. A new method of intralesional bleomycin therapy in the treatment of recalcitrant warts. *Br J Dermatol* 1996; **135**: 969–71.

38 Kubeyinje EP. Evaluation of the efficacy and safety of 0.05% tretinoin cream in the treatment of plane warts in Arab children. *J Dermatol Treat* 1996; **7**: 21–2.

39 Boyle J, Dick DC, MacKie RM. Treatment of extensive virus warts with etretinate (Tigason) in a patient with sarcoidosis. *Clin Exp Dermatol* 1983; **8**: 33–6.

40 Gross C, Pfister H, Hagedorn M *et al.* Effect of oral aromatic retinoid (Ro 10-9359) on human papilloma virus-2-induced common warts. *Dermatologica* 1983; **166**: 48–53.

41 Gelmetti C, Cerri D, Schiuma AA *et al.* Treatment of extensive warts with etretinate; a clinical trial in 20 children. *Pediatr Dermatol* 1987; **4**: 254–8.

42 Shah KC, Patel RM, Umrigar DD. Dinitrochlorobenzene treatment of verrucae plana. *J Dermatol* 1991; **18**: 639–42.

43 Iijima S, Otsuka F. Contact immunotherapy with squarid acid dibutylester for warts. *Dermatology* 1993; **187**: 115–8.

44 Rampen FH, Steijlen PM. Diphencyprone in the managment of refractory palmoplantar and periungual warts: an open study. *Dermatology* 1996; **193**: 236–8.

45 Buckley DA, Keane FM, Munn SE *et al.* Recalcitrant viral warts treated by diphencyprone immunotherapy. *Br J Dermatol* 1999; **141**: 292–6.

46 Bett WR. 'Wart, I bid thee begone'. *Practitioner* 1951; **166**: 77–80.

47 Spannos NP, Williams V, Gwynn MI. *Psychosom Med* 1990; **52**: 109–14.

48 Stern P, Levine N. Controlled localized heat therapy in cutaneous warts. *Arch Dermatol* 1992; **128**: 945–8.

49 Gibson JR, Harvey SG, Kemmett D *et al.* Treatment of common and plantar warts with human lymphoblastoid interferon-α – pilot studies with intralesional, intramuscular and dermojet injections. *Br J Dermatol* 1986; **115**: 76–9.

50 Hengge UR, Esser S, Schultewolter T, Behrendt C, Meyer T, Stockfleth E, Goos M. Self-administered topical 5% imiquimod for the treatmetn of common warts and molluscum contagiousum. *Br J Dermatol* 2000; **143**: 1026-31.

51 Hengge UR, Arndt R. Topical treatment of warts and mollusca with imiquimod. *Ann Int Med* 2000; **132**: 95.

http://bad.org.uk/Portals/_Bad/Guidelines/Clinical
%20Guidelines/Cutaneous%20Warts.pdf

Comment

The cutaneous wart guideline [1] published in 2001 has been updated by the 2006 Cochrane review [2], which concluded:

> There is a considerable lack of evidence on which to base the rational use of topical treatments for common warts. The reviewed trials are highly variable in method and quality. Cure rates with placebo preparations are variable but nevertheless considerable. There is certainly evidence that simple topical treatments containing salicylic acid have a therapeutic effect. There is less evidence for the efficacy of cryotherapy, but reasonable evidence that it is only of equivalent efficacy to simpler and safer treatments. The benefits and risks of topical dinitrochlorobenzene and 5-fluorouracil, intralesional bleomycin and interferons, photodynamic therapy and other miscellaneous treatments remain to be determined.

In the UK, purchasers of healthcare generally do not commission secondary care treatment of cutaneous warts unless there are functional problems.

A possible beneficial side effect of human papillomavirus vaccines may be cross-reactions against cutaneous types [3]. Further studies are needed to determine this.

REFERENCES

1 Sterling JC, Handfield-Jones S, Hudson PM. Guidelines for the management of cutaneous warts. *Brit J Dermatol* 2001; 144: 4–11.

2 Gibbs S, Harvey I. Topical treatments for cutaneous warts. *Cochrane Database Syst Rev* 2006; Issue 3: CD001781 (http://www.mrw.interscience.wiley.com/cochrane/clsysrev/articles/CD001781/frame.html).

3 Medeiros LR, Rosa DD, da Rosa MI, *et al.* Efficacy of human papillomavirus vaccines: a systematic quantitative review. *Int J Gynecol Cancer* 2009; 19: 1166–76.

Additional professional resources

Related to anogenital warts

United Kingdom national guideline on the management of anogenital warts, 2007. British Association for Sexual Health and HIV 2007 (http://www.bashh.org/documents/86/86.pdf).

http://www.cks.nhs.uk/warts_and_verrucae
http://www.cks.nhs.uk/warts_anogenital

BAD patient information leaflet

Plantar warts

http://www.bad.org.uk/site/859/Default.aspx

Other patient resources

http://www.dermnet.org.nz/viral/viral-warts.html
http://www.aad.org/pamphlets/warts.html
http://www.emedicine.com/emerg/topic641.htm
http://www.emedicinehealth.com/articles/20312-1.asp
http://www.lib.uiowa.edu/hardin/md/plantarwarts.html

Guidelines for treatment of onychomycosis

D.T.ROBERTS, W.D.TAYLOR* AND J.BOYLE†

Southern General Hospital, Glasgow G51 4TF, U.K.
*James Cook University Hospital, Middlesbrough, Cleveland TS4 3BW, U.K.
†Taunton and Somerset Hospital, Taunton TA1 5DA, U.K.

Accepted for publication 9 October 2002

Summary   These guidelines for management of onychomycosis have been prepared for dermatologists on behalf of the British Association of Dermatologists. They present evidence-based guidance for treatment, with identification of the strength of evidence available at the time of preparation of the guidelines, and a brief overview of epidemiological aspects, diagnosis and investigation.

Disclaimer

These guidelines have been prepared for dermatologists on behalf of the British Association of Dermatologists and reflect the best data available at the time the report was prepared. Caution should be exercised in interpreting the data; the results of future studies may require alteration of the conclusions or recommendations in this report. It may be necessary or even desirable to depart from the guidelines in the interests of specific patients and special circumstances. Just as adherence to guidelines may not constitute defence against a claim of negligence, so deviation from them should not necessarily be deemed negligent.

Introduction

Onychomycosis is one of the commonest dermatological conditions. A large questionnaire survey of 10 000 people suggested a prevalence of 2·71% in the U.K.[1,2] More recent mycologically controlled surveys in Finland[3] and in the U.S.A.[4] indicate a prevalence of between 7 and 10%. Increasing publicity about disease prevalence, and the advent of new and more effective antifungal drugs, has led to a greater enthusiasm

Correspondence: D.T.Roberts.
E-mail: dai.roberts@sgh.scot.nhs.uk

These guidelines were commissioned by the British Association of Dermatologists Therapy Guidelines and Audit subcommittee. Members of the committee are N.H.Cox (Chairman), A.V.Anstey, C.B.Bunker, M.J.D.Goodfield, A.S.Highet, D.Mehta, R.H.Meyrick Thomas, A.D.Ormerod, J.K.Schofield and C.H.Smith.

among sufferers to seek treatment and among medical practitioners to institute therapy. However, treatment is often prescribed without mycological confirmation of infection, there may be confusion as to whether fungi isolated on culture are primary or secondary pathogens, the relative efficacy of different antifungal agents against different fungi is not completely understood and drugs are often prescribed for inappropriate treatment durations.

Definition

Onychomycosis is an infection of the nail apparatus by fungi that include dermatophytes, nondermatophyte moulds and yeasts (mainly *Candida* species). The toenails are affected in 80% of all cases of onychomycosis; dermatophyte infection, mostly due to *Trichophyton rubrum*, is the cause in over 90% of cases.[5]

Onychomycosis is classified clinically as distal and lateral subungual onychomycosis (DLSO), superficial white onychomycosis (SWO), proximal subungual onychomycosis (PSO), candidal onychomycosis and total dystrophic onychomycosis.

Distal and lateral subungual onychomycosis

DLSO accounts for the majority of cases and is almost always due to dermatophyte infection. It affects the hyponychium, often at the lateral edges initially, and spreads proximally along the nail bed resulting in subungual hyperkeratosis and onycholysis although the nail plate is not initially affected. DLSO may be confined to one side of the nail or spread sideways to involve the whole of the nail bed, and progresses relentlessly until it reaches the posterior nail fold. Eventually the nail plate becomes friable and may break up, often due to trauma, although nail destruction may be related to invasion of the plate by dermatophytes that have keratolytic properties. Examination of the surrounding skin will nearly always reveal evidence of tinea pedis. Toenail infection is an almost inevitable precursor of fingernail dermatophytosis, which has a similar clinical appearance although nail thickening is not as common.

Superficial white onychomycosis

SWO is also nearly always due to a dermatophyte infection, most commonly *T. mentagrophytes*. It is much less common than DLSO and affects the surface of the nail plate rather than the nail bed. Discoloration is white rather than cream and the surface of the nail plate is noticeably flaky. Onycholysis is not a common feature of SWO and intercurrent foot infection is not as frequent as in DLSO.

Proximal subungual onychomycosis

PSO, without evidence of paronychia, is an uncommon variety of dermatophyte infection often related to intercurrent disease. Immunosuppressed patients, notably those who are human immunodeficiency virus-positive, may present with this variety of dermatophyte infection; conditions such as peripheral vascular disease and diabetes also may present in this way. Evidence of intercurrent disease should therefore be considered in a patient with PSO.

Candidal onychomycosis

Infection of the nail apparatus with *Candida* yeasts may present in one of four ways: (i) chronic paronychia with secondary nail dystrophy; (ii) distal nail infection; (iii) chronic mucocutaneous candidiasis; and (iv) secondary candidiasis.

Chronic paronychia of the fingernails generally only occurs in patients with wet occupations. Swelling of the posterior nail fold occurs secondary to chronic immersion in water or possibly due to allergic reactions to some foods, and the cuticle becomes detached from the nail plate thus losing its water-tight properties. Microorganisms, both yeasts and bacteria, enter the subcuticular space causing further swelling of the posterior nail fold

and further cuticular detachment, i.e. a vicious circle. Infection and inflammation in the area of the nail matrix eventually lead to a proximal nail dystrophy.

Distal nail infection with *Candida* yeasts is uncommon and virtually all patients have Raynaud's phenomenon or some other form of vascular insufficiency. It is unclear whether the underlying vascular problem gives rise to onycholysis as the initial event or whether yeast infection causes the onycholysis. Although candidal onychomycosis cannot be clinically differentiated from DLSO with certainty, the absence of toenail involvement and typically a lesser degree of subungual hyperkeratosis are helpful diagnostic features.

Chronic mucocutaneous candidiasis has multifactorial aetiology leading to diminished cell-mediated immunity. Clinical signs vary with the severity of immunosuppression, but in more severe cases gross thickening of the nails occurs, amounting to a *Candida* granuloma. The mucous membranes are almost always involved in such cases.

Secondary candidal onychomycosis occurs in other diseases of the nail apparatus, most notably psoriasis.

Total dystrophic onychomycosis

Any of the above varieties of onychomycosis may eventually progress to total nail dystrophy where the nail plate is almost completely destroyed.

Diagnosis

This section follows the criteria set out by Evans and Gentles.[6] Treatment should not be instituted on clinical grounds alone. Although 50% of all cases of nail dystrophy are fungal in origin it is not always possible to identify such cases accurately. Treatment needs to be administered long-term and enough time must elapse for the nail to grow out completely before such treatment can be designated as successful. Toenails take around 12 months to grow out and fingernails about 6 months. This is far too long to await the results of therapeutic trial and, in any case, treatment is not always successful. If the diagnosis is not confirmed, and improvement does not occur, it is impossible to tell whether this represents treatment failure or an initial incorrect diagnosis. Although the cost of diagnostic tests may be deemed high at times of budgetary constraint, the cost is always small relative to inappropriate and unnecessary treatment.

Laboratory diagnosis consists of microscopy to visualize fungal elements in the nail sample and culture to identify the species concerned. The success or otherwise of such tests depends upon the quality of the sample, the experience of the microscopist and the ability of the laboratory to discriminate between organisms that are likely pathogens, organisms growing in the nail as saprophytes, and contamination of the culture plate.

Given that dermatophyte onychomycosis is primarily a disease of the nail bed rather than of the nail plate, subungual debris taken from the most proximal part of the infection is likely to yield the best results. In DLSO material can be obtained from beneath the nail: a small dental scraper is most useful for this purpose. If the nail is onycholytic then this can be cut back and material can be scraped off the underside of the nail as well as from the nail bed. As much material as possible should be submitted to the laboratory because of the relative paucity of fungal elements within the specimen. In SWO the surface of the infected nail plate can be scraped and material examined directly. PSO is rare and again should be scraped with a scalpel blade. However, punch biopsy to obtain a sample of the full thickness of nail together with the nail bed may be necessary. Some of the material obtained is placed on a glass slide and 20% potassium hydroxide added. Fifteen to 20 min should be allowed to elapse before examining the sample by direct microscopy. The addition of Parker's blue/black ink may enhance visualization of the hyphae. An inexperienced observer may very well misdiagnose cell walls as hyphae and care should be taken to examine all of the specimen as fungal elements within the material may be very scanty.

The remaining material should be cultured on Saboraud's glucose agar, usually with the addition of an antibiotic. The culture plate is incubated at 28 °C for at least 3 weeks before it is declared negative, as dermatophytes tend to grow slowly.

Direct microscopy can be carried out by the clinician, and higher specialist training includes teaching of this technique. However, nail microscopy is difficult and should only be carried out by those who do it on a regular basis. Fungal culture should always be carried out in a laboratory experienced in handling mycology specimens, because of potential pitfalls in interpretation of cultures. It must be remembered that the most common cause of treatment failure in the U.K. is incorrect diagnosis, which is usually made on clinical grounds alone. This should not be further compounded by incorrect laboratory interpretation of results.

Histology is almost never required and its use is usually confined to other causes of nail dystrophy.

Such dystrophies, notably psoriasis, regularly yield *Candida* yeasts on culture but they are rarely causal in aetiology of fungal nail infection.

Reasons for treatment

Although dermatophyte onychomycosis is relentlessly progressive there remains a view among some practitioners that it is a trivial cosmetic problem that does not merit treatment. In the elderly the disease can give rise to complications such as cellulitis and therefore further compromise the limb in those with diabetes or peripheral vascular disease. While these complications may not be common they are certainly serious. The high prevalence of the disease is the result of heavy contamination of communal bathing places[7] by infected users; disinfecting the floors of such facilities is very difficult because fungal elements are protected in small pieces of keratin. It is therefore logical to try to reduce the number of infected users by effective treatment and thus reduce disease prevalence. Finally, onychomycosis is a surprisingly significant cause of medical consultation and of absence from work.[8]

Onychomycosis should not therefore be considered a trivial disease, and there is a sound case for treatment on the grounds of complications, public health considerations and effect on quality of life.

Treatment

Introduction

Both topical and oral agents are available for the treatment of fungal nail infection. The primary aim of treatment is to eradicate the organism as demonstrated by microscopy and culture. This is defined as the primary end-point in almost all properly conducted studies. Clinical improvement and clinical cure are secondary end-points based on a strict scoring system of clinical abnormalities in the nail apparatus. It must be recognized that successful eradication of the fungus does not always render the nails normal as they may have been dystrophic prior to infection. Such dystrophy may be due to trauma or nonfungal nail disease; this is particularly likely in cases where yeasts or nondermatophyte moulds (secondary pathogens and saprophytes, respectively) are isolated.[9]

Invariably mycological cure rates are about 30% better than clinical cure rates in the majority of studies, the clinical cure rates often being below 50%. Publications of clinical trials in onychomycosis are often criticized for quoting mycological cure rates and thus overemphasizing the efficacy of treatment. While it is understood that the patient is more concerned with improvement in the clinical appearance of the nail rather than eradication of the organism, questions regarding patients' satisfaction at the end of a study usually mirror very closely the mycological cure rate. This suggests that eradication of the organism does restore the nail to its previous state prior to infection even though that state may not be completely 'normal' as defined by a scoring system.

Systemic therapy is almost always more successful than topical treatment, which should only be used in SWO, possibly very early DLSO or when systemic therapy is contraindicated.

Topical therapy

There are several topical antifungal preparations available both as prescription-only medicines and on an over-the-counter basis. The active antifungal agent in these preparations is either an imidazole, an allylamine or a polyene, or a preparation that contains a chemical with antifungal, antiseptic and sometimes keratolytic properties such as benzoic acid, benzyl peroxide, salicylic acid or an undecenoate. Products that are specifically indicated for nail infection are available as a paint or lacquer that is applied topically. There are four such preparations (Table 1).

There are no published studies on the efficacy of salicylic acid (Phytex®; Pharmax, Bexley, U.K.) and methyl undecenoate (Monphytol®; LAB, London, U.K.) in fungal nail infection and their use cannot be recommended.

Amorolfine (Loceryl®; Galderma, Amersham, U.K.) nail lacquer has been shown to be effective in around 50% of cases of both fingernail and toenail infection in a large study where only cases with infections of the distal portion of the nail were treated.[10] There are several published studies examining the efficacy of tioconazole (Trosyl®; Pfizer, Sandwich, U.K.) nail solution, with very variable results ranging from cure rates of around 20% up to 70%.[11] While it is clearly possible to achieve clinical and mycological cure with topical nail preparations, these cure rates do not compare favourably with those obtained with systemic drugs. Currently, topical therapy can only be recommended for the treatment of SWO and in very early cases of DLSO where the infection is confined to the distal edge of the nail.

A combination of topical and systemic therapy may improve cure rates still further or possibly shorten the duration of therapy with the systemic agent. Thus far the results of such studies are inconclusive. A study comparing terbinafine and amorolfine with terbinafine alone produced somewhat idiosyncratic results[12] and was not properly blinded, so further evidence from well-controlled double-blind studies is required before combination therapy can be advocated.

Although there are no studies comparing one topical preparation with another in a properly controlled fashion, it is likely that amorolfine nail lacquer (Loceryl®) is the most effective preparation of those available.

Systemic therapy

The three drugs currently licensed for general use in onychomycosis are listed in Table 2. The two other systemic agents available for oral use, ketoconazole and fluconazole, are not licensed for nail infection. Ketoconazole may be used in some recalcitrant cases of yeast infection affecting the nails but cannot be prescribed for dermatophyte onychomycosis because of problems with hepatotoxicity. The use of fluconazole thus far has concentrated on vaginal candidiasis and systemic yeast infections although it is active against dermatophytes. There are some published studies of its use in nail infection but the dose and duration of treatment are not yet clear and it is not licensed for this indication in the U.K., nor does it appear likely to be so in the near future.

Griseofulvin. Griseofulvin (Fulcin®; Grisovin®; GlaxoSmithKline, Uxbridge, U.K.) is weakly fungistatic, and acts by inhibiting nucleic acid synthesis, arresting cell

Table 1. Topical agents for onychomycosis, with strength of recommendation and quality of evidence grading

Agent	Strength of recommendation and quality of evidence
Amorolfine (Loceryl®; Galderma, Amersham, U.K.) nail lacquer	*Strength of recommendation B, Quality of evidence II-ii*
Tioconazole (Trosyl®; Pfizer, Sandwich, U.K.) nail solution	*Strength of recommendation C, Quality of evidence II-iii*
Salicylic acid (Phytex®; Pharmax, Bexley, U.K.) paint	*Strength of recommendation E, Quality of evidence IV*
Undecenoates (Monphytol®; LAB, London, U.K.) paint	*Strength of recommendation E, Quality of evidence IV*

Table 2. Systemic agents for onychomycosis, with major advantages and disadvantages, and strength of recommendation and quality of evidence grading

Drug	Advantages	Disadvantages	Main drug interactions	Strength of recommendation, quality of evidence
Griseofulvin	Licensed in both adults and children, inexpensive, extensive experience	Lengthy treatment necessary in both fingernail and toenail infection; poor cure rates; high relapse rates; no paediatric formulation currently available; contraindicated in lupus erythematosus, porphyria and severe liver disease	Warfarin, ciclosporin, oral contraceptive pill	B-I
Terbinafine[a]	Fungicidal; high cure rates (compared with griseofulvin); short duration of therapy; good compliance	No U.K. licence for children; no suspension formulation; idiosyncratic liver and skin reactions; reversible taste disturbance in 1 : 400 patients	Plasma concentrations reduced by rifampicin, increased by cimetidine	A-I
Itraconazole[a]	Active against *Candida albicans*; pulsed treatment regimens are possible	Less effective in dermatophyte onychomycosis than terbinafine; monitoring of liver function required for treatment durations of longer than 1 month; not licensed for use in children and contraindicated in pregnancy	Enhanced toxicity of anticoagulants (warfarin), antihistamines (terfenadine and astemizole), antipsychotics (sertindole), anxiolytics (midazolam), digoxin, cisapride, ciclosporin and simvastatin (increased risk of myopathy); reduced efficacy of itraconazole with concomitant use of H2 blockers, phenytoin and rifampicin	A-I

[a]Terbinafine has better cure rate and lower relapse rate than itraconazole for dermatophytes (A-I).

division and inhibiting fungal cell wall synthesis.[13–15] It is available in tablet form and is the only antifungal agent licensed for use in children with onychomycosis, with a recommended dose for age groups of 1 month and above of 10 mg kg^{-1} daily. It requires to be taken with fatty food to increase absorption and aid bioavailability. In adults the recommended dose is 500 mg daily given for 6–9 months in fingernail infection and 12–18 months in toenail infection. Mycological cure rates in fingernail infection are reasonably satisfactory at around 70% but griseofulvin is a disappointing drug in toenail disease where cure rates of only 30–40% can be expected.[16]

It is generally recognized that 500 mg daily is too small a dose for nail infection and 1 g daily is most often prescribed, but there is no certain evidence that this improves cure rates in toenail infection. Although the cost of griseofulvin is very low, its poor cure rate, often necessitating further treatment, suggests that its cost/efficacy ratio is relatively high. Both direct and historical comparison with studies of the newer antifungal agents terbinafine[17–19] and itraconazole[20–22] suggest that griseofulvin is no longer the treatment of choice for dermatophyte onychomycosis.

Side-effects include nausea and rashes in 8–15% of patients. In adults, it is contraindicated in pregnancy and the manufacturers caution against men fathering a child for 6 months after therapy.

Terbinafine. Terbinafine (Lamisil®; Novartis, Camberley, U.K.), an allylamine, inhibits the enzyme squalene epoxidase thus blocking the conversion of squalene to squalene epoxide in the biosynthetic pathway of ergosterol, an integral component of the fungal cell wall.[23] Its action results in both a depletion of ergosterol, which has a fungistatic effect, together with an accumulation of squalene, which appears to be directly fungicidal. The minimum inhibitory concentration (MIC) of terbinafine is very low, approximately 0.004 µg mL^{-1}. This is equivalent to the minimal fungicidal concentration (MFC), demonstrating that this drug is truly fungicidal *in vitro*. It is the most active currently available antidermatophyte agent *in vitro* and clinical studies strongly suggest that this is also the case *in vivo*.[24]

Itraconazole. Itraconazole (Sporonox®; Janssen-Cilag, High Wycombe, U.K.) is active against a range of fungi including yeasts, dermatophytes and some nondermatophyte moulds. It is not as active *in vitro* against dermatophytes as terbinafine, its MIC being 10 times greater. Although it is generally felt to be a fungistatic agent it can achieve fungicidal concentrations, although its MFC is about 10 times higher than its MIC.[25]

Both terbinafine and itraconazole persist in the nail for a considerable period after elimination from the plasma.[26] This property has given rise to a novel intermittent ('pulsed') treatment regimen using itraconazole in nail infection.

Terbinafine vs. itraconazole in dermatophyte onychomycosis. Both of these drugs have been shown to be more effective than griseofulvin in dermatophyte onychomycosis and therefore the optimum choice of treatment lies between terbinafine and itraconazole.

Terbinafine is licensed at a dose of 250 mg daily for 6 weeks and 12 weeks in fingernail and toenail infection, respectively. Itraconazole is licensed at a dose of 200 mg daily for 12 weeks continuously, or alternatively at a dose of 400 mg daily for 1 week per month. It is recommended that two of these weekly courses, 21 days apart, are given for fingernail infections and three courses for toenail disease.

There have been numerous open and placebo-controlled studies of both drugs in dermatophyte nail infection. However, historical comparisons of such studies do not provide evidence of equivalent quality as that achieved by directly comparative double-blind trials, as even in properly conducted studies the results can be influenced by variation in the criteria for mycological or clinical cure, or by the period of follow-up. It is generally accepted that patients entered into such studies should be both microscopy- and culture-positive for fungus and that mycological cure should be defined as microscopy and culture negativity at completion. Clinical criteria for cure are difficult to interpret as the appearance of the nail prior to infection is generally unknown and, especially in the case of toenails, because trauma can affect their appearance. Short follow-up periods after cessation of therapy are unlikely to allow interpretation of which is the superior drug; a follow-up period of at least 48 weeks (preferably 72 weeks) from the start of treatment should be allowed both in order to allow the most effective preparation to become apparent and to identify relapse as far as possible.

There are various published studies comparing terbinafine with continuous itraconazole therapy,[27–29] most of which demonstrate terbinafine to be the more effective agent. Thus far there are only two studies comparing terbinafine with intermittent itraconazole

therapy. The first compared terbinafine 250 mg daily for 16 weeks with four 'pulses' of itraconazole 400 mg daily for 1 week in every 4 weeks for 16 weeks and also with terbinafine 500 mg daily for 1 week in every 4 weeks for 16 weeks.[30] As only approximately 20 patients were recruited in each study group, this was a very small study; the regimens used were not those of the U.K. product licences, and the results comparing the groups were not significantly different. A more recent and much larger study has been completed comparing terbinafine 250 mg daily for both 3 and 4 months with itraconazole 400 mg daily for 1 week × 3 and 1 week × 4. One hundred and twenty patients were recruited to each group and the follow-up period was 72 weeks.[31] The study was carried out in double-blind, double-placebo fashion and demonstrated terbinafine 250 mg daily for both 3 and 4 months to be very significantly superior to both three and four 'pulses' of itraconazole (*Strength of recommendation A, Quality of evidence I*; see Appendix 1).

The 151 patients in the Icelandic arm of this study were further studied for long-term effectiveness of treatment during a 5-year blinded prospective follow-up study.[32] At the end of the study mycological cure without a second therapeutic intervention was found in 46% of the 74 terbinafine-treated subjects but in only 13% of the 77 itraconazole-treated subjects. Mycological and clinical relapse was significantly higher in the itraconazole group (53% and 48%) than the terbinafine group (23% and 21%) (*Strength of recommendation A, Quality of evidence I*).

The superiority of terbinafine has recently been supported by a systematic review of oral treatments for toenail onychomycosis;[33] this reference documents many additional studies and also the varied and often incompletely presented criteria that have been used to describe a 'clinical cure'.

Treatment of yeast infections

Most yeast infections can be treated topically, particularly those associated with paronychia. Antiseptics can be applied to the proximal part of the nail and allowed to wash beneath the cuticle, thus sterilizing the subcuticular space. Ideally, such antiseptics should be broad spectrum, colourless and nonsensitizing. They require to be applied until the integrity of the cuticle has been restored, which may be several months. An imidazole lotion alternating with an antibacterial lotion is usually effective.

Itraconazole (Sporonox®) is the most effective agent for the treatment of candidal onychomycosis where the nail plate is invaded by the organism.[34] It is used in the same dosage regimen as for dermatophytes, i.e. 400 mg daily for 1 week per month repeated for 2 months in fingernail infection. *Candida* infection of toenails is much less common but can be treated as above using three or four pulses.

Treatment of nondermatophyte moulds

Many varieties of saprophytic moulds can invade diseased nail. *Scopulariopsis brevicaulis* is the commonest of these and may be a secondary pathogen. Its response to systemic antifungal agents is variable, although terbinafine is probably the drug of choice in that the primary nail disease is quite likely to be a dermatophyte infection that is masked by the *Scopulariopsis*. There is little categorical evidence to support the choice of one drug.[35] In the U.S.A. and Europe cyclopirox nail lacquer has its advocates but it is not available in the U.K. Nail avulsion followed by an oral agent during the period of regrowth is probably the best method of restoring the nail to normal.

Treatment failure

Although terbinafine is demonstrably the most effective agent in dermatophyte onychomycosis a consistent failure rate of 20–30% is found in all studies. If the most obvious causes of treatment failure, notably poor compliance, poor absorption, immunosuppression, dermatophyte resistance and zero nail growth are excluded, the commonest cause of failure is likely to be kinetic.[36] Subungual dermatophytoma has been described[37] and it is likely that this tightly packed mass of fungus prevents penetration of the drug in adequate concentrations. In such cases partial nail removal is indicated. It is been demonstrated that cure rates of close to 100% can always be achieved if all affected nails are avulsed under ring block prior to commencement of treatment. However, this is neither feasible nor necessary in most cases and the best approach is to try to identify those individual nails that are likely to fail and to remove the offending area.

Reports of long-term follow-up of treated patients have recently been presented, suggesting that positive mycology at 12 and 24 weeks after commencement of therapy are poor prognostic signs and may indicate a need for retreatment or for a change of drug. However, this work remains to be confirmed.

Cure rates, both short- and long-term, may be influenced by correction of associated orthopaedic and podiatric factors to avoid, as much as possible, trauma that particularly affects the great toenails.

Summary of conclusions

1 Treatment should not be commenced before mycological confirmation of infection.
2 Dermatophytes are by far the commonest causal organisms.
3 Culture of yeasts and nondermatophyte moulds should be interpreted carefully in each individual case. In the majority, yeasts are likely to be a secondary infection and nondermatophyte moulds to be saprophytic in previously damaged nails.
4 Topical treatment is inferior to systemic therapy in all but a small number of cases of very distal infection or in SWO.
5 Terbinafine is superior to itraconazole both *in vitro* and *in vivo* for dermatophyte onychomycosis, and should be considered first-line treatment, with itraconazole as the next best alternative.
6 Cure rates of 80–90% for fingernail infection and 70–80% for toenail infection can be expected. In cases of treatment failure the reasons for such failure should be carefully considered. In such cases either an alternative drug or nail removal in combination with a further course of therapy to cover the period of regrowth should be considered.

Audit points

1 Has a positive culture been obtained before commencing systemic therapy for onychomycosis?
2 Has an appropriate agent been chosen, based on the type of organism cultured?
3 Are arrangements in place for adequate duration of treatment to be supplied from hospital or general practitioner?
4 Has immunosuppression been considered in cases of PSO?

Declaration of interest

David T.Roberts is a member of the Dermatology Advisory Board of Novartis Pharmaceuticals Ltd. He has given advice to almost all other manufacturers of antifungal agents and has spoken at symposia organized by a number of these companies. The other authors have no conflict of interest.

References

1 Roberts DT. Prevalence of dermatophyte onychomycosis in the United Kingdom: results of an omnibus survey. *Br J Dermatol* 1992; **126** (Suppl. 39): 23–7.

2 Sais G, Jucgla J, Peyri J. Prevalence of dermatophyte onychomycosis in Spain: a cross-sectional study. *Br J Dermatol* 1995; **132**: 758–61.

3 Heikkila H, Stubb S. The prevalence of onychomycosis in Finland. *Br J Dermatol* 1995; **133**: 699–703.

4 Elewski BE, Charif MA. Prevalence of onychomycosis in patients attending a dermatology clinic in north eastern Ohio for other conditions. *Arch Dermatol* 1997; **133**: 1172–3.

5 Summerbell RC, Kane J, Krajden S. Onychomycosis, tinea pedis and tinea manuum caused by non dermatophyte filamentous fungi. *Mycoses* 1989; **32**: 609–19.

6 Evans EGV, Gentles JC. *Essentials of Medical Mycology*. Edinburgh: Churchill Livingstone, 1985.

7 Detandt M, Nolard M. Fungal contamination of the floors of swimming pools, particularly subtropical swimming paradises. *Mycoses* 1995; **38**: 509–13.

8 Drake LA, Sher RK, Smith EB *et al*. Effect of onychomycosis on quality of life. *J Am Acad Dermatol* 1998; **38**: 702–4.

9 English MP, Atkinson E. Nail mycology in chiropody patients. *Br J Dermatol* 1974; **91**: 67–72.

10 Zaug M, Bergstraesser M. Amorolfine in onychomycosis and dermatomycosis. *Clin Exp Dermatol* 1992; **17** (Suppl. 1): 61–70.

11 Hay RJ, MacKie RM, Clayton YM. Tioconazole nail solution – an open study of its efficacy in onychomycosis. *Clin Exp Dermatol* 1985; **10**: 111–15.

12 Baran R. Topical amorolfine for 15 months combined with 12 weeks of oral terbinafine, a cost effective treatment for onychomycosis. *Br J Dermatol* 2001; **145** (Suppl. 60): 15–19.

13 Roobol A, Gull K, Pogson CI. Griseofulvin-induced aggregation of microtubule protein. *Biochem J* 1977; **167**: 39–43.

14 Wehland DJ, Herzoy W, Weber K. Interaction of griseofulvin with microtubules, microtubular proteins and tubulin. *J Mol Biol* 1977; **111**: 329–42.

15 Roobol A, Gull K, Pogson CI. Evidence that griseofulvin binds to a microtubular protein. *FEBS Lett* 1977; **29**: 149–53.

16 Davies RR, Everall JD, Hamilton E. Mycological and clinical evaluation of griseofulvin for chronic onychomycosis. *Br Med J* 1967; **iii**: 464–8.

17 Faergemann J, Anderson C, Hersle K *et al*. Double-blind, parallel group comparison of terbinafine and griseofulvin in treatment of toenail onychomycosis. *J Am Acad Dermatol* 1995; **32**: 750–3.

18 Haneke E, Tausch I, Brautigam M *et al*. Short duration treatment of fingernail dermatophytosis: a randomised double-blind study with terbinafine and griseofulvin. *J Am Acad Dermatol* 1995; **32**: 72–7.

19 Hofmann H, Brautigam M, Weidinger G *et al*. Treatment of toenail onychomycosis. A randomised, double-blind study with terbinafine and griseofulvin. *Arch Dermatol* 1995; **131**: 919–22.

20 Walsoe I, Stangerup M, Svejgaard E. Itraconazole in onychomycosis. Open and double-blind studies. *Acta Derm Venereol (Stockh)* 1990; **70**: 137–40.

21 Korting HC, Schafer-Korting M, Zienicke H *et al*. Treatment of tinea unguium with medium and high doses of ultramicrosize griseofulvin compared with that with itraconazole. *Antimicrob Agents Chemother* 1993; **37**: 2064–8.

22 Cribier BJ, Paul C. Long-term efficacy of antifungals in toenail onychomycosis: a critical review. *Br J Dermatol* 2001; **145**: 446–52.

23 Ryder NS, Favre B. Antifungal activity and mechanism of action of terbinafine. *Rev Contemp Pharmcother* 1997; **8**: 275–88.

24 Ryder NS, Leitner I. *In vitro* activity of terbinafine; an update. *J Dermatol Treat* 1998; **9** (Suppl. 1): S23–8.

25 Clayton YM. Relevance of broad spectrum and fungicidal activity of antifungals in the treatment of dermatomycoses. *Br J Dermatol* 1994; **130** (Suppl. 43): 7–8.

26 Faergemann J. Pharmacokinetics of terbinafine. *Rev Contemp Pharmacother* 1997; **8**: 289–97.

27 Brautigam M, Nolting S, Schopf RE *et al*. German randomized double-blind multicentre comparison of terbinafine and itraconazole for the treatment of toenail tinea infection. *Br Med J* 1995; **311**: 919–22.

28 de Backer M, de Keyser P, de Vroey C *et al*. 12 week treatment for dermatophyte toenail onychomycosis: terbinafine 250 mg vs itraconazole 200 mg per day: a double-blind comparative trial. *Br J Dermatol* 1996; **134** (Suppl. 46): 16–17.

29 Arenas R, Dominguez-Cherit J, Fernandez LM. Open randomised comparison of itraconazole versus terbinafine in onychomycosis. *Int J Dermatol* 1995; **34**: 138–43.

30 Tosti A, Piraccini BM, Stinchi C *et al*. Treatment of dermatophyte nail infections: an open randomised study comparing intermittent terbinafine therapy with continuous terbinafine treatment and intermittent intraconazole therapy. *J Am Acad Dermatol* 1996; **34**: 595–600.

31 Evans EGV, Sigurgeirsson B, Billstein S. European multicentre study of continous terbinafine vs intermittent itraconazole in the treatment of toenail onychomycosis. *Br Med J* 1999; **318**: 1031–5.

32 Sigurgeirsson B, Olaffson JH, Steinssen JB *et al*. Long-term effectiveness of treatment with terbinafine vs itraconazole in onychomycosis: a 5-year blinded prospective follow-up study. *Arch Dermatol* 2002; **138**: 353–7.

33 Crawford F, Young P, Godfrey C *et al*. Oral treatments for toenail onychomycosis. A systematic review. *Arch Dermatol* 2002; **138**: 811–16.

34 Gupta AK, Shear NJ. The new oral antifungal agents for onychomycosis of the toenails. *J Eur Acad Dermatol Venereol* 1999; **13**: 1–3.

35 Gupta AK, Gregurek-Novak T. Efficacy of itraconzole, terbinafine, fluconazole, griseofulvin and ketoconazole in the treatment of *Scopulariopsis brevicaulis* causing onychomycosis of the toes. *Dermatology* 2001; **202**: 235–8.

36 Gupta AK, Daniel CR. Factors that may affect the response of onychomycosis to oral antifungal therapy. *Australas J Dermatol* 1998; **39**: 222–4.

37 Roberts DT, Evans EGV. Subungual dermatophytoma complicating dermatophyte onychomycosis. *Br J Dermatol* 1998; **138**: 189–90.

38 Griffiths CEM. The British Association of Dermatologists guidelines for the management of skin disease. *Br J Dermatol* 1999; **141**: 396–7.

39 Cox NH, Williams HC. The British Association of Dermatologists therapeutic guidelines: can we AGREE? *Br J Dermatol*, in press.

Appendix 1

The consultation process and background details for the British Association of Dermatologists guidelines have been published elsewhere.[38,39]

Strength of recommendations

A There is good evidence to support the use of the procedure.

B There is fair evidence to support the use of the procedure.

C There is poor evidence to support the use of the procedure.

D There is fair evidence to support the rejection of the use of the procedure.

E There is good evidence to support the rejection of the use of the procedure.

Quality of evidence

I Evidence obtained from at least one properly designed, randomized controlled trial.

II-i   Evidence obtained from well-designed controlled trials without randomization.

II-ii Evidence obtained from well-designed cohort or case-control analytical studies, preferably from more than one centre or research group.

II-iii Evidence obtained from multiple time series with or without the intervention. Dramatic results in uncontrolled experiments (such as the introduction of penicillin treatment in the 1940s) could also be regarded as this type of evidence.

III   Opinions of respected authorities based on clinical experience, descriptive studies or reports of expert committees.

IV   Evidence inadequate owing to problems of methodology (e.g. sample size, or length or comprehensiveness of follow-up or conflicts of evidence).

http://www.bad.org.uk/Portals/_Bad/Guidelines/Clinical
%20Guidelines/Onychomycosis.pdf

Comment

The Roberts *et al* guidelines [1] concluded that oral anti-fungals were superior to topical agents for the treatment of onychomycosis. The 2007 Cochrane review [2] found that topical antifungal agents were effective for skin infections but not so effective for onychomycosis. Amorolfine nail lacquer has been shown to be effective in around 50% of cases of both fingernail and toenail infection in a large study where only cases with infections of the distal portion of the nail were treated [1, 2]. A recent reasonably large study has shown the lack of utility of surgical nail avulsion and topical therapy for single nail infection [3]. Further research into newer topical therapies and effectiveness of current treatments for rare causes of onychomycosis and systemic treatment failures is needed.

REFERENCES

1 Roberts DT, Taylor WD, Boyle J. Guidelines for treatment of onychomycosis. *Brit J Dermatol* 2003; 148: 402–10.
2 Crawford F, Hollis S. Topical treatments for fungal infections of the skin and nails of the foot. *Cochrane Database Syst Rev* 2007; Issue 3: CD001434 (http://mrw.interscience.wiley.com/cochrane/clsysrev/articles/CD001434/frame.html).
3 Grover C, Bansal S, Nanda S, *et al*. Combination of surgical avulsion and topical therapy for single nail onychomycosis: a randomized controlled trial. *Brit J Dermatol* 2007; 157: 364–8.

Additional professional resources

Health Protection Agency. Fungal skin and nail infections: diagnosis and laboratory investigation – quick reference guide for primary care. http://www.hpa.org.uk/web/HPAwebFile/HPAweb_C/1240294785726.
Systematic review. Fungal toenail infections; definitions and results.http://www.medicine.ox.ac.uk/bandolier/band68/b68-8.html.
Fungal nail infection (onychomycosis). Clinical Knowledge Summary 2009. http://www.cks.nhs.uk/fungal_nail_infection.
Crawford F, Young P, Godfrey C, Bell-Syer SE, Hart R, Brunt E, Russell I. Oral treatments for toenail onychomycosis: a systematic review. *Arch Dermatol* 2002; 138(6): 811–16.
http://www.dermnetnz.org/fungal/onychomycosis.html

BAD patient information leaflet

http://www.bad.org.uk/site/820/Default.aspx

Other patient resources

http://www.aafp.org/afp/20010215/663.html
http://www.emedicine.com/derm/topic300.htm
http://www.nhs.uk/conditions/Fungal-nail-infection/Pages/Introduction.aspx?url=Pages/What-is-it.aspx
http://www.patient.co.uk/pdf/pilsL213.pdf
http://www.cks.nhs.uk/patient_information_leaflet/fungal_nail_infection

Guidelines for the management of tinea capitis

E.M.HIGGINS,*† L.C.FULLER* AND C.H.SMITH‡

*King's College Hospital, London SE5 9RS, U.K.
†Orpington Hospital, Kent BR6 9SU, U.K.
‡Lewisham Hospital, London SE13 6LH, U.K.

Accepted for publication 15 April 2000

Summary   These guidelines for the management of tinea capitis have been prepared for dermatologists on behalf of the British Association of Dermatologists. They present evidence-based guidance for treatment, with identification of the strength of evidence available at the time of preparation of the guidelines, and a brief overview of epidemiological aspects, diagnosis and investigation.

Key words: guidelines, tinea capitis

Disclaimer

These guidelines have been prepared for dermatologists on behalf of the British Association of Dermatologists and reflect the best data available at the time the report was prepared. Caution should be exercised in interpreting the data; the results of future studies may require alteration of the conclusions or recommendations in this report. It may be necessary or even desirable to depart from the guidelines in the interests of specific patients and special circumstances. Just as adherence to the guidelines may not constitute defence against a claim of negligence, so deviation from them should not necessarily be deemed negligent.

Definition

Tinea capitis is an infection caused by dermatophyte fungi (usually species in the genera *Microsporum* and *Trichophyton*) of scalp hair follicles and the surrounding skin.

Epidemiology

Tinea capitis is predominantly a disease of preadolescent children, adult cases being rare.[1] Although world-wide in distribution, its prevalence in the U.K. has been relatively low in the past. An increase in

These guidelines were commissioned, developed and edited by the Therapy Guidelines and Audit Sub-Committee of the British Association of Dermatologists, C.E.M.Griffiths (Chairman), A.V.Anstey, C.B.Bunker, N.H.Cox, K.L.Dalziel, M.R.Judge, H.C.Williams, D.K.Metha and S.M.Burge. These guidelines are planned to be updated by January 2001.

prevalence has recently been reported in urban areas, particularly in children of Afro-Caribbean extraction.[1-3] The main pathogens are anthropophilic organisms with *Trichophyton tonsurans* now accounting for > 90% of cases in the U.K. and North America.[2,4,5] These infections frequently spread among family members and classmates.[5,6] Certain hairdressing practices such as shaving of the scalp, plaiting or the use of hair oils may promote disease transmission, but their precise role remains the subject of study. In non-urban communities, sporadic infections acquired from puppies and kittens are due to *M. canis*, which, however, accounts for less than 10% of cases in the U.K. Occasional infection from other animal hosts (e.g. *T. verrucosum* from cattle) occur in rural areas.

Pathogenesis

There are three recognized patterns: endothrix, ectothrix and favus. The latter, a pattern of hair loss caused by *T. schoenleinii*, is rarely seen in the U.K. being largely confined to eastern Europe and Asia and is not considered further here. Endothrix infections are characterized by arthroconidia (spores) within the hair shaft. The cuticle is not destroyed. Ectothrix infections are characterized by hyphal fragments and arthroconidia outside the hair shaft, which leads eventually to cuticle destruction.

Clinical diagnosis of scalp ringworm

A variety of clinical presentations are recognized as being either inflammatory or non-inflammatory and

Table 1. Summarizing the clinical patterns of tinea capitis

Clinical patterns	Clinical description	Differential diagnosis
Diffuse scale	Generalized diffuse scaling of the scalp	Seborrhoeic and atopic dermatitis, psoriasis
Grey patch	Patchy, scaly alopecia	Seborrhoeic and atopic dermatitis, psoriasis
Black dot	Patches of alopecia studded with broken-off hair stubs	Alopecia areata, trichotillomania
Diffuse pustular	Scattered pustules associated with alopecia scaling ± associated lymphadenopathy	Bacterial folliculitis, dissecting folliculitis
Kerion	Boggy tumour studded with pustules ± associated lymphadenopathy	Abscess, neoplasia

are usually associated with patchy alopecia (Table 1). However, the infection is so widespread, and the clinical appearances can be so subtle, that in urban areas, tinea capitis should be considered in the diagnosis of any child over the age of 3 months with a scaly scalp, until dismissed by negative mycology. Infection may also be associated with painful regional lymphadenopathy, particularly in the inflammatory variants. A generalized eruption of itchy papules particularly around the outer helix of the ear may occur as a reactive phenomenon (an 'id' response). This may start with the introduction of systemic therapy and so be mistaken for a drug reaction.

Laboratory diagnosis of scalp ringworm

If tinea capitis is suspected, specimens should be taken to confirm the diagnosis as systemic therapy will be required.

Taking specimens

Affected areas should be scraped with a *blunt* scalpel to harvest affected hairs, broken-off hair stubs and scalp scale. This is preferable to plucking, which may remove uninvolved hairs. Scrapings should be transported in a folded square of paper preferably fastened with a paper clip, but commercial packs are also available (e.g. Dermapak, Dermaco, Toddington, Bedfordshire, U.K. and Mycotrans, Biggar, Lanarkshire, U.K.). It is easier to see affected hairs on white paper rather than black. Alternatively, the area can be rubbed with a moistened gauze swab[7,8] or brushed gently 10 times with a plastic, sterile, single use toothbrush [BR8 (unpasted), Brushaway Products, Chislehurst Railway Station, Station Approach, Chislehurst, Kent BR7 5NN, U.K.]. The brush can then be sent in the container provided to the laboratory for culture.[9] (*Strength of recommendation = A; quality of evidence III.*)

Microscopy and culture

Samples should be sent to laboratories with a particular interest and expertise in mycology.

Microscopy provides the most rapid means of diagnosis, but is not always positive. Scalp scales and broken off hair stumps containing the root section (rather than intact hairs) are mounted in a 10–30% potassium hydroxide solution and viewed under the light microscope. Positive microscopy (when the hairs or scales are seen to be invaded by spores or hyphae) confirms the diagnosis and allows treatment to commence at once.

Scales, hairs or samples obtained with a sterile single use brush are often not suitable for microscopy, but are inoculated on to a suitable culture medium, e.g. Sabouraud's. Culture allows accurate identification of the organism involved, and this may alter the treatment schedule. Culture is more sensitive than microscopy; results may be positive even when microscopy is negative, but may take up to 4 weeks to become available.

Conventional sampling of a kerion can be difficult. In these cases negative results are not uncommon and the diagnosis and decision to treat may need to be made clinically. A moistened standard bacteriological swab taken from the pustular areas and inoculated on to the culture plate may yield a positive result.[8]

Wood's light examination

This is useful for certain ectothrix infections, e.g. those caused by *M. canis*, *M. rivalieri* and *M. audouinii*, which cause the hair to fluoresce bright green. However, as most of the current infections in the U.K. are endothrix and so negative under Wood's light, it is of limited value for screening and monitoring these infections.

Therapy of tinea capitis

The aim of treatment is to achieve a clinical and mycological cure as quickly as possible. Oral antifungal

Table 2. Dosing regimen for tinea capitis

Drug	Current standard dose	Duration
Griseofulvin	10–25 mg/kg daily taken with food divided dose	8–10 weeks
Terbinafine	< 20 kg 62·5 mg od: > 20 < 40 kg 125 mg od: > 40 kg 250 mg od	4 weeks[a]
Itraconazole	5 mg/kg per day	1–4 weeks

[a] Longer for *Microsporum* infections.

therapy is generally needed.[10] (*Strength of recommendation = A; quality of evidence IIi.*)

Topical

Topical treatment alone is not recommended for the management of tinea capitis.[10] (*Strength of recommendation = A; quality of evidence = III.*) It may however, reduce the risk of transmission to others in the early stages of systemic treatment. (*Strength of recommendation = B; quality of evidence = IIii.*) Selenium sulphide[11] and povidone iodine[12] shampoos, used twice weekly, reduce the carriage of viable spores and are assumed to reduce infectivity.

Oral

Griseofulvin. This is fungistatic, and inhibits nucleic acid synthesis, arresting cell division at metaphase and impairing fungal cell wall synthesis. It is also anti-inflammatory. It remains the only licensed treatment for scalp ringworm in U.K. It is available in tablet or suspension form. The recommended dose, for those older than 1 month is 10 mg/kg per day. Taking the drug with fatty food increases absorption and aids bioavailability.[13,14] Dosage recommendations vary according to the formulation used, with higher doses being recommended by some authors for micronized griseofulvin as opposed to ultramicronized griseofulvin, but up to 25 mg/kg may be required. The duration of therapy depends on the organism (e.g. *T. tonsurans* infections may require prolonged treatment schedules) but varies between 8 and 10 weeks. (*Strength of recommendation = A; quality of evidence = IIii.*) Shorter courses may lead to higher relapse rates.

Side-effects include nausea and rashes in 8–15%. The drug is contra-indicated in pregnancy and the manufacturers caution against men fathering a child for 6 months after therapy. (*Strength of recommendation = B; quality of evidence = III.*)

Advantages. Licensed; inexpensive; syrup formulation is more palatable; suspension allows accurate dosage adjustments in children; and extensive experience.

Disadvantages: Prolonged treatment required.

Contra-indicated in lupus erythematosus, porphyria and severe liver disease.

Drug interactions. Include warfarin, cyclosporin and the oral contraceptive pill.

Terbinafine. This acts on fungal cell membranes and is fungicidal. It is effective against all dermatophytes. It is not yet licensed for tinea capitis, although a licence for children of > 2 years is being considered. It is at least as effective as griseofulvin and is safe for the management of scalp ringworm due to *Trichophyton* sp. in children.[15–17] Its role in management of *Microsporum* sp. is debatable.[18] Early evidence suggests that higher doses or longer therapy (> 4 weeks) may be required in microsporum infections.[19,20] Dosage depends on the weight of the patient, but lie between 3 and 6 mg/kg per day (see Table 2). Side-effects include; gastro-intestinal disturbances and rashes in 5% and 3% of cases, respectively.[21] (*Strength of recommendation = A/B; quality of evidence = I/IIi.*)

Advantages. Fungicidal so shorter therapy required (cf. griseofulvin) so increased compliance more likely.

Disadvantages. No suspension formulation and no U.K. licence for tinea capitis.

Drug interactions. Plasma concentrations are reduced by rifampicin and increased by cimetidine.

Itraconazole. Itraconazole exhibits both fungistatic and fungicidal activity depending on the concentration of drug in the tissues, but like other azoles, the primary mode of action is fungistatic, through depletion of cell membrane ergosterol, which interferes with membrane permeability. 100 mg/day for 4 weeks or 5 mg/kg per day in children is as effective as griseofulvin[22] and terbinafine.[23] (*Strength of recommendation = B; quality of evidence = I.*) Small studies suggest that shorter or pulsed regimens may also be effective.[24] (*Strength of recommendation = B; quality of evidence = I.*) Itraconazole is currently unlicensed in the U.K. for use in tinea capitis and for use in children and there are no plans to change this.

Advantage. Pulsed shorter treatment regimens are possible.

Disadvantage. Lack of U.K. licence to treat tinea capitis and possible side-effects. Potential drug interactions. More studies needed to confirm paediatric requirements.

Drug interactions. Enhanced toxicity of anticoagulants (warfarin), antihistamines (terfenadine and astemizole), antipsychotics (sertindole), anxiolytics (midazolam), digoxin, cisapride, cyclosporin and simvastatin (increased risk of myopathy). Reduced efficacy of itraconazole with concomitant use of H_2-blockers, phenytoin and rifampacin.

Fluconazole. Has occasionally been assessed for tinea capitis but its use has mainly been limited by side-effects. Doses of 3–5 mg/kg per day for 4 weeks are effective in children with tinea capitis.[25] There are no large published series of its use and it is not licensed for the treatment of tinea capitis in the U.K. (*Strength of recommendation = C; quality of evidence = I.*)

Ketoconazole. Has occasionally been assessed for tinea capitis but its use has mainly been limited by side-effects. Doses of between 3·3 and 6·6 mg/kg per day. Resolution is comparable with griseofulvin but the response may be slower. However, side-effects are arguably sufficiently significant to lead to the recommendation by some authors that it should not to be used in children.[26] Studies have not shown it to be consistently superior to griseofulvin and its use in children is limited by hepatotoxicity. Not licensed for the treatment of tinea capitis in the U.K. (*Strength of recommendation = D; quality of evidence = I.*)

Additional measures

Exclusion from school. Although there is a risk of the transmission of infection from patients to unaffected class-mates, for practical reasons children should be allowed to return to school once they have been commenced on appropriate systemic and adjuvant topical therapy.[3,12] (*Strength of recommendation = B; quality of evidence IIiii.*)

Familial screening. Index cases due to the anthropophilic *T. tonsurans* are highly infectious. Family members[27] as well as other close contacts should be screened (both for tinea capitis and corporis) and appropriate mycological samples taken preferably using the brush technique, even in the absence of clinical signs. (*Strength of recommendation = B; quality of evidence = III.*)

Cleansing of fomites. Viable spores have been isolated from hairbrushes and combs. For all anthropophilic species these should be cleansed with disinfectant.[28] (*Strength of recommendation = B; quality of evidence = IV.*) Proprietary phenolic disinfectants are no longer available, but simple bleach or Milton should be suitable alternatives. (*Strength of recommendation = B; quality of evidence = III.*)

Soaking off crust from kerions or pustules. This is recommend by some authors. Although this is not necessary, it is often soothing.[29] (*Strength of recommendation = C; quality of evidence III.*)

Steroids. The use of corticosteroids (both oral and topical) for inflammatory varieties, e.g. kerions and severe id reactions is controversial, but may help to reduce itching and general discomfort.[30] Although in the past steroids have been thought to minimize the risk of permanent alopecia secondary to scarring, current evidence does not suggest any reduction in clearance time compared with griseofulvin alone.[29,30] (*Strength of recommendation = C; quality of evidence = I.*)

Treatment failures

Some individuals are not clear at follow-up. The reasons for this include:

1 Lack of compliance with the long courses of treatment.
2 Suboptimal absorption of the drug.
3 Relative insensitivity of the organism.
4 Reinfection.

T. tonsurans and *Microsporum* sp. are typical culprits in persistently positive cases. If fungi can still be isolated at the end of treatment, but the clinical signs have improved, the authors recommend continuing the original treatment for a further month.

If there has been no clinical response and signs persist at the end of the treatment period, then the options include:

1 Increase the dose or duration of the original drug: both griseofulvin (in doses up to 25 mg/kg for 8–10 weeks) and terbinafine have been used successfully and safely at higher doses or for longer courses to clear resistant infections. (*Strength of recommendation = C; quality of evidence = IV.*)
2 Change to an alternative antifungal, e.g. switch from

griseofulvin to terbinafine or itraconazole. (*Strength of recommendation = C; quality of evidence = IV.*)

Carriers

The optimal management of symptom-free carriers (i.e. individuals without overt clinical infection, but who are culture positive) is unclear. In those with a heavy growth/high spore count on brush culture, systemic antifungal therapy may be justified as these individuals are especially likely to develop an overt clinical infection, are a significant reservoir of infection[3] and are unlikely to respond to topical therapy alone.[5,31] Alternatively, they may represent a missed overt clinical infection. For those with light growth/low spore counts on brush culture, twice weekly selenium sulphide or povidone iodine shampoo is probably adequate.[11,12] (*Strength of recommendation = B; quality of evidence = IV.*)

Follow-up

The definitive end-point for adequate treatment is not clinical response but mycological cure; therefore, follow-up with repeat mycology sampling is recommended at the end of the standard treatment period and then monthly until mycological clearance is documented. (*Strength of recommendation = A.*) Treatment should, therefore, be tailored for each individual patient according to response.

Acknowledgments

Thanks to G.Midgley for advice on mycology.

References

1 Bronson DM, Desai DR, Barsky S, McMillen Foley S. An epidemic of infection with *Trichophyton tonsurans* revealed in a 20-year survey of fungal infections I Chicago. *J Am Acad Dermatol* 1983; **8**: 322–30.

2 Fuller LC, Child FC, Higgins EM. Tinea capitis in southeast London: an outbreak of *Trichophyton tonsurans* infection. *Br J Dermatol* 1997; **136**: 139.

3 Hay RJ, Clayton YM, de Silva N, Midgley G, Rosser E. Tinea capitis in south east London—a new pattern of infection with public health implication. *Br J Dermatol* 1996; **135**: 955–8.

4 Leeming JG, Elliott TSJ. The emergence of *Trichophyton tonsurans* tinea capitis in Birmingham, U.K. *Br J Dermatol* 1995; **133**: 929–31.

5 Williams JV, Honig PJ, McGinley KJ, Leyden JJ. Semiquantitative study of tinea capitis and asymptomatic carrier state in inner-city school children. *Pediatrics* 1995; **96**: 265–7.

6 Kligman AM, Constant ER. Family epidemic of tinea capitis due to *Trichophyton tonsurans* (variety sulfureum). *Arch Dermatol* 1951; **63**: 493–9.

7 Borchers SW. Moistened gauze technique to aid diagnosis of tinea capitis. *J Am Acad Dermatol* 1985; **13**: 672–3.

8 Head ES, Henry JC, Macdonald EM. The cotton swab technique for the culture of dermatophyte infections—its efficacy and merit. *J Am Acad Dermatol* 1984; **11**: 797–801.

9 Fuller LC, Child FJ, Midgely G, Hay RJ, Higgins EM A practical method for mycological diagnosis of tinea capitis: validation of the toothbrush technique. *J Eur Acad Dermatol Venereol* 1997; **9** (Suppl. 1): S209.

10 Elewski BE. Cutaneous mycoses in children. *Br J Dermatol* 1996; **134** (Suppl.46): 7–11.

11 Allen HB, Honig PJ, Leyden JJ, McGinley KJ. Selenium sulphide: adjunctive therapy for tinea capitis. *Pediatrics* 1982; **69**: 81–3.

12 Neil G, Hanslo D. Control of the carrier state of scalp dermatophytes. *Pediatr Infect Dis J* 1990; **9**: 57–8.

13 Anonymous. *Alder Hey Book of Children's Doses*, 6th edn. Liverpool: Royal Liverpool Children's Hospital Academy, 1994

14 Crounse RG. Human pharmacology of Griseofulvin: the effect of fat intake on gastrointestinal absorption. *J Invest Dermatol* 1961; **37**: 529–33.

15 Hussain H. Randomised double blind controlled comparative study of terbinafine versus griseofulvin in tinea capitis. *J Dermatol Treat* 1995; **6**: 167–9.

16 Jones TC. Overview of the use of terbinafine (Lamisil) in children. *Br J Dermatol* 1995; **132**: 683–9.

17 Filho ST, Cuce LC, Foss NT, Marques SA, Santamaria JR. Efficacy, safety and tolerability of terbinafine for tinea capitis in children: Brazilian multicentric study with daily oral tablets for, 1, 2 and 4 weeks. *J Eur Acad Dermatol Venereol* 1998; **11**: 141–6.

18 Baudrez-Rosselet F, Monod M, Jaccoud S, Frenk E. Efficacy of terbinafine treatment of tinea capitis in children varies according to the dermatophyte species. *Br J Dermatol* 1996; **135**: 1011–12.

19 Mock M, Monod M, Baudraz-Rosselet F, Panizzon RG. Tinea capitis dermatophytes: susceptibility to antifungal drugs tested *in vitro* and *in vivo*. *Dermatology* 1998; **197**(4): 361–7.

20 Bruckbauer HR, Hofman H. Systemic antifungal treatment of children with terbinafine. *Dermatology* 1997; **195**: 134–6.

21 O'Sullivan DP, Needham CA, Bangs A *et al*. Post marketing surveillance of oral terbinafine in UK. report of large cohort study. *Br J Clin Pharmacol* 1996; **42**: 559–65.

22 Lopez Gomez S, Del-Palacio A, Van-Cutsem J *et al*. Itraconazole verses Griseofulvin in the treatment of tinea capitis: a double blind randomized study in children. *Int J Dermatol* 1994; **33**(10): 743–7.

23 Jahangir M, Hussain I, Ul Hasan M, Haroon TS. A double-blind randomized comparative trial of itraconazole versus terbinafine for 2 weeks in tinea capitis. *Br J Dermatol* 1998; **139**: 672–4.

24 Gupta AK, Alexis ME, Raboobee N *et al*. Itraconazole pulse therapy is effective in the treatment of tinea capitis in children: an open multicentre study. *Br J Dermatol* 1997; **137**: 251–4.

25 Solomon BA, Collins R, Sharma R *et al*. Fluconazole for the treatment of tinea capitis in children. *J Am Acad Dermatol* 1997; **37**: 274–5.

26 Gan VN, Petruska M, Ginsburg CM. Epidemiology and treatment of tinea capitis. ketoconazole vs griseofulvin. *Paediatr Infect Dis J* 1987; **6**: 46–9.

27 Babel DE, Baughman SA. Evaluation of the adult carrier state in juvenile tinea capitis caused by *Trichophyton tonsurans*. *J Am Acad Dermatol* 1989; **21**: 1209–12.

28 Mackenzie DWR. Hairbrush diagnosis in detection and

eradication of non-fluorescent scalp ringworm. *Br Med J* 1963;
10: 363–5.

29 Anonymous. Management of scalp ringworm. *Drug Ther Bull*
1996 Jan; **34** (1): 5–6.

30 Honig PJ, Caputo GL, Leyden JJ, McGinley K, Selbst SM,
McGravey AR. Treatment of kerions. *Pediatr Dermatol* 1994;
11: 69–71.

31 Midgley G, Clayton YM. Distribution of dermatophytes and
candida spores in the environment. *Br J Dermatol* 1972; **86**:
69–77.

Appendix

Strength of recommendations

A There is good evidence to support the use of the
procedure.

B There is fair evidence to support the use of the
procedure.

C There is poor evidence to support the use of
the procedure.

D There is fair evidence to support the rejection of
the use of the procedure.

E There is good evidence to support the rejection of the
use of the procedure.

Quality of evidence

I Evidence obtained from at least one properly
designed, randomized control trial.

II-i Evidence obtained from well designed, controlled
trials without randomization.

II-ii Evidence obtained from well designed cohort or
case–control analytical studies, preferably from more
than one centre or research group.

II-iii Evidence obtained from multiple time series with
or without the intervention. Dramatic results in
uncontrolled experiments (e.g. the introduction of
penicillin treatment in the 1940s) could also be
regarded as this type of evidence.

III Opinions of respected authorities based on clinical
experience, descriptive studies or reports of expert
committees.

IV Evidence inadequate owing to problems of
methodology (e.g. sample size, length or comprehensiveness of follow-up or conflicts of evidence)

http://bad.org.uk/Portals/_Bad/Guidelines/Clinical
%20Guidelines/Tinea%20Capitis.pdf

Comment

Updated information, since the BAD guidelines [1] were
published, has been provided by the Cochrane review in
2007 [2]. The Cochrane review confirms that the newer
antifungal agents such as terbinafine are as effective as
griseofulvin. The advantage of the newer agents is that
shorter courses can be given; however, paediatric preparations are not always available and are usually more expensive. With greater migration and ease of air travel, more
exotic (rarer) forms of scalp ringworm are being seen
in Europe [3, 4]. Fortunately, they seem to respond to
terbinafine [5].

REFERENCES

1 Higgins EM, Fuller LC, Smith CH. Guidelines for the management of tinea capitis. *Brit J Dermatol* 2000; 143: 53–8.
2 González U, Seaton T, Bergus G, Jacobson J, Martínez-
Monzón C. Systemic antifungal therapy for tinea capitis in
children. *Cochrane Database Syst Rev* 2007; Issue 4: CD004685
(http://mrw.interscience.wiley.com/cochrane/clsysrev/articles/
CD004685/frame.html).
3 Alexander CL, Brown L, Shankland GS. Epidemiology of fungal scalp infections in the West of Scotland 2000–2006. *Scott
Med J* 2009; 54: 13–16.
4 Fuller LC. Changing face of tinea capitis in Europe. *Curr Opin
Infect Dis* 2009; 22: 115–18.
5 Ghannoum MA, Wraith LA, Cai B, *et al*. Susceptibility
of dermatophyte isolates obtained from a large worldwide
terbinafine tinea capitis clinical trial. *Brit J Dermatol* 2008;
159: 711–13.

Additional professional resources

Fungal skin infection – scalp. Clinical Knowledge
Summary 2009. http://www.cks.nhs.uk/fungal_skin_
infection_scalp.
Tinea capitis in the United Kingdom: a report on
its diagnosis, management and prevention. Health
Protection Agency 2007. http://www.hpa.org.uk/web/
HPAwebFile/HPAweb_C/1194947321499.
Fuller LC, Child FJ, Midgley G, Higgins EM. Diagnosis
and management of scalp ringworm. *Brit Med J* 2003;
326: 539–41.

Other patient resources

http://www.patient.co.uk/pdf/pilsL500.pdf

3 Neoplasms

With an ageing population and ease of travel to sunnier climes, skin cancer management is an increasing part of a dermatologist's workload [1,2]. Therefore, it is essential that care be given in the most efficient and effective ways in order not to waste valuable medical resources and to give swift reassurance or treatment to patients. Patient satisfaction runs high in skin cancer clinics as they receive appointments within 2 weeks of referral and are very relieved that they are not suffering from skin cancer. Cancer networks and multidisciplinary teams (MDTs) composed of dermatologists, plastic surgeons, oncologists and pathologists have probably improved adherence to guidance and improved standards. A recent study has shown that primary care management of skin cancers was poor compared with the management of skin cancers by dermatologists in secondary care [3]. Their data presented a strong case for dermatologists to retain the responsibility for diagnosing skin lesions, and to continue to provide the lead in selection and execution of dermatological surgical procedures.

REFERENCES

1 Hoey SEH, Devereux CEJ, Murray L, *et al.* Skin cancer trends in Northern Ireland and consequences for provision of dermatology services. *Brit J Dermatol* 2007; 156: 1301–7.
2 Benton EC, Kerr OA, Fisher A, *et al.* The changing face of dermatological practice: 25 years' experience. *Brit J Dermatol* 2008; 159: 413–18.
3 Goulding JMR, Levine S, Blizard RA, *et al.* Dermatological surgery: a comparison of activity and outcomes in primary and secondary care. *Brit J Dermatol* 2009; 161: 110–14.

ADDITIONAL PROFESSIONAL RESOURCES AND REFERENCES

Uncertainties and recommendations for research. http://www.library.nhs.uk/duets/SearchResults.aspx?catID=14863.

Guidance on cancer services: improving outcomes for people with skin tumours including melanoma – the manual. NICE, 2006. http://www.nice.org.uk/nicemedia/pdf/CSG_Skin_Manual.pdf.

Manual for Cancer Services, 2008: skin measures. UK Department of Health. http://www.dh.gov.uk/en/Healthcare/Cancer/index.htm?IdcService=GET_FILE&dID=176743&Rendition=Web.

Referral guidelines for suspected cancer. NICE, 2005, pp 34–6. http://www.nice.org.uk/nicemedia/pdf/cg027niceguideline.pdf.

Skin cancer – suspected. Clinical Knowledge Summaries 2009. http://www.cks.nhs.uk/skin_cancer_suspected.

Minimum dataset for the histopathological reporting of common skin cancers. Royal College of Pathologists 2002. http://www.rcpath.org/resources/pdf/skincancers2802.pdf.

National Comprehensive Cancer Network (USA) (requires free registration). http://www.nccn.org/.

Skin cancer evidence collection. NHS evidence – cancer (regularly updated systematic review). http://www.library.nhs.uk/skin/ViewResource.aspx?resID=122061&tabID=289&catID=9775.

Saraiya M, Glanz K, Briss PA, *et al.* Interventions to prevent skin cancer by reducing exposure to ultraviolet radiation: a systematic review. *Am J Prevent Med* 2004; 27: 422–66.

Preventing skin cancer: findings of the task force on community preventive services on reducing exposure to ultraviolet light. Centers for Disease Control and Prevention 2003. http://www.cdc.gov/mmwr/preview/mmwrhtml/rr5215a1.htm.

Screening for skin cancer. Agency for Health Care Policy and Research, USA 2009. http://www.uspreventive servicestaskforce.org/uspstf/uspsskca.htm.

Photodynamic therapy for non-melanoma skin tumours (including premalignant and primary non-metastatic skin lesions). NICE 2006. http://www.nice.org.uk/nicemedia/pdf/ip/IPG155guidance.pdf.

GENERAL PATIENT INFORMATION ON SKIN CANCERS AND TREATMENTS

http://www.cks.nhs.uk/patient_information_leaflet/cancer_of_the_skin

http://www.dermnetnz.org/lesions/ (includes benign lesions and self-examination)

http://www.cancerresearchuk.org

http://www.cancerbackup.org.uk

http://www.cancerhelp.org.uk

http://www.patient.co.uk/pdf/pilsL726.pdf (preventing skin cancer)

http://www.cancerbackup.org.uk/Cancertype/Skin/Treatment/Cryotherapy

http://www.cancerbackup.org.uk/Cancertype/Skin/Treatment/Radiotherapy

http://www.cancerbackup.org.uk/Cancertype/Skin/Treatment/Photodynamictherapy

Guidelines for the management of actinic keratoses

D. de Berker, J.M. McGregor* and B.R. Hughes† on behalf of the British Association of Dermatologists
Therapy Guidelines and Audit Subcommittee

Bristol Dermatology Centre, Bristol Royal Infirmary, Bristol BS2 8HW, U.K.

*Department of Dermatology, St Bartholomew's and the London NHS Trust, London E1 1BB, U.K.

†Portsmouth Dermatology Centre, St Mary's Hospital, Milton Road, Portsmouth PO3 6AD, U.K.

Summary

These guidelines stemmed from a consensus meeting held by the British Photo-biology Group (BPG) in 1999. Following this meeting one of the authors (J.M.M.) was invited to draw up guidelines for the management of actinic keratoses by the British Association of Dermatologists Therapy Guidelines and Audit Subcommittee. Relevant evidence was sought using the search terms 'solar keratosis' and 'actinic keratosis' in Medline from 1966 onwards. Additional and earlier literature was reviewed on the basis of references within post-1966 publications. All articles of apparent relevance were reviewed independently of the nature of the publication. The quality of the evidence elicited has been indicated. The National Ambulatory Medical Care Survey (U.S.A.) was used for further data on topical chemotherapy. Papers were reviewed and discussed by the contributors to the BPG Workshop (see Acknowledgments). Recommendations are evidence based where possible. Strength of recommendation is coupled with quality of evidence. Strength of recommendation includes consideration of apparent cost-benefit and practical considerations. Quality of evidence reflects the nature of the trial structure that provides data of efficacy.

Disclaimer

These guidelines have been prepared for dermatologists on behalf of the British Association of Dermatologists (BAD) and reflect the best data available at the time the report was prepared. Caution should be exercised in interpreting the data; the results of future studies may require alteration of the conclusions or recommendations in this report. It may be necessary or even desirable to depart from the guidelines in the interests of specific patients and special circumstances. Just as adherence to the guidelines may not constitute defence against a claim of negligence, so deviation from them should not necessarily be deemed negligent.

Methodology

These guidelines stemmed from a consensus meeting held by the British Photobiology Group (BPG) in 1999. Following this meeting one of the authors (J.M.M.) was invited to draw up guidelines for the management of actinic keratoses (AKs) by the BAD Therapy Guidelines and Audit Subcommittee. Medline (1966–2004) was the main source of references for this review. Relevant evidence was sought using the search terms 'solar keratosis' and 'actinic keratosis'. Additional and earlier literature was reviewed on the basis of references within post-1966 publications. All articles of apparent relevance were reviewed independently of the nature of the publication. The National Ambulatory Medical Care Survey (U.S.A.) was used for further data on topical chemotherapy. Papers were reviewed and discussed by the contributors to the BPG Workshop (see Acknowledgments).

Definition and introduction to the guideline

Actinic (syn. solar) keratoses are keratotic lesions occurring on chronically light-exposed adult skin. They represent focal areas of abnormal keratinocyte proliferation and differentiation that carry a low risk of progression to invasive squamous cell carcinoma (SCC). A spectrum of histology is seen but the cardinal feature of an AK is epithelial dysplasia. This may be restricted to the basal layer or may extend to full-thickness atypia at which point differentiation from Bowen's disease can be difficult. There is disorderly arrangement and maturation of epithelial cells. Multiple buds of epithelial cells may occur at the membrane zone but no invasion is seen. Histological variants of AK have been described, including hypertrophic, bowenoid, lichenoid, acantholytic and pigmented.

AKs are widely considered to be premalignant lesions with low individual potential for invasive malignancy and higher potential for spontaneous regression. They present as discrete, sometimes confluent, patches of erythema and scaling on predominantly sun-exposed skin, usually in middle-aged and elderly individuals. They are often asymptomatic but may occasionally be sore or itch. Lesions may be single or multiple. The epidemiology, risk factors, disease associations and demographics of the 'at-risk' population are all pertinent to patient management. They are discussed together with the available treatment options.

Epidemiology

Evidence suggests that most AKs are the result of chronic exposure to ultraviolet (UV) radiation. They occur predominantly on chronically sun-exposed skin, such as that of the face and dorsa of hands, in fair-skinned individuals.[1] In addition, UVB-specific p53 mutations have been demonstrated in AKs, providing molecular evidence in support of a role for sunlight.[2] There is a high prevalence in those receiving chronic immunosuppression

Table 1 Factors determining choice of active therapy from six main alternatives. The scoring is based on the authors' evaluation of efficacy, ease of use, morbidity and cost-benefit

	Cryosurgery	5-FU	Diclofenac	Imiquimod[a]	Curettage	PDT	Comments
Main characteristic of AKs							
Low number of AKs	••••	••••	••	••	•	•	
High number of AKs	•••	••••	•••	•••	•	•••	
Thin AKs	•••	••••	•••	•••	•	••	Thin lesions may not always require treatment
Hypertrophic AKs	••	•	•	•	••••	•	Histology may be required. Formal excision may be preferred
Isolated lesions failing to respond to other therapies	••	•	•	•	••••	•	Histology may be required. Formal excision may be preferred
Confluent recalcitrant AKs, failing other treatments	•••	•••	•	•••	•	•••	Certain lesions within a resistant field may require histological assessment
Location							
Scalp, ears, nose, cheeks, forehead, perioral	••••	••••	•••	••••	•••	•••	
Periorbital	•••	•	•	•	•••	•••	Topical therapies can be difficult to use near mouth and eyes
Confluent scalp	•••	••••	•••	••••	•	••••	Pretreatment with 5% salicylic acid ointment may improve outcome
Below the knee	•••	•	••	•	••••	••••	Poor healing is a particular concern at this site. All modalities can lead to ulceration. Treatment may be combined with advice on elevation and compression bandaging where possible
Back of hands	••••	••••	••	•	•••	•••	Courses of topical therapy may need to be extended and pretreatment with 5% salicylic acid ointment may improve outcome
Characteristics of patient (rating may be considered in context of clinical need indicated by characteristic of AK and location)							
Medically dependent or senile	•••	••	•••	•	•	•••	Morbidity of treatment may dictate choice of modality
Self-reliant	•••	••••	•••	••••	•	•	5-FU may be repeated at sites of relapse or new lesions in primary care
One-off treatment	••••	••••	•	••••	•••	•••	
Lives far from hospital	•••	••••	•••	••••	–	–	May favour treatment that allows monitoring in primary care
Part of continuous management plan	••••	••••	•••	•	•	•••	

5-FU, 5-fluorouracil; PDT, photodynamic therapy; AKs, actinic keratoses; ••••, good treatment; •••, fair treatment, ••, can be used depending on circumstances; •, rarely used in these circumstances. [a]Imiquimod is not currently licensed for use in the treatment of AKs.

as organ transplant recipients.[3] Other possible risk factors include exposure to arsenic[4,5] and chronic sun bed use.[6–8]

Incidence and prevalence

In Ireland and the U.K., 24%, 23% and 19% of individuals aged over 60 years were found to have at least one AK in studies from Galway, South Wales and Merseyside, respectively.[9–11] There was a linear increase in the prevalence with age (from 60 to 80 years) in men but not in women, and the rate of new AKs was estimated to be 149 per 1000 person-years.[10] AKs were also present in 3·6% of men aged between 40 and 49 years.[11]

Natural history: spontaneous regression and malignant transformation

Studies indicate a high spontaneous regression rate in the order of 15–25% for AKs over a 1-year period,[10,12] and a low rate of malignant transformation, less than one in 1000 per annum.[13] None the less, mathematical models derived from this study predict that for an individual with an average of 7·7 AKs, the probability of at least one transforming within a 10-year period is approximately 10%.[14]

When 918 adults (mean age 61 years) with AKs but no previous history of skin cancer were followed prospectively for 5 years, the incidence rate for basal cell carcinoma (BCC) and SCC was estimated at 4106 and 3198 per 100 000 person-years, respectively, representing a substantial excess incidence compared with the general population.[15] These data suggest that even though the risk of malignant transformation for any given AK is very low, the probability of an individual with AKs presenting subsequently with skin cancer is none the less high compared with the population at large.

Investigation and diagnosis

Patients with AKs may present to dermatologists in various circumstances: they may be referred by the general practitioner (GP) because of diagnostic uncertainty or concern about malignant risk or for further management, and AKs may be detected incidental to referral for another problem, or detected during follow up of a skin cancer patient. Diagnosis is frequently made on clinical appearance alone but as the differential diagnosis includes superficial BCC, Bowen's disease, invasive SCC and even amelanotic melanoma, a skin biopsy may be indicated in selected cases where there is clinical doubt or suspicion of invasive malignancy.

Management

Many options are open to patients with AKs. The natural history of individual lesions studied in the U.K. suggests that treatment is not universally required on the basis of preventing progression into SCC.[10] However, others feel that prevention of SCC is the main reason for therapy.[16]

Some AKs have histological features within the spectrum of in-situ skin cancer. They can also represent a cause of symptoms and disfigurement which may be the main determinant of treatment choices. Clinical judgement should discern which lesions are more likely to represent a risk to the patient's health, but where the likelihood is low, options include no therapy or palliation with emollient or keratolytic agent such as low-strength salicylic acid ointment.

Where active treatment is sought, many modalities of therapy are available (Table 1). Good-quality data on the outcome of these different therapies are available in only a few instances. Treatment of an individual lesion may have a therapeutic effect on surrounding skin, with an effect on overall progression of actinic damage, but this potential benefit has not been quantified. Given the low morbidity and risk of the majority of AKs, the *Strength of recommendation* (see Appendix 1) made for treatments by the authors has an element of cost-benefit and risk-benefit included. This is derived from clinical experience in addition to the published evidence.

No therapy (*Strength of recommendation A, quality of evidence II-ii*)

Harvey et al.[10] reported in a study of 560 individuals from Wales that 21% of AKs resolved spontaneously over a 12-month period and none progressed into SCC. Marks et al.[13] reported the evolution of AKs in an Australian cohort, where malignant transformation was quoted at 0·075–0·096% of AKs per year.

Topical therapies

- No therapy (*A, II-ii*) or emollient (*A, I*) is a reasonable option for mild AKs
- Sun block applied twice daily for 7 months may protect against development of AKs (*A, I*)
- 5-Fluorouracil cream used twice daily for 6 weeks is effective for up to 12 months in clearance of the majority of AKs. Due to side-effects of soreness, less aggressive regimens are often used, which may be effective, but have not been fully evaluated (*A, I*)
- Diclofenac gel has moderate efficacy with low morbidity in mild AKs. There are few follow-up data to indicate the duration of benefit (*B, I*)
- Imiquimod 5% cream is not licensed for AKs, but has been demonstrated to be effective over a 16-week course of treatment but only 8 weeks of follow up. By weight, it is 19 times the cost of 5-fluorouracil. They have similar side-effects (*B, I*)

Emollient (*Strength of recommendation A, quality of evidence I*)

There are no trials dedicated to the study of palliative therapy of AKs but emollient has been employed in the placebo arm of a double-blind trial of masoprocol cream.[17] Forty subjects were in the vehicle placebo group, with an average of 13·4 AKs each falling to 11·1 after 28 days of emollient twice a day. This represented improvement in the global evaluation score in 44% of subjects, with only 2·4% showing a deterioration. The vehicle limb of a randomized trial of diclofenac gel in hyaluronan vehicle described resolution of the target lesion in 44% of subjects using the vehicle after 60 days.[18] Follow-up data are lacking and it is likely that the treatment is managing the clinical manifestations of mild AKs rather than reversing biological processes.

Sun block (*Strength of recommendation A, quality of evidence I*)

Sun block has a combined emollient and photoprotective effect. A randomized placebo-controlled trial of sun block with factor 17 protection applied twice daily to the face for 7 months showed sun block to be superior to emollient in terms of total number of AKs and new lesions at the end of the trial.[19] A single daily application of sun block (sun protection factor 16) in Queensland, Australia, showed it to be superior to discretionary use of the same sun block over a 2-year period in the reduction of AKs.[20] A similar approach in the same setting also reduced the incidence of cutaneous SCCs.[21]

Salicylic acid ointment (*Strength of recommendation A, quality of evidence III*)

Salicylic acid ointment is sometimes used as a preliminary to topical 5-fluorouracil (5-FU) to remove overlying keratin. Fifty per cent salicylic acid in croton oil has been described as a treatment for AKs when used in combination with 20% tri-chloroacetic acid (TCA) and pretreatment with topical tretinoin as a serial regimen for facial peel.[22] Acting primarily as an emollient for mild keratoses[17,18] (see above under Emollient), it may provide a small additional benefit based on the keratolytic effect. Thus 2% salicylic acid ointment BP may be used for its combined emollient and mild keratolytic effects, either alone or as pretreatment for topical 5-FU.

5-Fluorouracil (*Strength of recommendation A, quality of evidence I*)

The majority of the data on topical therapies relates to 5-FU. A wide range of open trials, dose-ranging studies and manipulations of the vehicle has been reported over the last 35 years, as well as two randomized controlled trials (RCTs), confirming efficacy. 5-FU works by the inhibition of thymidylate synthetase, which is needed for DNA synthesis. It may also interfere with the formation and function of RNA.[23]

Nine of the trials were controlled, where a right/left comparison (n 6) was the most common design, but only five were randomized. Numbers in the studies were generally small, with a mean of 26 patients per trial and fewer than 15 patients in 50% of trials. Minimum follow up was 12 months or more in only two studies. Many open studies appeared to demonstrate the efficacy of 5-FU in a range of potencies and different vehicles in the treatment of AKs when used on the face twice daily for 3 weeks. Only two trials studied the use of 5-FU in the currently available formulation of a 5% cream in a well-constructed, controlled manner.[24,25] Kurwa et al.[25] examined the lesional area of AKs on the back of the hands before and after treatment with 5% 5-FU cream twice daily for 3 weeks in a randomized right/left comparison with a single treatment with photodynamic therapy (PDT). Of the 14 patients evaluable at 6 months, there was a mean reduction in lesional area of 70% (5-FU) and 73% (PDT), with no statistically significant difference between them. Open studies have suggested that this regimen is not sufficiently long for effective treatment of AKs on the hands,[26] but is adequate for those on the face.[24] Witheiler et al.[24] used 5% 5-FU cream on the face as control in a right/left comparison with a single application of Jessner's solution (14% lactic acid, 14% salicylic acid, 14% resorcinol in ethanol) followed by a 35% TCA peel. There was a mean reduction in AKs on both sides of the face from 18 to four (78% reduction with 5-FU and 79% reduction with TCA). This benefit was sustained for 12 months. The third follow up at 32 months demonstrated that the number of AKs had risen again to 10 (5-FU) and 15 (TCA) in the eight evaluable patients. These differences were not statistically significant.

The results of using the same formulation of 5-FU less frequently, but for prolonged periods, are conflicting. An open trial of 10 patients reported clearance of 96% of AKs after a mean of 6·7 weeks applying treatment twice daily, once or twice per week.[27] Six patients were followed for 9 months and showed an 86% clearance rate that was maintained. Epstein[28] followed this study with a similar protocol and sample size, except that evaluation was done by dermatologists given a series of photographs and blinded as to the sequence. Eight of 13 patients failed to show any improvement, with the conclusion that pulsing 5-FU over a period of < 10 weeks is not effective. The small numbers of patients in both these studies leave the matter unresolved. Five per cent 5-FU cream was used alone or in combination with topical tretinoin to the back of the hands at night for 3 months in a blinded right/left comparison with a 3-month follow-up period.[29] Both sides produced a reduction of > 70% in AKs, with a statistically significant advantage to the side treated with additional tretinoin.

Imiquimod 5% cream (*Strength of recommendation B, quality of evidence I*)

Imiquimod 5% cream is a topical immune response modifier. A small early RCT against vehicle placebo[30] demonstrated clearance rates of 84% when used up to three times per week for 12 weeks. There have been two RCTs[31,32] with regimens of three times per week for 16 weeks and follow up 8 weeks later. These have classified responses in terms of complete or partial (> 75%) clinical clearance or histological clearance.

Results indicated 47% of patients with complete clearance (vs. 7·2% with placebo) increasing to 64% when adding those with partial clearance (vs. 13·6% with placebo).[31] Histological responses were 57% (vs. 2·2% for placebo) and 72% (vs. 4·3% for placebo) for the same categories.[32] The side-effects are similar to 5-FU with severe erythema (30·6%), scabbing and crusting (29·9%) and erosions or ulceration (10·2%).[32] The extent of side-effects is not wholly predictable, with some patients manifesting an extreme reaction and others very little. The clinical response is largely in proportion to the side-effects and those terminating treatment early due to extreme soreness may still get a good response. There are limited long-term data on relapse after treatment. The product is not currently licensed for this indication and imiquimod is more expensive than 5-FU, gram for gram, by a factor of 19.[33]

Diclofenac gel (*Strength of recommendation B, quality of evidence I*)

There are two vehicle-controlled studies of 3% diclofenac in a 2·5% hyaluronic gel in the treatment of mild AKs. In the first, patients were treated for a mean of 60 days, with a resolution of 70% of target lesions in the treatment group in comparison with 44% in those using the vehicle.[18] In the second study treatment was for 90 days, with 50% of those using active treatment achieving a target lesion number score of zero, vs. 20% of those treated with vehicle alone (P < 0·001).[34] Assessment was limited to 30 days post-treatment in both studies. These data provide indication of moderate efficacy with low morbidity in mild AKs. Treatment was well tolerated and side-effects were mainly pruritus (41% estimated after 30 days of treatment) and rash (40% estimated after 60 days).[18]

Tretinoin cream (*Strength of recommendation B, quality of evidence I*)

Topical tretinoin cream has been studied at different concentrations. There is a dose response; Bollag and Ott[35] reported complete clearance of AKs in 55% of subjects treated with 0·3% ointment vs. 35% of subjects with the same response when using 0·1%. Misiewicz et al.[36] undertook a right/left comparison of tretinoin cream with arotinoid methyl sulphone on the face, revealing a reduction of AKs on the tretinoin-treated skin by 30·3% (P < 0·01) after twice-daily use for 16 weeks. At between 3 and 9 weeks there was a deterioration of clinical appearance to below baseline before benefit was seen. This reflects the potential benefit from currently available formulations of tretinoin. In a multicentre open trial, published in nonpeer-reviewed literature, there was a reduction of facial AKs from a mean of 11·2 to 8·9 (11% reduction) after 6 months' use of 0·05% once or twice daily (P = 0·001). This changed to a reduction by 47% after 15 months' use (P = 0·001).[37] These figures do not illustrate a significant advantage over emollient and sun block. The product is licensed for photodamage in the U.K., but not specifically for the treatment of AKs.

Masoprocol cream (*Strength of recommendation C, quality of evidence I*)

A single RCT for masoprocol[17] suggested that this reduced AKs to 71% of the baseline number after a 28-day course of therapy. There was only a 1-month follow-up period. The product is not available in the U.K.

In conclusion, there is good evidence that 5% 5-FU cream used twice daily for 3 weeks is effective at reducing AKs on the face and back of hands by about 70% for up to 12 months. There is insufficient RCT evidence to support or refute the efficacy of alternative regimens and formulations, although one RCT suggests that a single night-time application for 3 months for AKs on the back of the hands is effective.[29] Imiquimod has been more rigorously assessed with modern RCT design and may produce a similar pattern of side-effects and response to 5-FU. Diclofenac gel is a relatively mild agent that reduces the AK count but there are no follow-up data beyond 1 month. Topical tretinoin has some efficacy on the face, with partial clearance of AKs, but may need to be used for up to a year at a time to optimize benefit. Sun block, emollient and 2% salicylic acid ointment BP may reduce the AK count by a similar amount.

Other treatments

- Cryosurgery is effective for up to 75% of lesions in trials comparing it with photodynamic therapy. It may be particularly superior for thicker lesions, but may leave scars (A, I)
- Photodynamic therapy is effective in up to 91% of AKs in trials comparing it with cryotherapy, with consistently good cosmetic result. It may be particularly good for superficial and confluent AKs, but is likely to be more expensive than most other therapies. It is of particular value where AKs are numerous or when located at sites of poor healing such as the lower leg (B, I)
- There are no studies of curettage or excisional surgery, but both are of value in determining the exact histological nature of proliferative or atypical AKs unresponsive to other therapies, where invasive squamous cell carcinoma is possible

Surgery

There are no trials of surgical therapy for AKs. The nature of the pathology makes it likely that a surgical procedure able to remove an area of diseased skin represents an effective therapy. It is unlikely that this would be a first line of treatment unless there was diagnostic uncertainty. A curettage specimen may make it difficult to determine whether a lesion has an element of dermal invasion. In some instances a deep shave or formal excision with histological examination might be preferred. If curettage is used for a hyperkeratotic AK, it may be warranted to employ two or three cycles of therapy. This will ensure that if the histology is that of invasive SCC, or if it is equivocal, the curettage is likely to still represent adequate treatment. Exceptions would be where the size, histological type or location of an SCC would make curettage an unacceptable treatment.[38]

In the U.S.A., surgical therapies, including electrodesiccation, are the preferred treatment of AKs provided by dermatologists according to medical insurance data, where 75% are treated by 'either local excision or destruction of lesion or tissue'.[39]

Cryosurgery (*Strength of recommendation A, quality of evidence I*)

A randomized study comparing cryosurgery with PDT in 193 patients indicated an overall 75% complete response rate for cryosurgery in contrast to 69% in those treated with PDT at 3 months.[40] The differential success of the two therapies was more marked for thick lesions, with 69% showing complete response to cryosurgery vs. 52% to PDT. A double freeze–thaw cycle was used in this study in contrast to a single cycle which, when used in a different study, yielded a 68% response.[41]

Extensive cryosurgery over large areas has been referred to as cryopeeling and can be used for treating fields of AKs and background damage.[42] Cryosurgery has been described in combination with topical 5-FU, where the duration of treatment and consequent side-effects of both modalities could be reduced while maintaining efficacy.[43] No data were presented to support this method. Cryosurgery is a flexible therapy that requires skill in administration. With larger doses it is likely to result in loss of pigment and scarring. Patient counselling is important concerning short- and long-term side-effects.

Photodynamic therapy (*Strength of recommendation B, quality of evidence I*)

PDT requires a dedicated light source in combination with the application of a photosensitizing cream. Photosensitizing agents include 5-aminolaevulinic acid (5-ALA) and a methyl ester of 5-ALA, 5-methylaminolaevulinate. The BPG published guidelines for the use of PDT in 2002,[44] and concluded that optimal irradiance, wavelength and dose for the treatment of AKs have yet to be established. For most situations, superficial crust or keratin is first removed with light curettage and the photosensitizing cream then applied under occlusion for 3 h prior to irradiation. Treatment can be painful but the BPG guidelines[44] describe the treatment as intrinsically safe.

Response rates to two cycles of PDT mainly on the scalp and face range from 69% to 91% in three randomized trials.[40,41,45] Studies had a 3[40,45] to 4[41] month follow-up period. In two studies where comparison was made with cryotherapy, one showed a higher clearance rate for cryotherapy (69% PDT vs. 75% cryotherapy)[40] and one showed a lower clearance rate

(91% PDT vs. 68% cryotherapy).[41] Cryotherapy appeared to be superior for thicker lesions (PDT response 52·2% vs. cryotherapy 69%) and lesions of the face and scalp (PDT response 75·8% vs. cryotherapy 91·7%). Local adverse reactions were reported by 44% of those receiving PDT and 26% of those given cryotherapy, although the cosmetic outcome in all studies was consistently rated higher by patients for PDT (98%) than for cryotherapy (91%).[40]

A right/left comparison of AK treatment on the back of the hands by PDT and 5-FU showed a similar response to both therapies,[25] clearing 73% and 70%, respectively. Responses remained similar at 6 months.

The cost-effectiveness of PDT is not established but its use is likely to be limited by the cost of the photosensitizing cream.

Laser, chemical peels and dermabrasion (*Strength of recommendation C, quality of evidence III*)

In principle, carbon dioxide laser or other destructive energy sources should be able to treat AKs.[46] Chemical peels and dermabrasion should have a similar effect, where skin is destroyed to a controlled depth. Spira *et al.*[47] reported a poorly controlled comparison of AKs of the face treated with a phenolic peel, dermabrasion or topical 5-FU. All therapies worked initially, but patients developed further AKs within a month of treatment with phenolic peel, within 6 months of dermabrasion and some time after 6 months following 5-FU. The nonblinded right/left comparison by Witheiler *et al.*[24] of a 35% TCA peel and 5-FU on the face suggested that they were of similar efficacy, with improvement sustained up to 12 months, waning considerably by 32 months. TCA can be combined with 70% glycolic acid[48] or with manual dermabrasion with silicon carbide sandpaper.[49]

In an open study of facial dermabrasion alone, 22 of 23 subjects (96%) remained free of AKs at 1 year and the mean period to development of a further AK was 4·5 years.[50] Treatment of scalp actinic damage and keratoses with dermabrasion has been reported as effective.[51]

Systemic retinoids (*Strength of recommendation B, quality of evidence I*)

Systemic retinoids have been assessed for their potential role in suppression or treatment of multiple AKs. Early studies employed etretinate and demonstrated in double-blind crossover trials the efficacy of this drug.[52] Anecdotal evidence over the last 20 years suggests that there can be some considerable morbidity employing this treatment. In addition, there may be a rebound effect once the systemic therapy is stopped. However, these effects were not observed at 4 months follow up in the one available report on this subject.[53]

Use of systemic retinoid may be justified in very high-risk patients, such as organ transplant recipients, where there is a presumed increased risk of progression from AK to SCC.[54] Low-dose acitretin is currently given as a treatment option in

'European best practice guidelines' for renal transplant patients with multiple dysplastic skin lesions.[55]

Site-specific treatments

The data from available treatments indicate that some treatments are more adaptable than others and that morbidity varies with location. The balance of issues determined by location, characteristics of the AKs and nature of the patient are summarized in Table 1. The scoring is based on the authors' evaluation of efficacy, ease of use, morbidity and cost-benefit.

Other considerations

Should actinic keratoses be treated?

There is inadequate evidence to justify treatment of all AKs to try to prevent malignant change. Treatment should be considered on an individual basis according to signs, symptoms and history. There will be instances where excision is undertaken for diagnostic purposes.

Overall, the data comparing individual treatments are not good enough to justify making a single recommendation. Decisions for an individual patient will be based on the clinical presentation, the efficacy, morbidity, availability and cost of relevant treatments and patient preference.

However, treatment of small numbers of AKs with cryotherapy is currently widely practised by dermatologists, while more extensive AKs are commonly treated with 5-FU. Due to expense and inconvenience PDT is probably best reserved for patients with extensive AKs that cannot be controlled with other therapies.

Is there a role for prevention and what works?

AKs are a marker for sun damage and therefore are an indication to increase sun-avoidance measures. There is some evidence that regular use of sunscreen reduces the number of AKs[19,20] and the risk of SCC.[21]

Should patients with actinic keratoses have follow up?

There are no data concerning the benefit of follow up in patients with AKs. Patients and their carers should be educated regarding changes that suggest malignancy. Those at high risk of nonmelanoma skin cancer, e.g. organ transplant recipients, may warrant follow up; the presence of numerous AKs is an indicator of this risk.

Are there high-risk groups and is their management different?

Patients with multiple and confluent AKs are likely to be at higher risk of nonmelanoma skin cancer, particularly patients with organ transplants who are estimated to have 50–100 times the risk of an age- and sex-matched control population.[56,57] Anecdotal and limited trial data suggest that treatments for AKs in transplant patients are less effective than in the general population,[58] perhaps because AKs are more proliferative and hyperkeratotic in this group, or because new lesions rapidly appear in the treated site. One study in transplant recipients failed to demonstrate a reduction in the development of subsequent skin cancers in those areas of skin previously treated for AKs with PDT.[57]

Cost-benefit of treatment

Most AKs result in few or no symptoms and are not dangerous. Where there is a wide range of treatments it is necessary to balance the benefits of treatment against side-effects. In many health care systems this calculation will have some element of cost-benefit, where the cost is to the state and the indication must justify the expense. These guidelines are not able to give details on the complex matter of cost-benefit, but it is apparent that some treatments are considerably more expensive than others. Where outcomes are comparable and morbidity of treatment tolerable, we have tended to give a higher strength of recommendation to the cheaper treatment or one that is more easily used in primary care.

Summary of recommendations

AKs represent a spectrum of clinical complaint and pathology. Most patients can be diagnosed and managed in primary care. In many instances, management may entail little or no medical treatment other than advice on sun avoidance and self-monitoring. Where there is clinical concern or the patient specifically wants treatment, cryosurgery or one of the many topical therapies can be employed taking into consideration the specifics of the situation. If there is diagnostic concern or failure to respond to first-line treatment, a histological specimen, such as obtained at curettage with cautery or formal excision, may be both diagnostic and curative. Where AKs are multiple or confluent, at sites of poor healing or with poor response to standard therapies, PDT may be helpful. Such patients may also warrant long-term follow up for the associated increased risk of nonmelanoma skin cancer.

Audit points

AKs are a biological marker of sun damage and hence patients with AKs are at a greater risk of skin cancer than those with no AKs. Patients with AKs need to be educated on self-monitoring and the need to seek a medical opinion if they detect new lesions or changes in old lesions on their skin.

• Evidence that the patient was provided with information about AKs and sun damage
• Evidence that the patient is adequately informed concerning the nature of any treatment when given
• Evidence that the GP is provided with advice concerning how to evaluate and manage further AKs when they develop

- Evidence that high-risk patients and their GPs are aware of their status. This includes organ transplant recipients, those with multiple large AKs or previous SCCs. Such patients need a low threshold of referral for lesions of an actinic nature or unclear diagnosis.

Acknowledgments

Contributions towards this were made by the British Photobiology Group, London, 1999: Dan Creamer, Jane McGregor, David de Berker, Colin Morton, David Bilsland, Kevin McKenna, Helene du Peloux-Menagé and Charlotte Proby.

References

1 Freeman RG. Carcinogenic effect of solar radiation and prevention measures. *Cancer* 1968; **21**:11114–20.

2 Zeigler A, Jonason AS, Leffell DJ et al. Sunburn and p53 in the onset of skin cancer. *Nature* 1994; **372**:773–6.

3 Barr BB, Benton EC, McLaren K et al. Papillomavirus infection and skin cancer in renal allograft recipients. *Lancet* 1989; **ii**:224–5.

4 Baudouin C, Charveron M, Tarroux R, Gall Y. Environmental pollutants and skin cancer. *Cell Biol Toxicol* 2002; **18**:341–8.

5 Wong ST, Chan HL, Teo SK. The spectrum of cutaneous and internal malignancies in chronic arsenic toxicity. *Singapore Med J* 1998; **39**:171–3.

6 Norris JF. Sun-screens, suntans and skin cancer. Local councils should remove sunbeds from leisure centres. *BMJ* 1996; **313**:941–2.

7 Bajdik CD, Gallagher RP, Astrakianakis G et al. Non-solar ultraviolet radiation and the risk of basal and squamous cell skin cancer. *Br J Cancer* 1996; **73**:1612–14.

8 Roest MA, Keane FM, Agnew K et al. Multiple squamous cell carcinomas following excess sunbed use. *J R Soc Med* 2001; **94**:636–7.

9 O'Beirn SFO, Judge P, Maccon CF, Martin CF. Skin cancer in County Galway, Ireland. In: *Proceedings of the Sixth National Cancer Conference*, sponsored by the American Cancer Society Inc. and the National Cancer Institute, September 1968. Philadelphia: Lippincott, 1970: 489–500.

10 Harvey I, Frankel S, Marks R et al. Non-melanoma skin cancer and solar keratoses. 1. Methods and descriptive results of the South Wales skin cancer study. *Br J Cancer* 1996; **74**:1302–7.

11 Memon AA, Tomenson JA, Bothwell J, Friedmann PS. Prevalence of solar damage and actinic keratosis in a Merseyside population. *Br J Dermatol* 2000; **142**:1154–9.

12 Marks R, Foley P, Goodman G et al. Spontaneous remission of solar keratoses: the case for conservative management. *Br J Dermatol* 1986; **155**:649–55.

13 Marks R, Rennie G, Selwood TS. Malignant transformation of solar keratoses to squamous cell carcinoma. *Lancet* 1988; **i**:795–7.

14 Dodson JM, DeSpain J, Hewett JE, Clark DP. Malignant potential of actinic keratoses and the controversy over treatment. *Arch Dermatol* 1991; **127**:1029–31.

15 Foote JA, Harris RB, Giuliano AR et al. Predictors for cutaneous basal- and squamous-cell carcinoma among actinically damaged adults. *Int J Cancer* 2001; **95**:7–11.

16 Callen JP, Bickers DR, Moy RL. Actinic keratoses. *J Am Acad Dermatol* 1997; **36**:650–3.

17 Olsen EA, Abernathy L, Kulp-Shorten C et al. A double blind, vehicle controlled study evaluating masoprocol cream in the treatment of actinic keratoses of the head and neck. *J Am Acad Dermatol* 1991; **24**:738–43.

18 Rivers JK, Arlette J, Shear N et al. Topical treatment of actinic keratoses with 3·0% diclofenac in 2·5% hyaluronan gel. *Br J Dermatol* 2002; **146**:94–100.

19 Thompson SC, Jolley D, Marks R. Reduction of solar keratoses by regular sunscreen use. *N Engl J Med* 1993; **329**:1147–51.

20 Darlington S, Williams G, Neale R et al. A randomized controlled trial to assess sunscreen application and beta carotene supplementation in the prevention of solar keratoses. *Arch Dermatol* 2003; **139**:451–5.

21 Green A, Williams G, Neale R et al. Daily sunscreen application and betacarotene supplementation in prevention of basal-cell and squamous-cell carcinomas of the skin: a randomised controlled trial. *Lancet* 1999; **354**:723–9.

22 Swinehart JM. Salicylic acid ointment peeling of the hands and forearms. Effective nonsurgical removal of pigmented lesions and actinic damage. *J Dermatol Surg Oncol* 1992; **18**:495–8.

23 Eaglstein WH, Weinstein GD, Frost P. Fluorouracil: mechanism of action in human skin and actinic keratoses. *Arch Dermatol* 1970; **101**:132–9.

24 Witheiler DD, Lawrence N, Cox SE et al. Long-term efficacy and safety of Jessner's solution and 35% trichloroacetic acid vs. 5% fluorouracil in the treatment of widespread facial actinic keratoses. *Dermatol Surg* 1997; **23**:191–6.

25 Kurwa HA, Yong Gee SA, Seed P et al. A randomized paired comparison of photodynamic therapy and topical 5-fluorouracil in the treatment of actinic keratoses. *J Am Acad Dermatol* 1999; **41**:414–18.

26 Robinson TA, Kligman AM. Treatment of solar keratoses of the extremities with retinoic acid and 5-fluorouracil. *Br J Dermatol* 1975; **92**:703–6.

27 Pearlman DL. Weekly pulse dosing: effective and comfortable topical 5-fluorouracil treatment of multiple facial actinic keratoses. *J Am Acad Dermatol* 1991; **25**:665–7.

28 Epstein E. Does intermittent 'pulse' topical 5-fluorouracil therapy allow destruction of actinic keratoses without significant inflammation? *J Am Acad Dermatol* 1998; **38**:77–80.

29 Bercovitch L. Topical chemotherapy of actinic keratoses of the upper extremity with tretinoin and 5-fluorouracil: a double-blind controlled study. *Br J Dermatol* 1987; **116**:549–52.

30 Stockfleth E, Meyer T, Benninghoff B et al. A randomized, double-blind, vehicle-controlled study to assess 5% imiquimod cream for the treatment of multiple actinic keratoses. *Arch Dermatol* 2002; **138**:1498–502.

31 Korman N, Moy R, Ling M et al. Dosing with 5% imiquimod cream 3 times per week for the treatment of actinic keratosis: results of two phase 3, randomized, double-blind, parallel-group, vehicle-controlled trials. *Arch Dermatol* 2005; **141**:467–73.

32 Szeimies RM, Gerritsen MJ, Gupta G et al. Imiquimod 5% cream for the treatment of actinic keratosis: results from a phase III, randomized, double-blind, vehicle-controlled, clinical trial with histology. *J Am Acad Dermatol* 2004; **51**:547–55.

33 Stockfleth E, Christophers E, Benninghoff B, Sterry W. Low incidence of new actinic keratoses after topical 5% imiquimod cream treatment: a long-term follow-up study. *Arch Dermatol* 2004; **140**:1542 [Letter].

34 Wolf JR, Taylor JR, Tschen E. Topical 3% diclofenac in 2·5% hyaluronan gel in the treatment of actinic keratoses. *Int J Dermatol* 2001; **40**:709–13.

35 Bollag W, Ott F. Retinoic acid: topical treatment of senile or actinic keratoses and basal cell carcinomas. *Agents Actions* 1970; **1**:172–5.

36 Misiewicz J, Sendagorta E, Golebiowska A et al. Topical treatment of multiple actinic keratoses of the face with arotinoid methyl sulfone cream vs. tretinoin cream: a double blind comparative study. *J Am Acad Dermatol* 1991; **24**:448–51.

37 Kligman AL, Thorne EG. Topical therapy of actinic keratoses with tretinoin. In: *Retinoids in Cutaneous Malignancy* (Marks R, ed.), Oxford: Blackwell Scientific Publications, 1991; 66–73.

38 Motley R, Kersey P, Lawrence C, on behalf of the British Association of Dermatologists, the British Association of Plastic Surgeons & the Faculty of Clinical Oncology of the Royal College of Radiologists. Multiprofessional guidelines for the management of the patient with primary cutaneous squamous cell carcinoma. Br J Dermatol 2002; **146**:18–25.

39 Feldman SR, Fleischer AB, Williford PM, Jorrizo JL. Destructive procedures are the standard of care for treatment of actinic keratoses. J Am Acad Dermatol 1999; **40**:43–7.

40 Szeimies RM, Karrer S, Radakovic-Fijan S et al. Photodynamic therapy using topical methyl 5-aminolevulinate compared with cryotherapy for actinic keratosis: a prospective, randomized study. J Am Acad Dermatol 2002; **47**:258–62.

41 Freeman M, Vinciullo C, Francis D et al. A comparison of photodynamic therapy using topical methyl aminolevulinate (Metvix) with single cycle cryotherapy in patients with actinic keratosis: a prospective, randomized study. Dermatolog Treat 2003; **14**:99–106.

42 Chiarello SE. Cryopeeling (extensive cryosurgery) for treatment of actinic keratoses: an update and comparison. Dermatol Surg 2000; **26**:728–32.

43 Abadir DM. Combination of topical 5-fluorouracil with cryotherapy for treatment of actinic keratoses. J Dermatol Surg Oncol 1983; **9**:403–4.

44 Morton CA, Brown SB, Collins S et al. Guidelines for topical photodynamic therapy: report of a workshop of the British Photodermatology Group. Br J Dermatol 2002; **146**:552–67.

45 Pariser DM, Lowe NJ, Stewart DM et al. Photodynamic therapy with topical methyl aminolevulinate for actinic keratosis: results of a prospective randomized multicenter trial. J Am Acad Dermatol 2003; **48**:227–32.

46 Trimas SJ, Ellis DA, Metz RD. The carbon dioxide laser. An alternative for the treatment of actinically damaged skin. Dermatol Surg 1997; **23**:885–9.

47 Spira M, Freeman R, Arfai P et al. Clinical comparison of chemical peeling, dermabrasion, and 5-FU for senile keratoses. J Plast Reconstr Surg 1970; **46**:61–6.

48 Tse Y, Ostad A, Lee HS et al. A clinical and histologic evaluation of two medium-depth peels. Glycolic acid vs. Jessner's trichloroacetic acid. Dermatol Surg 1996; **22**:781–6.

49 Cooley JE, Casey DL, Kauffman CL. Manual resurfacing and trichloroacetic acid for the treatment of patients with widespread actinic damage. Clinical and histologic observations. Dermatol Surg 1997; **23**:373–9.

50 Coleman WP 3rd, Yarborough JM, Mandy SH. Dermabrasion for prophylaxis and treatment of actinic keratoses. Dermatol Surg 1996; **22**:17–21.

51 Winton GB, Salasche SJ. Dermabrasion of the scalp as a treatment for actinic damage. J Am Acad Dermatol 1986; **14**:661–8.

52 Moriarty M, Dunn J, Darragh A et al. Etretinate in treatment of actinic keratosis. A double-blind crossover study. Lancet 1982; **i**:364–5.

53 Watson AB. Preventative effect of etretinate therapy on multiple actinic keratoses. Cancer Detect Prev 1986; **9**:161–5.

54 McNamara IR, Muir J, Galbraith AJ. Acitretin for prophylaxis of cutaneous malignancies after cardiac transplantation. J Heart Lung Transplant 2002; **21**:1201–5.

55 EBPG Expert Group on Renal Transplantation. European best practice guidelines for renal transplantation. Section IV. Long-term management of the transplant recipient. IV.6.2. Cancer risk after renal transplantation. Skin cancers: prevention and treatment. Nephrol Dial Transplant 2002; **17** (Suppl. 4):31–6.

56 Euvrard S, Kanitakis J, Claudy A. Skin cancers after organ transplantation. N Engl J Med 2003; **348**:1681–91.

57 de Graaf Y, Kennedy C, Wolterbeek R et al. Photodynamic therapy does not prevent cutaneous squamous cell carcinoma in organ transplant recipients: results of a randomised-controlled trial. J Invest Dermatol 2006; **126**:569–74.

58 Dragieva G, Hafner J, Dummer R et al. Topical photodynamic therapy in the treatment of actinic keratoses and Bowen's disease in transplant recipients. Transplantation 2004; **77**:115–21.

59 Ormerod AD. Recommendations in British Association of Dermatologists guidelines. Br J Dermatol 2005; **153**:477–8.

Appendix 1

Strength of recommendations and quality of evidence[a]

Strength of recommendations	
A	There is good evidence to support the use of the procedure
B	There is fair evidence to support the use of the procedure
C	There is poor evidence to support the use of the procedure
D	There is fair evidence to support the rejection of the use of the procedure
E	There is good evidence to support the rejection of the use of the procedure
Quality of evidence	
I	Evidence obtained from at least one properly designed, randomized controlled trial
II-i	Evidence obtained from well-designed controlled trials without randomization
II-ii	Evidence obtained from well-designed cohort or case–control analytical studies, preferably from more than one centre or research group
II-iii	Evidence obtained from multiple time series with or without the intervention. Dramatic results in uncontrolled experiments (such as the results of the introduction of penicillin treatment in the 1940s) could also be regarded as this type of evidence
III	Opinions of respected authorities based on clinical experience, descriptive studies or reports of expert committees
IV	Evidence inadequate owing to problems of methodology (e.g. sample size, or length of comprehensiveness of follow up, or conflicts in evidence)

[a]A new system of evidence grading and recommendations has been adopted for new guidelines,[59] but these were introduced after the inception of this guideline.

http://bad.org.uk/Portals/_Bad/Guidelines/Clinical
%20Guidelines/Actinic%20Keratoses.pdf

Comment

The guidelines for the management of actinic keratosis
(AK) [1] list as no treatment as a reasonable option for
AK; however, general practitioners probably 'over' refer
patients with AKs as they have difficulty determining
when progression to Bowen's disease (BD) or invasive
squamous cell carcinoma (SCC) will occur. Common
sense would dictate that when there are many AKs of
varying shapes and sizes then the bigger and more hyperkeratotic lesions would be more likely to progress to BD
and invasive SCC. These are the patients for whom perhaps preventative measures such as photodynamic therapy (PDT) or topical 5 fluorouracil and sunscreens should
be tried [2,3]. A recently published industry-sponsored
study of PDT versus cryotherapy showed PDT to be inferior on the face [4]. With the drive to care nearer to
home a recent study has demonstrated effectiveness of
home-based PDT [5]. Further studies of cryotherapy versus immunomodulators (imiquimod-like drugs) versus
topical 5 fluorouracil versus PDT versus resurfacing lasers
in the long-term management of AKs are needed.

REFERENCES

1 de Berker D, McGregor JM, Hughes BR. Guidelines for the
   management of actinic keratoses. *Brit J Dermatol* 2007; 156:
   222–30.
2 Apalla Z, Sotiriou E, Chovarda E, *et al.* Skin cancer: preventive photodynamic therapy in patients with face and scalp
   cancerization. A randomized placebo-controlled study. *Brit J
   Dermatol* 2010; 162: 171–5.
3 Ulrich C, Jürgensen JS, Degen A, *et al.* Prevention of non-
   melanoma skin cancer in organ transplant patients by regular
   use of a sunscreen: a 24 months, prospective, case–control
   study. *Brit J Dermatol* 2009; 161: 78–84.
4 Kaufmann R, Spelman L, Weightman W, *et al.* Multicentre intraindividual randomized trial of topical methyl
   aminolaevulinate–photodynamic therapy vs. cryotherapy for
   multiple actinic keratoses on the extremities. *Brit J Dermatol*
   2008; 158: 994–9.
5 Wiegell SR, Hædersdal M, Eriksen P, Wulf HC. Photodynamic
   therapy of actinic keratoses with 8% and 16% methyl aminolaevulinate and home-based daylight exposure: a double-
   blinded randomized clinical trial. *Brit J Dermatol* 2009; 160:
   1308–14.

Additional professional resources

Actinic (solar) keratosis – primary care treatment path-
way. Primary Care Dermatology Society 2006. http://
www.pcds.org.uk/images/stories/actinic_(solar)_
keratoses.pdf.
Helfand M, Gorman A K, Mahon S, Chan B K, Swanson
N. Actinic keratoses: final report. Portland, OR, USA:
Oregon Health and Science University, Evidence-Based
Practice Center, 2001.

BAD patient information leaflet

http://www.bad.org.uk/site/794/Default.aspx

Other patient resources

http://www.skincarephysicians.com/actinickeratosesnet
http://www.emedicine.com/derm/topic9.htm
http://www.aadassociation.org/Guidelines/actkeratoses.
html

Guidelines for the management of basal cell carcinoma

N.R. Telfer, G.B. Colver* and C.A. Morton†

Dermatology Centre, Salford Royal Hospitals NHS Foundation Trust, Manchester M6 8HD, U.K.
*Chesterfield Royal Hospital NHS Foundation Trust, Chesterfield, U.K.
†Stirling Royal Infirmary, Stirling, U.K.

Summary

This article represents a planned regular updating of the previous British Association of Dermatologists guidelines for the management of basal cell carcinoma. These guidelines present evidence-based guidance for treatment, with identification of the strength of evidence available at the time of preparation of the guidelines, and a brief overview of epidemiological aspects, diagnosis and investigation.

There are several effective modalities available to treat basal cell carcinoma (BCC).[1,2] Guidelines aim to aid selection of the most appropriate treatment for individual patients. Careful assessment of both the individual patient and certain tumour-specific factors are key to this process.

Definition

BCC is a slow-growing, locally invasive malignant epidermal skin tumour predominantly affecting caucasians. The tumour infiltrates tissues in a three-dimensional fashion[3] through the irregular growth of subclinical finger-like outgrowths which remain contiguous with the main tumour mass.[4,5] Metastasis is extremely rare[6,7] and morbidity results from local tissue invasion and destruction particularly on the face, head and neck. Clinical appearances and morphology are diverse, and include nodular, cystic, superficial, morphoeic (sclerosing), keratotic and pigmented variants. Common histological subtypes include nodular (nBCC), superficial (sBCC) and pigmented forms in addition to morphoeic, micronodular, infiltrative and basosquamous variants which are particularly associated with aggressive tissue invasion and destruction.[8] Perivascular or perineural invasion are features associated with the most aggressive tumours.

Incidence and aetiology

BCC is the most common cancer in Europe, Australia[9] and the U.S.A.,[10] and is showing a worldwide increase in incidence.

Inconsistent data collection unfortunately means that accurate figures for the incidence of BCC in the U.K. are difficult to obtain.[11] The age shift in the population has been accompanied by an increase in the total number of skin cancers, and a continued rise in tumour incidence in the U.K. has been predicted up to the year 2040.[12]

The most significant aetiological factors appear to be genetic predisposition and exposure to ultraviolet radiation.[13] The sun-exposed areas of the head and neck are the most commonly involved sites.[14,15] Sun exposure in childhood may be especially important.[16] Increasing age, male sex, fair skin types I and II, immunosuppression and arsenic exposure are other recognized risk factors[17] and a high dietary fat intake may be relevant.[18] Multiple BCCs are a feature of basal cell naevus (Gorlin's) syndrome (BCNS).[19] Following development of a BCC, patients are at significantly increased risk of developing subsequent BCCs at other sites.

Diagnosis and investigation

Dermatologists can make a confident clinical diagnosis of BCC in most cases. Diagnostic accuracy is enhanced by good lighting and magnification and the dermatoscope may be helpful in some cases.[20] Biopsy is indicated when clinical doubt exists or when patients are being referred for a subspecialty opinion, when the histological subtype of BCC may influence treatment selection and prognosis[8] (Table 1). The use of exfoliative cytology has been described.[21] Imaging techniques such as computed tomography or magnetic resonance imaging

Table 1 Factors influencing prognosis of basal cell carcinoma

Tumour size (increasing size confers higher risk of recurrence)
Tumour site (lesions on the central face, especially around
 the eyes, nose, lips and ears, are at higher risk of recurrence)
Definition of clinical margins (poorly defined lesions are at
 higher risk of recurrence)
Histological subtype (certain subtypes confer higher risk of
 recurrence)
Histological features of aggression (perineural and/or perivascular
 involvement confers higher risk of recurrence)
Failure of previous treatment (recurrent lesions are at higher
 risk of further recurrence)
Immunosuppression (possibly confers increased risk of recurrence)

scanning are indicated in cases where bony involvement is suspected or where the tumour may have invaded major nerves,[22] the orbit[23,24] or the parotid gland.[25] Other techniques, such as ultrasound, spectroscopy and teraherz scanning, are of academic interest but currently have little or no proven clinical role.

'Low-risk' and 'high-risk' tumours, patient factors and treatment selection

The likelihood of curing an individual BCC strongly correlates with a number of definable prognostic factors (Table 1). These factors[26,27] should strongly influence both treatment selection and the prognostic advice given to patients. The presence or absence of these prognostic factors allows clinicians to assign individual lesions as being at low or high risk of recurrence following treatment.

The recent development of more effective topical and nonsurgical therapies has increased the treatment options for many low-risk lesions, although surgery and radiotherapy (RT) remain the treatments of choice for the majority of high-risk lesions.[28]

Patient-specific factors which may influence the choice of treatment include general fitness, coexisting serious medical conditions, and the use of antiplatelet or anticoagulant medication. A conservative approach to asymptomatic, low-risk lesions will prevent treatment causing more problems than the lesion itself. Even when dealing with high-risk BCC aggressive management may be inappropriate for certain patients, especially the very elderly or those in poor general health, when a palliative rather than a curative treatment regimen may be in the best interests of the patient.

Finally, factors including patient choice, local availability of specialized services, together with the experience and preferences of the specialist involved may influence treatment selection.

Management

A wide range of different treatments has been described for the management of BCC,[29] and both the British Association of

Dermatologists (BAD)[30] and the American Academy of Dermatology[31] have published professional guidelines on their appropriate use. Usually the aim of treatment is to eradicate the tumour in a manner likely to result in a cosmetic outcome that will be acceptable to the patient. Some techniques [e.g. cryosurgery, curettage, RT, photodynamic therapy (PDT)] do not allow histological confirmation of tumour clearance. These techniques are generally used to treat low-risk tumours, although RT also has an important role in the management of high-risk BCC. Surgical excision with either intraoperative or postoperative histological assessment of the surgical margins is widely used to treat both low- and high-risk BCC, and is generally considered to have the lowest overall failure rate in BCC treatment.[28] In rare advanced cases, where tumour has invaded facial bones or sinuses, major multidisciplinary craniofacial surgery may be necessary.[32]

There are few randomized controlled studies comparing different skin cancer treatments, and much of the published literature on the treatment of BCC consists of open studies, some with low patient numbers and relatively short follow-up periods.[33]

Broadly, the available treatments for BCC can be divided into surgical and nonsurgical techniques, with surgical techniques subdivided into two categories: excision and destruction.

Surgical techniques

Excision with predetermined margins

The tumour is excised together with a variable margin of clinically normal surrounding tissue. The peripheral and deep surgical margins of the excised tissue can be examined histologically using intraoperative frozen sections[34] or, more commonly, using postoperative vertical sections taken from formalin-fixed, paraffin-embedded tissue.[35] This approach may be used with increasingly wide surgical margins for primary, incompletely excised and recurrent lesions.

Primary basal cell carcinoma

Surgical excision is a highly effective treatment for primary BCC,[35,36] with a recurrence rate of < 2% reported 5 years following histologically complete excision in two different series.[35,37] The overall cosmetic results are generally good,[36] particularly when excision and wound repair are performed by experienced practitioners. The use of curettage prior to excision of primary BCC may increase the cure rate by more accurately defining the true borders of the BCC.[38,39] The size of the peripheral and deep surgical margins should correlate with the likelihood that subclinical tumour extensions exist (Table 1). Although few data exist on the correct deep surgical margin, as this will depend upon the local anatomy, excision through subcutaneous fat is generally advisable. Studies using horizontal [Mohs micrographic surgery (MMS)] sections which can accurately detect BCC at any part of the surgical margin suggest that excision of small (< 20 mm) well-defined lesions with a 3-mm peripheral surgical margin will clear the tumour in 85% of cases. A 4–5-mm peripheral margin will increase the peripheral clearance rate to approximately 95%, indicating that approximately 5% of small, well-defined BCCs extend over 4 mm beyond their apparent clinical margins.[4,40,41] Morphoeic and large BCCs require wider surgical margins in order to maximize the chance of complete histological resection. For primary morphoeic lesions, the rate of complete excision with increasing peripheral surgical margins is as follows: 3-mm margin, 66%; 5-mm margin, 82%; 13–15-mm margin, > 95%.[4] Standard vertical section processing of excision specimens allows the pathologist only to examine representative areas of the peripheral and deep surgical margins, and it has been estimated that at best 44% of the entire margin can be examined in this fashion, which may partly explain why tumours which appeared to have been fully excised do occasionally recur.[42]

Evidence level: *Surgical excision is a good treatment for primary BCC.* (*Strength of recommendation A, quality of evidence I – see Appendix 1*).

Incompletely excised basal cell carcinoma

Incomplete excision, where one or more surgical margins are involved with (or extremely close to) tumour, has been reported in 4·7%[43] and 7%[44] of cases reported from British plastic surgical units and 6·3%[45,46] in two retrospective studies from Australia. This usually reflects the unpredictable extent of subclinical tumour spread beyond the apparent clinical margins. However, other relevant factors associated with incomplete excision include operator experience, the anatomical site and histological subtype of the tumour[43] and the excision of multiple tumours during one procedure.[47]

When the surgical margins are examined intraoperatively (excision under frozen section control, MMS), further resection of any involved margins can take place prior to wound repair. Using standard surgery, one approach to minimize the risk of incomplete excision is to excise tumours and delay wound repair until an urgent pathology report is received. In the more common situation, when surgical margins are examined routinely postoperatively, the wound has usually been repaired and the only options are further treatment or prolonged follow up to monitor for tumour recurrence.[48]

Various prospective and retrospective reviews of incompletely excised BCC suggest that not all tumours will recur. Studies using approximately 2–5 years of follow up have reported recurrence rates following histologically incomplete excision of 30%,[46] 38%,[49] 39%[50] and 41%.[51]

In a follow-up study of 140 incompletely excised BCCs 21% of lesions recurred; however, as 31% of the cohort died of other causes during the (minimum 5-year) follow-up period this figure could have been significantly higher.[47] Re-excision of incompletely excised lesions revealed the presence of residual tumour in 45%[47] and 54%[44] of cases when the tissue was examined using standard (vertical) tissue sectioning and in 55% of cases re-excised using MMS.[52]

The risk of recurrence seems highest in those lesions where both lateral and deep margins were involved with BCC and when the incomplete excision was performed to remove recurrent BCCs, especially those recurrent following radiation therapy.[49] BCCs incompletely excised at the deep margin were considered especially difficult to cure with re-excision.[49] One study calculated the probability of recurrence of incompletely excised BCC and found that it varied according to which margins were involved. When only the lateral margins were involved there was a 17% risk of recurrence, rising to a 33% risk of recurrence if the deep margins were involved.[53]

There is good evidence to support a policy of re-treatment of incompletely excised lesions[44,49,51,52,54–56] especially when they involve critical midfacial sites, where the deep surgical margin is involved, the surgical defect has been repaired using skin flaps or skin grafts[49,57] and where histology shows an aggressive histological subtype. It has been suggested that some incompletely excised lesions may demonstrate a more aggressive histological subtype when the lesion recurs, especially on the central face.[58] If the decision is made to re-treat rather than observe, re-excision (with or without frozen section control) or MMS are the treatments of choice (Table 2). Although there are limited data on the subject, RT appears to have a role in preventing the recurrence of incompletely excised BCC.[53]

Evidence level: *Tumours which have been incompletely excised, especially (i) high-risk lesions; and (ii) lesions incompletely excised at the deep margin, are at high risk of recurrence.* (*Strength of recommendation A, quality of evidence II-i*).

Recurrent basal cell carcinoma

Recurrent BCC is more difficult to cure than primary disease – the results of all published series on the surgical excision of BCC show cure rates following treatment of recurrent disease that are inferior to those for primary lesions.[59] Recurrent lesions generally require wider peripheral surgical margins than primary lesions with or without standard (non-Mohs) frozen section control.[34] Peripheral excision margins for recurrent BCC of 5–10 mm have been suggested.[60]

Evidence level: *Recurrent tumours, especially on the face, are at high risk of further recurrence following surgical excision even with wide surgical margins.* (*Strength of recommendation A, quality of evidence II-ii*).

Table 2 Indications for Mohs micrographic surgery

Tumour site (especially central face, around the eyes, nose, lips and ears)
Tumour size (any size, but especially > 2 cm)
Histological subtype (especially morphoeic, infiltrative, micronodular and basosquamous subtypes)
Poor clinical definition of tumour margins
Recurrent lesions
Perineural or perivascular involvement

Mohs micrographic surgery

This specialized surgical procedure was pioneered (as chemosurgery) by Frederic Mohs in the 1940s and later refined into the modern technique of MMS.[61] MMS combines staged resection with comprehensive surgical margin examination and results in extremely high cure rates for even the most high-risk lesions together with maximal preservation of normal tissues.[62,63] The technique, which is generally reserved for high-risk facial lesions, is based upon the principle that all traces of infiltrating BCC must be identified and excised in order to achieve complete cure.[64,65] The indications for using MMS are summarized in Table 2. A review of studies published since the mid-1940s suggested an overall 5-year cure rate of 99% following MMS for primary BCC[66] and 94·4% for recurrent disease.[59] Two prospective studies have been reported from Australia: in one, 5-year cure rates of 100% and 92·2% for primary and recurrent tumours, respectively, were reported in 819 patients with periocular BCC;[67] in the other, 3370 BCCs on the head and neck treated wth MMS resulted in 5-year cure rates of 98·6% for primary BCC and 96% for recurrent disease.[68] A retrospective review of 620 patients with 720 lesions gave estimated 5-year cure rates of 98·8% for primary BCC and 93·3% for recurrent disease.[69] Five-year cure rates of 93·5% for primary BCC and 90% for recurrent disease have been reported.[64]

MMS for BCC performed under local anaesthesia in an outpatient or day-case setting has a good safety record[70,71] and Mohs surgical defects can be repaired by the Mohs surgeon or by facial reconstructive specialists including plastic,[72] otolaryngeal[73] and oculoplastic[74,75] surgeons. The technique is performed using either frozen tissue sections,[76] when resection can take place over a matter of hours, or with formalin-fixed, paraffin-embedded tissues, when the procedure takes place over a number of days.[77,78] Variations of the technique, based upon different techniques of pathological processing of tissue excised in a standard fashion, have been described.[79-82] Both maxillofacial[83] and ophthalmic[84,85] surgeons have reported good results with staged excision of high-risk BCC using standard vertical (non-Mohs) permanent sections and delayed wound repair, as an alternative to MMS which one group felt was too 'labour-intensive'.[84] Several studies have looked at the comparative cost of MMS,[86-89] which (to produce tumour-free margins) has a similar cost to traditional excision[87] but is less expensive than excision using intraoperative frozen section control.[86] A study from the Netherlands found MMS to be more expensive than traditional surgery; however, as MMS is likely to produce extremely high cure rates, it remains cost-effective. The only study to date which tried to compare cure rates following standard excision and MMS[89] appeared to show little difference between the two treatment modalities. However, a failure to adhere to the study design (with 24 of 301 patients randomized to have standard surgical excision being moved into the MMS treatment group) raises concerns about the conclusions of this study.[90]

Evidence levels: *Mohs micrographic surgery is a good treatment for high-risk primary BCC. (Strength of recommendation A, quality of evidence I).*

Mohs micrographic surgery is a good treatment for high-risk recurrent BCC. (Strength of recommendation A, quality of evidence I).

Destructive techniques: surgical

Destructive surgical and nonsurgical techniques are best used for low-risk disease. Unless a confident clinical diagnosis and assessment has been made, a preoperative biopsy is indicated to confirm the diagnosis and to determine the histological subtype. This advice is especially important for facial lesions.

Curettage and cautery

Curettage and cautery (C&C, also known as electrodesiccation and curettage)[91-93] and curettage alone[91,94,95] are traditional methods of BCC removal. Successful outcomes rely heavily on careful selection of appropriate lesions (ideally small nodular or superficial)[94,96] as well as the skill and experience of the operator.[96,97] In a survey of 166 U.K. consultant dermatologists in 1995, 24% of 1597 lesions presenting for the first time were treated by C&C, making it the second most common form of treatment after surgical excision (58%).[98] Variations in technique include the use of different types of curette and the number of cycles of treatment;[93] however, the exact protocol is often unclear in published studies. Curettage and cautery is generally suitable for the treatment of low-risk lesions.[94,96,97,99] Curettage and cautery of high-risk facial lesions is associated with a high risk of tumour recurrence[97,100,101] and is generally contraindicated.

In a study of 69 C&C wounds that were immediately re-excised using MMS, residual tumour was found in 33% of cases overall, with striking differences seen in different body sites (47% of head and neck sites and 8·3% of trunk and limb sites contained residual BCC).[102] This may be one reason why C&C is generally less successful in the treatment of facial lesions. The relatively high incidence of residual BCC but an apparently low incidence of recurrence following C&C has led to suggestions that unidentified wound healing processes following C&C may play a part in tumour destruction, although at least two studies have failed to confirm this theory.[103,104] Tumour debulking by curettage has been combined with various treatment modalities such as imiquimod (IMQ)[105,106] and PDT[107] in attempts to increase efficacy. Curettage has also been combined with cryosurgery – a 5-year follow-up study of 70 noninfiltrative auricular BCCs (not involving the external auditory meatus) treated in this way resulted in one recurrence.[108]

A literature review of all studies published since 1947 suggested an overall 5-year cure rate of 92·3% following C&C for selected primary BCC.[66] Curettage is much less useful for recurrent BCC and a similar review suggested an overall 5-year cure rate of 60%.[59]

Evidence levels: *Curettage and cautery is a good treatment for low-risk BCC. (Strength of recommendation A, quality of evidence II-iii).*

Curettage and cautery is a poor treatment for high-risk BCC. (Strength of recommendation D, quality of evidence II-iii).

Curettage and cautery is a poor treatment for recurrent BCC. (Strength of recommendation D, quality of evidence II-ii).

Cryosurgery

Liquid nitrogen cryosurgery for the destruction of BCC uses the effects of extreme cold (tissue temperatures of −50 to −60 °C) to effect deep destruction of the tumour and surrounding tissues. Individual treatment techniques vary considerably, with both open and closed spray techniques and single or multiple cycles of freezing (freeze/thaw cycles).[109,110] Double freeze/thaw cycles are generally recommended for the treatment of facial BCC, although superficial truncal lesions may require only a single treatment cycle.[111] One report describes the use of 'fractional cryosurgery' where large lesions are treated on multiple separate occasions.[112] The success of cryosurgery relies upon careful selection of appropriate lesions[113] and the experience of the operator.

In one study 12 small nonfacial nBCCs were treated with single freeze-thaw cryosurgery to a monitored temperature of between −50 and −60 °C. When each treatment site was subsequently excised and examined with horizontal step sections, no residual tumour was detected.[114] Cryosurgery is most useful in the treatment of low-risk BCC.[115,116] Five-year cure rates of 99% have been reported by the same author in both 1991[117] and 2004.[118]

In expert hands, cryosurgery also has a role in the management of high-risk lesions, either as the sole treatment[118] or following curettage.[108,119] A follow-up study of 171 high-risk BCCs treated with combined curettage/cryotherapy reported a 8% recurrence rate after a mean follow up of 5·2 years (range 6 months–9·1 years).[119] Although cryosurgery is less useful for the treatment of recurrent BCC,[59] selected lesions may also respond to aggressive expert treatment.[120]

Some authors consider cryosurgery to be an appropriate treatment for selected periocular BCC[121–124] and one series of 158 periocular BCCs treated with double-cycle cryosurgery reported a 8% recurrence rate after a mean 5-year follow-up period. Careful lesion selection was crucial, as factors associated with recurrence included large size, morphoeic histology and involvement of the lid margin.[123] Other than tumour recurrence, adverse results of cryosurgery to eyelid and periocular BCC include conjunctival hypertrophy and ectropion which may require corrective surgery.[123] Cryosurgery (double 25–30-s treatment cycles) has been compared with 5-aminolaevulinic acid (ALA)-PDT in the treatment of low-risk BCC.[125] Histologically verified recurrence rates in the two groups were statistically comparable: 25% (11 of 44) for PDT and 15% (six of 39) for cryosurgery. Additional treatments had to be performed in 30% of the lesions in the PDT group although the healing time was shorter and the cosmetic outcome better with PDT. Pain and discomfort during and after treatment were the same. Additional studies using methylaminolaevulinic acid (MAL)-PDT with longer follow-up periods and

including comparison with surgical excision are detailed in the later section on PDT.

Cryosurgery wounds generally heal with minimal tissue contraction, resulting in good cosmetic results;[113,115,119] however, one study comparing the cosmetic results (but not efficacy) of cryosurgery with excisonal surgery for head and neck found that excision generally gave superior cosmetic results.[126]

Evidence level: Cryosurgery is a good treatment for low-risk BCC. (Strength of recommendation A, quality of evidence II-ii).

Carbon dioxide laser

Carbon dioxide (CO_2) laser ablation remains an uncommon form of treatment and there are few published data. When combined with curettage, CO_2 laser surgery may be useful in the treatment of large or multiple low-risk sBCCs. In one small series, the Ultrapulse CO_2 laser appeared effective in treating small BCCs in low-risk areas with minimal post-treatment scarring in three patients with BCNS.[127]

Evidence level: Carbon dioxide laser ablation may be effective in the treatment of low-risk BCC. (Strength of recommendation C, quality of evidence III).

Destructive techniques: nonsurgical

Topical immunotherapy with imiquimod

IMQ is an immune-response modifier which acts through toll-like receptors, predominantly expressed on dendritic cells and monocytes, to induce production of cytokines and chemokines which promote both innate and adaptive cell-mediated immune responses.[128] Several studies have reported the efficacy of topical 5% IMQ cream in the treatment of sBCC and dose–response studies indicate that the highest response rates are associated with more frequent or prolonged dosing, together with a significant inflammatory reaction.[129,130]

Pooled results from two randomized vehicle-controlled studies of 5% IMQ cream in the treatment of small sBCC in 724 patients have been reported. Twelve weeks following a 6-week treatment period the histological clearance rates were 82% (application five times weekly, 5x/week), 79% (application seven times weekly, 7x/week) and 3% (vehicle only). An increasing severity of local inflammatory reactions was associated with higher clearance rates. Moderate to severe local site reactions occurred in 87%, including erosion (36%) and ulceration (22%) in subjects in the 5x/week group, with higher figures for the 7x/week group. Rest periods were requested by 10% and 22% of patients in the 5x/week and 7x/week groups, respectively, with resumption of treatment when the reaction had resolved. Eleven patients withdrew from the study due to adverse events.[131]

A multicentre randomized study of the treatment of sBCC with 5% IMQ cream vs. vehicle alone in 84 patients reported similar results. Histological clearance rates following once-daily application for 6 weeks were 80% (IMQ) and 6% (vehicle).[132]

Topical IMQ is approved by the European Medicines Agency for the treatment of small sBCC, using the 5x/week regimen for 6 weeks. This regimen balances therapeutic efficacy with patient tolerability of the common inflammatory reactions.

Long-term data on clinical recurrence rates are limited. An on-going multicentre open-label study of 182 small sBCCs using the 5x/week regimen resulted in 10% of patients failing to respond at 12 weeks. The 90% who did respond then entered a 5-year follow-up phase. Interim results after 2 years of follow up reported an estimated recurrence rate of 20·6% in this group.[133]

Data on the treatment of nBCC using IMQ are limited. Two randomized dose–response studies (reported in the same paper) each evaluated four dosing regimens over a 6- or 12-week application period. Six weeks following treatment the entire treated areas were excised. Histologically confirmed complete response rates were highest in the groups receiving a once-daily dose, with clearance rates of 71% (25 of 35) and 76% (16 of 21) in the 6- and 12-week studies, respectively. Increasing response rates were associated with increasing frequency of dosing over all regimens, and there was a significant correlation between the most intense inflammatory reactions and complete response rate.[134]

A further randomized trial reported complete clinical clearance in 78% of 90 evaluable patients with nBCC following thrice-weekly application of IMQ for 8 or 12 weeks (no difference in outcome between protocols). The treated areas were excised 8 weeks following treatment, and residual BCC was found in 36% of cases, including 12 of 90 (13%) patients considered to have shown complete clinical clearance.[135]

There are currently limited published data on the long-term recurrence rates following IMQ treatment of nBCC. During 5-year follow up of 55 lesions in an open study of different types of BCC treated with IMQ, the long-term clearance rate for the intention-to-treat dataset was 100% (four of four) for sBCC, 75% (six of eight) for nBCC and 60% (26 of 43) for infiltrative BCC.[136]

Two pilot studies investigated the combination of curettage of nBCC prior to the use of topical IMQ.[105,106] In the first, following a single cycle of curettage, IMQ was applied daily for 6–10 weeks and this produced histological clearance of 94% (32 of 34) when the treatment sites were excised 12 weeks after treatment.[105] In the second study, 20 patients received three cycles of C&C followed by IMQ or vehicle once daily for 1 month. Histological examination revealed residual tumour in 10% (one of 10) in the IMQ group and 40% (four of 10) in the vehicle group.[106]

Occlusion of the treatment site does not appear to be beneficial as no difference in efficacy was demonstrated when 5% IMQ cream with and without occlusion was used to treat both sBCC and nBCC.[137] Three separate studies of topical IMQ in a total of seven patients with BCNS have suggested clinical benefit in treating multiple sBCC and nBCC.[138–140]

To date, there are no published randomized trials comparing topical IMQ with an existing standard therapy. One small study compared the efficacy and tolerability of topical IMQ (three times weekly for 3 weeks followed by a 1-week rest period, repeated for a total of 3 months) with MAL-PDT therapy (one cycle of two treatments). Histological clearance in the IMQ group was reported in six of eight (all sBCC) vs. 12 of 13 (sBCC and nBCC) in the PDT group 12 weeks after treatment. Cosmetic results in both groups were similar, although patients tolerated IMQ therapy less well.[141]

On the basis of the currently available data, topical 5% IMQ cream appears to have a role in treating small sBCC, although 5-year follow-up data are awaited. The role of IMQ in the treatment of nBCC remains unclear, as its use has been studied in only small numbers of patients and there are currently limited long-term follow-up data.

Evidence levels: *Topical imiquimod appears effective in the treatment of primary small superficial BCC. (Strength of recommendation A, quality of evidence I).*

Topical imiquimod may possibly have a role in the treatment of primary nodular BCC. (Strength of recommendation C, quality of evidence I).

Photodynamic therapy

Previous BAD guidelines have rated topical PDT using ALA as suitable for the treatment of low-risk sBCC, but a relatively poor option for the treatment of high-risk lesions.[30,142]

ALA-PDT has been compared with cryosurgery in the treatment of both sBCC and nBCC.[125] Clinical recurrence rates at 12 months of 5% (PDT) and 13% (cryotherapy) were underestimates, as histology demonstrated residual BCC in 25% (PDT) and 15% (cryotherapy) of cases, raising concerns both over clinical observation rather than histology as proof of tumour clearance and over the long-term efficacy of PDT. Two further studies of double-cycle ALA-PDT treatment of sBCC reported initial clinical clearance rates of 95% (60 of 62)[143] and 90% (76 of 87),[144] with subsequent recurrence rates of 18%[143] and 4·8%,[144] respectively, after 12 months of follow up.

Since the last BAD guidelines were published,[30] studies have increasingly reported the use of topical MAL, a more lipophilic methyl ester of ALA, which may demonstrate better tumour selectivity. There are currently limited data comparing these two agents, with no difference in tumour response (by histology) in one study of patients with nBCC receiving either ALA-PDT (n = 22) or MAL-PDT (n = 21) using identical regimens including surgical debulking of half of the tumours in each group prior to treatment.[145] MAL-PDT is currently the only licensed form of topical PDT for the treatment of BCC.

The use of MAL-PDT has been compared with both cryotherapy and surgery in the treatment of BCC. Clinical clearance at 3 months of 97% of 102 sBCCs treated by MAL-PDT compared with 95% of 98 lesions treated with cryotherapy in a randomized multicentre study was described in a review article.[146] The cosmetic outcome was superior following PDT, with a good or excellent outcome reported in 89% (PDT) and 50% (cryotherapy). During 48 months of follow up, recurrence rates of 22% (PDT) and 19% (cryotherapy) were reported. In another study previously mentioned in the curettage section, 91% of 131 sBCCs cleared following MAL-PDT, with 9% of these recurring during 35 months of follow up.[107] The same study also treated nBCCs with MAL-PDT (following curette debulk), with initial clearance of 89% of 168 lesions. Subsequently, 12 thick and six thin tumours (14% and 7%, respectively) recurred during 35 months of follow up.

MAL-PDT (following nonpainful superficial curette or scalpel surface preparation) has been compared with surgical excision (> 5 mm margin) in the treatment of 105 nonfacial nBCCs in a multicentre randomized study. Clearance rates at 3 months were 91% (PDT) and 98% (surgery), and cosmetic outcome rated as good/excellent in 83% (PDT) and 33% (surgery).[147] The same researchers reported long-term (60 months) recurrence rates of 14% (PDT) and 4% (surgery).[148]

A multicentre study of patients considered to be at high risk of complications, poor cosmesis, disfigurement and/or recurrence reported histologically confirmed initial (3 months) clearance rates following MAL-PDT treatment of 85% (40 of 47) for sBCCs and 75% (38 of 51) for nBCCs, with long-term (24 months) recurrence rates of 22% and 18%, respectively.[149] In a similar multicentre study, 148 sBCCs and nBCCs regarded by the authors as 'difficult-to-treat' (defined as large and/or central facial lesions, or patients at increased risk of surgical complications) received MAL-PDT treatment.[150] Histologically confirmed clearance rates at 3 months were 93% (sBCC) and 82% (nBCC). The authors used a time-to-event approach to estimate sustained lesion clearance rates of 82% (sBCC) and 67% (nBCC) at 24 months. These data suggest that MAL-PDT may be an option for high-risk disease when other more effective treatments are either contraindicated or unacceptable to patients.

Some patients with BCNS responded to PDT using either red (~630 nm) or blue (~417 nm) light sources, but experience is limited to case reports.[151,152] To date, there is no good evidence to support the use of PDT for infiltrative or recurrent BCC. Topical PDT can be a time-consuming procedure, especially if performed on multiple occasions. Pain during the illumination phase is significant for some patients and ranges from a stinging or burning sensation to occasionally severe discomfort. A number of measures can reduce this pain, including the use of fans, directed cool air, simple analgesia or local anaesthesia. Following PDT the area tends to swell and then form a crust which takes a few weeks to separate.[153]

Evidence levels: *Photodynamic therapy is a good treatment for primary superficial BCC. (Strength of recommendation A, quality of evidence I).*

Photodynamic therapy is a reasonable treatment for primary low-risk nodular BCC. (Strength of recommendation B, quality of evidence I).

Radiotherapy

RT is effective in the treatment of primary BCC,[154–158] surgically recurrent BCC,[159] as adjuvant therapy, and is probably the treatment of choice for high-risk disease in patients who are unwilling or unable to tolerate surgery.[159,160] RT is a complex mix of different techniques including superficial RT (generated at up to 170 kV) which is suitable for lesions up to ~6 mm in depth, electron beam therapy (generated at higher energies) which penetrates deeper tissues, and brachytherapy which is useful for lesions arising on curved surfaces. Due to the expensive nature of the equipment involved, RT is usually available only at major hospital centres. RT can be used in an adjuvant role, for example following incomplete excision of high-risk BCC. Poor long-term cosmetic results which were once a significant problem are much less likely following treatment using modern techniques. Fractionated treatment regimens (which repeatedly exploit the difference in radiosensitivity between malignant and normal tissues) generally produce superior cosmetic outcomes compared with single-fraction treatment, although this obviously requires multiple hospital visits. In the elderly, infirm patient, single-fraction regimens are still used, as the long-term cosmetic result of treatment is less of a concern. All RT treatments are a careful compromise between the likelihood of tumour destruction and an acceptable risk of radionecrosis (a 5% level being generally accepted as a maximum, and most clinical oncologists aiming for a much lower level). Different anatomical areas have different RT tolerances, with the head and neck generally tolerating RT well. However, certain areas such as the upper eyelid can be difficult to treat. The bridge of the nose, where thin skin overlies bone and is often subjected to repeated minor trauma from spectacles, is an area historically associated with a particularly high risk of radionecrosis. However, RT can be used successfully on many facial sites and studies have reported good outcomes following treatment of BCC on the nose,[155,158,159,161] lip,[162] ear[155,163] and periorbital[155,164] skin.

Unfortunately, some studies of RT for facial BCC report treatment of all nonmelanoma cancers (BCC, squamous cell carcinoma and basosquamous cancer), and do not clearly differentiate tumour-specific outcomes. However, in all these studies, BCC was generally the single largest tumour group and consequently some of these studies are referenced in these guidelines.

Review articles have reported overall 5-year cure rates following RT of 91·3%[66] for primary BCC and 90·2%[59] for recurrent disease. Other studies suggest long-term (> 4 years) local control rates of 84%,[165] 86%,[157] 88%,[166] 92·5%[167] and 96%.[158]

Attempts have been made to compare RT with other treatment modalities. A randomized comparison trial of RT against cryotherapy (93 patients) resulted in 2-year cure rates of 96% and 61%, respectively.[168]

Surgical excision (91% with frozen section margin control) of 174 primary facial BCCs < 4 cm in diameter has been compared with RT (mix of interstitial brachytherapy, contact therapy and conventional RT) for 173 lesions.[167] The 4-year recurrence rates were 0·7% (surgery) and 7·5% (RT). Cosmetic outcome at 4 years was significantly superior following surgery (good cosmesis in 79%) compared with RT (good cosmesis in 40%), with altered pigmentation and telangiectasia in over 65% of RT patients, and radiodystrophy in 41%.[169]

RT is contraindicated in the re-treatment of BCC that has recurred following previous RT. RT may promote the growth of new BCC in patients with BCNS, and consequently should either be avoided or used with extreme caution in this patient group.[170]

Evidence levels: *Radiotherapy is a good treatment for primary BCC.* (*Strength of recommendation A, quality of evidence I*).

Radiotherapy is a good treatment for recurrent (but not radiorecurrent) BCC. (*Strength of recommendation A, quality of evidence I*).

Follow up

Following treatment of a BCC, all patients are at some degree of risk of both local recurrence (treatment failure) and the development of further primary BCC at other sites (new lesions). These risks form the basis of the arguments both for and against long-term specialist follow up.

The risk of local recurrence is an individual risk, based upon the tumour characteristics and the treatment used. However, for primary BCC treated appropriately by experienced practitioners, the recurrence rate should be low. This is not true for recurrent BCC, where recurrence rates are universally higher than for primary BCC. Patients who have had recurrent (especially multiply recurrent) lesions treated are particularly worthy of follow up in view of their relatively high risk of further recurrence. The timing of follow-up visits should take into account the generally slow growth rate of BCC. Evidence suggests that recurrent disease may take up to 5 years to present clinically, and that up to 18% of recurrent BCC may present even later.[100] In a review of all studies published since 1947 looking at the treatment of primary BCC by various modalities, less than one third of all recurrences presented in the first year of follow up, 50% presented within 2 years, and 66% within 3 years.[66]

The risk of developing further BCC has been studied in a number of ways. Marcil and Stern[171] conducted an English language literature review and meta-analysis and found seven studies assessing the risk of developing a second BCC. Overall, the 3-year cumulative risk ranged from 33% to 70% (mean 44%), representing an approximately 10-fold increase over the rate expected in a comparable general population. The highest rates (60–70%) came from studies including large populations of patients with at least two (sometimes more than two) previous BCCs, suggesting that as the number of BCC lesions increases, so does the risk of developing more. In contrast, patients with only their index BCC who remain disease free for 3 years appear to have a decreased ongoing risk of further BCC. There was no general agreement on particular risk factors which might confer a higher risk of subsequent BCC.

The findings have been supported by the results of a prospective study of two cohorts (total 1183) of private patients in Denmark[172] in whom 299 (25·3%) developed at least 777 new skin cancers during 2 years of follow up, 89·5% of these being BCC. A study based upon data stored by the Swiss Cancer Registry[173] suggested the risk of a second BCC was 8·45

times higher (measured over an unlimited time period) than expected in a comparable general population.

Various authors have tried to identify specific risk factors which might be associated with an increased risk of developing further BCC. Van Iersel et al.[174] confirmed an overall increase of subsequent BCC over a 5-year period and identified a possible higher risk in older patients, those with multiple BCC at first presentation, and those with an index tumour > 1 cm in size.

A clinical study of 1200 patients also suggested that the presence of multiple BCC at presentation was associated with increased risk of further BCC[175] and the same group also reported that an index BCC arising on the trunk appeared strongly associated with the development of further (usually also truncal) BCC;[176] this group has suggested that different mechanisms may determine the development of truncal BCC and head and neck BCC.[177]

Two studies have looked at current U.K. practice regarding BCC follow up. Dermatologists in Belfast[178] offered follow up at 12 and 24 months following surgical excision of midfacial primary BCC. They reported attendance rates of 78% at 12 months, falling to 53% at 2 years. A recurrence rate of < 2% (two of 121) over 2 years was reported, and new BCCs were detected in 11·6% of patients during the first year and 6·3% during the second year of follow up. In 2001 a survey of British dermatologists (68% response) asked about routine follow-up practice following the excision of a primary midfacial BCC. No follow up at all was offered by 27% of responders, 37% would offer one follow-up clinic visit, while 36% would offer more than one hospital-based review.[179]

Clearly, within the British healthcare system it is not possible to offer long-term follow up to all patients who have had their first and only primary BCC treated. Provided treatment has been selected appropriately and performed competently, these patients should, by definition, be at low risk of local recurrence and would benefit from sensible sun protection advice and counselling on the significant (possibly up to 44%) 3-year risk of the development of a second primary lesion. Such patients are probably suitable (with appropriate education and advice) for self-monitoring or follow up in primary care.[50] The case for follow up in either a primary or secondary care setting is stronger for patients who have been treated for recurrent disease (increased risk of further recurrence following all types of treatment) and those with a history of multiple BCCs (significantly increased risk of further BCC), although this would possibly need to be for at least 3 years, to reflect the available evidence base.

Conclusions

Many treatments are known to be effective in the treatment of BCC, ranging from topical therapy (e.g. IMQ) and minimally invasive procedures (e.g. PDT), through destructive modalities (e.g. C&C, cryosurgery) to more specialized treatments such as RT, wide surgical excision and MMS. An assessment of the relative risk of recurrence of an individual lesion will generally

Table 3 Primary basal cell carcinoma (BCC): influence of tumour type, size (large = > 2 cm) and site on the selection of treatment

BCC type: histology, size and site	PDT	Topical imiquimod	Curettage and cautery	Radiation therapy	Cryosurgery	Excision	Mohs surgery
Superficial, small and low-risk site	**	**	**	?	**	?	X
Nodular, small and low-risk site	*	–	**	?	**	***	X
Infiltrative, small and low-risk site	X	X	*	*	*	***	?
Superficial, large and low-risk site	***	**	**	*	**	*	?
Nodular, large and low-risk site	–	–	**	**	**	***	?
Infiltrative, large and low-risk site	X	X	–	*	*	***	**
Superficial, small and high-risk site	*	*	*	**	*	**	*
Nodular, small and high-risk site	–	–	*	**	**	***	**
Infiltrative, small and high-risk site	X	X	–	*	*	**	***
Superficial, large and high-risk site	*	*	–	*	*	**	**
Nodular, large and high-risk site	–	X	X	–	*	**	**
Infiltrative, large and high-risk site	X	X	X	X	X	*	***

PDT, photodynamic therapy; ***, probable treatment of choice; **, generally good choice; *, generally fair choice; ?, reasonable, but not often needed; –, generally poor choice; X, probably should not be used.

Table 4 Recurrent basal cell carcinoma (BCC): influence of tumour type, size (large = > 2 cm) and site on the selection treatment

BCC type: histology, size and site	PDT	Topical imiquimod	Curettage and cautery	Radiation therapy	Cryosurgery	Excision	Mohs surgery
Superficial, small and low-risk site	**	*	*	*	**	**	–
Nodular, small and low-risk site	–	X	**	**	**	***	–
Infiltrative, small and low-risk site	X	X	–	**	**	***	*
Superficial, large and low-risk site	**	*	*	**	**	*	*
Nodular, large and low-risk site	X	X	–	*	*	***	*
Infiltrative, large and low-risk site	X	X	–	*	*	**	**
Superficial, small and high-risk site	?	X	*	*	*	**	**
Nodular, small and high-risk site	X	X	*	*	*	***	**
Infiltrative, small and high-risk site	X	X	X	*	*	**	***
Superficial, large and high-risk site	?	X	X	*	–	**	**
Nodular, large and high-risk site	X	X	X	–	–	**	***
Infiltrative, large and high-risk site	X	X	X	–	–	*	***

PDT, photodynamic therapy; ***, probable treatment of choice; **, generally good choice; *, generally fair choice; ?, reasonable, but not often needed; –, generally poor choice; X, probably should not be used.

be a useful way of identifying the most appropriate treatment modalities. For example, low-risk disease is generally suitable for topical therapy, C&C, cryotherapy, simple excision and PDT, while high-risk BCC is generally better managed with wide surgical excision, RT and MMS.

An indication of the relative value of the various treatment modalities covered in these guidelines is summarized in Table 3 (primary BCCs) and Table 4 (recurrent BCCs). While heavily based upon the overall likelihood of cure, these recommendations also take into account practicality of use, side-effects, cosmetic outcomes, and patient acceptability.

Disclaimer

These guidelines have been prepared for dermatologists on behalf of the British Association of Dermatologists and are based on the best data available at the time the report was prepared. Caution should be exercised when interpreting the data where there is a limited evidence base. The results of future studies may require alteration of the conclusions or recommendations in this report. It may be necessary to depart from the guidelines in the interests of specific patients and special circumstances. Just as adherence to guidelines may not constitute defence against a claim of negligence, so deviation from them should not necessarily be deemed negligent.

References

1 Kuijpers DI, Thissen MR, Neumann MH. Basal cell carcinoma: treatment options and prognosis, a scientific approach to a common malignancy. Am J Clin Dermatol 2002; **3**:247–59.

2 Thissen MR, Neumann MH, Schouten LJ. A systematic review of treatment modalities for primary basal cell carcinomas. Arch Dermatol 1999; **135**:1177–83.

3 Braun RP, Klumb F, Girard C et al. Three-dimensional reconstruction of basal cell carcinomas. Dermatol Surg 2005; 31:562–6.

4 Breuninger H, Dietz K. Prediction of subclinical tumor infiltration in basal cell carcinoma. J Dermatol Surg Oncol 1991; 17:574–8.

5 Hendrix JD Jr, Parlette HL. Duplicitous growth of infiltrative basal cell carcinoma: analysis of clinically undetected tumor extent in a paired case–control study. Dermatol Surg 1996; 22:535–9.

6 Lo JS, Snow SN, Reizner GT et al. Metastatic basal cell carcinoma: report of twelve cases with a review of the literature. J Am Acad Dermatol 1991; 24:715–19.

7 Ting PT, Kasper R, Arlette JP. Metastatic basal cell carcinoma: report of two cases and literature review. J Cutan Med Surg 2005; 9:10–15.

8 Costantino D, Lowe L, Brown DL. Basosquamous carcinoma – an under-recognized, high-risk cutaneous neoplasm: case study and review of the literature. J Plast Reconstr Aesthet Surg 2006; 59:424–8.

9 Gilbody JS, Aitken J, Green A. What causes basal cell carcinoma to be the commonest cancer? Aust J Public Health 1994; 18:218–21.

10 Miller DL, Weinstock MA. Nonmelanoma skin cancer in the United States: incidence. J Am Acad Dermatol 1994; 30:774–8.

11 Goodwin RG, Holme SA, Roberts DL. Variations in registration of skin cancer in the United Kingdom. Clin Exp Dermatol 2004; 29:328–30.

12 Diffey BL, Langtry JA. Skin cancer incidence and the ageing population. Br J Dermatol 2005; 153:679–80.

13 Gailani MR, Leffell DJ, Ziegler A et al. Relationship between sunlight exposure and a key genetic alteration in basal cell carcinoma. J Natl Cancer Inst 1996; 88:349–54.

14 Roenigk RK, Ratz JL, Bailin PL, Wheeland RG. Trends in the presentation and treatment of basal cell carcinomas. J Dermatol Surg Oncol 1986; 12:860–5.

15 Lindgren G, Diffey BL. Basal cell carcinoma of the eyelids and solar ultraviolet radiation exposure. Br J Ophthalmol 1998; 82:1412–15.

16 Corona R, Dogliotti E, D'Errico M et al. Risk factors for basal cell carcinoma in a Mediterranean population: role of recreational sun exposure early in life. Arch Dermatol 2001; 137:1162–8.

17 Zak-Prelich M, Narbutt J, Sysa-Jedrzejowska A. Environmental risk factors predisposing to the development of basal cell carcinoma. Dermatol Surg 2004; 30:248–52.

18 McNaughton SA, Marks GC, Green AC. Role of dietary factors in the development of basal cell cancer of the skin. Cancer Epidemiol Biomarkers Prev 2005; 14:1596–607.

19 Gorlin RJ. Nevoid basal cell carcinoma (Gorlin) syndrome. Genet Med 2004; 6:530–9.

20 Felder S, Rabinovitz H, Oliviero M, Kopf A. Dermoscopic differentiation of a superficial basal cell carcinoma and squamous cell carcinoma in situ. Dermatol Surg 2006; 32:423–5.

21 Bakis S, Irwig L, Wood G, Wong D. Exfoliative cytology as a diagnostic test for basal cell carcinoma: a meta-analysis. Br J Dermatol 2004; 150:829–36.

22 Williams LS, Mancuso AA, Mendenhall WM. Perineural spread of cutaneous squamous and basal cell carcinoma: CT and MR detection and its impact on patient management and prognosis. Int J Radiat Oncol Biol Phys 2001; 49:1061–9.

23 Leibovitch I, McNab A, Sullivan T et al. Orbital invasion by periocular basal cell carcinoma. Ophthalmology 2005; 112:717–23.

24 Meads SB, Greenway HT. Basal cell carcinoma associated with orbital invasion: clinical features and treatment options. Dermatol Surg 2006; 32:442–6.

25 Farley RL, Manolidis S, Ratner D. Aggressive basal cell carcinoma with invasion of the parotid gland, facial nerve, and temporal bone. Dermatol Surg 2006; 32:307–15.

26 Randle HW. Basal cell carcinoma: identification and treatment of the high-risk patient. Dermatol Surg 1996; 22:255–61.

27 Batra RS, Kelley LC. A risk scale for predicting extensive subclinical spread of nonmelanoma skin cancer. Dermatol Surg 2002; 28:107–12.

28 Bath-Hextall F, Perkins W, Bong J, Williams H. Interventions for basal cell carcinoma of the skin. Cochrane Database Syst Rev 2007; 1:CD003412.

29 Ceilley RI, Del Rosso JQ. Current modalities and new advances in the treatment of basal cell carcinoma. Int J Dermatol 2006; 45:489–98.

30 Telfer NR, Colver GB, Bowers PW. Guidelines for the management of basal cell carcinoma. Br J Dermatol 1999; 141:415–23.

31 Drake LA, Ceilley RI, Cornelison RL et al. Guidelines of care for basal cell carcinoma. The American Academy of Dermatology Committee on Guidelines of Care. J Am Acad Dermatol 1992; 26:117–20.

32 Backous DD, DeMonte F, El-Naggar A et al. Craniofacial resection for nonmelanoma skin cancer of the head and neck. Laryngoscope 2005; 115:931–7.

33 Smeets N. Little evidence available on treatments for basal cell carcinoma of the skin. Cancer Treat Rev 2005; 31:143–6.

34 Cataldo PA, Stoddard PB, Reed WP. Use of frozen section analysis in the treatment of basal cell carcinoma. Am J Surg 1990; 159:561–3.

35 Walker P, Hill D. Surgical treatment of basal cell carcinomas using standard postoperative histological assessment. Australas J Dermatol 2006; 47:1–12.

36 Marchac D, Papadopoulos O, Duport G. Curative and aesthetic results of surgical treatment of 138 basal-cell carcinomas. J Dermatol Surg Oncol 1982; 8:379–87.

37 Griffiths RW, Suvarna SK, Stone J. Do basal cell carcinomas recur after complete conventional surgical excision? Br J Plast Surg 2005; 58:795–805.

38 Johnson TM, Tromovitch TA, Swanson NA. Combined curettage and excision: a treatment method for primary basal cell carcinoma. J Am Acad Dermatol 1991; 24:613–17.

39 Chiller K, Passaro D, McCalmont T, Vin-Christian K. Efficacy of curettage before excision in clearing surgical margins of nonmelanoma skin cancer. Arch Dermatol 2000; 136:1327–32.

40 Wolf DJ, Zitelli JA. Surgical margins for basal cell carcinoma. Arch Dermatol 1987; 123:340–4.

41 Kimyai-Asadi A, Goldberg LH, Peterson SR et al. Efficacy of narrow-margin excision of well-demarcated primary facial basal cell carcinomas. J Am Acad Dermatol 2005; 53:464–8.

42 Kimyai-Asadi A, Goldberg LH, Jih MH. Accuracy of serial transverse cross-sections in detecting residual basal cell carcinoma at the surgical margins of an elliptical excision specimen. J Am Acad Dermatol 2005; 53:469–74.

43 Kumar P, Orton CI, McWilliam LJ, Watson S. Incidence of incomplete excision in surgically treated basal cell carcinoma: a retrospective clinical audit. Br J Plast Surg 2000; 35:563–6.

44 Griffiths RW. Audit of histologically incompletely excised basal cell carcinomas: recommendations for management by re-excision. Br J Plast Surg 1999; 52:24–8.

45 Dieu T, Macleod AM. Incomplete excision of basal cell carcinomas: a retrospective audit. Aust NZ J Surg 2002; 72:219–21.

46 Sussman LA, Liggins DF. Incompletely excised basal cell carcinoma: a management dilemma? Aust NZ J Surg 1996; 66:276–8.

47 Wilson AW, Howsam G, Santhanam V et al. Surgical management of incompletely excised basal cell carcinomas of the head and neck. Br J Oral Maxillofac Surg 2004; 42:311–14.

48 Grabski WJ, Salasche SJ. Positive surgical excision margins of a basal cell carcinoma. Dermatol Surg 1998; 24:921–4.

49 Richmond JD, Davie RM. The significance of incomplete excision in patients with basal cell carcinoma. Br J Plast Surg 1987; 40:63–7.

50 Park AJ, Strick M, Watson JD. Basal cell carcinomas: do they need to be followed up? J R Coll Surg Edinb 1994; 39:109–11.

51 De Silva SP, Dellon AL. Recurrence rate of positive margin basal cell carcinoma: results of a five-year prospective study. J Surg Oncol 1985; 28:72–4.

52 Bieley HC, Kirsner RS, Reyes BA, Garland LD. The use of Mohs micrographic surgery for determination of residual tumor in incompletely excised basal cell carcinoma. J Am Acad Dermatol 1992; 26:754–6.

53 Liu FF, Maki E, Warde P et al. A management approach to incompletely excised basal cell carcinomas of skin. Int J Radiat Oncol Biol Phys 1991; 20:423–8.

54 Hauben DJ, Zirkin H, Mahler D, Sacks M. The biologic behavior of basal cell carcinoma: part I. Plast Reconstr Surg 1982; 69:103–9.

55 Robinson JK, Fisher SG. Recurrent basal cell carcinoma after incomplete resection. Arch Dermatol 2000; 136:1318–24.

56 Berlin J, Katz KH, Helm KF, Maloney ME. The significance of tumor persistence after incomplete excision of basal cell carcinoma. J Am Acad Dermatol 2002; 46:549–53.

57 Koplin L, Zarem HA. Recurrent basal cell carcinoma: a review concerning the incidence, behavior, and management of recurrent basal cell carcinoma, with emphasis on the incompletely excised lesion. Plast Reconstr Surg 1980; 65:656–64.

58 Boulinguez S, Grison-Tabone C, Lamant L et al. Histological evolution of recurrent basal cell carcinoma and therapeutic implications for incompletely excised lesions. Br J Dermatol 2004; 151:623–6.

59 Rowe DE, Carroll RJ, Day CL. Mohs surgery is the treatment of choice for recurrent (previously treated) basal cell carcinoma. J Dermatol Surg Oncol 1989; 15:424–31.

60 Burg G, Hirsch RD, Konz B, Braun-Falco O. Histographic surgery: accuracy of visual assessment of the margins of basal-cell epithelioma. J Dermatol Surg Oncol 1975; 1:21–4.

61 Mohs FE. Chemosurgery for skin cancer: fixed tissue and fresh tissue techniques. Arch Dermatol 1976; 112:211–15.

62 Lawrence CM. Mohs' micrographic surgery for basal cell carcinoma. Clin Exp Dermatol 1999; 24:130–3.

63 Nelson BR, Railan D, Cohen S. Mohs' micrographic surgery for nonmelanoma skin cancers. Clin Plast Surg 1997; 24:705–18.

64 Wennberg AM, Larko O, Stenquist B. Five-year results of Mohs' micrographic surgery for aggressive facial basal cell carcinoma in Sweden. Acta Derm Venereol (Stockh) 1999; 79:370–2.

65 Williford PM, Feldman SR. Surgery for basal-cell carcinoma of the face. Lancet 2004; 364:1732–3.

66 Rowe DE, Carroll RJ, Day CL Jr et al. Long-term recurrence rates in previously untreated (primary) basal cell carcinoma: implications for patient follow-up. J Dermatol Surg Oncol 1989; 15:315–28.

67 Malhotra R, Huilgol SC, Huynh NT, Selva D. The Australian Mohs database, part II: periocular basal cell carcinoma outcome at 5-year follow-up. Ophthalmology 2004; 111:631–6.

68 Leibovitch I, Huilgol SC, Selva D et al. Basal cell carcinoma treated with Mohs surgery in Australia II. Outcome at 5-year follow-up. J Am Acad Dermatol 2005; 53:452–7.

69 Smeets NW, Kuijpers DI, Nelemans P et al. Mohs' micrographic surgery for treatment of basal cell carcinoma of the face – results of a retrospective study and review of the literature. Br J Dermatol 2004; 151:141–7.

70 Kimyai-Asadi A, Goldberg LH, Peterson SR et al. The incidence of major complications from Mohs micrographic surgery performed in office-based and hospital-based settings. J Am Acad Dermatol 2005; 53:628–34.

71 Cook JL, Perone JB. A prospective evaluation of the incidence of complications associated with Mohs micrographic surgery. Arch Dermatol 2003; 139:143–52.

72 Dobke MK, Miller SH. Tissue repair after Mohs surgery. A plastic surgeon's view. Dermatol Surg 1997; 23:1061–6.

73 Stein JM, Hrabovsky S, Schuller DE, Siegle RJ. Mohs micrographic surgery and the otolaryngologist. Am J Otolaryngol 2004; 25:385–93.

74 Inkster C, Ashworth J, Murdoch JR et al. Oculoplastic reconstruction following Mohs surgery. Eye 1998; 12:214–18.

75 Sciscio A, Stewart K, Grewal J et al. Periocular Mohs micrographic surgery: results of a dual-site day-surgery service. Orbit 2001; 20:209–15.

76 Breuninger H. Micrographic surgery of malignant skin tumors: a comparison of the frozen technique with paraffin sectioning. Facial Plast Surg 1997; 13:79–82.

77 der Plessis PJ, Dahl MG, Malcolm AJ et al. Mohs' surgery of periocular basal cell carcinoma using formalin-fixed sections and delayed closure. Br J Dermatol 1998; 138:1003–8.

78 Skaria AM, Salomon D. Mohs' surgery of periocular basal cell carcinoma using formalin-fixed sections and delayed closure. Br J Dermatol 1999; 140:775.

79 Wong VA, Marshall JA, Whitehead KJ et al. Management of periocular basal cell carcinoma with modified en face frozen section controlled excision. Ophthal Plast Reconstr Surg 2002; 18:430–5.

80 Strong JW, Worsham GF, Hagerty RC. Peripheral in-continuity tissue examination: a modification of Mohs' micrographic surgery. Clin Plast Surg 2004; 31:1–4.

81 Boztepe G, Hohenleutner S, Landthaler M, Hohenleutner U. Munich method of micrographic surgery for basal cell carcinomas: 5-year recurrence rates with life-table analysis. Acta Derm Venereol (Stockh) 2004; 84:218–22.

82 Bentkover SH, Grande DM, Soto H et al. Excision of head and neck basal cell carcinoma with a rapid, cross-sectional, frozen-section technique. Arch Facial Plast Surg 2002; 4:114–19.

83 Niederhagen B, von Lindern JJ, Berge S et al. Staged operations for basal cell carcinoma of the face. Br J Oral Maxillofac Surg 2000; 38:477–9.

84 Hsuan JD, Harrad RA, Potts MJ, Collins C. Small margin excision of periocular basal cell carcinoma: 5 year results. Br J Ophthalmol 2004; 88:358–60.

85 David DB, Gimblett ML, Potts MJ, Harrad RA. Small margin (2 mm) excision of peri-ocular basal cell carcinoma with delayed repair. Orbit 1999; 18:11–15.

86 Cook J, Zitelli JA. Mohs micrographic surgery: a cost analysis. J Am Acad Dermatol 1998; 39:698–703.

87 Bialy TL, Whalen J, Veledar E et al. Mohs micrographic surgery vs traditional surgical excision: a cost comparison analysis. Arch Dermatol 2004; 140:736–42.

88 Essers BA, Dirksen CD, Nieman FH et al. Cost-effectiveness of Mohs micrographic surgery vs surgical excision for basal cell carcinoma of the face. Arch Dermatol 2006; 142:187–94.

89 Smeets NW, Krekels GA, Ostertag JU et al. Surgical excision vs Mohs' micrographic surgery for basal-cell carcinoma of the face: randomised controlled trial. Lancet 2004; 364:1766–72.

90 Otley CC. Mohs' micrographic surgery for basal-cell carcinoma of the face. Lancet 2005; 365:1226–7.

91 Reymann F. 15 years' experience with treatment of basal cell carcinomas of the skin with curettage. Acta Derm Venereol (Stockh) 1985; 120 (Suppl.):56–9.

92 Sheridan AT, Dawber RP. Curettage, electrosurgery and skin cancer. Australas J Dermatol 2000; 41:19–30.

93 Edens BL, Bartlow GA, Haghighi P et al. Effectiveness of curettage and electrodesiccation in the removal of basal cell carcinoma. J Am Acad Dermatol 1983; **9**:383–8.

94 Barlow JO, Zalla MJ, Kyle A et al. Treatment of basal cell carcinoma with curettage alone. J Am Acad Dermatol 2006; **54**:1039–45.

95 McDaniel WE. Therapy for basal cell epitheliomas by curettage only. Further study. Arch Dermatol 1983; **119**:901–3.

96 Spiller WF, Spiller RF. Treatment of basal cell epithelioma by curettage and electrodesiccation. J Am Acad Dermatol 1984; **11**:808–14.

97 Kopf AW, Bart RS, Schrager D et al. Curettage-electrodesiccation treatment of basal cell carcinomas. Arch Dermatol 1977; **113**:439–43.

98 Motley RJ, Gould DJ, Douglas WS, Simpson NB. Treatment of basal cell carcinoma by dermatologists in the United Kingdom. British Association of Dermatologists Audit Subcommittee and the British Society for Dermatological Surgery. Br J Dermatol 1995; **132**:437–40.

99 Carlson KC, Connolly SM, Winkelmann RK. Basal cell carcinoma on the lower extremity. J Dermatol Surg Oncol 1994; **20**:258–9.

100 Silverman MK, Kopf AW, Grin CM et al. Recurrence rates of treated basal cell carcinomas. Part 2: curettage-electrodesiccation. J Dermatol Surg Oncol 1991; **17**:720–6.

101 Salasche SJ. Curettage and electrodesiccation in the treatment of midfacial basal cell epithelioma. J Am Acad Dermatol 1983; **8**:496–503.

102 Suhge d'Aubermont PC, Bennett RG. Failure of curettage and electrodesiccation for removal of basal cell carcinoma. Arch Dermatol 1984; **120**:1456–60.

103 Spencer JM, Tannenbaum A, Sloan L, Amonette RA. Does inflammation contribute to the eradication of basal cell carcinoma following curettage and electrodesiccation? Dermatol Surg 1997; **23**:625–30.

104 Nouri K, Spencer JM, Taylor JR et al. Does wound healing contribute to the eradication of basal cell carcinoma following curettage and electrodesiccation? Dermatol Surg 1999; **25**:183–7.

105 Wu JK, Oh C, Strutton G, Siller G. An open-label, pilot study examining the efficacy of curettage followed by imiquimod 5% cream for the treatment of primary nodular basal cell carcinoma. Australas J Dermatol 2006; **47**:46–8.

106 Spencer JM. Pilot study of imiquimod 5% cream as adjunctive therapy to curettage and electrodesiccation for nodular basal cell carcinoma. Dermatol Surg 2006; **32**:63–9.

107 Soler AM, Warloe T, Berner A, Giercksky KE. A follow-up study of recurrence and cosmesis in completely responding superficial and nodular basal cell carcinomas treated with methyl 5-aminolaevulinate-based photodynamic therapy alone and with prior curettage. Br J Dermatol 2001; **145**:467–71.

108 Nordin P, Stenquist B. Five-year results of curettage-cryosurgery for 100 consecutive auricular non-melanoma skin cancers. J Laryngol Otol 2002; **116**:893–8.

109 Graham G. Statistical data on malignant tumors in cryosurgery: 1982. J Dermatol Surg Oncol 1983; **9**:238–9.

110 Zacarian SA. Cryosurgery of cutaneous carcinomas. An 18 year study of 3,022 patients with 4,228 carcinomas. J Am Acad Dermatol 1983; **9**:947–56.

111 Mallon E, Dawber R. Cryosurgery in the treatment of basal cell carcinoma. Assessment of one and two freeze-thaw cycle schedules. Dermatol Surg 1996; **22**:854–8.

112 Goncalves JC. Fractional cryosurgery. A new technique for basal cell carcinoma of the eyelids and periorbital area. Dermatol Surg 1997; **23**:475–81.

113 Holt PJ. Cryotherapy for skin cancer: results over a 5-year period using liquid nitrogen spray cryosurgery. Br J Dermatol 1988; **119**:231–40.

114 Giuffrida TJ, Jimenez G, Nouri K. Histologic cure of basal cell carcinoma treated with cryosurgery. J Am Acad Dermatol 2003; **49**:483–6.

115 Kokoszka A, Scheinfeld N. Evidence-based review of the use of cryosurgery in treatment of basal cell carcinoma. Dermatol Surg 2003; **29**:566–71.

116 Bernardeau K, Derancourt C, Cambie M et al. [Cryosurgery of basal cell carcinoma: a study of 358 patients]. Ann Dermatol Venereol 2000; **127**:175–9.

117 Kuflik EG, Gage AA. The five-year cure rate achieved by cryosurgery for skin cancer. J Am Acad Dermatol 1991; **24**:1002–4.

118 Kuflik EG. Cryosurgery for skin cancer: 30-year experience and cure rates. Dermatol Surg 2004; **30**:297–300.

119 Jaramillo-Ayerbe F. Cryosurgery in difficult to treat basal cell carcinoma. Int J Dermatol 2000; **39**:223–9.

120 Kuflik EG, Gage AA. Recurrent basal cell carcinoma treated with cryosurgery. J Am Acad Dermatol 1997; **37**:82–4.

121 Buschmann W. A reappraisal of cryosurgery for eyelid basal cell carcinomas. Br J Ophthalmol 2002; **86**:453–7.

122 Anders M, Sporl E, Krantz H et al. [Cryotherapy of malignant eyelid tumors]. Ophthalmologe 1995; **92**:787–92.

123 Tuppurainen K. Cryotherapy for eyelid and periocular basal cell carcinomas: outcome in 166 cases over an 8-year period. Graefes Arch Clin Exp Ophthalmol 1995; **233**:205–8.

124 Gunnarson G, Larko O, Hersle K. Cryosurgery of eyelid basal cell carcinomas. Acta Ophthalmol (Copenh) 1990; **68**:241–5.

125 Wang I, Bendsoe N, Klinteberg CA et al. Photodynamic therapy vs. cryosurgery of basal cell carcinomas: results of a phase III clinical trial. Br J Dermatol 2001; **144**:832–40.

126 Thissen MR, Nieman FH, Ideler AH et al. Cosmetic results of cryosurgery vs. surgical excision for primary uncomplicated basal cell carcinomas of the head and neck. Dermatol Surg 2000; **26**:759–64.

127 Nouri K, Chang A, Trent JT, Jimenez GP. Ultrapulse CO_2 used for the successful treatment of basal cell carcinomas found in patients with basal cell nevus syndrome. Dermatol Surg 2002; **28**:287–90.

128 Stockfleth E, Trefzer U, Garcia-Bartels C et al. The use of toll-like receptor-7 agonist in the treatment of basal cell carcinoma: an overview. Br J Dermatol 2003; **149** (Suppl. 66):53–6.

129 Marks R, Gebauer K, Shumack S et al. Imiquimod 5% cream in the treatment of superficial basal cell carcinoma: results of a multicenter 6-week dose–response trial. J Am Acad Dermatol 2001; **44**:807–13.

130 Geisse JK, Rich P, Pandya A et al. Imiquimod 5% cream for the treatment of superficial basal cell carcinoma: a double-blind, randomized, vehicle-controlled study. J Am Acad Dermatol 2002; **47**:390–8.

131 Geisse J, Caro I, Lindholm J et al. Imiquimod 5% cream for the treatment of superficial basal cell carcinoma: results from two phase III, randomized, vehicle-controlled studies. J Am Acad Dermatol 2004; **50**:722–33.

132 Schulze HJ, Cribier B, Requena L et al. Imiquimod 5% cream for the treatment of superficial basal cell carcinoma: results from a randomized vehicle-controlled phase III study in Europe. Br J Dermatol 2005; **152**:939–47.

133 Gollnick H, Barona CG, Frank RG et al. Recurrence rate of superficial basal cell carcinoma following successful treatment with imiquimod 5% cream: interim 2-year results from an ongoing 5-year follow-up study in Europe. Eur J Dermatol 2005; **15**:374–81.

134 Shumack S, Robinson J, Kossard S et al. Efficacy of topical 5% imiquimod cream for the treatment of nodular basal cell carcinoma: comparison of dosing regimens. Arch Dermatol 2002; **138**:1165–71.

135 Eigentler TK, Kamin A, Weide BM et al. A phase III, randomized, open label study to evaluate the safety and efficacy of imiquimod

5% cream applied thrice weekly for 8 and 12 weeks in the treatment of low risk nodular basal cell carcinoma. *J Am Acad Dermatol* 2007; **57**:616–21.

136 Vidal D, Matias-Guiu X, Alomar A. Fifty-five basal cell carcinomas treated with topical imiquimod: outcome at 5-year follow-up. *Arch Dermatol* 2007; **143**:266–8.

137 Sterry W, Ruzicka T, Herrera E *et al.* Imiquimod 5% cream for the treatment of superficial and nodular basal cell carcinoma: randomized studies comparing low-frequency dosing with and without occlusion. *Br J Dermatol* 2002; **147**:1227–36.

138 Kagy MK, Amonette R. The use of imiquimod 5% cream for the treatment of superficial basal cell carcinomas in a basal cell nevus syndrome patient. *Dermatol Surg* 2000; **26**:577–8.

139 Stockfleth E, Ulrich C, Hauschild A *et al.* Successful treatment of basal cell carcinomas in a nevoid basal cell carcinoma syndrome with topical 5% imiquimod. *Eur J Dermatol* 2002; **12**:569–72.

140 Micali G, De Pasquale R, Caltabiano R *et al.* Topical imiquimod treatment of superficial and nodular basal cell carcinomas in patients affected by basal cell nevus syndrome: a preliminary report. *J Dermatolog Treat* 2002; **13**:123–7.

141 Nikkels AF, Pierard-Franchimont C, Nikkels-Tassoudji N *et al.* Photodynamic therapy and imiquimod immunotherapy for basal cell carcinomas. *Acta Clin Belg* 2005; **60**:227–34.

142 Morton CA, Brown SB, Collins S *et al.* Guidelines for topical photodynamic therapy: report of a workshop of the British Photodermatology Group. *Br J Dermatol* 2002; **146**:552–67.

143 Varma S, Wilson H, Kurwa HA *et al.* Bowen's disease, solar keratoses and superficial basal cell carcinomas treated by photodynamic therapy using a large-field incoherent light source. *Br J Dermatol* 2001; **144**:567–74.

144 Clark C, Bryden A, Dawe R *et al.* Topical 5-aminolaevulinic acid photodynamic therapy for cutaneous lesions: outcome and comparison of light sources. *Photodermatol Photoimmunol Photomed* 2003; **19**:134–41.

145 Kuijpers D, Thissen MR, Thissen CA, Neumann MH. Similar effectiveness of methyl aminolevulinate and 5-aminolevulinate in topical photodynamic therapy for nodular basal cell carcinoma. *J Drugs Dermatol* 2006; **5**:642–5.

146 Braathen LR, Szeimies R-M, Basset-Seguin N *et al.* Guidelines on the use of photodynamic therapy for nonmelanoma skin cancer. An international consensus. *J Am Acad Dermatol* 2007; **56**:125–43.

147 Rhodes LE, de Rie M, Enström Y *et al.* Photodynamic therapy using topical methyl aminolevulinate vs surgery for nodular basal cell carcinoma. Results of a multicenter randomized prospective trial. *Arch Dermatol* 2004; **140**:17–23.

148 Rhodes LE, de Rie MA, Leifsdottir R *et al.* Five year follow-up of a randomized, prospective trial of methyl aminolevulinate photodynamic therapy vs surgery for nodular basal cell carcinoma. *Arch Dermatol* 2007; **143**:1131–6.

149 Horn M, Wolf P, Wulf HC *et al.* Topical methyl aminolevulinate photodynamic therapy in patients with basal cell carcinoma prone to complications and poor cosmetic outcome with conventional treatment. *Br J Dermatol* 2003; **149**:1242–9.

150 Vinciullo C, Elliott T, Francis D *et al.* Photodynamic therapy with topical methyl aminolaevulinate for 'difficult-to-treat' basal cell carcinoma. *Br J Dermatol* 2005; **152**:765–72.

151 Oseroff AR, Shieh S, Frawley NP *et al.* Treatment of diffuse basal cell carcinomas and basaloid follicular hamartomas in nevoid basal cell carcinoma syndrome by wide-area 5-aminolevulinic acid photodynamic therapy. *Arch Dermatol* 2005; **141**:60–7.

152 Itkin A, Gilchrest BA. delta-Aminolevulinic acid and blue light photodynamic therapy for the treatment of multiple basal cell carcinomas in two patients with nevoid basal cell carcinoma syndrome. *Dermatol Surg* 2004; **30**:1054–61.

153 Morton CA. Methyl aminolevulinate (Metfix) photodynamic therapy – practical pearls. *J Dermatolog Treat* 2003; **14** (Suppl. 3):23–6.

154 Al-Othman MO, Mendenhall WM, Amdur RJ. Radiotherapy alone for clinical T4 skin carcinoma of the head and neck with surgery reserved for salvage. *Am J Otolaryngol* 2001; **22**:387–90.

155 Rio E, Bardet E, Ferron C *et al.* Interstitial brachytherapy of periorificial skin carcinomas of the face: a retrospective study of 97 cases. *Int J Radiat Oncol Biol Phys* 2005; **63**:753–7.

156 Guix B, Finestres F, Tello J *et al.* Treatment of skin carcinomas of the face by high-dose-rate brachytherapy and custom-made surface molds. *Int J Radiat Oncol Biol Phys* 2000; **47**:95–102.

157 Kwan W, Wilson D, Moravan V. Radiotherapy for locally advanced basal cell and squamous cell carcinomas of the skin. *Int J Radiat Oncol Biol Phys* 2004; **60**:406–11.

158 Childers BJ, Goldwyn RM, Ramos D *et al.* Long-term results of irradiation for basal cell carcinoma of the skin of the nose. *Plast Reconstr Surg* 1994; **93**:1169–73.

159 Caccialanza M, Piccinno R, Grammatica A. Radiotherapy of recurrent basal and squamous cell skin carcinomas: a study of 249 re-treated carcinomas in 229 patients. *Eur J Dermatol* 2001; **11**:25–8.

160 Finizio L, Vidali C, Calacione R *et al.* What is the current role of radiation therapy in the treatment of skin carcinomas? *Tumori* 2002; **88**:48–52.

161 Caccialanza M, Piccinno R, Moretti D, Rozza M. Radiotherapy of carcinomas of the skin overlying the cartilage of the nose: results in 405 lesions. *Eur J Dermatol* 2003; **13**:462–5.

162 Huynh NT, Veness MJ. Basal cell carcinoma of the lip treated with radiotherapy. *Australas J Dermatol* 2002; **43**:15–19.

163 Silva JJ, Tsang RW, Panzarella T *et al.* Results of radiotherapy for epithelial skin cancer of the pinna: the Princess Margaret Hospital experience, 1982–1993. *Int J Radiat Oncol Biol Phys* 2000; **47**:451–9.

164 Morrison WH, Garden AS, Ang KK. Radiation therapy for nonmelanoma skin carcinomas. *Clin Plast Surg* 1997; **24**:719–29.

165 Zagrodnik B, Kempf W, Seifert B *et al.* Superficial radiotherapy for patients with basal cell carcinoma; recurrence rates, histologic subtypes, and expression of p53 and Bcl-2. *Cancer* 2003; **98**:2708–14.

166 Caccialanza M, Piccinno R, Kolesnikova L, Gnecchi L. Radiotherapy of skin carcinomas of the pinna: a study of 115 lesions in 108 patients. *Int J Dermatol* 2005; **44**:513–17.

167 Avril MF, Auperin A, Margulis A *et al.* Basal cell carcinoma of the face: surgery or radiotherapy? Results of a randomized study. *Br J Cancer* 1997; **76**:100–6.

168 Hall VL, Leppard BJ, McGill J *et al.* Treatment of basal-cell carcinoma: comparison of radiotherapy and cryotherapy. *Clin Radiol* 1986; **37**:33–4.

169 Petit JY, Avril MF, Margulis A *et al.* Evaluation of cosmetic results of a randomized trial comparing surgery and radiotherapy in the treatment of basal cell carcinoma of the face. *Plast Reconstr Surg* 2000; **105**:2544–51.

170 Caccialanza M, Percivalle S, Piccinno R. Possibility of treating basal cell carcinomas of nevoid basal cell carcinoma syndrome with superficial X-ray therapy. *Dermatology* 2004; **208**:60–3.

171 Marcil I, Stern RS. Risk of developing a subsequent nonmelanoma skin cancer in patients with a history of nonmelanoma skin cancer: a critical review of the literature and meta-analysis. *Arch Dermatol* 2000; **136**:1524–30.

172 Veien K, Veien NK. Risk of developing subsequent nonmelanoma skin cancers. *Arch Dermatol* 2001; **137**:1251.

173 Levi F, Randimbison L, Maspoli M *et al.* High incidence of second basal cell skin cancers. *Int J Cancer* 2006; **119**:1505–7.

174 van Iersel CA, van de Velden HV, Kusters CD et al. Prognostic factors for a subsequent basal cell carcinoma: implications for follow up. Br J Dermatol 2005; **153**:1078–80.

175 Ramachandran S, Fryer AA, Smith AG et al. Basal cell carcinoma. Cancer 2000; **89**:1012–18.

176 Lear JT, Smith AG, Bowers B et al. Truncal tumor site is associated with high risk of multiple basal cell carcinoma and is influenced by glutathione S-transferase, GSTT1, and cytochrome P450, CYP1A1 genotypes, and their interaction. J Invest Dermatol 1997; **108**:519–22.

177 Ramachandran S, Fryer AA, Smith A et al. Cutaneous basal cell carcinomas: distinct host factors are associated with the development of tumors on the trunk and head and neck. Cancer 2001; **92**:354–8.

178 Mc Loone NM, Tolland J, Walsh M, Dolan OM. Follow up of basal cell carcinomas: an audit of current practice. J Eur Acad Dermatol Venereol 2006; **20**:698–701.

179 Bower CP, Lear JT, de Berker DA. Basal cell carcinoma follow-up practices by dermatologists: a national survey. Br J Dermatol 2001; **145**:949–56.

180 Griffiths CEM. The British Association of Dermatologists guidelines for the management of skin disease. Br J Dermatol 1999; **141**:396–7.

181 Cox NH, Williams HC. The British Association of Dermatologists therapeutic guidelines: can we AGREE? Br J Dermatol 2003; **148**:621–5.

Appendix 1

The consultation process and background details for the British Association of Dermatologists guidelines have been published elsewhere.[180,181]

Strength of recommendations

A There is good evidence to support the use of the procedure.
B There is fair evidence to support the use of the procedure.
C There is poor evidence to support the use of the procedure.
D There is fair evidence to support the rejection of the use of the procedure.
E There is good evidence to support the rejection of the use of the procedure.

Quality of evidence

I Evidence obtained from at least one properly designed, randomized controlled trial.
II-i Evidence obtained from well-designed controlled trials without randomization.
II-ii Evidence obtained from well-designed cohort or case–control analytical studies, preferably from more than one centre or research group.
II-iii Evidence obtained from multiple time series with or without the intervention. Dramatic results in uncontrolled experiments (such as the introduction of penicillin treatment in the 1940s) could also be regarded as this type of evidence.
III Opinions of respected authorities based on clinical experience, descriptive studies or reports of expert committees.
IV Evidence inadequate owing to problems of methodology (e.g. sample size, or length or comprehensiveness of follow-up or conflicts of evidence).

http://bad.org.uk/Portals/_Bad/Guidelines/Clinical %20Guidelines/BCC%20Guidelines%20BJDJul08.pdf

Comment

The main additions to the 2008 basal cell carcinoma (BCC) guidelines [1] have been the further developments of PDT (see PDT guideline), topical immunomodulators (imiquimod) for low-risk tumours and the acceptance of many departments in the UK of Moh's micrographic surgery for high-risk tumours. Imiquimod is a recent development and was not available for use in BCCs in 1999 [2]. It is finding its place in low-risk tumours [1,3], but whether it is better than surgery is being tested by a randomised control trial (SINS trial) [4], which has finished recruiting patients but the results not yet published. As there are usually several treatment options for BCCs, choice of treatment modality has to be a concordant agreement with the patient and doctor. Further studies are needed on genetics [5], prevention [6] and management of BCCs.

REFERENCES

1 Telfer NR, Colver GB, Morton CA. Guidelines for the management of basal cell carcinoma. *Brit J Dermatol* 2008; 159: 35–48.
2 Telfer NR, Colver GB, Bowers PW. Guidelines for the management of basal cell carcinoma. *Br J Dermatol* 1999; 141:415–23.
3 Love WE, Bernhard JD, Bordeaux JS. Topical imiquimod or fluorouracil therapy for basal and squamous cell carcinoma: a systematic review. *Arch Dermatol* 2009; 145: 1431–8.
4 http://www.ukdctn.org/ongoing/
5 Madan V, Hoban P, Strange RC, *et al.* Genetics and risk factors for basal cell carcinoma. *Brit J Dermatol* 2006; 154: 5–7.
6 Ulrich C, Jürgensen JS, Degen A, *et al.* Prevention of non-melanoma skin cancer in organ transplant patients by regular use of a sunscreen: a 24 months, prospective, case–control study. *Brit J Dermatol* 2009; 161: 78–84.

Additional professional resources

Bath-Hextall FJ, Perkins W, Bong J, Williams HC. Interventions for basal cell carcinoma of the skin. *Cochrane Database Syst Rev* 2007; Issue 1: CD003412 (update of *Cochrane Database Syst Rev* 2003 (Issue 2): CD003412) (http://mrw.interscience.wiley.com/cochrane/clsysrev/articles/CD003412/frame.html).
Bath-Hextall FJ, Bong J, Perkins W, Williams HC. Interventions for basal cell carcinoma of the skin: systematic review. *Brit Med J* 2004; 329: 705 (http://www.ncbi.nlm.nih.gov/pmc/articles/PMC518891/?tool=pubmed).
National Comprehensive Cancer Network (USA) (requires free registration). http://www.nccn.org/professionals/physician_gls/PDF/nmsc.pdf (covers basal and squamous cell carcinomas of skin 2009).
Miller SJ, Alam M, Andersen J, *et al.* Basal cell and squamous cell skin cancers. *J Natl Compr Canc Netw* 2007; 5: 506–29.

BAD patient information leaflet

http://www.bad.org.uk/site/800/default.aspx

Other patient resources

http://www.cancerbackup.org.uk

Guidelines for management of Bowen's disease: 2006 update

N.H. Cox, D.J. Eedy* and C.A. Morton† on behalf of the British Association of Dermatologists Therapy Guidelines and Audit Subcommittee

Department of Dermatology, Cumberland Infirmary, Carlisle CA2 7HY, U.K.
*Craigavon Area Hospital, Craigavon BT63 5QQ, U.K.
†Stirling Royal Infirmary, Stirling FK8 2AU, U.K.

Summary

This article represents a planned regular updating of the previous British Association of Dermatologists (BAD) guidelines for management of Bowen's disease. They have been prepared for dermatologists on behalf of the BAD. They present evidence-based guidance for treatment, with identification of the strength of evidence available at the time of preparation of the guidelines.

Disclaimer

These guidelines have been prepared for dermatologists on behalf of the British Association of Dermatologists (BAD) and are based on the best data available at the time the report was prepared. Caution should be exercised when interpreting data where there is a limited evidence base; the results of future studies may require alteration of the conclusions or recommendations in this report. It may be necessary or even desirable to depart from the guidelines in the interests of specific patients and special circumstances. Just as adherence to guidelines may not constitute defence against a claim of negligence, so deviation from them should not necessarily be deemed negligent.

Definition and introduction to the guideline

The scope, aims and methodology of the BAD guidelines process have been published elsewhere;[1,2] these references should be consulted for guideline validation purposes.

This article represents a planned regular updating of the previous BAD guidelines for management of Bowen's disease

(BD).[3] Those guidelines included discussion of epidemiology, predisposing factors, disease associations and risk of malignancy as well as the local treatment options for the disease itself. New information in these areas, other than that pertaining to issues that influence therapeutic decisions, will only be briefly summarized in this update. Similarly, detailed evidence for therapies discussed in the previous paper will not be repeated except where comparison with other evidence is necessary. It should be recognized that this may entail a disproportionate weight being given to referencing newer therapies. Where there are direct comparisons between therapies, these are generally discussed in the section relating to those deemed to be most efficacious. Recommendations take into account simplicity, cost and healing as well as the type and validity of the published evidence base; for any treatment, there may be site-specific differences in the recommended option. The abbreviation RCT is used for randomized controlled trial throughout.

BD is a form of intraepidermal (in situ) squamous cell carcinoma (SCC), originally described in 1912.[4] Genital lesions which have the histology of BD include erythroplasia of Queyrat (males), some vulval intraepithelial neoplasia (VIN) and bowenoid papulosis (either sex). There is a strong association of genital or perianal intraepithelial neoplasia in either sex with human papillomavirus (HPV) infection, although many such cases do not have the clinical morphology of BD. The association between BD and HPV is briefly discussed and we have included some brief comments in relation to therapy and outcomes (especially for erythroplasia of Queyrat, as this is often referred to as penile BD), but a detailed therapeutic review of HPV-related epidermal dysplasia, VIN, vaginal intraepithelial neoplasia and penile intraepithelial neoplasia (PIN) is beyond the scope of this guideline. Perianal BD is not commonly treated by dermatologists but is briefly discussed as its therapy and outcome also often differ from those of BD at extragenital sites.

Clinical description, demographics and variants

Typical BD presents as a gradually enlarging well-demarcated erythematous plaque with an irregular border and surface crusting or scaling.[3,5,6] An annual incidence of 15 per 100 000 has been suggested in the U.K.;[6] however, this figure was derived from an American study that primarily examined internal neoplasia associated with BD,[7] and was the annual incidence rate for the 1980 U.S. white population – this may not be the same as in the less sun-exposed U.K. population.

In the U.K., the peak age group for BD is the seventh decade, it occurs predominantly in women (70–85% of cases), and about three-quarters of patients have lesions on the lower leg (60–85%).[8,9] Lesions are usually solitary but are multiple in 10–20% of patients. Less common sites or variants include pigmented BD, subungual/periungual, palmar, genital and perianal (see above) and verrucous BD.

The age group, number and size of lesions, and site(s) affected may all influence therapeutic choice.

Aetiology

Reported relevant aetiological factors were discussed in the 1999 guidelines,[3] but are briefly listed here in order to update the roles of HPV and immunosuppression. Aetiologies include:
1 Irradiation – solar, photochemotherapy, radiotherapy.
2 Carcinogens – arsenic.
3 Immunosuppression – therapeutic,[10,11] AIDS. For example, one study demonstrated that 23% of skin cancers in renal transplant recipients were BD.[11] This would suggest that educating immunosuppressed patients about sun exposure is important.
4 Viral – oncogenic HPV types such as HPV 16 are strongly implicated in the aetiology of VIN, but are also common in perianal BD, and in PIN. However, HPV DNA has also been demonstrated in some extragenital BD. A report of 28 biopsies from extragenital sites demonstrated in situ hybridization evidence of oncogenic HPV types in eight of 28 (29%); all had HPV 16/18 and two of these also had HPV 31/33/51. Of note, this study had a higher than average proportion of

lesions on hands and feet (eight of 28 cases) and these accounted for 50% of the positive results.[12] A further study of HPV in extragenital cutaneous BD detected HPV DNA in 58% of 69 samples from 50 patients, the percentage of HPV detection being similar in exposed (55%) and unexposed areas (65%), and also between immunosuppressed and immunocompetent patients.[13] A study of the cell proliferation activity between HPV-positive and HPV-negative BD showed similar results in each, suggesting that HPV infection alone does not induce cell proliferation in those lesions.[14] HPV 16 has been implicated in 60% of palmoplantar and periungual lesions.[15] Multiple lesions of BD may occur on the distal digits ('polydactylous BD'), consistent with aetiological involvement of HPV. This has therapeutic implications, as HPV-induced BD should be responsive to agents that have a combined antiviral and antitumour effect.
5 Others – chronic injury or dermatoses, pre-existing skin lesions such as seborrhoeic keratoses (rarely).

Association with other malignancy

Internal neoplasia

Several larger studies and meta-analysis of the association between BD and internal cancers were summarized in our previous guideline.[3] A further study of 1147 patients found the overall incidence of internal cancers in patients with BD to be slightly increased [115 cancers vs. 103 expected, the standardized incidence ratio (SIR) of 1·1 not being statistically significant].[16] However, there was an SIR of 3·2 for leukaemia in men and of 4·6 for lung cancer in men with BD before age 60 years (the overall lung cancer SIR for both sexes and all ages was 1·3). There are various sources of potential bias in many studies of this type, and available evidence would still suggest that routine investigation for internal malignancy in patients with BD is not justified (*Strength of recommendation* E, *Quality of evidence* I; Appendix 1).

Skin malignancy

Previous studies suggested that about 30–50% of subjects with BD may have previous or subsequent nonmelanoma skin cancer (NMSC), mainly basal cell carcinoma.[17,18] The NMSC risk after an index BD is probably similar to the overall risk of NMSC following any index NMSC (overall 35–60% 3-year risk[19]). In the study by Jaeger *et al.*, NMSC had an SIR of 4·3, and lip cancer of 8·2, in patients with BD.[16] These increased risks of further BD or of other NMSC probably reflect a common solar aetiology.

Risk of progression to squamous cell carcinoma

There is no new literature to inform this debate in terms of the overall risk – *ex vivo* research studies to identify individual lesional risk and differentiation from other NMSC are beyond the scope of this guideline.

Most studies suggest a risk of invasive carcinoma of about 3–5% for 'ordinary' BD[20,21] and perhaps 10% for erythroplasia of Queyrat.[3] Perianal BD also has higher risk of invasion and recurrence (Quality of evidence II-ii), and an association with cervical and vulval dysplasia.[22–24] However, these estimates are drawn from retrospective case series, may be biased by different referral patterns of lesions to different disciplines (dermatologists, surgeons etc.), and do not take account of subjects with BD who have either not requested medical advice or who have been treated in primary care. Indeed, it is unlikely that this question can be accurately answered as any group of patients who could be followed up without intervention are likely to be unrepresentative individuals (for example, elderly patients with small lesions). Risks of cervical intraepithelial carcinoma in affected women or in female sex partners of affected men with bowenoid papulosis, and of oral papillomas and tumours in association with HPV 16-positive bowenoid papulosis, were discussed previously.[3]

Treatments

Evaluation of treatment studies of BD is difficult due to potential selection bias to specific forms of treatment. Similarly, healing and success rate may vary with body site. Earlier studies used clinical appearance rather than histological assessment to determine the end-point of lesion clearance. Even for the same treatment modality, there is difficulty in directly comparing studies due to different lesion sites, sizes of lesions, and use/availability of different types of equipment and treatment regimens.[25] Retrospective studies in particular may have several inherent problems – in 'real world' treatment of BD, dermatologists may select several different types of treatment,[26] decisions potentially being influenced by several factors such as lesion size and thickness, equipment available, and the perceived potential for poor wound healing (e.g. at sites such as the lower leg[27]). Even in recent controlled trials in which older treatments are compared with newer

modalities, the regimen for the established treatment or the site at which it is applied may not concur with the approach used by all dermatologists.

Other than a small number of anecdotal or single series reports considered at the end of the therapeutic list, the therapeutic options have been listed in a sequence to include observation alone, topical treatments and surgical treatments; within this sequence, longer-established or less interventional treatments are considered first. This sequence does not necessarily reflect the frequency of use, importance, availability or strength of evidence for any treatment option – a summary of advice incorporating these issues and related to lesion sites and sizes is provided in Table 1. Current U.K. product licences for many drugs listed do not include treatment of BD; all recommendations in this guideline are extrapolated from literature on BD and knowledge of other neoplastic skin lesions, and are presented on the understanding that neither the authors nor the BAD can formally recommend an unlicensed treatment.

Treatments are presented in a sequence that discusses the least invasive and topical therapies first, surgical approaches, and finally treatments that require more complex or expensive equipment or that are not as widely available.

No treatment

In some patients with slowly progressive thin lesions, especially on the elderly lower leg where healing is poor, there is an argument for observation rather than intervention.

5-Fluorouracil (*Strength of recommendation B, Quality of evidence II-i*)

5-Fluorouracil (5-FU) has been used topically for treatment of BD in several studies as previously summarized.[3] Most of these are open trials or small case series; several used concentrations that are not commercially available in the U.K., and some do not specify the concentration or schedule. These suggest cure

Table 1 Summary of the main treatment options for Bowen's disease. The suggested scoring of the treatments listed takes into account the evidence for benefit, ease of application or time required for the procedure, wound healing, cosmetic result and current availability/costs of the method or facilities required. Evidence for interventions based on single studies or purely anecdotal cases is not included

Lesion characteristics	Topical 5-FU	Topical imiqumod[a]	Cryotherapy	Curettage	Excision	PDT	Radiotherapy	Laser[b]
Small, single/few, good healing site[c]	4	3	2	1	3	3	5	4
Large, single, good healing site[c]	3	3	3	5	5	2	4	7
Multiple, good healing site[c]	3	4	2	3	5	3	4	4
Small, single/few, poor healing site[c]	2	3	3	2	2	1–2	5	7
Large, single, poor healing site[c]	3	2–3	5	4	5	1	6	7
Facial	4	7	2	2	4[d]	3	4	7
Digital	3	7	3	5	2[d]	3	3	3
Perianal	6	6	6	6	1[e]	7	2–3	6
Penile	3	3	3	5	4[d]	3	2–3	3

5-FU, 5-fluorouracil; PDT, photodynamic therapy; 1, probably treatment of choice; 2, generally good choice; 3, generally fair choice; 4, reasonable but not usually required; 5, generally poor choice; 6, probably should not be used; 7, insufficient evidence available. [a]Does not have a product licence for Bowen's disease. [b]Depends on site. [c]Refers to the clinician's perceived potential for good or poor healing at the affected site. [d]Consider micrographic surgery for tissue sparing or if poorly defined/recurrent. [e]Wide excision recommended.

rates of 90–100%. In current clinical use, 5-FU is usually applied once or twice daily as a 5% cream for a variable period of time (between 1 week and 2 months in most studies using this concentration) to achieve disease control, and repeated if required at intervals. Lower concentrations are less effective.

Efficacy may be increased by application under occlusion, use of dinitrochlorobenzene as a vehicle (both previously referenced[3]), iontophoresis[28] (to improve follicular penetration) or pretreatment with a laser (to ablate the stratum corneum and thereby enhance penetration of 5-FU).[29] In the study of iontophoresis,[28] only one of 26 patients had histological evidence of residual disease at 3 months after eight treatments. More recently, the erbium:YAG laser was used as a pretreatment measure on half of each lesion in three lesions from a patient with multiple BD, who was subsequently treated with twice-daily application of 5-FU cream to both sides. The response (clinical and histological) was accelerated on the side pretreated with laser.[29]

Few studies provide details of the success rate for the currently available preparation in the U.K. (5% cream to be used once or twice daily for 3–4 weeks) as a first-line option for unselected lesions. However, in an RCT comparing 5-FU with photodynamic therapy (PDT) the initial response rate in the 5-FU limb, after one (or two if required) cycles of once-daily application for 1 week then twice daily for 3 weeks, repeated at 6 weeks if clinically indicated, was 67%, with only 48% remaining clear at 12 months.[30] (The comparative results are discussed in the section on PDT, below). By contrast, in a follow-up study (26 patients, clinical follow up of 2·4–204 months), recurrences had occurred at some point in just two patients (8%).[31] This study used 5% 5-FU twice daily for a planned 9 weeks (actual 3–13 weeks), with a repeat cycle for recurrences, and biopsy to confirm clearance in most cases, but is a small number collected given the 10-year overall period.

As 5-FU can be very irritant, less aggressive regimens have been used for disease control rather than cure. Two applications of 5% 5-FU on a single day of each week for 3 months improved lesions in 24 of 26 patients (92%) with BD of the leg (lesions were flat with less or no erythema, and with minor or absent scaling), although long-term clearance was achieved only in a minority with this regimen.[32]

Formal comparison with other modalities is limited to RCTs of PDT vs. 5-FU, only one of which is currently published and which showed that PDT was the more effective[30] (see section on PDT below).

In erythroplasia of Queyrat, application of 5% 5-FU cream twice daily for 4–5 weeks has been recommended but inflammation frequently limits this treatment regimen.

Imiquimod (*Strength of recommendation B, Quality of evidence I*)

Imiquimod is a topical immunomodulatory heterocyclic imidazoquinoline amide that has become available since the earlier BAD guideline.[3] It has been used as a 5% cream to treat BD, including larger diameter lesions, lower leg lesions and erythroplasia of Queyrat. It has both anti-HPV and antitumour

effects, and is therefore potentially useful for HPV-associated BD/bowenoid papulosis as well as for non-HPV-associated BD. The evidence base consists of a single small RCT, one open study plus some small case series (most two or three patients) and individual case reports.[33–40] The regimen used varies between reports. Such reports are not referenced at length as it is felt that stronger evidence is required before firm conclusions can be drawn. At the time of writing, the product licence for topical imiquimod in the U.K. is for small superficial basal cell carcinomas; it is not currently licensed for use in BD.

The best evidence currently available is a single small RCT that demonstrated 73% histologically proven resolution with imiquimod (once daily for 16 weeks; lesions untreated for at least a month) vs. zero response in the placebo group.[33] This study acknowledged that the ideal dosing regimen and cost-effectiveness require further investigation. An earlier 16-patient open study (15 having lower leg lesions; once daily application for up to 16 weeks; previously untreated lesions) documented that 14 of 15 patients (93%) who completed the study had clinical and pathological resolution of BD 6 weeks after the treatment period (one patient died of unrelated causes and was not analysed).[34] Five lesions had an area of 5 cm^2 or greater.

Single cases or small case series suggest that different regimens such as cyclical treatment[35] might be useful, and also that imiquimod may be useful for large facial lesions.[36] The latter, together with lower leg lesions,[34] are typically those that pose the greatest therapeutic challenge. Some studies suggest that shorter treatment periods may be adequate.[34,35] In the open study discussed above,[34] six of 16 patients discontinued treatment early due to side-effects but still had lesion clearance, and in the placebo-controlled trial, three of 15 in the active limb dropped out (two being withdrawn by the investigators due to local side-effects).[33] A few anecdotal reports and small open-label case series suggest that there may be a role for imiquimod in treatment of erythroplasia of Queyrat[37] and in basaloid VIN.

Benefit has also been reported in the treatment of BD in immunosuppressed patients,[38–40] although combining it with other modalities such as oral sulindac[39] or 5-FU[40] makes interpretation of the relative roles of the pairs of agents used difficult. Five renal transplant patients with BD have been treated with a combination of a local immune therapy, imiquimod cream, and a topical chemotherapeutic agent, 5% 5-FU, with clearing of the areas of SCC in situ. In addition, there is evidence that cytokines induced by imiquimod may improve the therapeutic efficacy of topical 5% 5-FU in BD.[40]

Cryotherapy (*Strength of recommendation B, Quality of evidence II-i*)

The results reported vary, probably reflecting differences between studies in the techniques and regimens used. As previously summarized,[3,6] the failure rate varies from zero to about 35%, the larger series suggesting a failure or recurrence rate in the order of 5–10% provided that adequate cryotherapy is used [e.g. liquid nitrogen (LN$_2$) cryotherapy, using a single freeze-thaw cycle (FTC) of 30 s, two FTCs of 20 s with a thaw period, or up to three single treatments of 20 s at intervals of several weeks].[41–44] Such doses do, however, cause discomfort and may cause ulceration, especially on the lower leg.

In an RCT of PDT vs. cryotherapy,[44] the latter produced 100% clearance in 20 patients with one to three treatments of LN$_2$ using one FTC of 20 s on each occasion (50% success after a single treatment). Ulceration was observed following cryotherapy in 25% of lesions. There were two (10%) recurrences following cryotherapy in the 1-year follow-up period. A single treatment of PDT was significantly more effective than cryotherapy.

A prospective, nonrandomized study comparing curettage vs. cryotherapy found better healing, less discomfort and a lower recurrence rate with curettage,[45] and cryotherapy had more complications (discussed below).

Cryotherapy appears to have a good success rate with adequate treatment (recurrences less than 10% at 12 months) but healing may be slow for broad lesions and discomfort may limit treatment of multiple lesions. Curettage and PDT both have higher success rates and less discomfort overall, but are more time-consuming and/or expensive to perform.

Curettage with cautery/electrocautery (*Strength of recommendation A, Quality of evidence II-ii*)

Previously summarized studies[3] suggested a wide range of cure rates without recurrence, larger series suggesting a recurrence rate of 20%.[17] These studies do not give details of the treatment regimens or equipment used (cautery vs. electrodesiccation, number of cycles etc.).

In a prospective but nonrandomized trial of curettage and cautery (44 lesions) compared with cryotherapy (36 lesions) involving 67 patients, curettage was preferable in terms of pain, healing and recurrence rate.[45] Seventy-four percent of lesions were on the lower leg. Median time to healing with cryotherapy was 46 days (90 days on the lower leg) compared with 35 days (lower leg 39 days) for curetted lesions, and reported pain was significantly greater with cryotherapy. Recurrences were more likely following cryotherapy (13 of 44) compared with curettage (four of 36) during a median 2 years' follow up, although the cryotherapy regimen was less aggressive than that used by authors in most studies of this technique (see above and comment in this Journal[25]).

Curettage followed by cryotherapy has also been used, but reports are anecdotal and it is impossible to determine the relative contribution of the two treatments or whether the combination is better than either alone.

Excision (*Strength of recommendation A, Quality of evidence II-iii*)

There are no substantive new data on simple excision since the last guidelines.[3] In retrospective studies of 65 and 155 patients, the reported recurrence rates were 4·5%[17] and 19%,[46] respectively. Even higher rates are recorded in some smaller studies, and at sites such as the perianal region. While it is logical that excision should be an effective treatment, the evidence base is limited. Additionally, lower leg excision wounds may be associated with considerable morbidity.[26]

A retrospective study of 47 cases of perianal BD[24] found a lower recurrence rate for wide excision (six of 26, 23%) than for local excision (eight of 15, 53%) or laser therapy (four of five, 80%) although this series did not include patients treated with radiotherapy (which has been recommended as a first-line treatment,[47] discussed below). Wide surgical excision is the most commonly used treatment for perianal BD;[48] a survey of American colorectal surgeons found that most are performing wide local excision for both small and large perianal BD lesions (96% for patients with small lesions and 87% for patients with large lesions). Prolonged follow up is recommended as late recurrences are common at this site (see the previous guideline[3]).

Mohs micrographic surgery has become the recommended treatment for digital BD and for some cases of genital (especially penile) BD for its tissue-sparing benefits. A large retrospective series of 270 patients has reported on micrographic surgery for tissue sparing at head and neck sites (this site comprised 252 of 270 patients).[49] This study included 128 cases of previously treated head and neck BD. Among the 270 cases analysed, 94 had had previous cryotherapy, 18 curettage and cautery, 44 excision (10 incomplete) and one radiotherapy (some had been treated with more than one modality); nearly all referrals cited poorly defined tumour, recurrent or incompletely excised tumour, or tumour site as the rationale for micrographic surgery, so it cannot be assumed to be routinely necessary or cost-effective (*Strength of recommendation B, Quality of evidence II-iii*). The mean and median number of excision levels for clearance was 2, range 1–7. Of 95 patients who had 5-year follow-up data there were six (6%) recurrences.

Photodynamic therapy (*Strength of recommendation A, Quality of evidence I*)

This modality requires the activation of a photosensitizer, usually a porphyrin derivative, by visible light. Systemic photosensitization, with various photosensitizers, was used with excellent results in early studies summarized previously.[3] A recent report using systemic verteporfin, which has a much shorter duration of photosensitivity than agents used in earlier studies, has confirmed the efficacy of this approach.[50] It has a particular role in patients with multiple BD lesions, in whom use of topical porphyrin derivatives may be expensive and time-consuming, although topical PDT is more practical for most BD.

These guidelines refer mainly to topical PDT using topical 5-aminolaevulinic acid (ALA) or its ester, methyl aminolaevulinate (MAL). Studies have included various illumination sources (e.g. filtered xenon arc, diode, halogen, laser), wavelengths (red, green, blue/violet light) and dosing schedules (both in duration of ALA application and total light energy delivered), hence comparisons between studies may be difficult to interpret. Most studies have used one or two treatments, depending on response (usually repeated at about 6 weeks if clinically necessary). Issues such as use of analgesia, and fluorescence detection, are not addressed here but details may be found in the British Photodermatology Group guidelines for topical PDT.[51]

The previously summarized studies[3] suggested an initial clinical clearance rate for ALA-PDT of 80–100% (most around 90%) with one or two treatments, and a recurrence rate of about 0–10% at 12 months. These figures remain valid. In a prospective open study, 44 of 50 lesions (88%) cleared after two treatments (30 of 50 after one treatment, 60%) although two patients failed to clear after four treatments; this study, which used a halogen red light source, had a 31% 12-month recurrence rate in the 48 initially responsive lesions.[52] Similarly, a departmental review documented that 117 of 129 lesions (91%) were cleared,[53] and a trial vs. 5-FU found that 29 of 33 lesions (88%) cleared after one or two treatments.[30]

An open study using ALA-PDT specifically for large diameter and multiple BD lesions showed that 35 (88%) of 40 large patches of BD, all with a maximum diameter > 20 mm, cleared following one to three treatments, although four patches recurred within 12 months. In 10 further patients with multiple (three or more) patches of BD, 44 (98%) of 45 patches cleared, although four lesions recurred over 12 months.[54]

Digital BD was treated with PDT in four patients, with good cosmetic and functional results (one recurrence at 8 months responded to retreatment);[55] the schedule was different from that in most studies (2% ALA solution, occluded for 16 h, two treatments of 240 J cm^{-2} 90 min apart using a 630-nm diode source). There are additional single case reports.

There are several comparative studies involving PDT, as follows.

Comparison with other treatments

ALA-PDT for BD has been compared with cryotherapy[45] and with 5-FU,[30] each in an RCT involving 40 patients. PDT proved superior in terms of efficacy and adverse events in comparison with 5-FU, as well as being less painful than cryotherapy. Both studies used a PDT schedule of 20% ALA applied 4 h before irradiation with narrowband red light. The cryotherapy study is discussed above and was summarized in the 1999 guideline.[3] In the comparison with 5-FU, this was applied as 5% cream once daily for a week and then twice daily for 3 weeks; either treatment was repeated at 6 weeks if necessary. Initial clearance rates (PDT vs. 5-FU) were 88% vs. 67%, and 12-month rates were 82% vs. 48%, with more short-term side-effects in the 5-FU group.[30]

Topical MAL-PDT has been compared with clinician's choice of cryotherapy or 5-FU in a 40-centre European trial of 225 patients with 275 lesions of BD:[56] MAL was applied for 3 h and sites illuminated with a broadband red light. Lesion complete response rates 3 months after last treatment were similar with MAL-PDT (107 of 124; 86%), cryotherapy (75 of 91; 82%) and 5-FU (30 of 36; 83%). PDT gave superior cosmetic results compared with cryotherapy or 5-FU. MAL-PDT is now

approved in many countries for the treatment of actinic keratoses, basal cell carcinomas and BD.

Comparison between wavelengths

Green light (29 patients) was compared with red light (32 patients) in an RCT using ALA-PDT for BD but was inferior in terms of initial clearance (94% vs. 72%) and 12-month clearance (88% vs. 48%) and had no advantages in terms of pain (which was the rationale for the investigation).[57] Violet light irradiation (10–20 J cm^{-2}, after application of ALA for 8 h) was used in six patients with BD, including one with multiple lesions involving 50% of the scalp, the rationale being the lower light dose required for production of phototoxicity.[58] Despite the theoretical risk of reduced light penetration compared with red light PDT, the solitary lesions responded in all four evaluable patients (one dropped out for unrelated reasons) and the large area of scalp involvement showed a 90% response, 50% of the remaining area responding to retreatment. However, there has been no direct comparison with other wavelengths.

PDT has been used specifically in immunosuppressed subjects, in an open trial involving 20 transplant recipients and 20 immunocompetent controls with histologically confirmed actinic keratoses or BD (one or two treatments, 20% ALA for 5 h, 75 J cm^{-2} of visible light delivered at 80 mW cm^{-2}). The cure rates in both patient groups were comparable at 4 weeks (86%) but were significantly lower in transplant recipients than in controls at 12 and 48 weeks (below 50%). Despite the poor long-term response, the authors concluded that PDT is particularly useful in transplant recipients because of the possibility for repeated treatment of large lesional areas (although subsequent responsiveness was not confirmed).[59]

Successful use of PDT has also been reported in two cases of bowenoid papulosis using ALA-PDT with a diode red light source.

Radiotherapy (*Strength of recommendation overall B, Quality of evidence II-iii* for most sites; *Strength of recommendation D, Quality of evidence II-iii* for lower leg)

Various radiotherapy techniques and regimens have been used to treat BD. The larger studies have suggested a complete response rate to X-irradiation of 100%, for example in 77 lesions treated by Blank and Schnyder[60] (in this study, two patients with genital lesions relapsed at 8 and 16 months) and in 59 patients treated by Cox and Dyson.[43]

The patients in the latter series all had lower leg lesions; poor healing, related to age, diameter of field and radiotherapy dose, was a feature in 12 of 59 (20%) of cases. Poor healing of lower legs was supported by a more recent but smaller retrospective series of 11 patients with 16 lower leg lesions in which 100% cure was obtained but with 25% failure to heal (median follow up 27·5 months, minimum 9 months), even though the fraction sizes used were relatively low.[61] Thus the high cure rate of radiotherapy may be offset by impaired healing on the lower leg, and it is best avoided for BD at this site (Strength of recommendation D, Quality of evidence II-iii).

To overcome some of the disadvantages of external beam X-irradiation, a skin patch coated with high-energy β-emitter holmium-166 (^{166}Ho patch) was used to treat 29 biopsy-confirmed BD lesions in eight patients [one with 22 sites, one with three sites but only one (palmar) treated with this method, the others solitary].[62] All lesions were 3 cm or larger (up to 7·2 cm); most lesions were on buttocks or thighs, or were acral in the patient with multiple lesions (no lower leg lesions were specifically identified in the report). The patches were applied to the surface of lesions for 30–60 min for a total radiation dose of 35 Gy. Acute radiation reactions healed within a month with mild fibrosis; there were good functional and cosmetic results with confirmed histological clearance at 5 months and without any late (10 months–2 years) recurrences or complications. This treatment may therefore be useful, at least at non-lower leg sites (Strength of recommendation B, Quality of evidence II-ii).

Radiotherapy has been advocated as the treatment of choice for anal margin epidermoid cancers, although without any strong evidence to support this viewpoint.[47]

Laser (*Strength of recommendation overall B, Quality of evidence II-iii* but may vary according to site)

Lasers have mainly been used to treat lesions at difficult sites such as the finger or genitalia. Results are generally stated to be good (Strength of recommendation B, Quality of evidence II-iii), but most published results are based on small numbers, or are considered with other epidermal neoplasia and are difficult to analyse. One retrospective review included six cases of digital BD treated with CO_2 laser, and reported good cosmetic results, no functional deficit and no recurrences (follow up 0·5–7·7 years),[63] although some failures for digital BD are reported by others (one of five cases).[64]

A study of 16 patients with 25 lower leg BD lesions treated with CO_2 laser demonstrated 100% healing at 2 months and no recurrences at 6 months. However, there was a 12% progression to invasive carcinoma within 12 months of discharge from follow up. This suggests that the depth of laser eradication may have been inadequate, and there are currently some reservations about use of this modality at this site (Strength of recommendation C, Quality of evidence II-iii).[65]

Results for perianal BD are poor[48] (Strength of recommendation D, Quality of evidence II-iii). CO_2 laser has been recommended for erythroplasia of Queyrat (Strength of recommendation B, Quality of evidence II-iii) but there is inadequate evidence to comment on other sites (Quality of evidence IV).

Other treatments

An ultrasonic surgical aspirator was used initially in an animal model (grafted areas of BD onto immunodeficient mice) and subsequently for 20 human lesions of BD where surgery had been considered inappropriate.[66] The rationale is that the aspirator removes epidermis but not dermis. It has a 2-mm diameter probe, and up to 300 μm oscillation at 28 kHz. An area of about 1 cm of normal skin was included in the treatment field, treatment taking 5–10 min under local anaesthesia. Follow up was monthly for 12 months, 3-monthly thereafter, for 12–26 (mean 20) months with no recurrences. Large lesions, lower leg lesions and lesions over joints were included.

Hyperthermic treatment was performed using disposable chemical pocket warmers applied under pressure each day throughout the patient's waking hours for 4–5 months.[67] There was initial complete clinical remission in six of eight patients (and partial remission in one) but absence of residual histological evidence of BD was achieved only in three of eight. Although of some benefit, this response compares poorly with other standard therapies (Strength of recommendation E, Quality of evidence IV).

Acitretin has been used alone or in conjunction with 5-FU in anecdotal cases but the relative merits of each are unclear in the combination approach. The same applies to combinations of topical bleomycin with LN_2 cryotherapy in a case of digital BD and isotretinoin with interferon-α in a patient with multiple lesions.

Summary of treatment modalities

All of the above treatments have some advantages and disadvantages, which are dictated by lesional factors (size, number, site, potential for healing or functional impairment), general health issues, availability and costs (both of the equipment or agent, and of the time to deliver the treatment or its aftercare). A cost-minimization analysis showed that, at the time, curettage or excision were the cheapest options, and PDT the most expensive (other treatments considered in this study were cryotherapy, 5-FU and laser).[68] However, changing costs of PDT and laser, the likely use of (relatively expensive) imiquimod in the future, and the fact that all of these therapies may not have equivalent efficacy, means that it is difficult to make a strong and currently applicable single recommendation on the basis of this study.

The relative status of the available treatment options is summarized in Table 1. This takes into account the evidence for benefit, ease of application and time required for the technique, wound healing, cosmetic result and availability of the method or facilities required.

Follow up

The required duration of follow up remains uncertain. Some treatments may need to be repeated, for example a second PDT treatment is typically needed in about 20–30% of patients, and a second cycle of 5-FU is needed in a similar proportion (although the latter may potentially be instituted by the patient or the primary care physician). Formal studies have generally used 12-month follow-up periods and clinical assessment for detection of recurrences.

On the basis that most of the treatments have about a 10% recurrence risk, a follow-up check for possible recurrence at 6–12 months is recommended. Different arrangements may be dictated in the shorter term by a likely need for a second cycle of treatment or to check on healing (in which case review at about 2–3 months to confirm clearance and healing may be more appropriate). The requirement for subsequent review should take into account the presence of multiple lesions, previous recurrence, high-risk lesions, other skin neoplasia, background risk factors such as immunosuppression, the reliability of the patient and the degree of primary care support. For treatments that are novel, outside product licence, or have a small evidence base, we suggest that follow up should be more frequent and should continue for at least 12–24 months in order to compare results with current literature on other therapies.

As a specific follow-up issue, the higher risk and the late timing of recurrences of perianal BD should be noted. In a series of 19 patients with perianal BD[23] the recurrence rate increased from 16% at 1 year to 31% at 5 years; in another series, the median time to recurrence for 26 radically excised lesions was 41·5 months.[24] Longer follow up may therefore be appropriate for BD at less common and less visible sites, or where HPV infection is likely to have been relevant.

Tools for guideline users

We have presented here:
1 A summary of the evidence and relevant aspects of the main management options.
2 A tabular summary of appropriate treatment for different lesional types, sizes and situations.
3 Suggestions for audit.

Summary of the main management recommendations

1 Routine investigation for internal malignancy in patients with BD is not justified (*Strength of recommendation E, Quality of evidence I*).
2 The risk of progression to invasive cancer is about 3%. This risk is greater in genital BD, and particularly in perianal BD. A high risk of recurrence, including late recurrence, is a particular feature of perianal BD and prolonged follow up is recommended for this variant (*Strength of recommendation A, Quality of evidence II-ii*).
3 There is reasonable evidence to support use of 5-FU (*Strength of recommendation B, Quality of evidence II-i*) but its use may be limited by irritancy and it was less effective than PDT in an RCT. It is more practical than surgery for large lesions, especially at potentially poor healing sites, and has been used for 'control' rather than cure in some patients with multiple lesions.
4 Topical imiquimod is likely to be used for BD (*Strength of recommendation B, Quality of evidence I*), especially for larger lesions or difficult/poor healing sites. However, it is costly, currently unlicensed for this indication, and the optimum regimen has yet to be determined.

5 Topical PDT has been shown to be equivalent or superior to cryotherapy and 5-FU, either in efficacy and/or in healing, in RCTs (*Strength of recommendation A, Quality of evidence I*). It may be of particular benefit for lesions that are large, on the lower leg or at otherwise difficult sites, but it is costly. PDT for NMSC and premalignant skin lesions has now been approved as an interventional procedure by the National Institute for Health and Clinical Excellence in the U.K.,[69] and MAL-PDT has been approved by the European Medicines Authority for treatment of BD.
6 Curettage has good evidence of efficacy, and time to healing is faster than with cryotherapy (*Strength of recommendation A, Quality of evidence II-ii*).
7 Cryotherapy has good evidence of efficacy (*Strength of recommendation B, Quality of evidence II-i*), but discomfort and time to healing are inferior to PDT (*Strength of recommendation A, Quality of evidence I*) or curettage (*Strength of recommendation A, Quality of evidence II-ii*).
8 Excision should be an effective treatment with low recurrence rates, but the evidence base is limited and for the most part does not allow comment on specific sites of lesions (*Strength of recommendation overall A, Quality of evidence II-iii*). Lower leg excision may be limited by lack of skin mobility. For perianal BD treated surgically, wide excision is recommended rather than narrow excision or laser treatment (*Strength of recommendation A, Quality of evidence II-iii*). Micrographic surgery is logical at sites such as digits or penis where it is important to limit removal of unaffected skin (*Strength of recommendation B, Quality of evidence III*) and is useful for poorly defined or recurrent head and neck BD (*Strength of recommendation B, Quality of evidence II-iii*).
9 Radiotherapy has good evidence of efficacy but poor healing on the lower leg suggests that it should be avoided at this site (*Strength of recommendation generally B, Quality of evidence II-iii; for lower leg lesions Strength of recommendation D, Quality of evidence II-iii*).
10 There is limited evidence on laser treatment, suggesting that it is a reasonable option for digital or genital lesions (*Strength of recommendation B, Quality of evidence II-iii*) but probably not for other sites (*Strength of recommendation mostly C or D, Quality of evidence II-iii to IV*); specifically, results for perianal BD are worse than those using wide surgical excision.

All therapeutic options have failure and recurrence rates at least in the order of 5–10%, and no treatment modality appears to be superior for all clinical situations. Direct comparison between treatment modalities is difficult as there are few randomized clinical trials with comparable patient subgroups. There is now increased choice for patients between clinic-based and home-applied therapies. For individual patients, factors such as treatment-related morbidity and the ease and availability of the treatment options may be a greater issue than the cure rate. As previously, we still feel that it is important that our BAD therapeutic guidelines reflect the fact that there is no single definite 'right way' to treat all patients with BD.

Summary of appropriate treatment for different lesional types, sizes and situations

See Table 1.

Possible audit points

Is a measure of patient acceptability linked with treatment? (may be indirect, e.g. willingness to repeat treatment if necessary)

For novel, unlicensed or small evidence-base treatments, has clinical cure rate been extended to 12 months? (and what are the results?)

For destructive therapies, has the dose, frequency etc. been recorded where applicable?

Conflicts of interest

Relevant product details are given in brackets for the first citation of any pharmaceutical company below.

N.H.C. has received support for attendance at non-product-related educational meetings from Valeant Pharmaceuticals (5-fluorouracil cream); has acted as an advisor regarding development of pathways of care for basal cell carcinoma, sponsored by 3M Pharmaceuticals (imiquimod); and has a performed a sponsored clinical trial for Photocure of photodynamic therapy (PDT) using methyl aminolaevulinic acid for Bowen's disease. He has performed unsponsored research on cryotherapy and radiotherapy for Bowen's disease.

D.J.E. has received fees for speaking and chairing meetings for 3M Pharmaceuticals, travelling expenses from Leo Pharmaceuticals and is an advisor to Novartis (U.K.).

C.A.M. has received sponsorship for speaking and chairing meetings from Galderma (Metvix®, a brand of methyl aminolaevulinic acid), and sponsorship from 3M and Leo Pharmaceuticals. He has performed sponsored as well as unsponsored research to evaluate the potential of topical PDT using various photosensitizers in dermatological indications.

References

1 Griffiths CEM. The British Association of Dermatologists guidelines for the management of skin disease. Br J Dermatol 1999; 141:396–7.

2 Cox NH, Williams HC. The British Association of Dermatologists therapeutic guidelines: can we AGREE? Br J Dermatol 2003; 148:621–5.

3 Cox NH, Eedy DJ, Morton CA. Guidelines for management of Bowen's disease. Br J Dermatol 1999; 141:633–41.

4 Bowen JT. Precancerous dermatoses: a study of two cases of chronic atypical epithelial proliferation. J Cutan Dis 1912; 30:241–55.

5 Lee M-M, Wick MM. Bowen's disease. CA Cancer J Clin 1990; 40:237–42.

6 Anonymous. Management of Bowen's disease of the skin. Drug Ther Bull 2004; 42:13–16.

7 Chute CG, Chuang TY, Bergstralh EJ, Su WP. The subsequent risk of internal cancer with Bowen's disease. A population-based study. JAMA 1991; 266:816–9.

8 Eedy DJ, Gavin AT. Thirteen-year retrospective study of Bowen's disease in Northern Ireland. Br J Dermatol 1987; 117:715–20.

9 Cox NH. Body site distribution of Bowen's disease. Br J Dermatol 1994; 130:714–6.

10 Eedy DJ. Summary of inaugural meeting of the Skin Care in Organ Recipients Group, UK, held at the Royal Society of Medicine, 7 October 2004. Br J Dermatol 2005; 153:6–10.

11 Bordea C, Wojnarowska F, Millard PR et al. Skin cancers in renal-transplant recipients occur more frequently than previously recognized in a temperate climate. Transplantation 2004; 77:574–9.

12 Derancourt C, Mougin C, Chopard-Lallier M et al. Oncogenic human papillomaviruses in extra-genital Bowen disease revealed by in situ hybridization. Ann Dermatol Venereol 2001; 128:715–8.

13 Quéreux G, N'Guyen JM, Dréno B. Human papillomavirus and extragenital in situ carcinoma. Dermatology 2004; 209:40–5.

14 Mitsuishi T, Kawana S, Kato T, Kawashima M. Human papillomavirus infection in actinic keratosis and Bowen's disease: comparative study with expression of cell-cycle regulatory proteins p21(Waf1/Cip1), p53, PCNA, Ki-67, and Bcl-2 in positive and negative lesions. Hum Pathol 2003; 34:886–92.

15 McGregor JM, Proby CM. The role of papillomaviruses in human non-melanoma skin cancer. Cancer Surv 1996; 26:219–46.

16 Jaeger AB, Gramkow A, Hjalgrim H et al. Bowen disease and risk of subsequent malignant neoplasms: a population-based cohort study of 1147 patients. Arch Dermatol 1999; 135:790–3.

17 Thestrup-Pedersen K, Ravnborg L, Reymann F. Morbus Bowen. Acta Derm Venereol (Stockh) 1988; 68:236–9.

18 Reizner GT, Chuang TY, Elpern DJ et al. Bowen's disease (squamous cell carcinoma in situ) in Kauai, Hawaii. A population-based incidence report. J Am Acad Dermatol 1994; 31:596–600.

19 Marcil I, Stern RS. Risk of developing a subsequent nonmelanoma skin cancer in patients with a history of nonmelanoma skin cancer: a critical review of the literature and meta-analysis. Arch Dermatol 2000; 136:1524–30.

20 Peterka ES, Lynch FW, Goltz RW. An association between Bowen's disease and cancer. Arch Dermatol 1961; 84:623–9.

21 Kao GF. Carcinoma arising in Bowen's disease. Arch Dermatol 1986; 122:1124–6.

22 Beck DE, Fazio VW, Jagelman DG, Lavery IC. Perianal Bowen's disease. Dis Colon Rectum 1988; 31:419–22.

23 Sarmiento JM, Wolff BG, Burgart LJ et al. Perianal Bowen's disease: associated tumors, human papillomavirus, surgery, and other controversies. Dis Colon Rectum 1997; 40:912–8.

24 Marchesa P, Fazio VW, Oliart S et al. Perianal Bowen's disease: a clinicopathological study of 47 patients. Dis Colon Rectum 1997; 40:1286–93.

25 Cox NH. Bowen's disease: where now with therapeutic trials? Br J Dermatol 2000; 143:699–700.

26 Bell HK, Rhodes LE. Bowen's disease – a retrospective review of clinical management. Clin Exp Dermatol 1999; 24:338–9.

27 Ball SB, Dawber RPR. Treatment of cutaneous Bowen's disease with particular emphasis on the problem of lower leg lesions. Australas J Dermatol 1998; 39:63–70.

28 Welch ML, Grabski WJ, McCollough ML et al. 5-Fluorouracil iontophoretic therapy for Bowen's disease. J Am Acad Dermatol 1997; 36:956–8.

29 Wang KH, Fang JY, Hu CH, Lee WR. Erbium:YAG laser pretreatment accelerates the response of Bowen's disease treated by topical 5-fluorouracil. Dermatol Surg 2004; 30:441–5.

30 Salim A, Leman JA, McColl JH et al. Randomized comparison of photodynamic therapy with topical 5-fluorouracil in Bowen's disease. Br J Dermatol 2003; 148:539–43.

31 Bargman H, Hochman J. Topical treatment of Bowen's disease with 5-fluorouracil. J Cutan Med Surg 2003; 7:101–5.

32 Stone N, Burge S. Bowen's disease of the leg treated with weekly pulses of 5% fluorouracil cream. Br J Dermatol 1999; 140:987–8.

33 Patel GK, Goodwin R, Chawla M et al. Imiquimod 5% cream monotherapy for cutaneous squamous cell carcinoma in situ

(Bowen's disease): a randomised, double-blind, placebo-controlled trial. *J Am Acad Dermatol* 2006; **54**:1025–32.

34 Mackenzie-Wood A, Kossard S, de Launey J et al. Imiquimod 5% cream in the treatment of Bowen's disease. *J Am Acad Dermatol* 2001; **44**:462–70.

35 Chen K, Shumack S. Treatment of Bowen's disease using a cycle regimen of imiquimod 5% cream. *Clin Exp Dermatol* 2003; **28** (Suppl. 1):10–12.

36 Kossard S. Treatment of large facial Bowen's disease: case report. *Clin Exp Dermatol* 2003; **28** (Suppl. 1):13–15.

37 Arlette JP. Treatment of Bowen's disease and erythroplasia of Queyrat. *Br J Dermatol* 2003; **149** (Suppl. 66):43–7.

38 Prinz BM, Hafner J, Dummer R et al. Treatment of Bowen's disease with imiquimod 5% cream in transplant recipients. *Transplantation* 2004; **77**:790–1.

39 Smith KJ, Germain M, Skelton H. Bowen's disease (squamous cell carcinoma in situ) in immunosuppressed patients treated with imiquimod 5% cream and a COX inhibitor, sulindac: potential applications for this combination of immunotherapy. *Dermatol Surg* 2001; **27**:143–6.

40 Smith KJ, Germain M, Skelton H. Squamous cell carcinoma in situ (Bowen's disease) in renal transplant patients treated with 5% imiquimod and 5% fluorouracil therapy. *Dermatol Surg* 2001; **27**:561–4.

41 Plaza de Lanza M, Ralphs I, Dawber RPR. Cryosurgery for Bowen's disease of the skin. *Br J Dermatol* 1980; **103** (Suppl. 18):14.

42 Holt PJ. Cryotherapy for skin cancer: results over a 5-year period using liquid nitrogen spray cryosurgery. *Br J Dermatol* 1988; **119**:231–40.

43 Cox NH, Dyson P. Wound healing on the lower leg after radiotherapy or cryotherapy of Bowen's disease and other malignant skin lesions. *Br J Dermatol* 1995; **133**:60–5.

44 Morton CA, Whitehurst C, Moseley H et al. Comparison of photodynamic therapy with cryotherapy in the treatment of Bowen's disease. *Br J Dermatol* 1995; **135**:766–71.

45 Ahmed I, Berth-Jones J, Charles-Holmes S et al. Comparison of cryotherapy with curettage in the treatment of Bowen's disease: a prospective study. *Br J Dermatol* 2000; **143**:759–66.

46 Graham JH, Helwig EB. Bowen's disease and its relationship to systemic cancer. *Arch Dermatol* 1961; **83**:76–96.

47 Papillon J, Chassard JL. Respective roles of radiotherapy and surgery in the management of epidermoid carcinoma of the anal margin. *Dis Colon Rectum* 1992; **35**:422–9.

48 Cleary RK, Schaldenbrand JD, Fowler JJ et al. Treatment options for perianal Bowen's disease: survery of American Society of Colon and Rectal Surgeons Members. *Am Surg* 2000; **66**:686–8.

49 Leibovitch I, Huilgol S, Selva D et al. Cutaneous squamous cell carcinoma in situ (Bowen's disease): treatment with Mohs' micrographic surgery. *J Am Acad Dermatol* 2005; **52**:997–1002.

50 Lui H, Hobbs L, Tope WD et al. Photodynamic therapy of multiple nonmelanoma skin cancers with verteporfin and red light-emitting diodes: two-year results evaluating tumor response and cosmetic outcomes. *Arch Dermatol* 2004; **140**:26–32.

51 Morton CA, Brown SB, Collins S et al. Guidelines for topical photodynamic therapy: report of a workshop of the British Photodermatology Group. *Br J Dermatol* 2002; **146**:552–67.

52 Varma S, Wilson H, Kurwa HA et al. Bowen's disease, solar keratoses and superficial basal cell carcinomas treated by photodynamic therapy using a large-field incoherent light source. *Br J Dermatol* 2001; **144**:567–74.

53 Clark C, Bryden A, Dawe R et al. Topical 5-aminolaevulinic acid photodynamic therapy for cutaneous lesions: outcome and comparison of light sources. *Photodermatol Photoimmunol Photomed* 2003; **19**:134–41.

54 Morton CA, Whitehurst C, McColl JH et al. Photodynamic therapy for large or multiple patches of Bowen disease and basal cell carcinoma. *Arch Dermatol* 2001; **137**:319–24.

55 Wong TW, Sheu HM, Lee JY, Fletcher RJ. Photodynamic therapy for Bowen's disease (squamous cell carcinoma in situ) of the digit. *Dermatol Surg* 2001; **27**:452–6.

56 Morton CA, Horn M, Leman J et al. Comparison of topical methylaminolevulinate photodynamic therapy with cryotherapy or fluorouracil for treatment of squamous cell carcinoma in situ: results of a multicenter randomized trial. *Arch Dermatol* 2006; **142**:729–735.

57 Morton CA, Whitehurst C, Moore JV, MacKie RM. Comparison of red and green light in the treatment of Bowen's disease by photodynamic therapy. *Br J Dermatol* 2000; **143**:767–72.

58 Dijkstra AT, Majoie IM, van Dongen JW et al. Photodynamic therapy with violet light and topical δ-aminolaevulinic acid in the treatment of actinic keratosis, Bowen's disease and basal cell carcinoma. *J Eur Acad Dermatol Venereol* 2001; **15**:550–4.

59 Dragieva G, Hafner J, Dummer R et al. Topical photodynamic therapy in the treatment of actinic keratoses and Bowen's disease in transplant recipients. *Transplantation* 2004; **77**:115–21.

60 Blank AA, Schnyder UW. Soft-X-ray therapy in Bowen's disease and erythroplasia of Queyrat. *Dermatologica* 1985; **171**:89–94.

61 Dupree MT, Kiteley RA, Weismantle K et al. Radiation therapy for Bowen's disease: lessons for lesions of the lower extremity. *J Am Acad Dermatol* 2001; **45**:401–4.

62 Chung YL, Lee JD, Bang D et al. Treatment of Bowen's disease with a specially designed radioactive skin patch. *Eur J Nucl Med* 2000; **27**:842–6.

63 Tantikun N. Treatment of Bowen's disease of the digit with carbon dioxide laser. *J Am Acad Dermatol* 2000; **43**:1080–3.

64 Gordon KB, Garden JM, Robinson JK. Bowen's disease of the distal digit. Outcome of treatment with carbon dioxide laser vaporization. *Dermatol Surg* 1996; **22**:723–8.

65 Dave R, Monk B, Mahaffey P. Treatment of Bowen's disease with carbon dioxide laser. *Lasers Surg Med* 2003; **32**:335.

66 Otani K, Ito Y, Sumiya N et al. Treatment of Bowen disease using the ultrasonic surgical aspirator. *Plast Reconstr Surg* 2001; **108**:68–72.

67 Hiruma M, Kawada A. Hyperthermic treatment of Bowen's disease with disposable chemical pocket warmers: a report of 8 cases. *J Am Acad Dermatol* 2000; **43**:1070–5.

68 Ramrakha-Jones VS, Herd RM. Treating Bowen's disease: a cost-minimization study. *Br J Dermatol* 2003; **148**:1167–72.

69 National Institute for Health and Clinical Excellence. IPG155 Photodynamic therapy for non-melanoma skin tumours – guidance (http://www.nice.org.uk/page.aspx?o IPG155guidance) (last accessed 10 July 2006).

70 Ormerod AD. Recommendations in British Association of Dermatologists guidelines. *Br J Dermatol* 2005; **153**:477–8.

Appendix 1 Strength of recommendations and quality of evidence[a]

Strength of recommendations

A There is good evidence to support the use of the procedure

B There is fair evidence to support the use of the procedure

C There is poor evidence to support the use of the procedure

D There is fair evidence to support the rejection of the use of the procedure

E There is good evidence to support the rejection of the use of the procedure

Quality of evidence

I Evidence obtained from at least one properly designed, randomized controlled trial

II-i Evidence obtained from well-designed controlled trials without randomization

II-ii Evidence obtained from well-designed cohort or case–control analytical studies, preferably from more than one centre or research group

II-iii Evidence obtained from multiple time series with or without the intervention. Dramatic results in uncontrolled experiments (such as the results of the introduction of penicillin treatment in the 1940s) could also be regarded as this type of evidence

III Opinions of respected authorities based on clinical experience, descriptive studies or reports of expert committees

IV Evidence inadequate owing to problems of methodology (e.g. sample size, or length of comprehensiveness of follow up, or conflicts in evidence)

[a]A different system of evidence grading and recommendations has been adopted for new guidelines,[70] but the Therapy Guidelines and Audit Committee has recommended use of the original grading system in this guideline update.

http://bad.org.uk/Portals/_Bad/Guidelines/Clinical
%20Guidelines/Bowens%20Disease%20update
%20January%202007.pdf

Comment

Greater knowledge of the different modalities for the treatment of BD has been gained in the 2007 guidelines [1] compared with the 1999 version [2]. There is a wide choice of modalities for treating BD or not. These include no treatment (watchful waiting), cryotherapy, topical 5 fluorouracil, imiquimod, curettage and cautery, and full excision. In the US, surgery is still probably favoured over topical therapies [3]. The choice of treatment method has to be tailored to the patients' wants and needs and expertise of the treating clinician. Good-quality studies comparing the different modalities are lacking [1,3].

REFERENCES

1 Cox NH, Eedy DJ, Morton CA. Guidelines for the management of Bowen's disease: 2006 update. *Brit J Dermatol* 2007; 156: 11–21.
2 Cox NH, Eedy DJ, Morton CA. Guidelines for management of Bowen's disease. *Br J Dermatol* 1999; 141: 633–41.
3 Love WE, Bernhard JD, Bordeaux JS. Topical imiquimod or fluorouracil therapy for basal and squamous cell carcinoma: a systematic review. *Arch Dermatol* 2009; 145: 1431–38.

Additional professional resources

http://www.dermnetnz.org/treatments/5-fluorouracil.html

BAD patient information leaflet

http://www.bad.org.uk/site/802/default.aspx

Other patient resources

http://www.emedicine.com/derm/topic59.htm

SQUAMOUS CELL CARCINOMA

Multi-professional guidelines for the management of the patient with primary cutaneous squamous cell carcinoma

R J Motley, P W Preston, C M Lawrence

SUMMARY

These guidelines for management of primary cutaneous squamous cell carcinoma present evidence-based guidance for treatment, with identification of the strength of evidence available at the time of preparation of the guidelines, and a brief overview of epidemiological aspects, diagnosis and investigation. These guidelines aim to ensure people with cutaneous squamous cell carcinoma receive the best possible treatment and care.

DISCLAIMER

These guidelines reflect the best published data available at the time the report was prepared. Caution should be exercised in interpreting the data; the results of future studies may require alteration of the conclusions or recommendations in this report. It may be necessary or even desirable to depart from the guidelines in the interests of specific patients and special circumstances. Just as adherence to the guidelines may not constitute defence against a claim of negligence, so deviation from them should not be necessarily deemed negligent.

DEFINITION

Primary cutaneous squamous cell carcinoma (SCC) is a malignant tumour which may arise from the keratinising cells of the epidermis or its appendages. It is locally invasive and has the potential to metastasize to other organs of the body. These guidelines are confined to the treatment of SCC of the skin and the vermilion border of the lip, and exclude SCC of the penis, vulva and anus, SCC in-situ (Bowen's disease), SCC arising from mucous membranes and keratoacanthoma.

INCIDENCE, AETIOLOGY AND PREVENTION

SCC is the second most common skin cancer and, in many countries, its incidence is rising.[1–7] Its occurrence is usually related to chronic ultra violet light exposure and is therefore especially common in people with sun-damaged skin, fair skin, albinism and xeroderma pigmentosum. It may develop *de-novo*, as a result of previous exposure to ultraviolet or ionising radiation, or arsenic, within chronic wounds, scars, burns, ulcers or sinus tracts and from pre-existing lesions such as Bowen's disease (intraepidermal SCC).[8–17] Individuals with impaired immune function, for example those receiving immunosuppressive drugs following allogeneic organ transplantation or for inflammatory disease, and those with lymphoma or leukaemia, are at increased risk of this tumour. The risk of SCC with the new wave of 'biologic' therapies (for inflammatory and haematological disease) has yet to be quantified, although reports identify cases of rapid-onset or reactivation of

The authors are grateful to Professor PJ Barrett-Lee (Radiotherapy), Dr DAL Morgan (Oncology) Dr DN Slater (Pathology), Mr M Schenker (Plastic Surgery) and Mr A Langford (Skin Care Campaign) for their expert advice and comments on the manuscript.

SCC in patients with risk factors or a past history of the disease.[18–27] Some SCCs are associated with human papilloma virus infection.[28–36] There is good evidence linking SCCs with chronic actinic damage, (including that from the use of tanning devices)[8] and to support sun avoidance, use of protective clothing and effective sunblocks[37] in the prevention of actinic keratoses and SCCs. These measures are particularly important for people receiving long term immunosuppressive medication.[38–41]

People with organ transplants are at high risk of developing cutaneous SCC. Skin surveillance to allow early detection and treatment, and measures to prevent SCC should be part of their routine care. In patients with multiple, frequent or high-risk SCCs consideration should be given to modifying immunosuppressive regimens[42,43] and the prophylactic use of systemic retinoids[44,45] which may also be valuable in other high risk groups.[46] Topical agents, such as imiquimod may have a useful role in preventing the development of skin dysplasia in high-risk renal transplant recipients but substantive evidence is awaited.[47]

CLINICAL PRESENTATION

SCC usually presents as an indurated nodular keratinising or crusted tumour that may ulcerate, or it may present as an ulcer without evidence of keratinisation. All patients where there is a possibility of a cutaneous SCC should be referred urgently to an appropriately trained specialist, usually in the local Dermatology Department, rapid access skin cancer clinic.[48]

DIAGNOSIS

The diagnosis is established histologically. The histology report should include the following: histopathological subtype (for example 'acantholytic', 'desmoplastic', 'spindle' or 'verrucous SCC'), degree of differentiation (well, moderately, poorly or un-differentiated; histological grades as described by Broders: Appendix 2), tumour depth (thickness in mm – excluding layers of surface keratin), the level of dermal invasion (as Clark's levels), and the presence or absence of perineural, vascular or lymphatic invasion.[49] The margins of the excised tissue can be stained prior to tissue preparation to allow their identification histologically and comment should be made on the peripheral and deep margins of excision.[50–64]

COMMUNICATION

Having a diagnosis of cancer can evoke many emotions within a person. It is essential that each person with SCC receives very clear and fully informed advice about his or her tumour. A Skin Cancer Clinical Nurse Specialist can provide invaluable information, support and advice. Some people may require additional psychological support and this can often be accessed through the multi-professional supportive and palliative care team. All clinicians working with people who have cancer should have advanced communication skills training.

PROGNOSIS

The accumulated experience of treating cutaneous SCC by various methods has allowed some predictions to be made about prognosis based on the original lesion.

Factors which influence metastatic potential include anatomical site, size, tumour thickness, level of invasion, rate of growth, aetiology, degree of histological differentiation and host immunosuppression. These details are frequently omitted from reported series of treated SCC and the conclusions of such series must therefore be interpreted with caution. Patient referral patterns may influence local experience of this condition, and series reported from office practices tend to suggest a more favourable prognosis than cases reported from hospital and tertiary centres.[61–72] Changes to the TNM staging system have been proposed to more accurately reflect the prognosis and natural history of cutaneous SCC.[73]

FACTORS AFFECTING METASTATIC POTENTIAL OF CUTANEOUS SCC

A   Site

Tumour location influences prognosis: sites are listed in order of increasing metastatic potential[65,74–77]

1 SCC arising at sun-exposed sites excluding lip and ear.
2 SCC of the lip.
3 SCC of the ear.
4 Tumours arising in non sun-exposed sites (e.g. perineum, sacrum, sole of foot).
5 SCC arising in areas of radiation or thermal injury, chronic draining sinuses, chronic ulcers, chronic inflammation or Bowen's disease.

B Size: Diameter

Tumours greater than 2 cm in diameter are twice as likely to recur locally (15.2% vs. 7.4%), and three times as likely to metastasize (30.3% vs. 9.1%) as smaller tumours.[61,65]

C Size: Depth and level of invasion

Tumours greater than 4 mm in depth (excluding surface layers of keratin) or extending into or beyond the subcutaneous tissue (Clark level V) are more likely to recur and metastasize (metastatic rate 45.7%) compared with thinner tumours. Tumours less than 2 mm in thickness rarely metastasise.[51,55,65] Recurrence and metastases are less likely in tumours confined to the upper half of the dermis and less than 4 mm in depth (metastatic rate 6.7%).[52,55,61,65]

D Histological differentiation and subtype

Poorly differentiated tumours (i.e. those of Broders grades 3 and 4) (Appendix 2) have a poorer prognosis, with more than double the local recurrence rate and triple the metastatic rate of better differentiated SCC.[52,53,65] Acantholytic, spindle and desmoplastic subtypes have a poorer prognosis, whereas the verrucous subtype has a better prognosis. Tumours with perineural involvement, lymphatic or vascular invasion are more likely to recur and to metastasize.[59,62,78]

E Host immunosuppression

Tumours arising in patients who are immunosuppressed have a poorer prognosis. Host cellular immune response may be important both in determining the local invasiveness of SCC and the host's response to metastases.[35,36,50]

F Previous treatment and treatment modality

The risk of local recurrence depends upon the treatment modality. Locally recurrent disease itself is a risk factor for metastatic disease. Local recurrence rates are considerably less with Mohs' micrographic surgery than with any other treatment modality.[65,75–77,79–82]

TREATMENT

In interpreting and applying guidelines for treatment of SCC, three important points should be noted:

- There is a lack of randomised controlled trials (RCTs) for the treatment of primary cutaneous SCC.
- There is widely varying malignant behaviour of tumours which fall within the histological diagnostic category of 'primary cutaneous SCC'.
- There are varied experiences among the different specialists treating these tumours, which are determined by referral patterns and interests. Plastic and maxillofacial surgeons may encounter predominantly high-risk, aggressive tumours, whereas dermatologists may deal predominantly with smaller and less aggressive lesions.

However, there are three main factors which influence treatment, which are:

- The need for complete removal or treatment of the primary tumour
- The possible presence of local 'in transit' metastases
- The tendency of metastases to spread by lymphatics to lymph nodes

The majority of SCC cases are low risk and amenable to various forms of treatment, but it is essential to identify the significant proportion which are high risk. These may be best managed by a multiprofessional team with experience of treating the most malignant tumours.[66,67,69,72,83–86]

The goal of treatment is complete (preferably histologically confirmed) removal or destruction of the primary tumour and of any metastases. In order to achieve this, the margins of the tumour must be identified. The gold standard for identification of tumour margins is histological assessment, but most treatments rely on clinical judgement. It must be recognised that this is not always an accurate predictor of tumour extent, particularly when the margins of the tumour are ill-defined.[60,87–90]

SCC may give rise to local metastases, which are discontinuous with the primary tumour. Such 'in-transit' metastases may be removed by wide surgical excision or destroyed by irradiation of a wide field around the primary lesion. Small margins may not remove metastases in the vicinity of the primary tumour. Locally recurrent tumour may arise either due to failure to treat the primary continuous body of tumour, or from local metastases.[50,52,66,67,69,84,91,92]

SCC usually spreads to local lymph nodes and clinically enlarged nodes should be examined histologically (for example by fine needle aspiration or excisional biopsy).

Tumour positive lymph nodes are usually managed by regional node dissection, but detailed discussion of the management of metastatic disease is beyond the scope of these guidelines.[74,93–96]

In the absence of clinically enlarged nodes, techniques such as high resolution ultrasound-guided fine needle aspiration cytology may be useful in evaluating regional lymph nodes in patients with high risk tumours.[97–100] The role of sentinel lymph node biopsy has yet to be established.[101–109]

Although there are many large series in which long-term outcome after treatment for cutaneous SCC has been reported (comprehensively summarised in Rowe *et al.*[65]), there are no large prospective randomised studies in which different treatments for this tumour have been compared.[66,90,110–112]

Guidelines for patient treatment

Conclusions from population-based studies do not necessarily indicate the best treatment for an individual patient. In particular, when choosing a treatment modality it is important to be aware of factors which may influence success. Curettage and cautery, cryosurgery, and to a lesser degree radiotherapy are all techniques in which the outcome depends of the experience of the physician. Although the same could be said of surgical excision and Mohs' micrographic surgery, these two modalities provide tissue for histological examination that allows the pathologist to assess the adequacy of treatment and for the physician to undertake further surgery if necessary. For this reason, where feasible, surgical excision (including Mohs' micrographic surgery where appropriate) should be regarded as the treatment of first choice for cutaneous SCC. The other techniques can yield excellent results in experienced hands, but the quality of treatment cannot be assured or audited contemporaneously by a third party.[50,65,70,88,89,94,96,110,113–115]

Surgical Excision

Surgical excision is the treatment of choice for the majority of cutaneous SCC. It allows full characterisation of the tumour and a guide to the adequacy of treatment through histological examination of the margins of the excised tissue.[52,65]

When undertaking surgical excision a margin of normal skin is excised from around the tumour. For clinically well-defined, low risk tumours less than 2 cm in diameter, surgical excision with a minimum 4-mm margin around

the tumour border is appropriate and would be expected to completely remove the primary tumour mass in 95% of cases[88] (*Strength of Recommendation A, Quality of Evidence II-iii*). Narrower margins of excision are more likely to leave residual tumour. In order to maintain the same degree of confidence of adequate excision, tumours more than 2 cm in diameter, tumours classified as moderately, poorly or undifferentiated, tumours extending into the subcutaneous tissue and those on the ear, lip, scalp, eyelids or nose should be removed with a wider margin (6 mm or more) and the tissue margins examined histologically, or with Mohs' micrographic surgery.[75–77,88]

It is only meaningful to consider such margins when the peripheral boundary of the tumour appears clinically well-defined. The concept of a 'surgical margin' (i.e. normal-appearing tissue around the tumour) is based upon an assumption that the clinically visible margin of the tumour bears a predictable relationship to the true extent of the tumour, and that excision of a margin of clinically normal-appearing tissue around the tumour will encompass any microscopic tumour extension. The wider the surgical margin the greater the likelihood that all tumour will be removed. Large tumours have greater microscopic tumour extension and should be removed with a wider margin. This concept is equally valid for non-surgical treatments such as radiotherapy and cryotherapy in which a margin of clinically normal-appearing tissue is treated around the tumour. Mohs' micrographic surgery, does not make this assumption but displays the margins of the tissue for histological examination, and allows a primary tumour mass, growing in-continuity to be excised completely with minimal loss of normal tissue. There are important lessons to be learnt from the experiences of micrographic surgery in treating cutaneous SCC (see below).[60,65,75–77,79,89]

Local Metastases

Microscopic metastases may be found around high-risk primary cutaneous SCC.[67,92,95] Under these circumstances a 'wide' surgical margin extending well beyond the primary tumour may include such metastases and thus have a higher cure rate than a narrower margin. Mohs' micrographic surgery removes tumour growing in-continuity but does not identify in-transit micro-metastases. For this reason some practitioners of Mohs' micrographic surgery will excise a further surgical margin when treating high risk tumours after the Mohs' surgical wound has been histologically confirmed to be clear of the primary tumour mass.[67,95]

Histological Assessment of Surgical Margins

Conventional histological examination of one or more transverse sections of excised tissue displays a cross-section of the tumour and tissue margins. This is the best way of assessing and categorising the nature of the tumour, and it is usual to comment on whether tumour extends to the tissue margin, or if not, to record the margin of uninvolved skin around the tumour.[49,60] The value of such comments depends on how closely the section examined reflects the excised tissue in general. If SCC appears to extend to the margin of the examined tissue, then it should be assumed, particularly if the true margin of the tissue has been stained prior to sectioning, that excision is incomplete. Orientating markers or sutures should be placed in the surgical specimen by the surgeon to allow the pathologist to report accurately on the location of any residual tumour. A pathologist, using the conventional 'breadloaf' technique for examining tissue, typically views only a small sample of the specimen microscopically,[60] and this may allow incompletely excised high-risk tumour to go undetected. There are several alternative tissue preparations that allow the peripheral margins of the excised tissue to be more comprehensively examined.[87] The clinician and pathologist must work closely together in order to ensure appropriate sampling and microscopic examination of excised tissue, particularly with high-risk tumours.[60,87]

Mohs' micrographic surgery differs because the tissue is not displayed in cross-section and, if the first level of excision is adequate, tumour may not be seen at all in the microscopic sections. There are technical factors that may occasionally hamper identification of SCC in frozen sections and under these circumstances final histological examination should be undertaken on formalin-fixed tissue.[116,117]

Mohs' Micrographic Surgery

Mohs' micrographic surgery allows precise definition and excision of primary tumour growing in-continuity, and as such would be expected to reduce errors in primary treatment which may arise due to clinically invisible tumour extension. There is good evidence that the incidence of local recurrent and metastatic disease are low after Mohs' micrographic surgery and it should therefore be considered in the surgical treatment of high-risk SCC, particularly at difficult sites where wide surgical margins may be technically difficult to achieve without functional impairment.[52,65] (*Strength of Recommendation B, Quality of Evidence II-iii*). The best cure rates for high risk SCCs are reported in series treated by Mohs' micrographic surgery.[65,81,82,116–118] Where Mohs' micrographic surgery is indicated but not available then one of the other histological techniques to examine the peripheral margin of the excised tissue should be employed.[87]

However, there are no prospective randomised studies comparing therapeutic outcome between conventional or wide surgical excision versus Mohs' micrographic surgery for cutaneous SCC.

It is firmly established that incomplete surgical excision is associated with a worse prognosis and, when doubt exists as to the adequacy of excision at the time of surgery, it is desirable, where practical, to delay or modify wound repair until complete tumour removal has been confirmed histologically.[50,65–69,78]

Curettage and Cautery

Excellent cure rates have been reported in several series and experience suggests that small (<1 cm) well-differentiated, primary, slow growing tumours arising on sun-exposed sites can be removed by experienced physicians with curettage.[65,90,110,114,119] There are few published data relating outcome after curettage of larger tumours and different clinical tumour types.

The high cure rates reported following curettage and cautery of cutaneous SCC (*Quality of Evidence II-iii*), may reflect case selection, with a greater proportion of small tumours treated by curettage than by other techniques, but also raise the question as to whether curettage per se has a therapeutic advantage. The experienced clinician undertaking curettage can detect tumour tissue by its soft consistency and this may be of benefit in identifying invisible tumour extension and ensuring adequate treatment. Conventionally, cautery or electrodesiccation is applied to the curetted wound and the curettage-cautery cycle then repeated once or twice. Curettage is routinely undertaken to 'debulk' the tumour prior to Mohs' micrographic surgery, but is of no proven benefit prior to standard surgical resection.[120] Curettage provides poorly orientated material for histological examination and no histological assessment of the adequacy of treatment is possible. Curettage and cautery is not appropriate treatment for locally recurrent disease or high risk tumours.

Cryosurgery

Good short term cure rates have been reported for small histologically confirmed SCC treated by cryosurgery in experienced hands. Prior biopsy is necessary to establish the diagnosis histologically. There is great variability in the use of liquid nitrogen for cryotherapy and significant transatlantic variations in practice. For this reason caution should be exercised in the use of cryotherapy for SCC although it may be an appropriate technique for selected cases in specialised centres.[65,113,121] Cryosurgery is not appropriate for locally recurrent disease or high risk tumours.

Radiotherapy

Radiotherapy is generally contraindicated in the younger patient because the scar from surgery is usually less noticeable than the pallor and telangiectases which develop as a late effect in irradiated skin. In some circumstances radiotherapy will give a better cosmetic effect, particularly where loss of tissue is likely to cause cosmetic or functional impairment. For example, the lower eyelid, the inner canthus of the eye, the lip, the tip of the nose and in some cases the ear. SCC can be cured by radiotherapy in more than 90% of cases.[52,65,110,122–125] Choice of radiotherapy modality (electrons or photons) dose and technique require experience and the involvement of a qualified clinical oncologist.

Some skin sites tolerate radiotherapy poorly, e.g. the back of the hand, the abdominal wall and the lower limb, and surgical excision is preferable at these sites. Any tumour invading cartilage or bone, e.g. over the ear or nose is best treated surgically to avoid radio-necrosis.

In all cases where there is debate about whether radiotherapy or surgery is the best option, close liaison should take place between the dermatologist, clinical oncologist and plastic surgeon ideally in a multi-disciplinary clinic.

Other Treatments

Other reported treatments include: topical Imiquimod, intralesional Interferon Alpha, intralesional 5-Fluorouracil, and photodynamic therapy.[126–135] Evidence for the role of these treatments is lacking and limited to isolated case reports (*Strength of Recommendation C, Quality of Evidence IV*).

Elective prophylactic lymph node dissection / sentinel lymph node biopsy

Elective prophylactic lymph node dissection has been proposed for SCC on the lip greater than 6 mm in depth and cutaneous SCC greater than 8 mm in depth, but evidence for this is weak[70,74] (*Strength of Recommendation C, Quality of Evidence II-iii*). Elective lymph node dissection is not routinely practised and there is no compelling evidence of benefit over morbidity.[51,56]

There has been recent interest in the application of sentinel lymph node biopsy in the management of high risk SCC. The procedure is technically feasible and may help avoid unnecessary lymph node dissection. However, the overall benefit of the technique in patients with SCC has yet to be determined.[101–109]

The multiprofessional oncology team

Patients with high risk SCC and those presenting with clinically involved lymph nodes should ideally be reviewed by a multiprofessional skin oncology team which includes a dermatologist, pathologist, appropriately trained surgeon (usually a plastic, ENT or maxillo-facial surgeon), clinical oncologist, radiologist and a clinical nurse specialist in skin cancer.[48] Some advanced tumours are not surgically resectable and these should be managed in a multiprofessional setting in order that other therapeutic options are considered. Patients should be provided with suitable written information concerning diagnosis, prognosis, self-examination and follow up support, local and national support organisations and, where appropriate, access to a multiprofessional palliative care team.

Follow-up

Early detection and treatment improves survival of patients with recurrent disease. All patients should be instructed in self-examination of the surgical scar site, local skin and lymph nodes and should receive written information sheets giving clear instructions and actions to take should they suspect recurrent disease. Elderly patients may have difficulty in undertaking adequate self-examination. A specialist or appropriately trained clinical nurse specialist or primary care physician may undertake regular follow-up examination for recurrent disease. Seventy five percent of local recurrences and metastases are detected within 2 years and 95% within 5 years.[52,65] It would therefore seem reasonable for the patient who has had a high-risk SCC to be kept under close medical observation for recurrent disease for at least 2 and up to 5 years (*Strength of Recommendation A, Quality of Evidence II-ii*; Table 1). The decision as to who follows the patient will depend upon the disease risk, local facilities and interests.[52,65]

Table 1 Risk Factors: Primary Cutaneous Squamous Cell Carcinoma

	Site	Diameter	Tumour Depth and level of invasion	Histological Features and subtype	Host Immune status
Low risk	SCC arising at sun-exposed sites excluding lip and ear	Tumours up to 20 mm in diameter	Tumours up to 4 mm in depth and confined to dermis	Well-differentiated tumour or Verrucous subtype	No evidence of immune dysfunction
High risk	SCC of lip or ear	Tumours more than 20 mm in diameter	Tumours more than 4 mm in depth or invading beyond dermis	Moderately-differentiated tumour	Immunosupressive therapy – such as Organ Transplant Recipients
	Recurrent SCC			Poorly-differentiated tumour	Chronic immuno-suppressive disease – e.g. CLL
	SCC arising in non exposed sites such as perineum, sacrum, sole of foot			Perineural invasion Acantholytic, Spindle, or Desmoplastic subtypes	
	SCC arising in radiation or thermal scars, chronic ulcers or inflammation or Bowen's disease			Incomplete excision	

Tumours with features confined to the first row are considered 'low risk' all others are 'high risk'.

Summary of treatment options for primary cutaneous squamous cell carcinoma

Please see Table 2 for recommendations.

AUDIT POINTS

1 Surgical excision margins: Are the margins of excision (recommended: 4 mm for well-defined, low risk tumours and 6 mm for high risk tumours) appropriate and clearly documented in the medical notes?

Table 2 Summary of Treatment Options for Primary Cutaneous Squamous Cell Carcinoma

Treatment	Indications	Contraindications	Notes
Surgical Excision	All resectable tumours	Where surgical morbidity is likely to be unreasonably high	General treatment of choice for SCC
Mohs Micrographic Surgery/Excision with histological control	High risk tumours	Where surgical morbidity is likely to be unreasonably high	High risk tumours need wide margins or histological margin control
Radiotherapy	Non-resectable tumours	Where tumour margins are ill-defined	
Curettage and Cautery	Small, well-defined, low-risk tumours	High risk tumours	Only suitable for experienced practitioners
Cryotherapy	Small, well-defined, low-risk tumours	High risk tumours, recurrent tumours	Only suitable for experienced practitioners

2 Are those involved in the care of patients with SCC able to show evidence of advanced communications skills training?

3 Has the prognosis of the tumour – low-risk or high-risk been documented in the notes?

4 Is there evidence of the patient being instructed in self-examination and being provided with written information sheets?

5 Is there evidence of appropriate follow up examination by suitably trained persons?

APPENDIX 1

STRENGTH OF RECOMMENDATIONS

A There is good evidence to support the use of the procedure.

B There is fair evidence to support the use of the procedure.

C There is poor evidence to support the use of the procedure.

D There is fair evidence to support the rejection of the use of the procedure.

E There is good evidence to support the rejection of the use of the procedure.

QUALITY OF EVIDENCE

I Evidence obtained from at least one properly designed, randomised control trial.

II-i Evidence obtained from well designed controlled trials without randomisation.

II-ii Evidence obtained from well designed cohort or case control analytic studies, preferably from more than one centre or research group.

II-iii Evidence obtained from multiple time series with or without the intervention. Dramatic results in uncontrolled experiments (such as the introduction of penicillin treatment in the 1940's) could also be regarded as this type of evidence.

III Opinions of respected authorities based on clinical experience, descriptive studies or reports of expert committees.

IV Evidence inadequate owing to problems of methodology (e.g. sample size, or length or comprehensiveness of follow-up or conflicts in evidence).

APPENDIX 2

BRODERS HISTOLOGICAL CLASSIFICATION OF DIFFERENTIATION IN SCC

Broders devised a classification system in which grades 1, 2 and 3 denoted ratios of differentiated to undifferentiated cells of 3:1, 1:1 and 1:3 respectively. Grade 4 denoted tumour cells having no tendency towards differentiation.

REFERENCES

1 Marks R. Squamous cell carcinoma. *Lancet* 1996; **347**: 735–38.

2 Bernstein SC, Lim KK, Brodland DG, Heidelberg KA. The many faces of squamous cell carcinoma. *Dermatol Surg* 1996; **22**: 243–54.

3 Glass AG, Hoover RN. The emerging epidemic of melanoma and squamous cell skin cancer. *JAMA* 1989; **262**: 2097–100.

4 Gray DT, Suman VJ, Su WP, Clay RP, Harmsen WS, Roenigk RK. Trends in the population-based incidence of squamous cell carcinoma of the skin first diagnosed between 1984 and 1992. *Arch Dermatol* 1997; **133**: 735–40.

5 Weinstock MA. The epidemic of squamous cell carcinoma. *JAMA* 1989; **262**: 2138–40.

6 Holme SA, Malinovszky K, Roberts DL. Changing trends in non-melanoma skin cancer in South Wales, 1988–98. *Br J Dermatol* 2000; **143**: 1224–9.

7 Hemminki K, Dong C. Subsequent cancers after in-situ and invasive squamous cell carcinoma of the skin. *Arch Dermatol* 2000; **136**: 647–51.

8 Karagas MR, Stannard VA, Mott LA *et al*. Use of tanning devices and risk of basal cell and squamous cell skin cancers. *J Natl Cancer Inst* 2002; **94**: 224–6.

9 Baldursson B, Sigurgeirsson B, Lindelof B. Leg ulcers and squamous cell carcinoma. An epidemiological study and review of the literature. *Acta Derm Venereol* 1993; **73**: 171–4.

10 Bosch RJ, Gallardo MA, Ruiz del Portal G *et al*. Squamous cell carcinoma secondary to recessive dystrophic epidermolysis bullosa: report of eight tumours in four patients. *J Eur Acad Dermatol Venereol* 1999; **13**: 198–204.

11 Keefe M, Wakeel RA, Dick DC. Death from metastatic cutaneous squamous cell carcinoma in autosomal recessive dystrophic epidermolysis bullosa despite permanent inpatient care. *Dermatologica* 1988; **177**: 180–4.

12 Chang A, Spencer JM, Kirsner RS. Squamous cell carcinoma arising from a nonhealing wound and osteomyelitis treated with Mohs' micrographic surgery: a case study. *Ostomy Wound Manage* 1998; **44**: 26–30.

13 Chowdri NA, Darzi MA. Postburn scar carcinomas in Kashmiris. *Burns* 1996; **22**: 477–82.

14 Dabski K, Stoll HL Jr, Milgrom H. Squamous cell carcinoma complicating late chronic discoid lupus erythematosus. *J Surg Oncol* 1986; **32**: 233–7.

15 Fasching MC, Meland NB, Woods JE, Wolff BG. Recurrent squamous cell carcinoma arising in pilonidal sinus tract – multiple flap reconstructions. Report of a case. *Dis Colon Rectum* 1989; **32**: 153–8.

16 Lister RK, Black MM, Calonje E, Burnand KG. Squamous cell carcinoma arising in chronic lymphoedema. *Br J Dermatol* 1997; **136**: 384–7.

17 Maloney ME. Arsenic in Dermatology. *Dermatol Surg* 1996; **22**: 301–4.

18 Moloney FJ, Comber H, O'Lorcain P *et al.* A population-based study of skin cancer incidence and prevalence in renal transplant recipients. *Br J Dermatol* 2006; **154**: 498–504.

19 Lindelof B, Jarnvik J, Ternesten-Bratel A *et al.* Mortality and Clinicopathological features of cutaneous squamous cell carcinoma in organ transplant recipients: A Study of the Swedish Cohort. *Acta Derm Venereol* 2006; **86**: 219–22.

20 Fogarty GB, Bayne M, Bedford P *et al.* Three cases of activation of cutaneous squamous cell carcinoma during treatment with prolonged administration of rituximab. *Clin Oncol (Royal College of Radiologists)* 2006; **18**: 155–6.

21 Baskaynak G, Kreuzer KA, Schwarz M *et al.* Squamous cutaneous epithelial cell carcinoma in two CML patients with progressive disease under imatinib treatment. *Eur J Haematol* 2003; **70**: 231–4.

22 Lebwohl M, Blum R, Berkowitz *et al.* No evidence for increased risk of cutaneous squamous cell carcinoma in patients with rheumatoid arthritis receiving etanercept therapy for up to 5 years. *Arch Dermatol* 2005; **141**: 861–4.

23 Smith KJ, Skelton HG. Rapid onset of cutaneous squamous cell carcinoma in patients with rheumatoid arthritis after starting tumor necrosis factor α receptor IgG1-Fc fusion complex therapy. *J Am Acad Dermatol* 2001; **45**: 953–6.

24 Burge D. Etanercept and squamous cell carcinoma. *J Am Acad Dermatol* 2003; **49**: 358–9.

25 Smith KJ, Skelton H. Etanercept and squamous cell carcinoma. Reply. *J Am Acad Dermatol* 2003; **49**: 359.

26 Mehrany K, Weenig RH, Lee KK *et al.* Increased metastasis and mortality from cutaneous squamous cell carcinoma in patients with chronic lymphatic leukaemia. *J Am Acad Dermatol* 2005; **53**: 1067–71.

27 Mehrany K, Weenig RH, Pittelkow MR *et al.* High recurrence rates of squamous cell carcinoma after Mohs' surgery in patients with chronic lymphocytic leukaemia. *Dermatol Surg* 2005; **31**: 38–42.

28 Moy R, Eliezri YD. Significance of human papillomavirus-induced squamous cell carcinoma to dermatologists. *Arch Dermatol* 1994; **130**: 235–8.

29 Bens G, Wieland U, Hofmann A *et al.* Detection of new human papillomavirus sequences in skin lesions of a renal transplant recipient and characterization of one complete genome related to epidermodysplasia verruciformis-associated types. *J Gen Virol* 1998; **79**: 779–87.

30 Harwood CA, McGregor JM, Proby CM, Breuer J. Human papillomavirus and the development of non-melanoma skin cancer. *J Clin Pathol* 1999; **52**: 249–53.

31 Harwood CA, Surentheran T, McGregor JM *et al.* Human papillomavirus infection and non-melanoma skin cancer in immunosuppressed and immunocompetent individuals. *J Med Virol* 2000; **61**: 289–97.

32 Glover MT, Niranjan N, Kwan JT, Leigh IM. Non-melanoma skin cancer in renal transplant recipients: the extent of the problem and a strategy for management. *Br J Plast Surg* 1994; **47**: 86–9.

33 Liddington M, Richardson AJ, Higgins RM, Endre ZH, Venning VA, Murie JA, Morris PJ. Skin cancer in renal transplant recipients. *Br J Surg* 1989; **76**: 1002–5.

34 Ong CS, Keogh AM, Kossard S *et al.* Skin cancer in Australian heart transplant recipients. *J Am Acad Dermatol* 1999; **40**: 27–34.

35 Veness MJ, Quinn DI, Ong CS *et al.* Aggressive cutaneous malignancies following cardiothoracic transplantation: the Australian experience. *Cancer* 1999; **85**: 1758–64.

36 Weimar VM, Ceilley RI, Goeken JA. Aggressive biologic behaviour of basal and squamous cell cancers in patients with chronic lymphocytic leukaemia or chronic lymphocytic lymphoma. *J Dermatol Surg Oncol* 1979; **5**: 609–14.

37 van der Pols JC, Williams GM, Pandeya N *et al.* Prolonged prevention of squamous cell carcinoma of the skin by regular sunscreen use. *Cancer Epidemiol Biomarkers Prev* 2006; **15**: 2546–8.

38 Green A, Williams G, Neale R *et al.* Daily sunscreen application and betacarotene supplementation in prevention of basal-cell and squamous-cell carcinomas of the skin: a randomised controlled trial. *Lancet* 1999; **354**: 723–9.

39 Marks R, Rennie G, Selwood TS. Malignant transformation of solar keratoses to squamous cell carcinoma in the skin: a prospective study. *Lancet* 1988, **9**: 795–7.

40 Naylor MF, Boyd *et al.* High sun protection factor sunscreens in the suppression of actinic neoplasia. *Arch Dermatol* 1995; **131**: 170–5.

41 Thompson SC, Jolley D, Marks R. Reduction of solar keratosis by regular sunscreen use. *New Engl J Med* 1993; **329**: 1147–51.

42 Moloney FJ, Kelly PO, Kay EW *et al.* Maintenance versus reduction of immunosuppression in renal transplant recipients with aggressive squamous cell carcinoma. *Dermatol Surg* 2004; **30**: 674–8.

43 Euvrard S, Ulrich C, Lefrancois N. Immunosuppressants and skin cancer in transplant patients; focus on rapamycin. *Dermatol Surg* 2004; **30**: 628–33.

44 Chen K, Craig JC, Shumack S. Oral retinoids for the prevention of skin cancers in solid organ transplant recipients: a systematic review of randomized controlled trials. *Br J Dermatol* 2005; **152**: 518–23.

45 Harwood CA, Leedham-Green M, Leigh IM, Proby CM. Low-dose retinoids in the prevention of cutaneous squamous cell carcinomas in organ transplant recipients. *Arch Dermatol* 2005; **141**: 456–64.

46 Nijsten TEC, Stern RS. Oral retinoid use reduces cutaneous squamous cell carcinoma risk in patients with psoriasis treated with psoralen-UVA; a nested cohort study. *J Am Acad Dermatol* 2003; **49**: 644–50.

47 Brown VL, Atkins CL, Ghali L *et al.* Safety and efficacy of 5% imiquimod cream for the treatment of skin dysplasia in high-risk renal transplant recipients. *Arch Dermatol* 2005; **141**: 985–93.

48 National Institute for Health and Clinical Excellence. *Improving Outcomes for People with Skin Tumours including Melanoma.* February 2006 (accessed 19 June 2007, at: http://guidance.nice.org.uk/csgstim/guidance/pdf/English/download.dspx">).

49 Royal College of Pathologists. *Minimum Dataset for the Histopathological Reporting of Common Skin Cancers.* February 2002 (accessed 19 June 2007, at: http://www.rcpath.org/resources/pdf/skincancers2802.pdf).

50 Barksdale SK, O'Connor N, Barnhill R. Prognostic factors for cutaneous squamous cell and basal cell carcinoma. Determinants of risk of recurrence, metastasis and development of subsequent skin cancers. *Surg Oncol Clin N Am* 1997; **6**: 625–38.

51 Breuninger H, Black B, Rassner G. Microstaging of squamous cell carcinomas. *Am J Clin Pathol* 1990: **94**: 624–7.

52 Breuninger H. Diagnostic and therapeutic standards in interdisciplinary dermatologic oncology. Published by the German Cancer Society 1998.

53 Broders AC. Squamous cell epithelioma of the lip. *JAMA* 1920: **74**: 656–64.

54 Broders AC. Squamous cell epithelioma of the skin. *Ann Surg* 1921: **73**: 141–60.

55 Friedman HI, Cooper PH, Wanebo HJ. Prognostic and therapeutic use of microstaging in cutaneous squamous cell carcinoma of the trunk and extremities. *Cancer* 1985: **56**: 1099–1105.

56 Frierson HF, Cooper PH. Prognostic factors in squamous cell carcinoma of the lower lip. *Hum Pathol* 1986: **17**: 346–54.

57 Heenan PJ, Elder DJ, Sobin LH. *WHO International histological classification of tumors.* Springer, Berlin, Heidelberg, New York, 1993.

58 Hermanek P, Heuson DE, Hutter RVP, Sobin LH. *UICC (International Union Against Cancer) TNM Supplement,* Springer, Berlin, Heidelberg, New York 1993.

59 Mendenhall WM, Parsons JT, Mendenhall NP, Brant TA, Stringer SP. Cassisi NJ, Million RR. Carcinoma of the skin of the Head and Neck with perineural invasion. *Head Neck* 1989; **11**: 301–8.

60 Abide JM, Nahai F, Bennett RG. The Meaning of Surgical Margins. *Plast Reconstr Surg* 1984: **73**: 492–496.

61 Clayman GL, Lee JJ, Holsinger C *et al.* Mortality risk from squamous cell carcinoma. *J Clin Oncol* 2005; **23**: 759–65.

62 Moore BA, Weber RS, Prieto V *et al.* Lymph node metastases from cutaneous squamous cell carcinoma of the head and neck. *Laryngoscope* 2005; **115**: 1561–7.

63 Veness MJ, Palme CE, Morgan GJ. High-risk cutaneous squamous cell carcinoma of the head and neck. Results from 266 treated patients with metastatic lymph node disease. *Cancer* 2006; **106**: 2389–96.

64 Mullen JT, Feng L, Xing Y *et al.* Invasive squamous cell carcinoma of the skin: defining a high-risk group. *Ann Surg Oncol* 2006; **13**: 902–9.

65 Rowe DE, Carroll RJ, Day CL. Prognostic Factors for local recurrence, metastasis and survival rates in squamous cell carcinoma of the skin, ear and lip. *J Am Acad Dermatol* 1992: **26**: 976–90.

66 Dzubow LM, Rigel DS, Robins P. Risk factors for local recurrence of primary cutaneous squamous cell carcinomas. *Arch Dermatol* 1982; **118**: 900–2.

67 Epstein E, Epstein NN, Bragg K, Linden G. Metastases from squamous cell carcinomas of the skin. *Arch Dermatol* 1968; **97**: 245–51.

68 Epstein E. Malignant sun-induced squamous cell carcinoma of the skin. *J Dermatol Surg Oncol* 1983; **9**: 505–6.

69 Eroglu A, Berberoglu U, Berberoglu S. Risk factors related to locoregional recurrence in squamous cell carcinoma of the skin. *J Surg Oncol* 1996; **61**: 124–30.

70 Friedman NR. Prognostic factors for local recurrence, metastases and survival rates in squamous cell carcinoma of the skin, ear and lip. *J Am Acad Dermatol* 1993; **28**: 281–2.

71 Katz AD, Urbach F, Lilienfeld AM. The frequency and risk of metastases in squamous cell carcinoma of the skin. *Cancer* 1957; **10**: 1162–6.

72 Kwa RE, Campana K, Moy RL. Biology of Cutaneous squamous cell carcinoma. *J Am Acad Dermatol* 1992: **26**: 1–26.

73 Dinehart SM, Peterson S. Evaluation of the American Joint Committee on cancer Staging System for cutaneous squamous cell carcinoma and proposal of a new staging system. *Dermatol Surg* 2005; **31**: 1379–84.

74 Afzelius LE, Gunnarsson M, Nordgren H. Guidelines for prophylactic radical lymph node dissection in cases of carcinoma of the external ear. *Head Neck Surg* 1980; **2**: 361–5.

75 Mohs FE, Snow SN. Microscopically controlled surgical treatment for squamous cell carcinoma of the lower lip. *Surg Gynecol Obstet* 1985; **160**: 37–41.

76 Mohs FE. Chemosurgical treatment of cancer of the ear: a microscopically controlled method of excision. *Surgery* 1947; **21**: 605–622.

77 Mohs FE. Chemosurgical treatment of cancer of the lip. *Archives of Surgery* 1944; **48**: 478–88.

78 Cottel WI. Perineural invasion by squamous cell carcinoma. *J Dermatol Surg Oncol* 1982; **8**: 589–600.

79 Glass RL, Spratt JS, Perez-Mesa C. The fate of inadequately excised epidermoid carcinoma of the skin. *Surg Gynecol Obstet* 1966; **122**: 245–8.

80 Mohs FE. Chemosurgery. *Clinics in Plastic Surgery.* 1980; **7**: 349–60.

81 Leibovitch I, Huilgol SC, Selva D *et al.* Cutaneous squamous cell carcinoma treated with Mohs micrographic surgery in Australia I. Experience over 10 years. *J Am Acad Dermatol* 2005; **53**: 253–6.

82 Leibovitch I, Huilgol SC, Selva D *et al.* Cutaneous squamous cell carcinoma treated with Mohs micrographic surgery in Australia II. Perineural invasion. *J Am Acad Dermatol* 2005; **53**: 261–6.

83 Immerman SC, Scanlon EF, Christ M, Knox KL. Recurrent squamous cell carcinoma of the skin. *Cancer* 1983; **51**: 1537–40.

84 Kraus DH, Carew JF, Harrison LB. Regional lymphnode metastasis from cutaneous squamous cell carcinoma. *Arch Otolaryngol Head Neck Surg.* 1998; **124**: 582–7.

85 Petter G, Haustein UF. Histologic subtyping and malignancy assessment of cutaneous squamous cell carcinoma. *Dermatol Surg* 2000; **26**: 521–30.

86 Tavin E, Persky M. Metastatic cutaneous squamous cell carcinoma of the head and neck region. *Laryngoscope* 1996; **106**: 156–8.

87 Rapini RP. Comparison of Methods for Checking Surgical Margins. *J Am Acad Dermatol* 1990; **23**: 288–94.

88 Brodland DG, Zitelli JA. Surgical margins for excision of primary cutaneous squamous cell carcinoma. *J Am Acad Dermatol* 1992: **27**: 241–8.

89 Fleming ID, Amonette R, Monaghan T, Fleming MD. Principles of management of basal and squamous cell carcinoma of the skin. *Cancer* 1995; **75**: 699–704.

90 Knox JM, Freeman RG, Duncan WC, Heaton CL. Treatment of skin cancer. *Southern Medical Journal* 1967; **60**: 241–6.

91 Lund HZ. Metastasis from sun-induced squamous cell carcinoma of the skin: an uncommon event. *J Dermatol Surg Oncol* 1984; **10**: 169–70.

92 Dinehart SM, Pollack SV. Metastases from squamous cell carcinoma of the skin and lip. *J Am Acad Dermatol* 1989; **21**: 241–8.

93 Nicolson GL. Organ specificity of tumor metastasis: role of preferential adhesion, invasion and growth of malignant cells at specific secondary sites. *Cancer Metastasis Rev* 1988; **7**: 143–88.

94 Weisberg NK, Bertagnolli MM, Becker DS. Combined sentinel lymphadenectomy and Mohs' micrographic surgery for high-risk cutaneous squamous cell carcinoma. *J Am Acad Dermatol* 2000; **43**: 483–8.

95 Brodland DG, Zitelli JA. Mechanisms of metastasis. *J Am Acad Dermatol* 1992; **27**: 1–8.

96 Geohas J, Roholt NS, Robinson JK. Adjuvant radiotherapy after excision of cutaneous squamous cell carcinoma. *J Am Acad Dermatol* 1994; **30**: 633–6.

97 van den Brekel MWM, Stel HV, Castelijns *et al.* Lymph node staging in patients with clinically negative neck examinations by ultrasound and ultrasound-guided aspiration cytology. *Am J Surg* 1991; **162**: 362–6.

98 Vassallo P, Wernecke K, Roos N, Peters PE. Differentiation of benign from malignant superficial lymphadenopathy: The role of high resolution US. *Radiology* 1992; **183**: 215–20.

99 Knappe M, Louw M, Gregor RT. Ultrasonography-guided fine-needle aspiration for the assessment of cervical metastases. *Arch Otolaryngol Head Neck Surg* 2000; **126**: 1091–6.

100 Sumi M, Ohki M, Nakamura T. Comparison of sonography and CT for differentiating benign from malignant cervical lymph nodes in patients with squamous cell carcinoma of the head and neck. *AJR Am J Roentgenol* 2001; **176**: 1019–24.

101 Civantos FJ, Moffat FL, Goodwin WJ. Lymphatic mapping and sentinel lymphadenectomy for 106 head and neck lesions: contrasts between oral cavity and cutaneous malignancy. *Laryngoscope* 2006; **116** (S109): 1–15.

102 Wagner JD, Evdokimow DZ, Weisberger E *et al.* Sentinel node biopsy for high-risk non-melanoma cutaneous malignancy. *Arch Dermatol* 2004; **140**: 75–9.

103 Nouri K, Rivas P, Pedroso F *et al.* Sentinel lymph node biopsy for high-risk cutaneous squamous cell carcinoma of the head and neck. *Arch Dermatol* 2004; **140**: 1284.

104 Reschly MJ, Messina JL, Zaulyanov LL *et al.* Utility of sentinel lymphadenectomy in the management of patients with high risk cutaneous squamous cell carcinoma. *Dermatol Surg* 2003; **29**: 135–40.

105 Altinyollar H, Berberoglu U, Celen O. Lymphatic mapping and sentinel lymph node biopsy in squamous cell carcinoma of the lower lip. *Eur J Surg Oncol* 2002; **28**: 72–4.

106 Weisberg NK, Bertagnolli MM, Becker DS. Combined sentinel lymphadenectomy and Mohs micrographic surgery for high risk cutaneous squamous cell carcinoma. *J Am Acad Dermatol* 2000; **43**: 483–8.

107 Eastman AL, Erdman WA, Lindberg GM *et al.* Sentinel lymph node biopsy identifies occult nodal metastases in patients with Marjolin's ulcer. *J Burn Care Rehabil* 2004; **25**: 241–5.

108 Ozcelik D, Tatlidede S, Hacikerim S *et al.* The use of sentinel lymph node biopsy in squamous cell carcinoma of the foot: a case report. *J Foot Ankle Surg* 2004; **43**: 60–3.

109 Perez-Naranjo L, Herrera-Saval A, Garcia-Bravo B *et al.* Sentinel lymph node biopsy in recessive dystrophic epidermolysis bullosa and squamous cell carcinoma. *Arch Dermatol* 2005; **141**: 110–1.

110 Freeman RG, Knox JM, Heaton CL. The treatment of skin cancer. A statistical study of 1,341 skin tumours comparing results obtained with irradiation, surgery and curettage followed by electrodesiccation. *Cancer* 1964; **17**: 535–8.

111 Macomber WB, Wang MKH, Sullivan JG. Cutaneous Epithelioma. *Plast Reconst Surgery* 1959; **24**: 545–62.

112 Stenbeck KD, Balanda KP, Williams MJ, Ring IT, MacLennan R, Chick JE, Morton AP. Patterns of treated

non-melanoma skin cancer in Queensland – the region with the highest incidence rates in the world. *Med J Aust.* 1990; **153**: 511–5.

113 Kuflik EG, Gage AA. The five-year cure rate achieved by cryosurgery for skin cancer. *J Am Acad Dermatol* 1991; **24**: 1002–4.

114 Tromovitch TA. Skin Cancer. Treatment by curettage and desiccation. *Calif Med* 1965: **103**: 107–8.

115 Karagas MR. Occurrence of cutaneous basal cell and squamous cell malignancies among those with a prior history of skin cancer. *J Invest Dermatol.* 1994; **102**: 10S-13S.

116 Telfer NR. Mohs' micrographic surgery for cutaneous squamous cell carcinoma: practical considerations. *Br J Dermatol* 2000; **142**: 631–3.

117 Turner RJ, Leonard N, Malcolm AJ, Lawrence CM, Dahl MGC. A retrospective study of outcome of Mohs' micrographic surgery for cutaneous squamous cell carcinoma using formalin fixed sections. *Br J Dermatol* 2000; **142**: 752–7.

118 Lawrence CM, Dahl MGC, Dickinson AJ, Turner RJ. Mohs' micrographic surgery for cutaneous squamous cell carcinoma: practical considerations. *Br J Dermatol* 2001; **144**: 186.

119 de Graaf YGL, Basdew VR, Van Der Zwan-Kralt N *et al.* The occurrence of residual or recurrent squamous cell carcinomas in organ transplant recipients after curettage and electrodesiccation. *Br J Dermatol* 2006; **154**: 493–7.

120 Chiller K, Passaro D, McCalmont T, Vin-Christian K. Efficacy of curettage before excision in clearing surgical margins of non-melanoma skin cancer. *Arch Dermatol* 2000; **136**: 1327–32.

121 Kuflik EG. Cryosurgery for skin cancer: 30 year experience and cure rates. *Dermatol Surg* 2004; **30**: 297–300.

122 Tsao MN, Tsang RW, Liu F-F *et al.* Radiotherapy management for squamous cell carcinoma of the nasal skin: the Princess Margaret Hospital experience. *Int J Radiation Oncology Biol Phys* 2002; **52**: 973–9.

123 Caccialanzi M, Piccinno R, Kolessnikova L, Gnecchi L. Radiotherapy of skin carcinomas of the pinna: a study of 115 lesions in 108 patients. *Int J Dermatol* 2005; **44**: 513–7.

124 Locke J, Karimpour S, Young G. Radiotherapy for epithelial skin cancer. *Int J Radiation Oncology Biol Phys* 2001; **51**: 748–55.

125 Schulte K-W, Lippold A, Auras C *et al.* Soft x-ray therapy for cutaneous basal cell and squamous cell carcinomas. *J Am Acad Dermatol* 2005; **53**: 993–1001.

126 Oster-Schmidt C. Two cases of squamous cell carcinoma treated with topical imiquimod 5%. *JEADV* 2004; **18**: 93–5.

127 Fernandez-Vozmediano J, Armario-Hita J. Infiltrative squamous cell carcinoma on the scalp after treatment with 5% imiquimod cream. *J Am Acad Dermatol* 2005; **52**: 716–7.

128 Peris K, Micantonio T, Concetta Fargnoli M *et al.* Imiquimod 5% cream in the treatment of Bowen's disease and invasive squamous cell carcinoma. *J Am Acad Dermatol* 2006; **55**: 324–7.

129 Hengge UR, Schaller J. Successful treatment of invasive squamous cell carcinoma using topical imiquimod. *Arch Dermatol* 2004; **140**: 404–6.

130 Florez A, Feal C, de la Torre C, Cruces M. Invasive squamous cell carcinoma treated with imiquimod 5% cream. *Acta Derm Venereol* 2004; **84**: 227–8.

131 Martin-Garcia RF. Imiquimod: an effective alternative for the treatment of invasive cutaneous squamous cell carcinoma. *Dermatol Surg* 2005; **31**: 371–4.

132 Kim KH, Yavel RM, Gross VL, Brody N. Intralesional interferon α-2b in the treatment of basal cell carcinoma and squamous cell carcinoma: revisited. *Dermatol Surg* 2004; **30**: 116–20.

133 Morse LG, Kendrick C, Hooper D *et al.* Treatment of squamous cell carcinoma with intralesional 5-fluorouracil. *Dermatol Surg* 2003; **29**: 1150–3.

134 Marmur ES, Schmults CD, Goldberg DJ. A review of laser and photodynamic therapy for the treatment of non-melanoma skin cancer. *Dermatol Surg* 2004; **30**: 264–71.

135 Rossi R, Puccioni M, Mavilia L *et al.* Squamous cell carcinoma of the eyelid treated with photodynamic therapy. *J Chemotherapy* 2004; **16**: 306–9.

http://www.bad.org.uk/Portals/_Bad/Guidelines/Clinical %20Guidelines/SCC%20Guidelines%20Final%20Aug %2009.pdf

Comment

The updated 2009 guidelines on the management of SCC [1], which were not published in the *British Journal of Dermatology*, highlight the lack of good-quality trials of different modalities of treatment and also for excision margins. The main recommended treatment is still wide local excision with or without Moh's micrographic surgery as this is a potentially metastasising tumour [1,2]. Further studies of immunmodulators (imiquimod-like drugs) versus surgery are needed to determine the place of them in the management of SCC [3]. More (some) evidence for radiotherapy and width of surgical margins is needed. In the UK, skin cancer networks and MDTs have helped in the collection of a minimum pathological data set that helps with prognosis and advice on management; however, the advice often does not rely on good-quality evidence.

REFERENCES

1 http://www.bad.org.uk/Portals/_Bad/Guidelines/Clinical %20Guidelines/SCC%20Guidelines%20Final%20Aug %2009.pdf.

2 Motley R, Kersey P, Lawrence C. Multiprofessional guidelines for the management of the patient with primary cutaneous squamous cell carcinoma. *Brit J Dermatol* 2002; 146: 18–25.

3 Love WE, Bernhard JD, Bordeaux JS. Topical imiquimod or fluorouracil therapy for basal and squamous cell carcinoma: a systematic review. *Arch Dermatol* 2009; 145: 1431–38.

Additional professional resources

Bath-Hextall FJ, Leonardi-Bee J, Somchand N, Webster AC, Delitt J, Perkins W. Interventions for preventing non-melanoma skin cancers in high-risk groups. *Cochrane Database Syst Rev* 2007; Issue 4: CD005414 (http://dx.doi.org/10.1002/14651858.CD005414).

National Comprehensive Cancer Network (USA) (requires free registration). http://www.nccn.org/professionals/physician_gls/PDF/nmsc.pdf (covers basal and squamous cell carcinomas of skin 2009).

Chen K, Craig J C, Shumack S. Oral retinoids for the prevention of skin cancers in solid organ transplant recipients: a systematic review of randomized controlled trials. *Brit J Dermatol* 2005; 152: 518–23.

BAD patient information leaflet

http://www.bad.org.uk/site/876/Default.aspx

Related topics

Keratoacanthoma: http://www.bad.org.uk/site/835/Default.aspx

Skin cancer in immunosuppression: http://www.bad.org.uk/site/879/default.aspx

Skin cancer prevention pre-transplant: http://www.bad.org.uk/site/880/Default.aspx

Prevention of further skin cancer: http://www.bad.org.uk/site/875/Default.aspx

Other patient resources

http://www.cancerbackup.org.uk
http://www.skincancer.org/content/view/23/81/
http://www.intelihealth.com/IH/ihtIH/WSIHW000/8297/24556/211186.html?d=dmtHealthAZ
http://www.aad.org/public/publications/pamphlets/sun_squamous.html
http://www.cancerresearchuk.org/sunsmart/

MELANOMA

Revised U.K. guidelines for the management of cutaneous melanoma 2010

J.R. Marsden, J.A. Newton-Bishop,* L. Burrows,† M. Cook,‡ P.G. Corrie,§ N.H. Cox,¶ M.E. Gore,** P. Lorigan,††
R. MacKie,‡‡ P. Nathan,§§ H. Peach,¶¶ B. Powell*** and C. Walker

University Hospital Birmingham, Birmingham B29 6JD, U.K.
*University of Leeds, Leeds LS9 7TF, U.K.
†Salisbury District Hospital, Salisbury SP2 8BJ, U.K.
‡Royal Surrey County Hospital NHS Trust, Guildford GU2 7XX, U.K.
§Cambridge University Hospitals NHS Foundation Trust, Cambridge CB2 2QQ, U.K.
¶Cumberland Infirmary, Carlisle CA2 7HY, U.K.
**Royal Marsden Hospital, London SW3 6JJ, U.K.
††The Christie NHS Foundation Trust, Manchester M20 4BX, U.K.
‡‡University of Glasgow, Glasgow G12 8QQ, U.K.
§§Mount Vernon Hospital, London HA6 2RN, U.K.
¶¶St James's University Hospital, Leeds LS9 7TF, U.K.
***St George's Hospital, London SW17 0QT, U.K.

Disclaimer

These guidelines reflect the best published data available at the time the report was prepared. Caution should be exercised in interpreting the data; the results of future studies may require alteration of the conclusions or recommendations in this report. It may be necessary or even desirable to depart from the guidelines in the interests of specific patients and special circumstances. Just as adherence to the guidelines may not constitute defence against a claim of negligence, so deviation from them should not necessarily be deemed negligent.

These guidelines for the management of cutaneous melanoma present evidence-based guidance for treatment, with identification of the strength of evidence available at the time of preparation of the guidelines, and a brief overview of epidemiology, diagnosis, investigation and follow up.

Contribution to these guidelines has been made by a large number of clinicians. They have also been endorsed by, or have had input from, representatives of the following groups or organizations: the U.K. Melanoma Study Group, the British Association of Dermatologists, the British Association of Plastic, Reconstructive and Aesthetic Surgeons, the Royal College of Physicians, London, the Association of Cancer Physicians, the Royal College of Radiologists, London, the Royal College of Surgeons of England, the Royal College of Pathologists (pathology section only), the Royal College of General Practitioners, London, and the Department of Health.

These consensus guidelines have been drawn up by a multidisciplinary working party with membership drawn from a variety of groups and coordinated by the U.K. Melanoma Study Group and the British Association of Dermatologists. The guidelines deal with aspects of the management of melanoma from its prevention, through the stages of diagnosis and initial treatment to palliation of advanced disease.

PubMed literature searches for this guidelines revision were carried out to identify publications from 2000 to April 2010, with search terms including: melanoma genetics, epidemiology, early diagnosis, risk factors, clinical features, pathology, surgery, chemotherapy and clinical trials. Relevant materials were also isolated from reviews and other publications identified from the PubMed searches, independent searches carried out by the authors, as well as materials collected by the authors as part of their ongoing professional interest in the latest developments in this clinical area. Levels of evidence to support the guidelines are quoted according to the criteria stated in Appendix 1. The consultation process for British Association of Dermatologists guidelines and their compliance with guideline recommendations have been published elsewhere.[1,2] There are arguments in favour of newer guideline grading methods, such as those of GRADE,[3] but the authors believe that the system used here allows greater potential for consensus in areas of conflicting evidence or where evidence sources are not directly comparable. In some instances, this is not due to an absence of high quality (Level Ib) trials but because different entry criteria or endpoints preclude direct comparison of results; in other cases interpretation of the clinical significance of results has been challenged. To assist production of unified guidelines taking account of these issues, the 'quality of evidence' grading used in these guidelines differs slightly from that used in other British Association of Dermatologists current guidelines; the 'strength of recommendations' grading is the same as used in many other publications. Where no level is quoted the evidence is to be regarded as representing Level IV (i.e. a consensus statement).

The intention of the working party was to agree best practice for the management of melanoma in the belief that this will promote good standards of care across the whole country. However, they are guidelines only. Care should be individualized wherever appropriate. These guidelines will be revised as necessary to reflect changes in practice in light of new evidence.

Integration with national cancer guidance

Multidisciplinary care of the patient is held to be the most desirable model, as recommended in the Calman/Hine report.[4] This has been defined by the National Institute for Health and Clinical Excellence (NICE) *Improving Outcomes for People with Skin Tumours including Melanoma*.[5] Core services will be provided within each Cancer Network by Local Skin Cancer Multidisciplinary Teams (LSMDTs). Specialist services will be provided by Specialist Skin Cancer Multidisciplinary Teams (SSMDTs). For melanoma there is a clear demarcation of care such that more advanced primary melanoma, rare subtypes of melanoma, melanoma in children, and patients eligible for trial entry or sentinel lymph node biopsy (SLNB) should be promptly referred for investigation and treatment from an LSMDT to an SSMDT (Table 1).

Prevention of melanoma

Individuals, and particularly children, should not get sunburnt (Level I).[6–9] Meta-analysis of case–control studies provides

Table 1 Melanoma patients who must be referred from a Local Skin Cancer Multidisciplinary Team to a Specialist Skin Cancer Multidisciplinary Team (SSMDT) (National Institute for Health and Clinical Excellence *Improving Outcomes for People with Skin Tumours including Melanoma*, 2006[5])

- Patients with melanoma managed by other site specialist teams, e.g. gynaecological, mucosal and head and neck (excluding ocular)
- Patients with stage IB or higher primary melanoma when sentinel lymph node biopsy (SLNB) is available within the Network. In the absence of SLNB then patients with stage IIB or higher should be referred to the SSMDT (American Joint Committee on Cancer staging system)
- Patients with melanoma at any stage who are eligible for clinical trials that have been approved at Cancer Network level
- Patients with multiple primary melanomas
- Children and young adults under 19 years with melanoma
- Any patient with metastatic melanoma diagnosed at presentation or on follow up
- Patients with giant congenital naevi where there is suspicion of malignant transformation
- Patients with skin lesions of uncertain malignant potential

good evidence that melanoma is caused predominantly by intermittent intense sun exposure; fair-skinned individuals should therefore limit their recreational exposure through life (Level I).[10] People with freckles, red or blond hair, skin which burns in the sun, increased numbers of naevi, and those with a family history of melanoma are at increased risk and should heed this advice.

Adequate sun exposure to allow vitamin D synthesis, or sufficient dietary intake of vitamin D_3, is essential to human health; insufficiency of vitamin D is now recognized to be common.[11] It would therefore be inappropriate to greatly limit sun exposure in people without the risk factors listed above. Recent studies have shown that in the U.K. vitamin D levels are often suboptimal in melanoma patients, and are lower in fair-skinned people.[12,13] Fair-skinned people who avoid the sun rigorously to reduce the risk of melanoma should consider supplementing their intake of vitamin D_3 in the absence of medical contraindications.

There is evidence from a recent meta-analysis that sunbed usage does increase the risk of melanoma, particularly under the age of 35 years, and therefore it is recommended that this should be avoided (Level Ia).[14]

Referral and clinical diagnosis

Melanoma remains relatively uncommon and therefore the opportunity to develop diagnostic skills is limited in primary care. All lesions suspicious of melanoma should be referred urgently under the 2-week rule to local screening services usually run by dermatologists. In England and Wales, this would be to an LSMDT. In Scotland, referral should be made to a local Rapid Access Cancer Clinic according to Scottish Cancer Referral Guidelines. The seven-point checklist or the

ABCD rule may be helpful in the identification of melanomas although they are more sensitive than specific.[15–18] Urgent referral to the LSMDT is indicated where there is:

• A new mole appearing after the onset of puberty which is changing in shape, colour or size
• A long-standing mole which is changing in shape, colour or size
• Any mole which has three or more colours or has lost its symmetry
• A mole which is itching or bleeding
• Any new persistent skin lesion especially if growing, if pigmented or vascular in appearance, and if the diagnosis is not clear
• A new pigmented line in a nail especially where there is associated damage to the nail
• A lesion growing under a nail

Lesions which are suspicious for melanoma should not be removed in primary care. This is because clinicopathological correlation is vital for diagnostic accuracy, which in turn determines prognosis and defines adjuvant treatment options, and because diagnostic surgery requires specialist training. Early recognition of melanoma presents the best opportunity for cure[15,19–22] (Level III, Grade A).

All patients presenting with an atypical melanocytic lesion or a large number of moles should have a complete skin examination and assessment of risk factors. The dermoscope is a useful tool for the trained clinician screening pigmented lesions, as it can increase diagnostic accuracy.[23] It is also useful for monitoring multiple pigmented lesions where photography of dermoscopic images provides a record of change (Level Ia, Grade A). Recommendations for LSMDT record keeping of clinical features are provided in Table 2.

Screening and surveillance of high-risk individuals

There are some individuals at higher risk of melanoma who should be considered for referral to specialist clinics. These

Table 2 Recommendations for Local Skin Cancer Multidisciplinary Team record keeping of clinical features

As a minimum the following should be included:
History (the presence or absence of these changes should be recorded)
• Duration of the lesion
• Change in size
• Change in colour
• Change in shape
• Symptoms (itching, bleeding etc.)
Examination
• Site
• Size (maximum diameter)
• Elevation (flat, palpable, nodular)
• Description (irregular margins, irregular pigmentation and if ulceration is present)
(Level III, Grade B)

individuals can be divided broadly into two groups based upon the degree of risk:

1 Individuals at moderately increased risk (approximately 8–10 times that of the general population) should be counselled about this risk and taught how to self-examine for changing naevi, but long-term follow up is not usual. Such patients are those with either a previous primary melanoma or large numbers of moles, some of which may be clinically atypical (Level Ia, Grade B).[24–28] Organ transplant recipients are also at this level of increased risk (Level III, Grade B).[29,30]

2 Those at greatly increased risk of melanoma (more than 10 times that of the general population). Patients with a giant congenital pigmented hairy naevus (definitions include '20 cm or more in diameter' and '5% of body surface area') should be monitored by an expert for their life time because of the risk of malignant change, which is significant but poorly quantified (Level III, Grade B).[31,32] Excision biopsy of suspicious areas in large congenital naevi may be necessary but requires expert histopathological review. Patients with a strong family history of melanoma are also at greatly increased risk. In some families, most clearly in mainland Europe and North America, families at risk of melanoma are also at increased risk of pancreatic cancer.[33] Those with three or more cases of melanoma or pancreatic cancer in the family should be referred to appropriate clinics managing inherited predisposition to cancer (involving dermatologists and/or clinical geneticists) for counselling. It is the consensus of the Melanoma Genetics Consortium (http://www.genomel.org) that it is premature to suggest gene testing routinely but this may change as more is known of the genes predisposing to melanoma.[34] The risk to families associated with the presence of two family members affected with melanoma is lower. In these families, if affected individuals also have the atypical mole syndrome, or if there is a history of multiple primary melanomas in an individual or pancreatic cancer, then referral should also be made for counselling; otherwise family members should probably be considered at moderately increased risk.

All of the above individuals at increased risk of melanoma should be advised on the specific changes that suggest melanoma and encouraged to undertake monthly skin self-examination (Level III, Grade B). Close-up and distant photography may be a useful adjunct to detecting early melanoma in either of these high-risk groups (Level III). They should be given written information and access to images of moles and melanomas. Such images are available at: http://www.genomel.org or http://www.rcplondon.ac.uk/pubs/contents/f36b1656-cc74-4867-8498-cc94b378312a.pdf. Recommendations for screening and surveillance of high-risk individuals are summarized in Table 3.

Biopsy of suspected melanoma

A lesion suspected to be melanoma, or where melanoma needs to be excluded, should be photographed, and then excised completely. The axis of excision should be orientated

Table 3 Recommendations for screening and surveillance of high-risk individuals

> - Patients who are at moderately increased risk of melanoma should be advised of this and taught how to self-examine. This includes patients with atypical mole phenotype, those with a previous melanoma, and organ transplant recipients (Level Ia, Grade B)
> - Patients with giant congenital pigmented naevi are at increased risk of melanoma and require long-term follow up (Level IIIa, Grade B)
> - Individuals with a family history of three or more cases of melanoma, or of pancreatic cancer, should be referred to a clinical geneticist or specialized dermatology services for counselling. Those with two cases in the family may also benefit, especially if one of the cases had multiple primary melanomas or the atypical mole phenotype (Level IIa, Grade B)

to facilitate possible subsequent wide local excision; generally on the limb this will be along the long axis. If uncertain, direct referral to the multidisciplinary team (MDT) will allow appropriate planning for future surgery. The excision biopsy should include the whole tumour with a clinical margin of 2 mm of normal skin, and a cuff of fat. This allows confirmation of the diagnosis by examination of the entire lesion, such that subsequent definitive treatment can be based on Breslow thickness.[35–37]

Diagnostic shave biopsies should not be performed as they may lead to incorrect diagnosis due to sampling error, and make accurate pathological staging of the lesion impossible (Level III). For the same reasons partial removal of naevi for diagnosis must be avoided and partial removal of a melanocytic naevus may result in a clinical and pathological picture very like melanoma (pseudomelanoma). This gives rise to needless anxiety and is avoidable. Incisional or punch biopsy is occasionally acceptable, for example in the differential diagnosis of lentigo maligna (LM) on the face or of acral melanoma, but there is no place for either incisional or punch biopsy outside the skin cancer MDT (Level III). It is acceptable in certain circumstances to excise the lesion entirely but without repair, and to dress the wound while awaiting definitive pathology.

Biopsies of possible subungual melanomas should be carried out by surgeons regularly doing so. The nail should be removed sufficiently for the nail matrix to be adequately sampled: clinically obvious tumour should be biopsied if present.

Prophylactic excision of naevi, or of small (< 5 cm diameter) congenital naevi in the absence of suspicious features is not recommended (Level III, Grade D).

Full clinical details should be supplied on the histopathology form, including history of the lesion, relevant previous history, site and differential diagnosis. All melanocytic lesions excised for whatever reason must be sent for histopathological review to the pathologist associated with the LSMDT or SSMDT.

The diagnosis of melanoma, both in situ and invasive, should be given or supervised by doctors who have received advanced communication skills training, following local policies for breaking bad news. A skin cancer trained nurse should be present to provide continuing support.

Histopathology

General comments

The Royal College of Pathologists has produced a minimum dataset which should be included in the histopathology report.[38] Double reporting is recommended for all melanomas and all naevi showing severe dysplasia if resources allow this to be achieved within 14 days.[5]

The histopathology report

The report should include the following:

Clinical information

- Site of the tumour
- Type of surgical procedure: excision or re-excision, incision biopsy, punch biopsy
- Any other relevant clinical information

Macroscopic description

Contour, colour and size of the tumour and the excised skin specimen in millimetres.

Microscopy – essential features

Presence or absence of ulceration Ulceration has prognostic value, and its presence should be confirmed microscopically as full-thickness loss of epidermis with reactive changes which include a fibrinous exudate and attenuation or acanthosis of the adjacent epidermis. These distinguish true ulceration from artefact.[39]

Thickness The tumour should be measured from the granular layer of the overlying epidermis to the deepest cells in the dermis judged to be malignant, to the nearest 0·1 mm. Ulcerated tumours should be measured from the base of the ulcer. Tumour forming a sheath around appendages should be excluded when measuring thickness except when the melanoma extends out into the adjacent reticular dermis when it should be measured in the conventional manner. In the presence of histological regression thickness measurements should be of the residual melanoma. Microsatellites should not be included in thickness measurements (Level III, Grade B).

Mitotic count The number of mitoses has prognostic value and is now included in the American Joint Committee on Cancer (AJCC) staging system for melanomas ≤ 1·0 mm.[40,41] It should be recorded as number of mitoses mm^{-2} in the area of greatest number of mitoses in the vertical growth phase (VGP). It has prognostic value at all thicknesses.

Histological subtypes Desmoplastic melanoma with or without neurotropism should be recorded because of its different biological behaviour and clinical outcome.[42] The subtypes superficial spreading, nodular, LM and acral lentiginous melanomas have good clinicopathological correlation, but their prognostic value has not been established.

Margins of excision This indicates whether excision is complete and the minimum margin of excision to peripheral and deep aspects measured in millimetres. If the excision or re-excision is not complete, whether the tumour is *in situ* or invasive at the resection margin should be indicated. When possible a statement should be made of whether the lesion is primary or secondary melanoma.

Pathological staging Staging using TNM and AJCC (Table 4), and coding, e.g. SNOMED, should be given.[41]

Microscopy – desirable features

Growth phase Invasive melanoma without a VGP is termed microinvasion.[43] The assessment of microstaging criteria should be applied to the VGP only.

Clark level of dermal invasion This is a less reliable indicator of prognosis than thickness and is subject to poor observer agreement. It is not used to define T1 melanomas in the 2009 AJCC staging system, except that Clark levels IV or V may be used for defining T1b melanoma in rare instances when mitotic count cannot be determined in a nonulcerated T1 melanoma.

Regression The presence or absence of tumour regression has not been shown consistently to affect long-term outcome. Until its relevance is clear it should be reported as segmental

Table 4 The 2009 American Joint Committee on Cancer (AJCC) staging system

Stage	Primary tumour (pT)	Lymph nodes (N)	Metastases (M)
IA	< 1 mm, no ulceration, mitoses < 1 mm^{-2}		
IB	< 1 mm, with ulceration or mitoses ≥ 1 mm$^{-2\ a}$		
	1·01–2 mm, no ulceration		
IIA	1·01–2 mm, with ulceration		
	2·01–4 mm, no ulceration		
IIB	2·01–4 mm, with ulceration		
	> 4 mm, no ulceration		
IIC	> 4 mm, with ulceration		
IIIA	Any Breslow thickness, no ulceration	Micrometastases 1–3 nodes	
IIIB	Any Breslow thickness, with ulceration	Micrometastases 1–3 nodes	
	Any Breslow thickness, no ulceration	1–3 palpable metastatic nodes	
	Any Breslow thickness, no ulceration	No nodes, but in-transit or satellite metastasis/es	
IIIC	Any Breslow thickness, with ulceration	Up to three palpable lymph nodes	
	Any Breslow thickness, with or without ulceration	Four or more nodes or matted nodes or in-transit disease + lymph nodes	
	Any Breslow thickness, with ulceration	No nodes, but in-transit or satellite metastasis/es	
IV, M1a			Skin, subcutaneous or distant nodal disease
IV, M1b			Lung metastases
IV, M1c			All other sites or any other sites of metastases with raised lactate dehydrogenase

[a]In the rare circumstances where mitotic count cannot be accurately determined, a Clark level of invasion of either IV or V can be used to define T1b melanoma. Every patient with melanoma should be accurately staged using the AJCC system; this may include performing a sentinel lymph node biopsy where this is provided by the Specialist Skin Cancer Multidisciplinary Team. Staging should be updated following relapse.

replacement of melanoma by fibrosis, as this is subject to less observer variation.[44]

Tumour-infiltrating lymphocytes It remains unclear whether tumour-infiltrating lymphocytes have prognostic value.[40] The categories absent, non-brisk and brisk are subject to wide observer variation. 'Absent' indicates no lymphocytes infiltrating among the tumour cells, but does not exclude lymphocytes in the surrounding dermis. 'Non-brisk' is a patchy or discontinuous infiltrate either among the peripheral cells or in the centre of the tumour, whereas 'brisk' is a continuous infiltrate but may be confined to peripheral cells. These are qualified as mild, moderate or severe in intensity.

Lymphatic or vascular invasion Vascular or lymphatic infiltration has prognostic value, and its presence should be recorded even though it is infrequently observed.[45]

Perineural infiltration Perineural infiltration occurring beyond the main bulk of the tumour correlates with increased local recurrence. It is most commonly associated with desmoplastic melanoma.[46]

Microsatellites These are defined as islands of tumour > 0·05 mm in the tissue beneath the main invasive mass of melanoma, but separated from it by 0·3 mm of normal collagen (i.e. not tumour stroma or sclerosis of regression).[47] Current AJCC staging also requires that satellites must be intralymphatic;[41] this may be subject to revision. Microsatellites are predictive of regional lymph node metastases; this is reflected by stage N2c.

Precursor naevus The presence of contiguous melanocytic naevus should be recorded.

Requirements for microscopy of melanoma

These are given in Table 5.

Equivocal lesions

It may not be possible to distinguish pathologically between a melanoma and a benign melanocytic lesion. Such patients

Table 5 Requirements for microscopy of melanoma

Essential features	Desirable features
• Ulceration	• Clark level
• Thickness	• Growth phase
• Mitotic count[a]	• Regression
• Histological subtype	• Tumour-infiltrating lymphocytes
• Margins of excision	• Lymphatic or vascular invasion
• Pathological staging	• Perineural invasion
	• Microsatellites[b]

[a]Mitotic count is included in the 2009 American Joint Committee on Cancer staging system. [b]Microsatellites are not included in thickness measurement.

must be referred to the SSMDT for clinical and pathological review. A decision to treat as a melanoma should be made by the SSMDT in discussion with the patient. Thickness should be measured as for melanoma.

Sentinel lymph node pathology

Pathological assessment

This needs to be done in a standardized way so that findings between centres are comparable (Level III, Grade B).

Dissection

The dissection should be either by bivalving or multiple slicing, although the former is recommended.[48–50] A minimum of six serial sections should be taken, but a higher incidence of metastases is detected by extended step sectioning with immunohistochemistry at each level. The clinical relevance of the smaller metastases detected by these extended procedures is still unclear.

Staining

Use of haematoxylin and eosin and immunohistochemistry is essential. S100 and Melan A are most favoured immunohistochemical stains but a composite method such as PanMel is also appropriate.

Assessment of tumour burden

This gives additional prognostic information. The following are recommended:

Assessing the depth of the metastasis from the inner aspect of the sentinel lymph node capsule; categorizing the metastasis according to its site, either subcapsular or parenchymal; measuring the maximum dimension of the largest confluent group of melanoma cells.[50–52]

Completion lymphadenectomy specimens

The pathological examination of regional nodes dissected following positive SLNB should include an attempt to examine all lymph nodes at least at one level, and count the number involved. The presence of extracapsular spread and involvement of perinodal fat should be recorded together with the size of the tumour-free margin. The use of immunohistochemistry such as S100 or Melan A facilitates this.

Investigations and imaging

Stage I and II melanoma

Routine investigations are not required for asymptomatic patients with primary melanoma. Blood tests are unhelpful.

Routine computed tomography (CT) is not recommended for patients with stage I and II melanoma as this has a very low incidence of true-positive and high incidence of false-positive findings. Patients with particularly high-risk primary melanoma may undergo staging investigations if deemed appropriate by the SSMDT and/or as a prerequisite to trial entry. There is no indication for routine imaging with any other modality including plain X-ray, positron emission tomography (PET)/CT and magnetic resonance imaging (MRI). PET/CT is not effective in detecting positive sentinel lymph nodes and/or distant metastases in patients with primary melanoma[53–58] (Level IIa, Grade E).

Sentinel lymph node biopsy and ultrasound/fine needle aspiration cytology

SLNB, as discussed later, has high sensitivity and specificity for diagnosing subclinical regional lymph node involvement.

Ultrasound and fine needle aspiration cytology (FNAC) is the next best method but quoted sensitivities range from 4·7% to 80%, with the higher sensitivities being achieved only by sentinel node mapping and FNAC of the sentinel node in all cases regardless of morphological appearance.[59–62] Further staging by CT imaging following a positive sentinel lymph node, and prior to completion lymphadenectomy, has a very low yield.[63–65] Consequently this should be done only after discussion with an informed patient and the SSMDT (Level IIa, Grade D).

Stage III and IV melanoma

In stage III and IV melanoma, imaging strategies will be planned by the SSMDT.

CT scanning of the head, chest, abdomen and pelvis will normally adequately exclude metastases, and is most relevant in stage III melanoma before planning regional lymph node dissection (LND) and regional chemotherapy. If patients are considering entry to an adjuvant study following lymphadenectomy, the timing of scans should be determined by the SSMDT to avoid duplication.

When stage IV disease is suspected clinically, CT scanning of the head and whole body should be considered. Further imaging will be determined by symptoms, clinical trial protocols, and for clarification or reassessment of previous imaging findings. Generally, the added yield of PET/CT is unlikely to be clinically relevant in established stage IV melanoma (Level III, Grade D). Where metastasectomy is planned, PET/CT may be useful in excluding disease that might make surgery inappropriate. Serum lactate dehydrogenase (LDH) should be measured in all patients with suspected stage IV melanoma.

There is no indication for a bone scan in staging except where symptoms point to possible bone disease. Staging investigations are summarized in Table 6.

Treatment of the primary lesion

Surgery is the only curative treatment for melanoma. Following excision for diagnosis and for measurement of micro-

Table 6 Staging investigations for melanoma

- Patients with stage I, II and IIIA melanoma should not routinely be staged by imaging or other methods as the true-positive pick-up rate is low and the false-positive rate is high (Level IIa, Grade E)
- Patients with stage IIIB or IIIC melanoma should be imaged by computed tomography of head, chest, abdomen and pelvis prior to surgery after SSMDT review (Level IIa, Grade A)
- Patients with stage IV melanoma should be imaged according to clinical need and SSMDT review. Lactate dehydrogenase should also be measured (Level III, Grade A)

SSMDT, Specialist Skin Cancer Multidisciplinary Team.

scopic Breslow thickness, a wider and deeper margin is taken to ensure complete removal of the primary lesion, and to remove any micrometastases. The depth of the therapeutic excision has conventionally been to the muscle fascia or deeper, and there is no evidence to support altering this approach.

Lateral surgical excision margins for invasive melanoma depend on Breslow thickness and are based on five randomized controlled trials (RCTs) including about 3300 patients, and a National Institutes of Health Consensus Panel.[66–73] However, only one of these studies is adequately powered, and two provide little scope for detecting reduced disease-free or overall survival due to narrow margins.[68,69,71] Most exclude melanoma on the head and neck and/or extremities.[74] A recent systematic review estimated overall survival in favour of wide excision (hazard ratio 1·04; 95% confidence interval 0·95–1·15; P = 0·40), although the difference was not significant. Therefore a small, but potentially important, difference in overall survival between wide and narrow excision margins cannot be confidently ruled out. Current randomized trial evidence is insufficient to address optimal excision margins for primary cutaneous melanoma.[75]

The recommended surgical margins are those measured clinically at the time of surgery, but adequacy of excision should be subsequently confirmed by review of re-excision histology, making an adjustment for average shrinkage of 20%.[76] The final decision about the size of the margin should be made by the MDT, after discussion with the patient. The recommendation should be made with consideration of functional and cosmetic implications of the margin chosen. All patients with primary melanoma stage IB and higher should be referred before treatment to an SSMDT when this provides an SLNB service. When the SSMDT does not provide this, all primary melanomas stage IIB or IIC should be referred. There are no RCT data for margin size for LM or other in situ melanoma.

Lentigo maligna and *in situ* superficial spreading melanoma

LM and other in situ melanomas have no potential for metastatic spread and the aim should be to excise the lesion completely with a clear histological margin, although margin size remains undefined. No further treatment is then required.

LM is best treated by complete excision because of the risk of subclinical microinvasion. This may be missed on incisional biopsy due to sampling error.[73] The risk of progression to invasive melanoma is poorly quantified, and in the very elderly may be unlikely within their lifespan. Therefore, for some particular clinical situations, treatment by other methods such as radiotherapy, or observation only may be appropriate.[77-81] There is little evidence to support the use of cryotherapy, and this treatment may make subsequent progression difficult to detect. Topical treatment with imiquimod is as yet of unproven value so should be used only in the context of a clinical trial.[82] If the patient with LM is treated by nonsurgical means then the reason for this choice should be discussed and clearly documented by the MDT.

Local recurrence of LM occurs in about 5% of patients by 2 years.[77] Excision with micrographic control of surgical margins should be considered, although histological clearance is often difficult to define.[83] In situ melanoma on acral and genital skin is also associated with a higher risk of local recurrence, but this is less common in other types of in situ melanoma. In theory, in situ melanoma should not metastasize, but occasional cases do recur. This may be due to histological regression obscuring a more advanced tumour, missed microinvasion, or progression after incomplete removal of in situ disease.

Melanoma up to 1·0 mm Breslow thickness

There have been three RCTs of patients with melanomas in this thickness band.[66,68,69,73] The recommended surgical margins are based on the World Health Organization (WHO) Melanoma Co-operative Group Trial 10.[66,73] This randomized trial compared 1 and 3 cm margins for melanomas up to 2 mm thick. No local metastases, and similar overall survival, were seen in patients with melanomas < 1 mm in depth with either excision margin. However, this was based on analysis of data from only 359 patients. The French and Swedish studies compared 2 cm with 5 cm margins, and the latter included only patients with melanomas 0·8 mm or more in thickness in this group.[68,69] A 1 cm margin is deemed safe for this group (Level Ib, Grade A).

Melanoma 1·01–2·0 mm Breslow thickness

There have been four randomized studies that have included patients in this category. The WHO study showed a small excess of local metastasis as first site of relapse in the 1 cm margins group.[66,73] There was no difference in overall survival between 1 and 3 cm margins but the study was inadequately powered to detect this. The Intergroup Melanoma Trial compared 2 vs. 4 cm margins of excision for lesions of 1–4 mm in thickness.[67,70] No difference was seen between the two groups in either local recurrence or survival. Two other studies have included patients with melanomas up to 2 mm, also treated with either 2 or 5 cm margins.[68,69] There was no difference in outcome between the groups. The 1 vs. 3 cm, 2 vs. 4 cm and 2 vs. 5 cm studies cannot be compared directly, but no study using 2 cm margins as one comparator has shown any advantage of wider margins than this. However, trials of narrower margins have either not been performed (e.g. 1 vs. 2 cm margins) or have been underpowered, and do not permit a definite conclusion that a 1 cm margin is adequate. Evidence to date shows that a minimum margin of 1 cm is required, although 2 cm margins are equally appropriate. The final decision will be determined by anatomical site, MDT review, and after discussion with an informed patient (Level Ib, Grade A).

Melanoma 2·01–4·0 mm Breslow thickness

The Intergroup Melanoma Trial showed no difference in rates of local metastasis between patients treated with 2 cm, and those treated with 4 cm margins.[67] However, longer follow up showed reduced overall survival in the 2 cm margins group, although this fell just short of reaching statistical significance.[70] The results of a randomized trial with 3 cm margins showed significantly increased rates of locoregional recurrence in patients treated with 1 cm margins, and a reduction in melanoma-specific survival, again just short of significance, although no difference in overall survival.[71] The significance of this is unclear, and the 2 vs. 4 cm and 1 vs. 3 cm trials cannot be directly compared. Until the resulting uncertainty is resolved, which may not happen as the number of patients required to detect a difference between 2 and 3 cm margins is considerable, the default position should be to minimize locoregional and distant metastatic risk. Therefore a minimum 2 cm margin is required in this group, although 3 cm margins are equally appropriate. The final decision will be determined by anatomical site, need for skin grafting, MDT review, and after discussion with an informed patient (Level Ib, Grade A).

Melanoma greater than 4 mm in thickness

The risk of locoregional and distant metastasis is 50% or more in this group. None the less, the same surgical objectives apply to minimize locoregional and distant metastatic risk. There is only one randomized study which includes melanomas thicker than 4 mm.[71] This trial compared 1 cm with 3 cm margins. The results show a significant increase in locoregional recurrence when 1 cm margins are used, and a reduction in melanoma-specific survival just short of significance, although no difference in overall survival. As there are no data that margins smaller than 3 cm are as effective, the evidence suggests 3 cm margins for this group. There is no evidence that margins > 3 cm are required. The final decision will be determined by anatomical site, need for skin grafting, MDT review, and after discussion with an informed patient (Level Ib, Grade B).

Recommended surgical excision margins are summarized in Table 7.

Table 7 Recommended surgical excision margins

Breslow thickness	Excision margins	Level of evidence	Grading of evidence
In situ	5-mm margins to achieve complete histological excision	III	B
< 1 mm	1 cm	Ib	A
1·01–2 mm	1–2 cm	Ib	A
2·1–4 mm	2–3 cm	Ib	A
> 4 mm	3 cm	Ib	B

Table 8 Recommendations for the management of clinically node-negative patients

- There is no role for elective lymph node dissection (Level I, Grade E)
- SLNB can be considered in stage IB melanoma and upwards in Specialist Skin Cancer Multidisciplinary Teams (Level Ia, Grade A)
- Patients should be introduced to the concept of SLNB as a staging procedure but should also understand that it has no proven therapeutic value
- Surgical risks of SLNB, the possibility of failure to find a sentinel lymph node, and of a false-negative result, should also be explained

SLNB, sentinel lymph node biopsy.

Management of lymph node basins

Investigation and management of lymph node basins in melanoma patients should be carried out by SSMDTs so that surgical treatment planning and investigations can run in parallel. There is no place for elective LND in the management of primary melanoma unless this is unavoidable because the primary melanoma lies over the lymph node basin (Level Ib, Grade A). Patients should have access to a skin cancer specialist nurse when relapse is suspected.

Clinically node-negative patients

SLNB was developed as a means of identifying the first lymph node draining the skin in which the melanoma arises.[84] The procedure is carried out at the same time as definitive wider excision of the primary melanoma.[85] SLNB gives information about prognosis, and is increasingly used in conjunction with adjuvant therapy clinical trials. Patients with melanoma of Breslow thickness 1·2–3·5 mm and a positive SLNB have a 75% 5-year survival compared with 90% if the SLNB is negative.[86] SLNB is normally considered for patients with melanoma ≥ 1 mm, when about 20% are positive; however, the risk of a positive SLNB in a melanoma < 1·0 mm is still 5%.[86,87] The procedure is associated with a 5% morbidity, which is less than that seen with complete nodal dissection. In patients with a positive SLNB, 20% have pathological evidence of metastases in additional regional nodes.[84] Patients with a positive SLNB usually choose to proceed to completion lymphadenectomy. In about 5% it is not possible to identify the sentinel node either on lymphoscintigraphy, at surgery, or both. Patients should be aware of this limitation. The relevance of increasingly detailed evaluation of the sentinel node and its correlation with prognosis remains to be defined.[88] MSLT-1 showed no overall 5-year survival benefit following SLNB and completion lymphadenectomy, and it is unclear whether SLNB improves local control of lymph node basins.[85,86] A final report with longer follow up is awaited.

Recommendations for the management of clinically node-negative patients are summarized in Table 8.

Management of patients with clinically or radiologically suspicious lymph nodes

FNAC of nodes is recommended when there is clinical doubt about the significance of the nodes. If there is a negative FNAC result but ongoing suspicion, then the fine needle aspiration should be repeated or an image-guided core biopsy arranged.

Open biopsy is recommended when there is clinical suspicion even in the presence of negative FNACs in which lymphocytes have been successfully aspirated. If open biopsy is performed, the incision must be such as to allow subsequent complete formal block dissection of the regional nodes without compromise. It should be done only by SSMDT members.[5]

Exploration or removal of a mass within a nodal basin which drains a known primary melanoma site, and prior to definitive surgical treatment, may increase the risk of melanoma recurrence in that basin.[89] Any melanoma patient who develops a mass in a nodal basin should be referred urgently to the SSMDT, and without prior investigation, for investigation and treatment planning (Level III, Grade B).

Management of patients with confirmed positive lymph node metastasis

Radical LND should be performed only by SSMDT members who do a combined minimum of 15 axillary and groin block dissections for skin cancer each year.[5,90]

Preoperative staging investigations should be carried out as already discussed for stage III melanoma. If such staging is not feasible prior to surgery, and surgery is considered necessary even if distant metastatic disease were to be detected, then a chest X-ray and LDH measurement is recommended.

The block dissection specimen should be marked and orientated for the pathologist. Axillary LND for melanoma should include all nodes in levels I–III, and this may require either resection or division of pectoralis minor. The management of inguinal lymph node metastases is controversial. Between 30% and 44% of patients with clinically involved superficial inguinal nodes will have involved pelvic nodes, and the risk increases with the number of involved superficial nodes.[91–97] If Cloquet's node is positive the risk of pelvic node involvement ranges from 44% to 90%.[93,96,97] There is no reported increased morbidity associated with combined pelvic and superficial node dissection.[94] Following ilioinguinal dissection for palpable inguinal disease 5-year survival varies with extent of pelvic involvement: 49% with one pelvic node, 28% with two to three nodes, and 7% with more than three nodes.[97–100]

A superficial inguinal LND should be considered in the presence of:

- A single clinically involved inguinal node or femoral triangle node
- A single positive superficial inguinal sentinel node (Level Ib, Grade A).

A pelvic lymph node dissection should be considered in the presence of:

- More than one clinically palpable inguinal and/or femoral triangle node/s
- CT or ultrasound evidence of more than one inguinal and/or femoral triangle node/s, or of pelvic node involvement
- More than one microscopically involved node at SLNB
- A conglomerate of inguinal or femoral triangle lymph nodes
- Microscopic or macroscopic involvement of Cloquet's node (Level III, Grade B).

Cervical nodal recurrence should be treated either by surgeons in the SSMDT specializing in head and neck skin cancer including melanoma or by a head and neck MDT with a special interest in melanoma.[5] A comprehensive, and not a selective, neck dissection should be performed (Level III, Grade A). The term 'comprehensive' allows either:

- A radical dissection of levels 1–5
- Modified radical – the above, sparing spinal accessory nerve, internal jugular vein and sternocleidomastoid muscle
- Extended radical – radical dissection including parotid and/or posterior occipital chain.

The risk of further locoregional recurrence is 16–32% despite comprehensive surgery.[101,102]

Locoregional recurrent melanoma: skin and soft tissues

Surgery is the treatment of choice for single local or regional metastases. Excision should be clinically and histologically complete, but a wide margin is not required. Multiple small (< 1 cm) dermal lesions respond well to treatment with the CO_2 laser.[103] Dermal disease which is progressing despite surgery or laser, and subcutaneous or deeper limb metastases, should be considered for regional chemotherapy with isolated limb infusion (ILI) with melphalan and actinomycin D, or with isolated limb perfusion (ILP)[104,105] (Level IIb, Grade B). ILI is less invasive than ILP, and can be more easily repeated,

Table 9 Recommendations for locoregional recurrent melanoma

- Nodes clinically suspicious for melanoma should be sampled using fine needle aspiration cytology (FNAC) prior to carrying out formal block dissection. If FNAC is negative although lymphocytes were seen, a core or open biopsy should be performed if suspicion remains (Level III, Grade B)
- Prior to lymph node dissection, performed by an expert,[5] staging by computed tomographic scan should be carried out other than where this would mean undue delay (Level III, Grade B)
- The treatment of locoregional recurrence in a limb is palliative. Surgical excision, CO_2 laser, or isolated limb infusion or perfusion may be considered (Level IIb, Grade B)

but may be less effective.[105] ILI is suitable for patients with low volume (< 5 cm) disease and those with comorbidities which prevent ILP. Patients with bulky disease (> 5 cm) may be more likely to benefit from ILP using melphalan with tumour necrosis factor (TNF), but a recent trial comparing this combination with melphalan alone did not confirm additional benefit from adding TNF.[106] Radiotherapy may be considered for disease which cannot otherwise be controlled. Selected patients suitable for ILI/ILP should be referred to specialized centres. The role of electrochemotherapy using intralesional or systemic bleomycin is still being evaluated. Recommendations for locoregional recurrent melanoma are given in Table 9.

Adjuvant therapy

There is no evidence of a survival benefit for adjuvant chemotherapy in patients with melanoma.[107] This includes adjuvant regional chemotherapy using ILP, and therefore ILI.[108]

Interferon has been evaluated in low-, intermediate- and high-risk patients using various doses and schedules. A recent individual patient data meta-analysis concluded that interferon was associated with a significant impact on relapse-free survival and a small effect on overall survival (5-year survival benefit 3%, $P < 0.05$).[109] However, the benefit was seen across all interferon regimens, and was greatest in those with ulcerated melanomas. There was no clear indication as to optimum dose or duration. The results are awaited of further analysis including more recent data. Interferon is not recommended as standard of care for adjuvant therapy of primary or stage III melanoma (Level Ia, Grade A). This is because its effect on disease-free survival is of uncertain clinical relevance, and although overall survival is improved in meta-analysis, the effect is small and is associated with significant drug toxicity. Prospective studies are required to establish whether a subset of patients who derive most benefit can be identified.

Clinical trials of adjuvant melanoma vaccines have not so far been successful.

Patients should be offered entry into adjuvant clinical trials approved by the local Cancer Network. They should have access to a melanoma specialist who is conversant with current melanoma adjuvant trials, and who is able to ensure their access to such studies. Details may be found on the websites of the National Cancer Research Network and the European Organization for Research and Treatment of Cancer.

Adjuvant radiotherapy

The Tasmanian Radiation Oncology Group has completed a randomized study of adjuvant radiotherapy to dissected nodal basins, 48 Gy in 20 fractions, in 250 patients with a high (> 25%) risk of local recurrence following lymphadenectomy.[110] Eligible patients had ≥ 1 parotid, ≥ 2 cervical or axillary or ≥ 3 groin nodes, or extranodal spread of tumour, or node diameter ≥ 3 cm in neck or axilla or ≥ 4 cm in the groin. Interim results show a 15% improvement in local control following radiotherapy, but there was no effect on overall survival. There are no data yet on morbidity following this treatment, and so at present the risk:benefit of adjuvant radiotherapy is unclear. If there is clinical or histological doubt about the adequacy of surgery following recurrence, or about the feasibility of salvage surgery, adjuvant radiotherapy may be considered by the SSMDT (Level Ib, Grade B).

Occult primary melanoma

Patients with occult primary melanoma may present with a solitary metastasis, lymph node disease, or systemic disease. Such patients should be referred promptly to the SSMDT for investigation and treatment planning. All patients should have a thorough examination of the skin. Occult primary uveal tract melanoma nearly always causes liver metastases before these are apparent at other sites; searching for a uveal tract primary in a patient with occult nodal disease is not appropriate. For patients presenting with inguinal lymphadenopathy, examination of the genital and urinary tracts and anorectum is especially relevant. All patients should be staged with CT scans of head, chest, abdomen and pelvis. Various reports from institution-based series suggest that patients presenting with stage III disease from an unknown primary have a better prognosis than patients with a similar stage and a known primary.[111,112] One published series suggested a survival advantage in patients with stage IV disease from an unknown primary compared with those with a declared primary.[113]

Patients presenting with lymph node disease from an occult primary involving a single lymph node basin should be presumed to have regional rather than distant metastasis, and treated as for stage III disease with lymph node block dissection.

Metastatic disease

All patients should have access to a skin cancer clinical nurse specialist and a palliative care team providing expertise in symptom control and psychosocial support. Links should be made with community cancer support networks as soon as possible. All patients with metastatic disease should have access to an oncologist specializing in melanoma for management advice.

Selected patients who relapse with oligometastatic disease may benefit from metastatectomy. Although this has not been evaluated in a prospective randomized trial, median survival of 21 months for selected surgically treated patients has been reported[114–119] (Level IIb, Grade B).

No systemic therapy has been shown to extend survival significantly. Dacarbazine is standard chemotherapy outside a clinical trial, although its benefits are limited, and it is ineffective in brain metastases (Level IIa, Grade C). The oral dacarbazine derivative temozolomide has greater central nervous system (CNS) penetration but has not shown significant clinical advantages over dacarbazine in two multicentre clinical trials.[120,121] Biochemotherapy (the addition of biologically active agents such as interferon-α and interleukin-2 to chemotherapy) increases response rates and toxicity but does not significantly increase overall survival.[122] The same is true for combination chemotherapy, and so this is not recommended other than in highly selected patients in whom palliation is dependent upon maximizing response in symptomatic deposits. High-dose interleukin-2 has not been evaluated in a randomized phase III trial although a small minority of patients may experience durable complete responses.[123]

Patients with elevated LDH have a reduced likelihood of benefiting from currently available systemic treatment. Given the limited benefits with standard systemic therapy, all patients with metastatic melanoma should be considered for entry into clinical trials of novel therapies.

Patients with CNS metastases have a poor prognosis. Surgery or stereotactic radiotherapy should be considered for selected patients with limited disease.[114,115,124–126] The benefits of treating patients with cerebral metastases with whole-brain radiotherapy are limited, but this may sometimes have palliative value. Supportive care is therefore the most appropriate strategy for many patients (Level IIb, Grade B).

Spinal cord compression should be treated surgically if feasible, but multiple sites of disease, poor prognosis and poor performance status may make this inappropriate. Radiotherapy may be useful for palliation of rapidly enlarging or painful metastases involving soft tissues and bones (Level IIb, Grade B).

Recommendations for metastatic disease are shown in Table 10.

Table 10 Recommendations for metastatic disease

- All patients should be managed by Specialist Skin Cancer Multidisciplinary Teams[5]
- Surgery should be considered for oligometastatic disease at sites such as the skin, brain or bowel (Level IIb, Grade B), or to prevent pain or ulceration
- Radiotherapy may have a palliative role in the treatment of metastases (Level II, Grade B)
- Standard chemotherapy is dacarbazine although its role is palliative (Level II, Grade C)
- Patients with stage IV melanoma should be considered for entry to clinical trials

Melanoma, hormone replacement therapy and pregnancy

There is no evidence that melanoma at or near the time of pregnancy adversely affects prognosis.[127] Breslow thickness, site and presence of ulceration are still the key determinants of outcome, and are not different from a control population.[128] The outcomes of pregnancy for both mother and baby are not worsened (Level IIa).[128,129]

Surgical treatment should be determined in the normal way, but the risks of exposure to ionizing radiation and blue dye during sentinel node biopsy will need special consideration.

There is no medical reason to justify delaying conception after a diagnosis of melanoma (Level IIa) but the social and family effects of developing recurrent melanoma during pregnancy or after birth are great.[127,130] It is proper therefore to counsel a woman in the reproductive age range about her risk of recurrence over time so that she and her partner can make their decision about conception with adequate information. These social or family considerations may also be relevant to a male patient whose partner is pregnant or if he and his partner are considering a pregnancy.

There is no evidence that the use of the oral contraceptive pill plays any role in the natural history of melanoma (Level Ia).[130–133] Decisions about use of the contraceptive pill should be made on the basis of health issues other than melanoma.

There is no evidence that hormone replacement therapy plays any role in the natural history of melanoma,[130,132] neither does it worsen prognosis in stage I and II melanoma (Level IIa).[133] Decisions about use of hormone replacement therapy should be made on the basis of health issues other than melanoma.

In pregnancy, staging using X-rays should be avoided where possible especially in the first trimester. MRI should be used in preference to CT scan, where feasible.

Because chemotherapy does not have a survival benefit in stage IV disease its use in pregnancy requires careful discussion. Use of chemotherapy agents in the first trimester should be avoided. There are case reports of the successful birth of normal babies who were exposed to dacarbazine in utero later in pregnancy, but this does not exclude later toxicity. Melanoma can metastasize to the placenta and to the fetus more frequently than any other solid tumour. This has a poor prognosis for both mother and baby. At delivery in patients with stage IV melanoma the placenta should be examined for melanoma.

Recommendations regarding pregnancy and hormone replacement therapy are summarized in Table 11.

Use of drugs in melanoma patients

There are theoretical reasons to suggest that L-DOPA may have an adverse effect on patients with melanoma. There are no data to support this idea, however, and such an association seems unlikely.[134] The use of immunosuppressants after melanoma is a cause for concern. The results of a recent cohort

Table 11 Recommendations regarding pregnancy and hormone replacement therapy

Pregnancy with primary melanoma
• No worsening of prognosis
• No increase in adverse outcomes for mother or baby
Pregnancy in advanced melanoma
• Placental and fetal metastases possible in stage IV disease
Oral contraceptives and melanoma
• No increased risk of melanoma
Hormone replacement therapy
• No increased risk of melanoma
• No worsening of prognosis

study of patients with rheumatoid arthritis treated with biologic agents showed an increased risk of melanoma (odds ratio 2·3, 95% confidence interval 0·9–5·4).[135] However, there is usually little that can be done to avoid these drugs without an unacceptable loss of quality of life. Their use after treatment of primary or secondary melanoma should be discussed between the prescribing doctors and patients, and the decision to continue their use and their dosage should be subject to ongoing review following a diagnosis of melanoma (Level III, Grade C).

Organ and blood donation

The decision about whether organs or tissue are suitable for transplant is made on an individualized basis, taking into account the patient's medical history.[136] A melanoma patient would not normally be considered as a donor.

Follow up

There are three main reasons for follow up after treatment of primary cutaneous melanoma. The first is to detect recurrence when further treatment can improve the prognosis, the second is to detect further primary melanomas and the third is to provide support, information and education. The proportion of patients with melanoma who have impaired health-related quality of life is comparable with other cancers, and their needs for psychosocial support are likely to be similar.[137] Provision of this is an important part of MDT management.[138] There are no RCTs which have formally evaluated follow up. Numerous follow-up regimens have been reviewed but few are evidence based.[139–141] Sixty-two per cent of all recurrences were detected by patients themselves in one review, but definition of patient or doctor detection is unclear and other series emphasize the importance of physician-detected recurrence.[134] Patient opinion was equally divided as to whether follow-up visits were reassuring or provoked further anxiety. There is little evidence of survival advantage following self-detection of metastases.[139–141] Most first relapses occur in the 5 years following diagnosis, but there is a significant risk of later first relapse; both patients and their doctors should be aware of this.

© British Association of Dermatologists

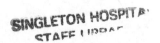

A primary melanoma follow-up clinic should be provided by an MDT of dermatologists and surgeons with clinical nurse specialist support, and there should be continuity of care. Patients should be taught to self-examine to detect locoregional recurrence and new primary melanoma. Photography can be useful for follow up of patients who also have atypical moles. Patients should routinely be examined for locoregional and distant metastases, and the whole skin should be checked for new primary melanomas. A defined rapid-access pathway must be provided to all patients and general practitioners for suspected recurrence. Suspected new primary melanoma should be referred as normal through the 2-week wait system. For Scotland this needs to be compliant with the 62-day rule. Follow up of patients with AJCC stage III and IV disease should be led by melanoma SSMDTs.

Follow-up intervals and duration should be tailored to the stage group of the primary melanoma and therefore to the risk of recurrence. The follow-up plan should be agreed between the patient and the responsible doctors.

Care can be shared with primary care, but only if the secondary care team have defined and explained to the primary care team what is required, and only if the primary care team are prepared to accept responsibility for this. In the event of suspected recurrence, even after discharge from follow up, it is recommended that the patient contact the secondary care team directly to avoid possible delay in diagnosis.

Screening asymptomatic clinically normal patients with lymph node ultrasound is sensitive and can detect nodal disease, but this has not been shown to be useful in primary melanoma follow up.[142] The same applies to CT and PET imaging. These investigations should not be used outside a clinical trial.

In situ melanoma

Patients with a surgically treated single *in situ* melanoma do not require follow up, as there is no risk of metastasis. They require a return visit after complete excision to explain the diagnosis, check the whole skin for further primary melanoma/s, and to teach self-examination for a new primary melanoma. Clinical nurse specialist support may be required despite the absence of metastatic risk.

Stage IA melanoma

Patients with invasive primary cutaneous melanoma < 1·0 mm have a 5-year disease-free survival of over 90% or better. A recent review of 430 patients with melanomas < 0·5 mm showed no recurrences at 5–15 years follow up but 4% of patients developed a second primary melanoma over this period.[143] Patients with invasive, nonulcerated primary tumours 0·5–1·0 mm thick have only slightly worse 5-year disease-free survival, and are in the same stage group. Therefore, for stage IA patients a series of two to four visits over up to 12 months is suggested to teach self-examination, and then they may be discharged from regular follow up (Level III, Grade B).

Stage IB and IIA melanoma

This group are at 15–35% risk of recurrence, but most of this risk is in years 2–4. Once they have learnt how to self-examine for locoregional metastasis and new primaries, and understand how to access the follow-up team promptly for suspected recurrence, they should be seen every 3 months for 3 years, then 6-monthly to 5 years. No routine investigations are required (Level III, Grade B).

Stage IIB and IIC melanoma

This group are at 40–70% risk of recurrence. Most of this risk is in years 2–4. They should be taught self-examination and be seen 3-monthly for 3 years, and 6-monthly to 5 years. No routine investigations are required (Level III, Grade B).

Sentinel lymph node biopsy

Patients who have had a negative SLNB should be followed up on the basis of Breslow thickness.

Most patients who have had a positive SLNB will have had a completion lymphadenectomy. As these patients now have at least stage IIIA disease, their follow up should be supervised by the SSMDT, and entry into appropriate trials considered. Risk of recurrence depends on extent of sentinel lymph node involvement, and may be less than for some with stage II melanoma. They should be followed up as for stage IB–IIC melanoma (Level III, Grade B).

Stage IIIB, IIIC, and resected stage IV melanoma

The risk of further metastasis in this group is high. Many will be eligible for adjuvant trials. Those outside trials should be seen 3-monthly for 3 years from the date of staging, 6-monthly to 5 years, then annually to 10 years by an SSMDT. Investigations should be carried out on the basis of clinical need, and may include CT surveillance if considered appropriate by the SSMDT. This might be used to monitor a site considered at high risk of relapse. The SSMDT will need to balance the use of follow-up investigations for this group against the need for early detection of further stage III and IV disease. Early detection facilitates both effective treatment and trial entry (Level III, Grade B).

Unresectable stage IV melanoma

These patients should be followed up and investigated by the SSMDT according to clinical need. They may be eligible for clinical trials.

Clinical trials

Many patients will be in clinical trials. These will have defined follow-up intervals which should be adhered to.

Follow up for melanoma is detailed in Table 12.

Table 12 Follow up for melanoma

- Patients with *in situ* melanomas do not require follow up
- Patients with invasive melanomas have differing risk of relapse according to their stage group
- Patients with stage IA melanoma should be seen two to four times over up to 12 months, then discharged
- Patients with stage IB–IIIA melanoma should be seen 3-monthly for 3 years, then 6-monthly to 5 years
- Patients with stage IIIB and IIIC and resected stage IV melanoma should be seen 3-monthly for 3 years, then 6-monthly to 5 years, then annually to 10 years
- Patients with unresectable stage IV melanoma are seen according to need
  (Level III, Grade B)

Audit points

The following are suggested points for audit:

1 Timeliness and appropriateness of referral from LSMDT to SSMDT (referenced to the standard described in the NICE *Improving Outcomes for People with Skin Tumours including Melanoma*, February 2006, available at: http://www.nice.org.uk/nicemedia/live/10901/28906/28906.pdf).

2 Comparison and appropriateness of stated clinical, and measured histological, surgical margins (referenced to the standards described in these guidelines).

3 Use of investigations at diagnosis in primary melanoma by stage grouping (referenced to the standards described in these guidelines).

Acknowledgments

The authorship team would like to acknowledge the contribution to these guidelines made by the late Dr Neil Cox. Neil worked tirelessly to improve care for patients, and his clear thinking, expert knowledge and generous nature were invaluable to us. We shall miss him greatly.

References

1 Griffiths CEM. The British Association of Dermatologists' guidelines for the management of skin disease. Br J Dermatol 1999; **141**:396–7.

2 Cox NH, Williams HC. The British Association of Dermatologists therapeutic guidelines: can we AGREE? Br J Dermatol 2003; **148**:621–5.

3 Guyatt GH, Oxman AD, Vist GE et al. GRADE: an emerging consensus on rating quality of evidence and strength of recommendations. BMJ 2008; **336**:924–6.

4 Calman K, Hine D. *Report by the Advisory Group on Cancer Services to the Chief Medical Officers of England and Wales*. Cardiff: Department of Health/Welsh Office, 1995.

5 National Institute for Health and Clinical Excellence. *Improving Outcomes for People with Skin Tumours including Melanoma*, 2006. Available at: http://www.nice.org.uk/nicemedia/live/10901/28906/28906.pdf (last accessed 25 May 2010).

6 Marks R, Whiteman D. Sunburn and melanoma: how strong is the evidence? BMJ 1994; **308**:75–6.

7 Whiteman D, Green A. Melanoma and sunburn. Cancer Causes Control 1994; **5**:564–72.

8 Armstrong BK. Epidemiology of malignant melanoma: intermittent or total accumulated exposure to the sun? J Dermatol Surg Oncol 1988; **14**:835–49.

9 Armstrong BK, Kricker A. Sun exposure causes both nonmelanocytic skin cancer and malignant melanoma. In: *Proceedings on Environmental UV Radiation and Health Effects*. Health Rep 1993; **5**:106–13.

10 Gandini S, Sera F, Cattaruzza MS et al. Meta-analysis of risk factors for cutaneous melanoma: III. Family history, actinic damage and phenotypic factors. Eur J Cancer 2005; **41**:2040–59.

11 Holick MF. High prevalence of vitamin D inadequacy and implications for health. Mayo Clin Proc 2006; **81**:353–73.

12 Newton-Bishop J, Beswick S, Randerson-Moor J et al. Serum 25-hydroxyvitamin D3 levels are associated with Breslow thickness at presentation, and survival from melanoma. J Clin Oncol 2009; **27**:5439–44.

13 Randerson-Moor JA, Taylor JC, Elliott F et al. Vitamin D receptor gene polymorphisms, serum 25-hydroxyvitamin D levels and melanoma: UK case–control comparisons and a meta-analysis of published VDR data. Eur J Cancer 2009; **45**:3271–81.

14 International Agency for Research on Cancer Working Group on Artificial Ultraviolet Light and Skin Cancer. The association of use of sunbeds with cutaneous melanoma and other skin cancers: a systematic review. Int J Cancer 2007; **120**:1116–22.

15 McGovern TW, Litaker MS. Clinical predictors of malignant pigmented lesions. A comparison of the Glasgow seven-point checklist and the American Cancer Society's ABCDs of pigmented lesions. J Dermatol Surg Oncol 1992; **18**:22–6.

16 Abbasi NR, Shaw HM, Rigel DS et al. Early diagnosis of cutaneous melanoma: revisiting the ABCD criteria. JAMA 2004; **292**:2771–6.

17 MacKie RM. *Clinical Dermatology*, 5th edn. Oxford: Oxford University Press, 2003; 345–6.

18 Du Vivier AWP, Williams HC, Brett JV et al. How do malignant melanomas present and does this correlate with the seven-point check-list? Clin Exp Dermatol 1991; **16**:344–7.

19 Cox NH, Madan V, Sanders T. The U.K. skin cancer 'two-week rule' proforma: assessment of potential modifications to improve referral accuracy. Br J Dermatol 2008; **158**:1293–8.

20 Melia J, Cooper EJ, Frost T et al. Cancer Research Campaign health education programme to promote the early detection of cutaneous malignant melanoma I. Work-load and referral patterns. Br J Dermatol 1995; **132**:405–13.

21 Melia J. Early detection of cutaneous malignant melanoma in Britain. Int J Epidemiol 1995; **24** (Suppl. 1):S39–44.

22 MacKie RM, Hole D, Hunter JAA et al. Cutaneous malignant melanoma in Scotland: incidence, survival, and mortality, 1979–94. The Scottish Melanoma Group. BMJ 1997; **315**:1117–21.

23 Braun RP, Oliviero M, Kolm I. Dermoscopy: what's new? Clin Dermatol 2009; **27**:26–34.

24 Melia J. Changing incidence and mortality from cutaneous malignant melanoma. BMJ 1997; **315**:1106–7.

25 Parkin DM, Muir CS. Cancer incidence in five continents: comparability and quality of data. IARC Sci Publ 1992; **120**:45–173.

26 Rhodes AR, Weinstock MA, Fitzpatrick TB et al. Risk factors for cutaneous melanoma. A practical method of recognizing predisposed individuals. JAMA 1987; **258**:3146–54.

27 Newton JA, Bataille V, Griffiths K et al. How common is the atypical mole syndrome phenotype in apparently sporadic melanoma? J Am Acad Dermatol 1993; **29**:989–96.

28 Bataille V, Newton Bishop JA, Sasieni P *et al.* Risk of cutaneous melanoma in relation to the numbers, types and sites of naevi: a case–control study. *Br J Cancer* 1996; **73**:1605–11.

29 Le Mire L, Hollowood K, Gray D *et al.* Melanomas in renal transplant recipients. *Br J Dermatol* 2006; **154**:472–7.

30 Brown VL, Matin RN, Cerio R *et al.* Melanomas in renal transplant recipients: the London experience and invitation to participate in a European study. *Br J Dermatol* 2007; **156**:165–7.

31 Marghoob AA, Schoenbach SP, Kopf AW *et al.* Large congenital melanocytic nevi and the risk for the development of malignant melanoma. A prospective study. *Arch Dermatol* 1996; **132**:170–5.

32 Illig L, Weidner F, Hundeiker M *et al.* Congenital nevi less than or equal to 10 cm as precursors to melanoma: 52 cases, a review, and a new conception. *Arch Dermatol* 1985; **121**:1274–81.

33 Goldstein AM, Chan M, Harland M *et al.* High-risk melanoma susceptibility genes and pancreatic cancer, neural system tumors, and uveal melanoma across GenoMEL. *Cancer Res* 2006; **66**:9818–28.

34 Leachman SA, Carucci J, Kohlmann W *et al.* Selection criteria for genetic assessment of patients with familial melanoma. *J Am Acad Dermatol* 2009; **61**:677.e1–14.

35 Lederman JS, Sober AJ. Does biopsy type influence survival in clinical stage I cutaneous melanoma? *J Am Acad Dermatol* 1985; **13**:983–7.

36 Lees VC, Briggs JC. Effect of initial biopsy procedure on prognosis in stage I invasive cutaneous malignant melanoma: review of 1086 patients. *Br J Surg* 1991; **78**:1108–10.

37 Austin JR, Byers RM, Brown WD, Wolf P. Influence of biopsy on the prognosis of cutaneous melanoma of the head and neck. *Head Neck* 1996; **18**:107–17.

38 Association of Directors of Anatomic and Surgical Pathology. Recommendations for the reporting of tissues removed as part of the surgical treatment of cutaneous melanoma. *Pathol Int* 1998; **48**:168–70.

39 Spatz A, Cook M, Elder D *et al.* Interobserver reproducibility of ulceration assessment in primary cutaneous melanomas. *Eur J Cancer* 2003; **39**:1861–5.

40 Gimotty PA, Guerry D, Ming ME *et al.* Thin primary cutaneous malignant melanoma: a prognostic tree for 10-year metastasis is more accurate than American Joint Committee on Cancer staging. *J Clin Oncol* 2004; **22**:3668–76.

41 Edge SE, Byrd DR, Compton CC *et al.* (eds). *Melanoma of the Skin. AJCC Cancer Staging Manual*, 7th edn. New York, NY: Springer, 2009.

42 Hawkins WG, Busam KJ, Ben-Porat L *et al.* Desmoplastic melanoma: a pathologically and clinically distinct form of cutaneous melanoma. *Ann Surg Oncol* 2005; **12**:207–13.

43 Elder DE, Murphy GF. Malignant tumors (melanoma and related lesions). In: *Melanocytic Tumors of the Skin. Atlas of Tumor Pathology* (Elder DE, Murphy GF, eds). Washington, DC: Armed Forces Institute of Pathology, 1990; 103–205.

44 Kaur C, Thomas RJ, Desai N *et al.* The correlation of regression in primary melanoma with sentinel lymph node status. *J Clin Pathol* 2008; **61**:297–300.

45 Straume O, Akslan LA. Independent prognostic importance of vascular invasion in nodular melanoma. *Cancer* 1996; **78**:1211–19.

46 Quinn MJ, Crotty KA, Thompson JF *et al.* Desmoplastic and desmoplastic neurotropic melanoma: experience with 280 patients. *Cancer* 1998; **83**:1128–35.

47 Harrist TJ, Rigel DS, Day CL Jr *et al.* Microscopic satellites are more highly associated with regional lymph node metastases than is primary melanoma thickness. *Cancer* 1984; **53**:2183–7.

48 Cook MG, Di Palma S. Pathology of sentinel lymph nodes for melanoma. *J Clin Pathol* 2008; **61**:897–902.

49 Cochran AJ. Surgical pathology remains pivotal in the evaluation of 'sentinel' lymph nodes. *Am J Surg Pathol* 1999; **23**:1169–72.

50 Starz H, Balda BR, Kramer KU *et al.* A micromorphometry-based concept for routine classification of sentinel lymph node metastases and its clinical relevance for patients with melanoma. *Cancer* 2001; **91**:2110–21.

51 Dewar DJ, Newell B, Green MA *et al.* The microanatomic location of metastatic melanoma in sentinel lymph nodes predicts nonsentinel lymph node involvement. *J Clin Oncol* 2004; **22**:3345–9.

52 van Akkooi AC, de Wilt JH, Verhoef C, Eggermont AM. The Rotterdam criteria for sentinel node tumor load: the simplest prognostic factor? *J Clin Oncol* 2008; **26**:6011.

53 Basseres N, Grob JJ, Richard MA *et al.* Cost-effectiveness of surveillance of stage I melanoma. A retrospective appraisal based on a 10-year experience in a dermatology department in France. *Dermatology* 1995; **191**:199–203.

54 Khansur T, Sanders J, Das SK. Evaluation of staging workup in malignant melanoma. *Arch Surg* 1989; **124**:847–9.

55 Yancovitz M, Finelt N, Warycha MA *et al.* Role of radiologic imaging at the time of initial diagnosis of stage T1b–T3b melanoma. *Cancer* 2007; **110**:1107–14.

56 Maubec E, Lumbroso J, Masson F *et al.* F-18 fluorodeoxy-D-glucose positron emission tomography scan in the initial evaluation of patients with a primary melanoma thicker than 4 mm. *Melanoma Res* 2007; **17**:147–54.

57 Clark PB, Soo V, Krass J *et al.* Futility of fluorodeoxyglucose F 18 positron emission tomography in initial evaluation of patients with T2 to T4 melanoma. *Arch Surg* 2006; **141**:284–8.

58 Wagner JD, Schauwecker D, Davidson D *et al.* Prospective study of fluorodeoxyglucose positron emission tomography imaging of lymph node basins in melanoma patients undergoing sentinel lymph node biopsy. *J Clin Oncol* 1999; **17**:1508–15.

59 van Rijk MC, Teertstra HJ, Peterse JL *et al.* Ultrasonography and fine-needle aspiration cytology in the preoperative assessment of melanoma patients eligible for sentinel node biopsy. *Ann Surg Oncol* 2006; **13**:1511–16.

60 Sibon C, Chagnon S, Tchakérian A *et al.* The contribution of high-resolution ultrasonography in preoperatively detecting sentinel-node metastases in melanoma patients. *Melanoma Res* 2007; **17**:233–7.

61 Starritt EC, Uren RF, Scolyer RA *et al.* Ultrasound examination of sentinel nodes in the initial assessment of patients with primary cutaneous melanoma. *Ann Surg Oncol* 2005; **12**:18–23.

62 Voit C, Kron M, Schäfer G *et al.* Ultrasound-guided fine needle aspiration cytology prior to sentinel node biopsy in melanoma patients. *Ann Surg Oncol* 2006; **13**:1682–9.

63 Aloia TA, Gershenwald JE, Andtbacka RH *et al.* Utility of computed tomography and magnetic resonance imaging staging before completion lymphadenectomy in patients with sentinel lymph node-positive melanoma. *J Clin Oncol* 2006; **24**:2858–65.

64 Horn J, Lock-Anderson J, Sjøstrand H, Loft A. Routine use of FDG-PET scans in melanoma patients with positive sentinel node biopsy. *Eur J Nucl Mol Imaging* 2006; **33**:887–92.

65 Constantinidou A, Hofman M, O'Doherty M *et al.* Routine positron emission tomography and emission tomography/computed tomography in melanoma staging with positive sentinel node biopsy is of limited benefit. *Melanoma Res* 2008; **18**:56–60.

66 Veronesi U, Cascinelli N, Adamus J *et al.* Thin stage I primary cutaneous malignant melanoma. Comparison of excision with margins of 1 or 3 cm. *N Engl J Med* 1988; **318**:1159–62.

67 Balch CM, Urist MM, Karakousis CP et al. Efficacy of 2 cm surgical margins for intermediate-thickness melanomas (1–4 mm): results of a multi-institutional randomized surgical trial. Ann Surg 1993; **218**:262–7.

68 Cohn-Cedermark G, Rutqvist LE, Andersson R et al. Long term results of a randomized study by the Swedish Melanoma Study Group on 2 cm versus 5 cm resection margins for patients with cutaneous melanoma with a tumor thickness of 0·8–2·0 mm. Cancer 2000; **89**:1495–501.

69 Khayat D, Rixe O, Martin G et al. Surgical margins in cutaneous melanoma (2 cm versus 5 cm for lesions measuring less than 2·1-mm thick). Long-term results of a large European multicentric phase III study. Cancer 2003; **97**:1941–6.

70 Balch C, Soong SJ, Smith T et al. Long term results of a prospective surgical trial comparing 2 cm vs. 4 cm excision margins for 740 patients with 1–4 mm melanomas. Ann Surg Oncol 2001; **8**:101–8.

71 Thomas J, Newton-Bishop J, A'Hern R et al. Excision margins in high-risk malignant melanoma. N Engl J Med 2004; **350**:757–66.

72 NIH Consensus Conference. Diagnosis and treatment of early melanoma. JAMA 1992; **268**:1314–19.

73 Veronesi U, Cascinelli N. Narrow excision (1 cm margin) – a safe procedure for thin cutaneous melanoma. Arch Surg 1991; **126**:438–41.

74 Lens M, Nathan P, Bataille V. Excision margins for primary cutaneous melanoma: updated pooled analysis of randomized controlled trials. Arch Surg 2007; **142**:885–91.

75 Sladden MJ, Balch C, Barzilai DA et al. Surgical excision margins for primary cutaneous melanoma. Cochrane Database Syst Rev 2009; **4**:CD004835.

76 Silverman MK, Golomb FM, Kopf AW et al. Verification of a formula for determination of pre-excision surgical margins from fixed-tissue melanoma specimens. J Am Acad Dermatol 1992; **27**:214–19.

77 Preston P, Matey P, Marsden JR et al. Surgical treatment of lentigo maligna using 2 mm excision margins. Br J Dermatol 2003; **149** (Suppl. 64):109–10.

78 Mahendran RM, Newton-Bishop JA. Survey of U.K. current practice in the treatment of lentigo maligna. Br J Dermatol 2001; **144**:71–6.

79 Schmid-Wendtner MH, Brunner B, Konz B et al. Fractionated radiotherapy of lentigo maligna and lentigo maligna melanoma in 64 patients. J Am Acad Dermatol 2000; **43**:477–82.

80 Tsang RW, Liu FF, Wells W et al. Lentigo maligna of the head and neck. Results of treatment by radiotherapy. Arch Dermatol 1994; **130**:1008–12.

81 Pitman GH, Kopf AW, Bart RS et al. Treatment of lentigo maligna and lentigo maligna melanoma. J Dermatol Surg Oncol 1979; **5**:727–37.

82 Rajpar S, Marsden JR. Imiquimod in the treatment of lentigo maligna. Br J Dermatol 2006; **155**:653–6.

83 Walling HW, Scupham RK, Bean AK, Ceilley RI. Staged excision versus Mohs micrographic surgery for lentigo maligna and lentigo maligna melanoma. J Am Acad Dermatol 2007; **57**:659–64.

84 Morton DL, Wen DR, Wong JH et al. Technical details of intraoperative lymphatic mapping for early stage melanoma. Arch Surg 1992; **127**:392–9.

85 Morton DL, Thompson JF, Cochran AJ et al. Sentinel-node biopsy or nodal observation in melanoma. N Engl J Med 2006; **355**:1307–17.

86 Morton DL, Cochran AJ, Thompson JF et al. Sentinel node biopsy for early stage melanoma – accuracy and morbidity in MSLT-1, an international multicentre trial. Ann Surg 2005; **242**:302–13.

87 Wright BE, Scheri RP, Ye X et al. Importance of sentinel lymph node biopsy in patients with thin melanoma. Arch Surg 2008; **143**:892–9.

88 Li W, Stall A, Shivers SC et al. Clinical relevance of molecular staging for melanoma: comparison of RT-PCR and immunohistochemistry staining in sentinel lymph nodes of patients with melanoma. Ann Surg 2000; **231**:795–803.

89 Nathansohn N, Schachter J, Gutman H. Patterns of recurrence in patients with melanoma after radical lymph node dissection. Arch Surg 2005; **140**:1172–7.

90 National Cancer Peer Review Programme. Manual for Cancer Services 2008: Skin Measures. Available at: http://www.library.nhs.uk/integratedSearch/viewResource.aspx?resID=299673 (last accessed 25 May 2010).

91 Karakousis CP, Emrich LJ, Rao U et al. Groin dissection in malignant melanoma. Am J Surg 1986; **152**:491–5.

92 Badgwell B, Xing Y, Gershenwald JE et al. Pelvic lymph node dissection is beneficial in subsets of patients with node-positive melanoma. Ann Surg Oncol 2007; **14**:2867–75.

93 Finck SJ, Giuliano AE, Mann BD, Morton DL. Result of ilioinguinal dissection for stage II melanoma. Ann Surg 1982; **196**:180–6.

94 Sterne GD, Murray DS, Grimley RP. Ilioinguinal block dissection for malignant melanoma. Br J Surg 1995; **82**:1057–9.

95 Essner R, Scheri R, Kavanagh M et al. Surgical management of the groin lymph nodes in melanoma in the era of sentinel lymph node dissection. Arch Surg 2006; **141**:877–82.

96 Shen P, Conforti A, Essner R et al. Is the node of Cloquet the sentinel node for the iliac/obturator node group? Cancer J 2000; **6**:93–7.

97 Hughes TMD, A'Hern R, Thomas J et al. Prognosis and surgical management of patients with palpable inguinal lymph node metastases from melanoma. Br J Surg 2000; **87**:892–901.

98 Karakousis CP, Driscoll DL. Positive deep nodes in the groin and survival in malignant melanoma. Am J Surg 1996; **171**:421–2.

99 Balch CM, Ross MI. Melanoma patients with iliac nodal metastases can be cured. Ann Surg Oncol 1999; **6**:230–1.

100 Strobbe LJA, Jonk A, Hart AA et al. Positive iliac and obturator nodes in melanoma: survival and prognostic factors. Ann Surg Oncol 1999; **6**:255–62.

101 O'Brien CJ, Coates AS, Petersen-Schaefer K et al. Experience with 998 cutaneous melanomas of the head and neck over 30 years. Am J Surg 1991; **162**:310–14.

102 Turkula LD, Woods J. Limited or selective nodal dissection for malignant melanoma of the head and neck. Am J Surg 1984; **148**:446–8.

103 Hill S, Thomas JM. Use of the carbon dioxide laser to manage cutaneous metastases from malignant melanoma. Br J Surg 1996; **83**:509–12.

104 Thompson JF, Kam PC. Current status of isolated limb infusion with mild hyperthermia for melanoma. Int J Hyperthermia 2008; **24**:219–25.

105 Beasley GM, Petersen RP, Yoo J et al. Isolated limb infusion of in-transit malignant melanoma of the extremity: a well-tolerated but less effective alternative to hyperthermic isolated limb perfusion. Ann Surg Oncol 2008; **15**:2195–205.

106 Cornett WR, McCall LM, Petersen RP et al. Randomized multicenter trial of hyperthermic isolated limb perfusion with melphalan alone compared with melphalan plus tumor necrosis factor: American College of Surgeons Oncology Group Trial Z0020. J Clin Oncol 2006; **24**:4196–201.

107 Veronesi U, Adamus J, Aubert C et al. A randomised trial of adjuvant chemotherapy and immunotherapy in cutaneous melanoma. N Engl J Med 1982; **307**:913–16.

108 Koops HS, Vaglini M, Suciu S et al. Prophylactic isolated limb perfusion for localized, high-risk limb melanoma: results of a multicenter randomized phase III trial. European Organization for Research and Treatment of Cancer Malignant Melanoma Cooperative Group Protocol 18832, the World Health Organization Melanoma Program Trial 15, and the North American Perfusion Group Southwest Oncology Group-8593. J Clin Oncol 1998; **16**:2906–12.

109 Wheatley K, Ives N, Eggermont A et al. Adjuvant therapy for melanoma: an individual patient meta-analysis of randomised trials. J Clin Oncol 2007; **25**:8526.

110 Henderson MA, Burmeister B, Thompson JF et al. Adjuvant radiotherapy and regional lymph node field control in melanoma patients after lymphadenectomy: results of an intergroup randomized trial. J Clin Oncol 2009; **27** (Suppl.): 18 (Abstract LBA9084).

111 Chang P, Knapper WH. Metastatic melanoma of unknown primary. Cancer 1982; **49**:1106–11.

112 Lee CC, Faries MB, Wanek LA, Morton DL. Improved survival after lymphadenectomy for nodal metastasis from an unknown primary melanoma. J Clin Oncol 2008; **26**:535–41.

113 Lee CC, Faries MB, Wanek LA, Morton DL. Improved survival for stage IV melanoma from an unknown primary site. J Clin Oncol 2009; **27**:3489–95.

114 Patchell RA, Tibbs PA, Walsh JW et al. A randomised trial of surgery in the treatment of single metastases of the brain. N Engl J Med 1990; **322**:494–500.

115 Miller JD. Surgical excision for single cerebral metastasis? Lancet 1993; **341**:1566.

116 Sondak V, Liu P, Warneke J et al. Surgical resection for stage IV melanoma: a Southwest Oncology Group Trial (S9430). J Clin Oncol 2006; **24** (Suppl.): 8019 (Abstract).

117 Overett TK, Shiu MH. Surgical treatment of distant metastatic melanoma. Indications and results. Cancer 1985; **56**: 1222–30.

118 Meyer T, Merkel S, Goehl J, Hohenberger W. Surgical therapy for distant metastases of malignant melanoma. Cancer 2000; **89**:1983–91.

119 Essner R, Lee JH, Wanek LA et al. Contemporary surgical treatment of advanced-stage melanoma. Arch Surg 2004; **139**:961–7.

120 Middleton MR, Grob JJ, Aaronson N et al. Randomized phase III study of temozolomide versus dacarbazine in the treatment of patients with advanced metastatic malignant melanoma. J Clin Oncol 2000; **18**:158–66.

121 Patel P, Suciu S, Mortier L et al. Extended schedule escalated dose temozolomide versus dacarbazine in stage IV malignant melanoma; final results of the randomised phase 3 study (EORTC 18032). Ann Oncol 2009; **19** (Suppl. 8):viii3.

122 Ives NJ, Stowe RL, Lorigan P, Wheatley K. Chemotherapy compared with biochemotherapy for the treatment of metastatic melanoma: a meta-analysis of 18 trials involving 2,621 patients. J Clin Oncol 2007; **25**:5426–34.

123 Tarhini AA, Kirkwood JM, Gooding WE et al. Durable complete responses with high-dose bolus interleukin-2 in patients with metastatic melanoma who have experienced progression after biochemotherapy. J Clin Oncol 2007; **25**:3802–7.

124 Zacest AC, Besser M, Stevens G et al. Surgical management of cerebral metastases from melanoma: outcome in 147 patients treated at a single institution over two decades. J Neurosurg 2002; **96**:552–8.

125 Mori Y, Kondziolka D, Flickinger JC et al. Stereotactic radiosurgery for cerebral metastatic melanoma: factors affecting local disease control and survival. Int J Radiat Oncol Biol Phys 1998; **42**:581–9.

126 Selek U, Chang E, Hassenbusch SJ III et al. Stereotactic radiosurgical treatment in 103 patients for 153 cerebral melanoma metastases. Int J Radiat Oncol Biol Phys 2004; **59**:1097–106.

127 Lens MB, Rosdahl I, Ahlbom A et al. Effect of pregnancy on survival in women with cutaneous malignant melanoma. J Clin Oncol 2004; **22**:4369–75.

128 O'Meara AT, Cress R, Xing G et al. Malignant melanoma in pregnancy. A population-based evaluation. Cancer 2005; **103**: 1217–26.

129 Daryanani D, Plukker JT, De Hullu JA et al. Pregnancy and early-stage melanoma. Cancer 2003; **97**:2248–53.

130 Naldi L, Altieri A, Imberti GL et al. Oncology study group of the Italian Group for Epidemiologic Research in Dermatology (GISED). Cutaneous malignant melanoma in women. Phenotypic characteristics, sun exposure, and hormonal factors: a case–control study from Italy. Ann Epidemiol 2005; **15**:545–50.

131 Karagas MR, Stukel TA, Dykes J et al. A pooled analysis of 10 case–control studies of melanoma and oral contraceptive use. Br J Cancer 2002; **86**:1085–92.

132 Lea CS, Holly EA, Hartge P et al. Reproductive risk factors for cutaneous melanoma in women: a case–control study. Am J Epidemiol 2007; **165**:505–13.

133 MacKie RM, Bray CA. Hormone replacement therapy after surgery for stage I or II cutaneous melanoma. Br J Cancer 2004; **90**:770–2.

134 Siple J, Schneider D, Wanlass W et al. Levodopa therapy and risk of malignant melanoma. Ann Pharmacother 2000; **34**:382–5.

135 Wolfe F, Michaud K. Biologic treatment of rheumatoid arthritis and the risk of malignancy: analyses from a large US observational study. Arthritis Rheum 2007; **56**:2886–95.

136 NHS Blood and Transplant. Organ Donation: How to Become a Donor. Available at: http://www.organdonation.nhs.uk/ukt/how_to_become_a_donor/how_to_become_a_donor.jsp (last accessed 25 May 2010).

137 Cornish D, Holterhues C, van der Poll-Franse L et al. A systematic review of health-related quality of life in cutaneous melanoma. Ann Oncol 2009; **20** (Suppl. 6):51–8.

138 Sollner W, Zschocke I, Augustin M. Melanoma patients: psychosocial stress, coping with illness and social support. A systematic review. Psychother Psychosom Med Psychol 1998; **48**:338–48.

139 Francken AB, Bastiannet E, Hoekstra HJ. Follow up in patients with localized primary melanoma. Lancet Oncol 2005; **6**:608–21.

140 Hofmann U, Szedlak M, Ritgen W et al. Primary staging and follow up in melanoma patients – monocenter evaluation of methods, costs and patient survival. Br J Cancer 2002; **87**: 151–7.

141 Garbe C, Hauschild A, Volkenandt M et al. Evidence and interdisciplinary consensus-based German guidelines: diagnosis and surveillance of melanoma. Melanoma Res 2007; **17**:393–9.

142 Balfounta ML, Beauchet A, Chagnon S et al. Ultrasonography or palpation for detection of melanoma nodal invasion: a meta-analysis. Lancet Oncol 2004; **5**:673–80.

143 Einwachter-Thompson J, MacKie RM. An evidence base for reconsidering current follow-up guidelines for patients with cutaneous melanoma less than 0.5 mm thick at diagnosis. Br J Dermatol 2008; **159**:337–41.

Summary of 2010 guidelines for management of melanoma

(See full manuscript for details of evidence and recommendation gradings)

Melanoma patients who must be referred from the Local Skin Cancer Multidisciplinary Team to the Specialist Skin Cancer Multidisciplinary Team

- Patients with stage IB or higher primary melanoma when sentinel lymph node biopsy (SLNB) is available within their Network. In the absence of SLNB then patients with stage IIB or higher should be referred to the Specialist Skin Cancer Multidisciplinary Team
- Patients with melanoma stage I or above who are eligible for clinical trials that have been approved at Cancer Network level
- Patients with melanoma managed by other site specialist teams, e.g. gynaecological, mucosal and head and neck (excluding ocular)
- Patients with multiple primary melanomas
- Children younger than 19 years with melanoma
- Any patient with metastatic melanoma diagnosed at presentation or on follow up
- Patients with giant congenital naevi where there is suspicion of malignant transformation
- Patients with skin lesions of uncertain malignant potential

Recommendations for Local Skin Cancer Multidisciplinary Team record keeping of clinical features

See National Institute for Health and Clinical Excellence *Improving Outcomes for People with Skin Tumours including Melanoma*, February 2006. Available at: http://www.nice.org.uk/nicemedia/live/10901/28906/28906.pdf

Recommendations for screening and surveillance of high-risk individuals

- Patients who are at moderately increased risk of melanoma should be advised of this and taught how to self-examine. This includes patients with atypical mole phenotype, those with a previous melanoma, and organ transplant recipients
- Patients with giant congenital pigmented naevi are at increased risk of melanoma and require long-term follow up
- The prophylactic excision of small congenital naevi is not recommended
- Individuals with a family history of three or more cases of melanoma should be referred to a clinical geneticist or specialized dermatology services for counselling. Those with two cases in the family may also benefit,

especially if one of the cases had multiple primary melanomas or the atypical mole syndrome

Requirements for microscopy of melanoma

Essential
- Ulceration
- Histological subtype

- Thickness
- Margins of excision

- Mitotic count
- Pathological staging

Desirable
- Level of dermal invasion
- Tumour-infiltrating lymphocytes
- Perineural invasion

- Growth phase
- Lymphatic or vascular invasion
- Microsatellites

- Regression

Surgical wider excision margins for primary melanoma

Breslow thickness	Lateral excision margins to muscle or muscle fascia
In situ	5-mm margins to achieve complete histological excision
< 1 mm	1 cm
1·01–2 mm	1–2 cm
2·1–4 mm	2–3 cm
> 4 mm	3 cm

Staging investigations for melanoma

- Patients with stage I, II and IIIA melanoma should not routinely be staged by imaging or other methods as the true-positive pick-up rate is low and the false-positive rate is high
- Patients with stage IIIB or IIIC melanoma should be imaged by computed tomography prior to surgery and with Specialist Skin Cancer Multidisciplinary Team (SSMDT) review
- Patients with stage IV melanoma should be imaged according to clinical need and SSMDT review; lactate dehydrogenase should also be measured

Recommendations for the management of clinically node-negative patients

- There is no role for elective lymph node dissection
- Sentinel lymph node biopsy (SLNB) can be considered in stage IB melanoma and upwards in Specialist Skin Cancer Multidisciplinary Teams
- SLNB is a staging procedure with no proven therapeutic value
- Surgical risks of SLNB, and of a false-negative result, should also be explained

Recommendations for locoregional recurrent melanoma

• All patients should be managed by Specialist Skin Cancer Multidisciplinary Teams
• Nodes clinically suspicious for melanoma should be sampled using fine needle aspiration cytology (FNAC) prior to carrying out formal block dissection. If FNAC is negative although lymphocytes were seen, a core or open biopsy should be performed if suspicion remains
• Prior to formal dissection, performed by an expert, staging by computed tomographic scan should be carried out other than where this would mean undue delay
• The treatment of locoregional limb recurrence is palliative and, depending on extent and response, includes excision or CO_2 laser, isolated limb infusion or perfusion

Recommendations for metastatic disease

• All patients should be managed by Specialist Skin Cancer Multidisciplinary Teams
• Surgery should be considered for oligometastatic disease at sites such as the skin, brain or gut, or to prevent pain or ulceration
• Radiotherapy may have a palliative role in the treatment of metastases
• Standard chemotherapy is dacarbazine although its role is palliative
• Patients with stage IV melanoma should be considered for entry to clinical trials

Pregnancy, oral contraceptives and hormone replacement therapy

Pregnancy in melanoma	Oral contraceptives	Hormone replacement therapy
• No worsening of prognosis • No increase in adverse outcomes for mother or baby • Placental metastases possible in stage IV disease	• No increased risk of melanoma	• No increased risk of melanoma • No worsening of prognosis

Follow up of melanoma patients

• Patients with in situ melanomas do not require follow up
• Patients with stage IA melanoma should be seen two to four times over up to 12 months, then discharged
• Patients with stage IB–IIIA melanoma should be seen 3-monthly for 3 years, then 6-monthly to 5 years
• Patients with stage IIIB and IIIC and resected stage IV melanoma should be seen 3-monthly for 3 years, 6-monthly to 5 years, then annually to 10 years
• Patients with unresectable stage IV melanoma are seen according to need

Appendix 1

Definition of the levels of evidence used in preparation of these guidelines

Level	Type of evidence
Ia	Evidence obtained from meta-analysis of randomized controlled trials, or meta-analysis of epidemiological studies
Ib	Evidence obtained from at least one randomized controlled trial
IIa	Evidence obtained from at least one well-designed controlled study without randomization
IIb	Evidence obtained from at least one other type of well-designed quasi-experimental study
III	Evidence obtained from well-designed nonexperimental descriptive studies, such as comparative studies, correlation studies and case studies
IV	Evidence obtained from expert committee reports or opinions and/or clinical experience of respected authorities
Grade of recommendation	
A	There is good evidence to support the use of the procedure
B	There is fair evidence to support the use of the procedure
C	There is poor evidence to support the use of the procedure
D	There is fair evidence to support the rejection of the use of the procedure
E	There is good evidence to support the rejection of the use of the procedure

http://bad.org.uk/Portals/_Bad/Guidelines/Clinical
%20Guidelines/Cutaneous%20Melanoma.pdf

Comment

The 2002 guidelines on the management of cutaneous melanoma [1] have been updated by a large multidisciplinary group who have published a very thorough update [2]. Over the past few decades, recommended excision margins have diminished from very wide local excision of 5 cm (dinner plate excisions) for all melanoma to a recommendation of 1–2 cm depending upon thickness [2,3]. Excision margins still remain a controversial area, as adequate trials have not been undertaken for the poorer prognosis lesions [4]. Sentinel lymph node biopsy has not been widely accepted as a useful practical intervention in the UK as it is still not standard practice in many cancer centres; controversy remains concerning this procedure [5]. Further studies of its day-to-day utility are needed. The updated guidelines [2] give information and advice regarding sunlight exposure and vitamin D as recent controversy has arisen with the sun protection leading to low levels of vitamin D and the potential for the development of rickets [6].

Legislation is being introduced to limit sunbed use. In Scotland, this has brought about an end to unmanned, coin-operated tanning salons and a ban on the sale or hire of sunbeds to those under 18 [7]. The rest of the UK will, hopefully, follow this sensible public health legislation. Further genetic studies are needed to identify risks of developing melanoma in different phenotypes. Both primary and secondary prevention are important with further studies needed [8]. More effective adjuvant therapies for poor prognosis melanoma and metastatic disease are desperately needed [9]. The national and international trials of various adjuvant therapies will take time to bear fruit.

REFERENCES

1 Roberts DLL, Anstey AV, Barlow RJ, *et al.* UK guidelines for the management of cutaneous melanoma. *Br J Dermatol* 2002: 146; 7–17.
2 Marsden JR, Newton-Bishop JA, Burrows L, *et al.* Guidelines for the management of cutaneous melanoma 2009. *Brit J Dermatol* 2010; xx: xx–xx.
3 Lens M B, Dawes M, Goodacre T, Bishop J A. Excision margins in the treatment of primary cutaneous melanoma: a systematic review of randomized controlled trials comparing narrow vs wide excision. *Arch Surg* 2002; 137: 1101–5.
4 Sladden MJ, Balch C, Barzilai DA, *et al.* Surgical excision margins for primary cutaneous melanoma. *Cochrane Database Syst Rev* 2009; Issue 4: CD004835 (http://mrw.interscience.wiley.com/cochrane/clsysrev/articles/CD004835/frame.html).
5 Medalie N, Ackerman AB. Sentinel node biopsy has no benefit for patients whose primary cutaneous melanoma has metastasized to a lymph node and therefore should be abandoned now. *Brit J Dermatol* 2004; 151: 298–307.
6 Reichrath J. Skin cancer prevention and UV-protection: how to avoid vitamin D-deficiency? *Brit J Dermatol* 2009; 161: 54–60.
7 Roberts DLL, Foley K. Sunbed use in children: time for new legislation? *Brit J Dermatol* 2009; 161: 193–4.
8 C. Sinclair, P. Foley. Skin cancer prevention in Australia. *Brit J Dermatol* 2009; 161: 116–23.
9 Lui P, Cashin R, Machado M, *et al.* Treatments for metastatic melanoma: synthesis of evidence from randomized trials. *Cancer Treatment Reviews* 2007; 33: 665–80.

Additional professional resources

Guidance on cancer services: improving outcomes for people with skin tumours including melanoma – the manual. National Institute for Clinical Evidence. http://www.nice.org.uk/nicemedia/pdf/CSG_Skin_Manual.pdf.

Cutaneous melanoma: a national clinical guideline. Scottish Intercollegiate Guidelines Network 2003. http://www.sign.ac.uk/pdf/sign72.pdf.

The prevention, diagnosis, referral and management of melanoma of the skin. Royal College of Physicians, British Association of Dermatologists 2007. http://www.rcplondon.ac.uk/pubs/contents/f36b1656-cc74-4867-8498-cc94b378312a.pdf.

Bataille V, de Vries E. Melanoma – Part 1: epidemiology, risk factors, and prevention. *Brit Med J* 2008; 337: 2249.

Thirlwell C, Nathan P. Melanoma – Part 2: management. *Brit Med J* 2008; 337: 2488.

National Comprehensive Cancer Network (USA) (requires free registration). http://www.nccn.org/professionals/physician_gls/PDF/melanoma.pdf.

BAD patient information leaflet

http://www.bad.org.uk/site/842/Default.aspx

Related to benign moles

http://www.bad.org.uk/site/840/default.aspx

Other patient resources

http://www.cancerbackup.org.uk

http://www.macmillan.org.uk

http://www.cancerhelp.org.uk/help/default.asp?page= 2788

http://www.patient.co.uk/pdf/pilsL725.pdf

http://www.skincancer.org/content/view/17/79/

http://www.wessexcancer.org

http://www.cks.nhs.uk/patient_information_leaflet/ malignant_melanoma

http://www.nhs.uk/conditions/Malignant-melanoma/Pages/Introduction.aspx?url=Pages/what-is-it.aspx

http://www.cks.nhs.uk/patient_information_leaflet/moles (benign moles)

http://www.dermnetnz.org/lesions/atypical-naevi.html (atypical naevi)

http://www.dermnetnz.org/procedures/mole-mapping.html ('mole mapping')

http://www.bad.org.uk/desktopDefault.aspx?TabId=1221 (British Association of Dermatologists vitamin D position statement)

Joint British Association of Dermatologists and U.K. Cutaneous Lymphoma Group guidelines for the management of primary cutaneous T-cell lymphomas

S.J.WHITTAKER, J.R.MARSDEN,* M.SPITTLE†† AND R.RUSSELL JONES†

St John's Institute of Dermatology, St Thomas' Hospital, Lambeth Palace Road, London SE1 7EH, U.K.
*Department of Dermatology, Selly Oak Hospital, Birmingham B29 6JD, U.K.
†Department of Dermatology, Ealing Hospital, Uxbridge Road, Southall UB1 3HW, U.K.
††Department of Oncology, Middlesex Hospital, Mortimer St, WIN 8AA, U.K.

Accepted for publication 9 July 2003

These guidelines were commissioned by the British Association of Dermatologists guidelines and therapeutics subcommittee. Members of the committee are N.H.Cox (Chairman), A.S.Highet, D.Mehta, R.H.Meyrick Thomas, A.D.Ormerod, J.K.Schofield, C.H.Smith and J.C.Sterling. Members of the U.K. Cutaneous Lymphoma Group who have contributed include C.Benton, R.Cowan, C.Deardon, B.Hancock, H.Lucraft and D.Slater.

Disclaimer   These guidelines have been prepared for dermatologists on behalf of the British Association of Dermatologists and the U.K. Cutaneous Lymphoma Group (UKCLG) and reflect the best data available at the time the report was prepared. Caution should be exercised in interpreting the data; the results of future studies may require alteration of the conclusions or recommendations in this report. It may be necessary or even desirable to depart from the guidelines in special circumstances. Just as adherence to guidelines may not constitute defence against a claim of negligence, so deviation from them should not be necessarily deemed negligent.

Summary   These guidelines for the management of cutaneous T-cell lymphoma have been prepared for dermatologists on behalf of the British Association of Dermatologists and the U.K. Cutaneous Lymphoma Group. They present evidence-based guidance for treatment, with identification of the strength of evidence available at the time of preparation of the guidelines, and a brief overview of epidemiological aspects, diagnosis and investigation.

Epidemiology

The incidence of cutaneous lymphomas is 0·4 per 100 000 per year but, because most are low-grade malignances with long survival, the overall prevalence is much higher. Approximately two-thirds of primary cutaneous lymphomas are of T-cell origin (cutaneous

Correspondence: Dr Sean J.Whittaker.
E-mail: sean.whittaker@kcl.ac.uk

Conflicts of interest by authors: Dr Sean J.Whittaker has previously acted as an expert witness for Ligand Pharmaceuticals with regard to European licensing applications for bexarotene gel and denileukin diftitox.

T-cell lymphoma, CTCL), of which the majority are mycosis fungoides. Studies suggest that the incidence is rising but this may reflect improved diagnosis and better registration. The disease is commoner in males and, in the U.S.A., in the black population. The European Organization for Research and Treatment of Cancer (EORTC) cutaneous lymphoma classification (Appendix A) defines several well characterized clinicopathological entities for primary CTCL and forms a useful basis for a rational approach to therapy.[1] Most of the CTCL entities defined by the EORTC have been recognized in the recent WHO classification for lymphoma,[2] shown in Appendix A. The staging systems are shown in Appendix B.

Initial assessment

This article is restricted to the management of primary CTCL, and specifically of mycosis fungoides and Sézary syndrome. Two sections devoted to primary cutaneous CD30+ lymphoproliferative disorders and rare CTCL variants are found towards the end of the article. It is recommended that all patients, possibly with the exception of those with early stages of mycosis fungoides (IA) or with lymphomatoid papulosis, should be reviewed by a multidisciplinary team (MDT) which should include a dermatologist, a clinical or medical (haemato)oncologist, and a dermatopathologist or pathologist with considerable experience of the diagnosis and management of primary CTCL. In addition, a central review of all pathology would be desirable, consistent with current recommendations from the Royal College of Pathologists for specialized pathology services. Subsequent management should ideally be shared between the cancer centre and the local referring physician in a cancer unit. The MDT should ideally be supported by an accredited laboratory for immunophenotypic and molecular diagnostic studies in lymphoma.

All patients should have adequate diagnostic biopsies for histology, immunophenotypic and preferably molecular studies. This is advised even for stage IA disease as studies have shown that patients with a detectable T-cell clone have a shorter duration of response and higher rate of failure to respond. These findings should be interpreted with the clinical features in order to make a specific diagnosis based on the WHO classification for primary CTCL. This is critical because treatment and prognosis can vary widely depending on the diagnostic category. Occasionally, multiple skin biopsies are required to make a diagnosis and often the opinion of other dermatopathologists experienced in cutaneous lymphoma is required. The patient should be examined fully and any bulky palpable peripheral nodes should be biopsied, preferably by excision rather than by core or fine needle biopsy. Staging computed tomographic (CT) scans of the chest, abdomen and pelvis are indicated in all those patients with non-mycosis fungoides CTCL variants or with stage IIA/B/III/IV mycosis fungoides, but not in those with stage IA/IB disease or lymphomatoid papulosis. Bone marrow aspirate or trephine biopsies are indicated in all patients with CTCL variants (except lymphomatoid papulosis), and should be considered in stage IIB/III/IV mycosis fungoides and also in patients with peripheral blood involvement (as indicated by the presence of Sézary cell

counts representing > 5% of the total lymphocyte count). Peripheral blood samples should be taken for routine haematology, biochemistry, serum lactate dehydrogenase (LDH), Sézary cells, lymphocyte subsets, CD4/CD8 ratio, human T-cell lymphotropic virus (HTLV)-I serology and T-cell receptor (TCR) gene analysis of peripheral blood mononuclear cells. These tests are necessary to distinguish patients with HTLV-I-associated adult T-cell leukaemia/lymphoma (ATLL) and other T-cell leukaemias such as T-prolymphocytic leukaemia (T-PLL), and also to identify those with T-cell clones in peripheral blood as a marker of tumour burden and as a prognostic indicator. On the basis of these findings a specific clinicopathological diagnosis should be established and all patients should be accurately staged, providing prognostic data (Table 1).[3–8]

Recommendations: initial assessment

- Repeated skin biopsies (ellipse rather than punch) are often required to confirm a diagnosis of CTCL
- Histology, immunophenotypic and preferably TCR gene analysis should be performed on all tissue samples (ideally molecular studies require fresh tissue)
- All patients (with the possible exception of early stage mycosis fungoides (stage IA) and lymphomatoid papulosis) should ideally be reviewed by an appropriate MDT for confirmation of the diagnosis and to establish a management strategy
- Initial staging CT scans are required in all patients with the exception of those with early stages of mycosis fungoides (stage IA/IB) and lymphomatoid papulosis
- At diagnosis peripheral blood samples should be analysed for total white cell, lymphocyte and Sézary cell counts, serum LDH, liver and renal function, lymphocyte subsets, CD4/CD8 ratios, HTLV-I serology and, preferably, TCR gene analysis
- Bone marrow aspirate or trephine biopsies are required for CTCL variants (with the exception of lymphomatoid papulosis) and may also be appropriate for those with late stages of mycosis fungoides (stage IIB or above). *Grade A/level III (Appendix C)*

Recommendations: histology

- The presence or absence of epidermotropism should be documented
- The depth of the infiltrate should be noted

Table 1. Prognosis in cutaneous T-cell lymphoma

Stage	IA	IB	IIA	IIB	III	IVA	IVB
OS at 5 y	96–100%	73–86%	49–73%	40–65%	40–57%	15–40%	0–15%
OS at 10 y	84–100%	58–67%	45–49%	20–39%	20–40%	5–20%	0–5%
DSS at 5 y	100%	96% (81%[a])	68%	80%		40%	0%
DSS at 10 y	97–98%	83% (36%[a])	68%	42%		20%	0%
Median survival	Not reached at 32 y	12·1–12·8 y	10·0 y	2·9 y	3·6–4·6 y	13 mo	13 mo
Disease progression at 5 y	4%	21%	65%	32%		70%	100%
Disease progression at 10 y	10%	39%	65%	60%		70%	100%
Overall disease progression	9%	20%	34%				
FFR at 5 y	50%	36%	9%				
FFR at 10 y		31%	3%				

OS, overall survival; DSS, disease-specific survival; FFR, freedom from relapse; y, years; mo, months. Based on data.[3–8] [a]Indicates DSS at 5 y and 10 y for stage IB patients with folliculotropic mycosis fungoides.[65]

- The morphology or cytology of the atypical cells and presence of large cell transformation, folliculotropism, syringotropism, granuloma formation, angiocentricity and subcutaneous infiltration should be mentioned
- Immunophenotypic studies should be performed on paraffin-embedded sections and include the T-cell markers CD2, CD3, CD4, CD8, B-cell marker CD20 and the activation marker CD30. Additional markers such as p53 may have prognostic significance in mycosis fungoides. Markers of cytotoxic function such as TIA-I, the monocyte/macrophage marker CD68 and natural killer (NK) cell marker CD56 may be useful for specific CTCL variants
- Ideally all pathology results should be reviewed by a central panel (usually within cancer centres) as recommended for specialized pathology services
- The histology, after correlation with the clinical features, should be classified according to an integration of the WHO and EORTC classification. (*Grade A/level III*)

Mycosis fungoides/Sézary syndrome

Therapeutic overview. There has been one pivotal randomized controlled trial in patients with CTCL at diagnosis and the majority of these patients had mycosis fungoides.[9] This study compared palliative therapy, consisting of topical mechlorethamine, superficial radiotherapy and phototherapy with combined total skin electron beam (TSEB) therapy and multiagent chemotherapy consisting of cyclophosphamide, adriamycin, vincristine and etoposide (CAVE). The complete response rate was higher in the chemotherapy group (38% compared with 18%) but morbidity was greater and, critically, there was no significant difference in disease-free or overall survival between the two groups after a median follow-up of 75 months.[9] This study provides the rationale for the management of mycosis fungoides which is based on a skin-directed palliative approach that varies according to the stage of the disease. There have been a large number of uncontrolled studies in CTCL with response data but virtually no other controlled studies with data on disease-free and overall survival.[10] This partly reflects the prolonged survival of patients with early stage disease.

Prognosis. Recent findings suggest that a patient's life expectancy is not adversely affected in stage IA disease.[3–5] Patients with stage IB/IIA disease have a 73–86% or 49–73% overall 5-year survival, respectively, while patients with stage IIB disease have a 40–65% 5-year survival.[3–5] The 5-year survival of patients with erythrodermic stage III disease is 45–57%, 15–40% for those with stage IVA and 0–15% for IVB disease.[3,4,7,8] Recent studies also suggest that stage A/B patients with thick plaques may have a worse prognosis but this depends on a histological assessment of plaque thickness and there are concerns that this might not be reproducible. The presence of a peripheral blood T-cell clone may indicate which patients with early stage disease are likely to develop disease progression.[11] Sézary syndrome patients by definition are staged as T4 N1–3 M0 B1 and have a poor prognosis with an overall median survival of 32 months from diagnosis.[1] Recent studies of erythrodermic CTCL have shown that the presence of peripheral nodal disease is the most important prognostic factor in a multivariate analysis although the degree of haematological involvement was also very close to significance.[12] Unfortunately most studies of erythrodermic CTCL have not staged erythrodermic patients adequately and therefore accurate comparisons of different therapies are difficult.

There are a number of clinical variants of mycosis fungoides including localized disease such as pagetoid reticulosis (Woringer Kolopp), folliculotropic mycosis fungoides (follicular mucinosis), poikilodermatous mycosis fungoides, hypopigmented mycosis fungoides and granulomatous slack skin.[1] Although there have been no specific therapeutic trials in these variants, these clinical variants appear to have a good prognosis and are often responsive to skin-directed therapies such as radiotherapy. The exception is folliculotropic mycosis fungoides which may have a worse prognosis.

Recommendations: prognosis

- Prognosis in mycosis fungoides (and clinical variants) is related to age at presentation (worse if > 60 years), to the stage of the disease and possibly to the presence of a peripheral blood T-cell clone; some mycosis fungoides clinical variants may have a better prognosis
- In Sézary syndrome the median survival is 32 months from diagnosis
- Primary cutaneous CD30+ lymphoproliferative disorders without peripheral nodal disease have an excellent prognosis (range 96–100% 5-year survival)
- The prognosis of other types of CTCL is generally poor with the frequent development of systemic disease. (*Grade A/level IIii*)

Therapy

Topical therapy

For patients with limited early stage mycosis fungoides life expectancy may not be adversely affected; it is acceptable simply to use emollients with or without moderate topical steroids. Potent topical corticosteroids can produce a clinical response although this is usually short-lived.[13]

Topical mechlorethamine (nitrogen mustard) 0·01% or 0·02%, either as an aqueous solution (in normal saline) or in an ointment base (emulsifying ointment), is effective for superficial disease with response rates of 51–80% for stage IA, 26–68% for IB and 61% for IIA

disease.[14–16] The aqueous solution is relatively unstable, and the ointment base, which is more irritant than the aqueous solution, can cause irritant or allergic dermatitis in sensitized individuals (35–58%), but its efficacy is similar. This product must not be used in pregnancy but other concerns about safety have not been realized. There is no consensus as to whether mechlorethamine should be applied to individual lesions or to the whole skin, daily or twice weekly, or about the duration of topical therapy after a clinical remission has been produced, but responses can be sustained for prolonged periods. (*Grade A/level IIii*)

Topical carmustine (BCNU) is an alternative topical chemotherapeutic agent in mycosis fungoides with similar efficacy to mechlorethamine as indicated by response rates of 86% in stage IA, 47% in stage IB and 55% in stage IIA patients.[17] Alternate day or daily treatment with 10 mg of BCNU in 60 mL of dilute alcohol (95%) or 20–40% BCNU ointment can be used. Hypersensitivity reactions occur less often (5–10%) than with mechlorethamine. All patients treated topically with BCNU should have regular monitoring of their full blood count; treatment is normally given for only a limited period, depending on the extent of the treated area (2–4 weeks for extensive areas), to avoid myelosuppression; maintenance therapy is contraindicated. (*Grade A/level IIii*)

Recently a novel retinoid, 1% targretin (bexarotene) gel, has been approved by the Federal Drug Administration (FDA) for topical therapy in stage I mycosis fungoides in patients who are resistant or intolerant of other topical therapies.[18] In open uncontrolled studies response rates of 63% with 21% complete response rates have been reported in 67 patients with early stage (IA–IIA) disease. Median time to and duration of response were 20 and 99 weeks, respectively.[18] This product is currently not licensed in Europe. (*Grade B/level IIii*)

There has been only one randomized placebo controlled trial of topical peldesine cream (BCX-34, an inhibitor of the purine nucleoside phosphorylase enzyme) in mycosis fungoides, which showed no benefit compared with vehicle, with complete responses of 28% and 24%, respectively, emphasizing the difficulties in interpretation of uncontrolled studies of topical therapy in early stages of mycosis fungoides.[19] (*Grade E/level I*)

Phototherapy

The clinical benefit of photochemotherapy [psoralen + ultraviolet A (PUVA)] was noted over 20 years ago and response rates of 79–88% in stage IA and

52–59% in stage IB disease have been reported.[20,21] Flexural sites ('sanctuary sites') often fail to respond completely and the duration of response varies. There is no significant response in tumour (IIB) stage disease. Maintenance therapy is rarely effective at preventing relapse[22] and therefore should be avoided if possible so as to limit the total cumulative dose as patients will often require repeated courses over many years. One study has shown that 56% of stage IA and 39% of stage IB complete PUVA responders had no recurrence of disease after 44 months, follow-up without maintenance therapy.[22] PUVA is an ideal therapy for patients with stage IB/IIA disease who are intolerant of or fail to respond to topical therapies such as mechlorethamine although both therapies can be complementary for some patients. Treatment schedules have varied in reported studies of PUVA in CTCL with twice to four times weekly and different protocols for incremental dosage but usually two to three times weekly treatment is acceptable until disease clearance or best partial response. Many patients will inevitably have a high total cumulative UVA dose and the risks of nonmelanoma skin cancer are consequently increased for these patients. Therefore efforts should be made to restrict the total PUVA dose to less than 200 treatment sessions or a total cumulative dose of 1200 J cm^{-2}. In some circumstances patients may receive a greater total dose, if clinically justified and with the consent of the patient. PUVA remains one of the most effective therapies for patients with early stage disease but surprisingly there are no data to establish if PUVA can improve overall survival. PUVA therapy is rarely tolerated in erythrodermic disease but some patients will respond repeatedly. (*Grade A/level IIii*)

Broadband and narrowband UVB and high-dose UVA1 phototherapy have also been used with benefit in mycosis fungoides.[23–25] There have been no adequate comparative studies of different phototherapy modalities or regimens in CTCL. (*Grade B/level III*)

Radiotherapy

Mycosis fungoides and other CTCL variants are very radiosensitive malignancies; individual thick plaques, eroded plaques or tumours can be treated successfully with low-dose superficial orthovoltage radiotherapy, often administered in several fractions (e.g. two or three fractions of 400 cGy at 80–120 kV). Large tumours may be treated by electrons, the choice of energy being dependent on tumour size and thickness.

Radiotherapy is often used with other therapeutic modalities such as PUVA; closely adjacent and overlapping fields can often be retreated because of the low doses used.[26] (*Grade A/level IIii*)

Whole body TSEB therapy has been evaluated extensively in CTCL although it is not widely available. Different field arrangements have been used in an attempt to treat the whole skin uniformly to a depth of 1 cm with various total doses administered and with additional radiotherapy to shielded areas. A systematic review of open uncontrolled and mostly retrospective studies of TSEB as monotherapy in 952 patients with CTCL has established that responses are stage-dependent with complete responses of 96% in stage IA, IB and IIA disease but disease relapse rates are very high, indicating that this approach is not curative even in early stage disease.[27] In stage IIB disease complete responses are less common (36%) but erythrodermic (stage III) disease shows complete responses of 60%. Greater skin surface dose (32–36 Gy) and higher energy (4–6 MeV electrons) are associated with a higher rate of complete response and 5-year relapse-free survivals of 10–23% were noted.[27] A retrospective study of erythrodermic disease has also shown 60% complete responses with 26% progression-free at 5 years.[28] In this study the overall median survival was 3·4 years with a median dose of 32 Gy given as five weekly fractions over 6–9 weeks. Patients with stage III disease did best compared with those with significant nodal or haematological (IVA/IVB) disease. The duration of response was also longer for those who received more than 20 Gy using 4–9 MeV.[28]

A comparative study of TSEB vs. topical mechlorethamine in early stage mycosis fungoides showed similar response rates and duration of response suggesting that TSEB therapy should be reserved for those who fail to respond to first- and second-line therapies.[29] Adverse effects of TSEB include temporary alopecia, telangiectasia and skin malignancies, and the treatment is only available in a limited number of centres.

Although TSEB is usually only given once in a lifetime, several reports have documented patients who have received two or three courses; however, the total doses tolerated and the duration of response have been lower with subsequent courses.[30,31] Consensus EORTC recommendations for the clinical use of TSEB have been published with technical modifications to optimize the efficacy of therapy in CTCL.[32] (*Grade A/level IIii*)

Immunotherapy

Different forms of immunotherapy have been evaluated in CTCL with the intention of enhancing antitumour host immune responses by promoting the generation of cytotoxic T cells and Th1 cytokine responses. Studies of α-interferon have shown overall response rates of 45–74% with complete responses of 10–27%.[33–35] Various dosage schedules have been employed (3 MU × 3 week^{-1} to 36 MU day^{-1}) and it appears that response rates are higher for larger doses (overall responses of 78% vs. 37% for the lower dose schedule).[34] Overall response rates are also higher in early (IB/IIA 88%) compared with late (III/IV 63%) stages of disease.[35] (*Grade A/level IIi*)

Combined α-interferon and retinoids produce similar response rates to interferon alone and are not recommended.[36] (*Grade D/level IIi*)

Studies comparing PUVA and α-interferon with α-interferon and acitretin in early-stage disease have shown complete response rates of 70% and 38%, respectively, but there are no data on duration of response.[37] Uncontrolled studies of combined PUVA and α-interferon (maximum tolerated dose 12 MU m^{-2} × 3 week^{-1}) in mycosis fungoides and Sézary syndrome have shown overall response rates of 100% with 62% complete response rates.[38] This combination may also be useful in patients with resistant early-stage disease such as those with thick plaques and folliculotropic disease. (*Grade A/level IIii*)

A recently completed randomized study comparing PUVA with PUVA and α-interferon in early-stage mycosis fungoides suggests that the response rates are similar but the cumulative dose is lower and the duration of response is more prolonged for the combined regimen (EORTC Annual Clinical Meeting, Helsinki June 2003). At present there are few data about the effect on disease-free and overall survival.

Other small pilot studies have shown that both interleukin (IL)-12 and γ-interferon can produce clinical responses in CTCL but their therapeutic value remains to be established.[39,40] (*Grade C/level III*)

Ciclosporin has been used in CTCL, particularly in erythrodermic variants to relieve severe pruritus, but there is some evidence that treatment may actually cause rapid disease progression and its use in CTCL is not recommended.[41] (*Grade D/level III*)

Chemotherapy

Mycosis fungoides and Sézary syndrome are relatively chemoresistant and responses are usually short-lived, as illustrated by the controlled study by Kaye *et al.*[9] This may reflect the low proliferative rate of tumour cells and a high prevalence of inactivating p53 mutations which produce a relative resistance to tumour cell apoptosis. A systematic review of published data on different regimens has shown a complete response rate of 33% in 526 patients treated with single agent chemotherapy with a median duration of 3–22 months.[42] Combination chemotherapy in 331 patients produced complete response rates of 38% with a median duration of 5–41 months.[42] CTCL patients are prone to infection and septicaemia is a common preterminal event.

Chemotherapy should not be used in patients with early stage IA, IB or IIA disease. (*Grade E/level I*) However, treatment of stage IIB and IVA disease remains problematic. Individual tumours and effaced peripheral lymph nodes will respond to superficial radiotherapy and additional chemotherapy should be considered in patients with a good performance status [Eastern Cooperative Oncology Group (ECOG), 0–2, where 0 is 'fully active' and 4 is 'completely disabled']. However, responses are likely to be short-lived, and patients should be entered into ongoing clinical trials. Single agent chemotherapy which has been shown to produce a clinical response in stage IIB–IVB disease includes oral chlorambucil (4–6 cycles of 0·15–0·2 mg kg^{-1} day^{-1} for 2–4 weeks), methotrexate and etoposide, and the intravenous use of the purine analogues 2-deoxycoformycin, 2-chlorodeoxyadenosine and fludarabine.[42] Open studies of 2-deoxycoformycin in mycosis fungoides and Sézary syndrome have reported response rates of 35–71% with complete response rates of 10–33%.[43,44] Methotrexate has been reported to produce a complete response rate of 41% in 29 patients with erythrodermic (stage III/T4) disease with a median survival of 8·4 years given as single weekly doses over a wide dose range of 5–125 mg, but this study was uncontrolled and it is unclear if the patients included represented an usually good prognostic group.[45] Recently, liposomal doxorubicin and gemcitabine have been used in CTCL[46,47] and EORTC phase II trials are due to start shortly. All patients with a good performance status (ECOG 0–2) and advanced stages of mycosis fungoides should if possible be entered into randomized controlled studies. (*Grade B/level IIii*)

Recent pilot studies assessing the use of TSEB combined with high-dose conditioning chemotherapy before autologous stem cell transplantation in patients with stage IIB–IVA disease have shown good clinical responses,[48] but there are no data available at present to indicate if this approach affects disease-free or overall survival. Patients with a poor prognosis and good performance status should be selected for existing clinical trials. Allogeneic stem cell or bone marrow transplantation has only been used in a few patients with encouraging results[49,50] but the associated mortality suggests that this approach is difficult to justify. However, a graft-versus-lymphoma effect may be therapeutically important and the future assessment of nonmyeloablative mini-allografts in CTCL would be appropriate. (*Grade C/level III*)

Monoclonal antibody therapy

A humanized chimeric anti-CD4 monoclonal antibody has been used to treat eight patients with CTCL; seven patients showed a clinical response but this was of short duration.[51] (*Grade C/level III*) A radiolabelled anti-CD5 antibody has also been used in mycosis fungoides with some objective results[52] and alemtuzumab (CAMPATH—anti-CD52) has also been administered to CTCL patients (stage III) with demonstrable but short-lived clinical responses.[53,54] At present these approaches are not considered standard treatment and remain potential options for future phase I/II studies. A current phase II study is assessing the therapeutic benefit of a fully humanized anti-CD4 antibody in both early and late stages of mycosis fungoides. (*Grade C/level III*)

Recently a novel antibody approach has been used in CTCL. Denileukin diftitox, a DAB_{389}–IL-2 fusion toxin (Onzar in Europe/Ontak in the U.S.A.) has completed phase I/II studies and has received provisional FDA approval for the treatment of resistant or recurrent CTCL, but this therapy has not yet received a license in Europe for late stages of mycosis fungoides or Sézary syndrome. Denileukin diftitox is a recombinant fusion protein consisting of peptide sequences for the enzymatically active domain (389) of diphtheria toxin and the membrane translocation domain of IL-2 and can inhibit protein synthesis in tumour cells that express high levels of the IL-2 receptor, thereby resulting in cell death. Phase III studies of 71 heavily pretreated patients with stage IB–IVA mycosis fungoides, and more than 20% CD25+ lymphocytes, showed an overall response rate (defined as lasting at least 6 months) of 30% including 10% with complete response.[55] The median duration of response was 6·9 months (range 2·7–46·1 months). The optimally tolerated dose $(18 \mu g \ kg^{-1} \ day^{-1})$ is given intravenously for 5 days and repeated every 21 days for four to eight cycles. Adverse effects include fever, chills, myalgia, nausea and vomiting, and a mild increase in transaminase levels. Acute hypersensitivity reactions occurred in 60%, invariably within 24 h and during the initial infusion. A vascular leak syndrome characterized by hypotension, hypoalbuminaemia and oedema was defined retrospectively within the first 14 days of a given dose in 25% of patients. Myelosuppression is rare. Five per cent of adverse effects are severe or life threatening. (*Grade A/level IIii.*) The clinical relevance of antibody responses to denileukin diftitox is unclear. The duration of clinical response has not yet been established and current studies are comparing different doses of denileukin diftitox and are also assessing the use of this therapy in CD25-negative tumours. This therapy is not likely to be appropriate for early-stage disease but may be useful in advanced disease. Patients should be treated with denileukin diftitox in the context of appropriate clinical trials.

Novel retinoids

Phase II and III studies of a novel synthetic retinoid in CTCL have recently been published.[56,57] Bexarotene (Targretin) is the only retinoid that selectively binds and activates the retinoid X receptor and has recently been approved in Europe for the treatment of advanced stages (IIB–IVB) of mycosis fungoides. Bexarotene has been shown to promote apoptosis and inhibit cell proliferation. It is relatively selective and therefore should have little effect on the retinoid A receptor (RAR) receptor involved in cell differentiation. In phase II and III studies of 152 patients with CTCL, response rates from 20% to 67% have been reported.[56,57] The most effective tolerated oral dose is 300 mg m^{-2} day^{-1} although responses improve with higher doses. Side-effects are transient and generally mild but most patients require treatment for hyperlipidaemia and central (hypothalamic) hypothyroidism while on therapy. At doses of 300 mg m^{-2} day^{-1} in early stage disease (IA/IB/IIA) response rates of 54% have been noted[56] whereas patients with advanced mycosis fungoides (stage IIB–IVB) have shown response rates of 45% with a notable reduction in pruritus in stage III disease.[57] (*Grade A/level IIii*)

EORTC studies due to start enrolment shortly include a phase III randomized study comparing PUVA alone with combined PUVA and oral bexarotene in stage IB and IIA disease. Future studies should also clarify the role of oral bexarotene in later stages of disease and specifically in erythrodermic patients. At the present time oral bexarotene can only be prescribed for early stages of mycosis fungoides in the context of clinical trials.

Extracorporeal photopheresis

Extracorporeal photopheresis (ECP) is licensed by the FDA for the treatment of CTCL; there are no randomized studies to clarify whether ECP has any effect on overall survival. The original open study of ECP in 29 erythrodermic CTCL patients reported a response rate of 73% but response rates in patients with earlier stages of mycosis fungoides were much lower (38%).[58] Subsequently a median survival of 62 months was reported in the original cohort of 29 erythrodermic patients, which compares favourably with historical controls (30 months).[59] A study of 33 patients with Sézary syndrome treated with ECP reported a median survival of 39 months, which was similar to historical controls from the same institution.[60] A systematic review of response rates in erythrodermic disease (stage III/IVA) with ECP has shown overall responses of 35–71%, with complete responses of 14–26%.[61] Other studies are more difficult to interpret because they have involved small numbers, patients with earlier stages of disease and in most studies many of the patients have been on other concurrent therapies. (*Grade A/level IIii*)

Randomized controlled trials of ECP are required to assess its effect on disease-free and overall survival. There have been claims that the CD8 count is critical in predicting whether patients will respond to ECP,[59] although others have provided evidence that the total baseline Sézary count is the only predictor of response.[62]

Recommendations in mycosis fungoides and Sézary syndrome (Table 2)

- Skin-directed therapy (topical therapy, superficial radiotherapy and phototherapy) is appropriate treatment for patients with early stages of mycosis fungoides (stages IA–IIA) with the choice of therapy dependent on the extent of cutaneous disease and plaque thickness (*Grade A/level I*)
- Combined PUVA and α-interferon therapy can be effective for patients with resistant early-stage disease (stage IB–IIA) (*Grade A/level IIi*)
- Patients with later stages of mycosis fungoides (stage IIB or higher) will require some form of systemic therapy (*Grade A/level IIii*)

- CTCL is a very radiosensitive malignancy and several fractions (2–3) of low energy (80–120 kV) superficial radiotherapy are appropriate for many patients (*Grade A/level IIii*)
- Chemotherapy regimens in advanced stages of mycosis fungoides generally achieve complete responses in the region of 30% but these are short-lived (*Grade B/level IIii*)
- Erythrodermic CTCL patients should be considered for immunotherapy and ECP as responses to chemotherapy are generally poor (*Grade A/level IIii*)
- TSEB therapy is an effective treatment for stage IB and stage III mycosis fungoides but is not sufficient alone for stage IIB disease or those with significant haematological involvement (*Grade A/level IIi*)
- New agents such as bexarotene and denileukin diftitox offer important therapeutic alternatives which are currently being evaluated (*Grade A/level IIii*)
- In treatment-resistant cases of late stage disease palliative radiotherapy and/or chemotherapy may produce a significant short-term benefit but the patient's quality of life should always be given priority (*Grade B Level III*)
- All patients and especially those with late stages of disease (> IIA) should be considered for entry into well designed randomized controlled clinical trials.

Primary cutaneous CD30+ T-cell lymphomas

The primary cutaneous CD30+ T-cell lymphomas represent a spectrum of disease in which lymphomatoid papulosis represents an indolent form characterized by recurrent crops of self-healing papules and nodules which may become necrotic and usually resolve to leave varioliform scars. Histologically, lymphomatoid papulosis shows a wedge-shaped polymorphic infiltrate consisting of atypical mononuclear cells with cerebriform, anaplastic (CD30+) and pleomorphic cytology. In contrast larger tumours which do not resolve spontaneously and which histologically show a monomorphic infiltrate of large anaplastic CD30+ mononuclear cells (> 80% of dermal infiltrate) represent primary cutaneous anaplastic large cell lymphomas. Both conditions have an excellent prognosis with 100% and 96% 5-year survival for lymphomatoid papulosis and primary large cell anaplastic lymphomas, respectively, and therefore skin-directed therapy is indicated.[63] Lymphomatoid papulosis is radiosensitive and both PUVA therapy and low-dose oral methotrexate are effective at preventing recurrent lesions.[63,64] (*Grade*

Table 2. Treatment of mycosis fungoides/Sézary syndrome

Stage	First line	Second line	Experimental	Not suitable
IA	SDT or no therapy	SDT or no therapy	Bexarotene gel	Chemotherapy
IB	SDT	α-interferon + PUVA, TSEB	Denileukin diftitox, bexarotene	Chemotherapy
IIA	SDT	α-interferon + PUVA, TSEB	Denileukin diftitox, bexarotene	Chemotherapy
IIB	Radiotherapy or TSEB, chemotherapy	α-interferon, denileukin diftitox, bexarotene	Autologous PBSCT mini-allograft	Cyclosporin
III	PUVA ± α-interferon, ECP ± α-interferon, methotrexate	TSEB, bexarotene, denileukin diftitox,* chemotherapy, alemtuzumab	Autologous PBSCT, mini-allograft	Cyclosporin
IVA	Radiotherapy or TSEB, chemotherapy	α-interferon, denileukin diftitox,* alemtuzumab bexarotene	Autologous PBSCT, mini-allograft	Cyclosporin
IVB	Radiotherapy, chemotherapy	Palliative therapy	Mini-allograft	

PBSCT, peripheral blood stem cell transplant; ECP, extracorporeal photopheresis; TSEB, total skin electron beam; PUVA, psoralen + ultraviolet A; SDT, skin-directed therapy including topical emollients, steroids, mechlorethamine, carmustine, bexarotene gel, UVB/PUVA, superficial radiotherapy. Stage III includes Sézary syndrome, although some cases of Sézary syndrome will be stage IVA. ECP ideal for those patients with peripheral blood involvement. *Not yet licensed in Europe.

A/level IIii) The use of high-dose chemotherapy is not indicated in the management of lymphomatoid papulosis. However, a small proportion of patients (4%) will develop other forms of lymphoma including mycosis fungoides, Hodgkin's disease and large cell anaplastic lymphoma. Skin-directed treatment of primary cutaneous large cell anaplastic lymphoma is also appropriate unless patients develop very extensive cutaneous involvement or systemic disease.[63]

Other primary cutaneous T-cell lymphomas

This group of primary cutaneous T-cell lymphomas are poorly defined in terms of clinicopathological features, but the CD30-negative large cell pleomorphic, anaplastic and immunoblastic variants all have a poor prognosis. There have been no significant therapeutic studies. When disease is restricted to the skin radiotherapy may be indicated, but systemic dissemination is likely and most patients will require some form of multiagent chemotherapy, although responses are likely to be poor. Primary cutaneous extranodal NK-like/T-cell lymphomas (nasal type) have a poor prognosis.[2] Primary subcutaneous panniculitis-like T-cell lymphomas are rare but also have a poor prognosis with a high incidence of systemic involvement and haemophagocytosis either at diagnosis or shortly afterwards.[2] Extranodal NK-like/T-cell, blastic NK-cell and subcutaneous T-cell lymphomas can have

a cytotoxic phenotype and may show angiocentricity. These categories of CTCL will invariably require systemic chemotherapy and skin-directed therapy alone is not indicated. (*Grade A/level III*)

Conclusions

The few randomized studies in CTCL so far clearly indicate that in early stage disease skin directed treatment represents the most appropriate therapy. Long-term cure may be achieved in localized disease such as pagetoid reticulosis but patients with multifocal early stage disease, as present in most cases of mycosis fungoides, are only likely to achieve a short-term clinical response with recurrent disease for many years and, in the majority of cases, a normal life expectancy. Therefore potentially toxic and aggressive therapies ought to be avoided.

In contrast, patients with later stages of mycosis fungoides have a poor prognosis and the absence of large well-designed randomized controlled studies at present is reflected by a lack of consensus regarding treatment. CTCL is a very radiosensitive tumour and both superficial radiotherapy and TSEB therapy are invaluable treatments for all patients and especially those with later stages of disease. A striking feature of the published studies of a wide variety of different therapies to date is an overall response rate of approximately 30% and a complete response rate of 10%. Single and multiagent chemotherapy regimens produce a higher complete response rate (approximately 30%) but this tends to be short-lived (median duration 3–41 months). This suggests that, for most patients, none of these therapies has so far had any significant impact on disease outcome and that the same minority of patients with responsive disease are benefiting. Ideally all patients with late-stage disease should be entered into appropriate clinical trials. It is also critical to ensure that the individual patient's quality of life is considered when therapeutic options are discussed and that patient expectations are realistic. Palliative care should be considered for all patients with resistant late-stage disease and those with poor performance status (ECOG > 2).

References

1 Willemze R, Kerl H, Sterry W *et al.* EORTC classification for primary cutaneous lymphomas: a proposal from the cutaneous lymphoma study group of the European Organisation for Research and Treatment of Cancer. *Blood* 1997; **90**: 354–71.

2 Harris NL, Jaffe ES, Diebold J *et al.* The World Health Organization classification of neoplastic diseases of the haematopoietic and lymphoid tissues: report of the clinical advisory committee meeting, Airlie House, Virginia, November 1997. *Histopathology* 2000; **36**: 69–86.

3 Zackheim HS, Amin S, Kashani-Sabet M, McMillan A. Prognosis in cutaneous T-cell lymphoma by skin stage: long term survival in 489 patients. *J Am Acad Dermatol* 1999; **40**: 418–25.

4 Van Doorn R, van Haselan CW, van Voorst Vader P *et al.* Mycosis fungoides: disease evolution and prognosis of 309 Dutch patients. *Arch Dermatol* 2000; **136**: 504–10.

5 Kim YH, Jensen RA, Watanabe GI *et al.* Clinical stage IA (limited patch and plaque) mycosis fungoides. *Arch Dermatol* 1996; **132**: 1309–13.

6 Kim YH, Chow S, Varghese A, Hoppe RT. Clinical characteristics and long-term outcome of patients with generalized patch and/or plaque (T2) mycosis fungoides. *Arch Dermatol* 1999; **135**: 26–32.

7 de Coninck EC, Kim YH, Varghese A, Hoppe RT. Clinical characteristics and outcome of patients with extracutaneous mycosis fungoides. *J Clin Oncol* 2001; **19**: 779–84.

8 Kim YH, Bishop K, Varghese A, Hoppe RT. Prognostic factors in erythrodermic mycosis fungoides and the Sézary syndrome. *Arch Dermatol* 1995; **131**: 1003–8.

9 Kaye FJ, Bunn PA Jr, Steinberg SM *et al.* A randomized trial comparing combination electron beam radiation and chemotherapy with topical therapy in the initial treatment of mycosis fungoides. *N Engl J Med* 1989; **321**: 1748–90.

10 Whittaker SJ. Primary cutaneous T-cell lymphomas. In: *Evidence-based Oncology* (Williams H, Bigby M, Diepgen T *et al.*, eds). London: BMJ Books, 2003; IX: 498–517.

11 Fraser-Andrews E, Woolford A, Russell Jones R, Whittaker SJ. Detection of a peripheral blood T-cell clone is an independent prognostic marker in mycosis fungoides. *J Invest Dermatol* 2000; **114**: 117–21.

12 Scarisbrick JJ, Whittaker SJ, Evans A *et al.* Prognostic significance of tumour burden in the blood of patients with erythrodermic primary cutaneous T-cell lymphoma. *Blood* 2001; **97**: 624–30.

13 Zackheim H, Kashani-Sabet M, Amin S. Topical corticosteroids for mycosis fungoides. *Arch Dermatol* 1998; **134**: 949–54.

14 Hoppe RT, Abel EA, Deneau DG, Price NM. Mycosis fungoides: management with topical nitrogen mustard. *J Clin Oncol* 1987; **5**: 1796–803.

15 Ramsey DL, Halperin PS, Zeleniuch-Jacquotte A. Topical mechlorethamine therapy for early stage mycosis fungoides. *J Am Acad Dermatol* 1988; **19**: 684–91.

16 Vonderheid EC, Tan ET, Kantor AF *et al.* Long term efficacy, curative potential and carcinogenicity of topical mechlorethamine chemotherapy in cutaneous T-cell lymphoma. *J Am Acad Dermatol* 1989; **20**: 416–28.

17 Zackheim H, Epstein E, Crain W. Topical carmustine (BCNU) for cutaneous T-cell lymphoma: a 15-year experience in 143 patients. *J Am Acad Dermatol* 1990; **22**: 802–10.

18 Breneman D, Duvic M, Kuzel T *et al.* Phase I and II trial of bexarotene gel for skin-directed treatment of patients with cutaneous T-cell lymphoma. *Arch Dermatol* 2002; **138**: 325–32.

19 Duvic M, Olsen E, Omura G *et al.* A phase III, randomized, double-blind, placebo-controlled study of peldesine (BCX-34) cream as topical therapy for cutaneous T-cell lymphoma. *J Am Acad Dermatol* 2001; **44**: 940–7.

20 Hermann JJ, Roenigk HH Jr, Hurria A *et al.* Treatment of mycosis fungoides with photochemotherapy (PUVA): long term follow-up. *J Am Acad Dermatol* 1995; **33**: 234–42.

21 Roenigk HH Jr, Kuzel TM, Skoutelis AP *et al.* Photochemotherapy alone or combined with interferon alfa in the treatment of cutaneous T-cell lymphoma. *J Invest Dermatol* 1990; **95** (Suppl.6): 198–205.

22 Honigsmann H, Brenner W, Rauschmeier W *et al.* Photochemotherapy for cutaneous T cell lymphoma. *J Am Acad Dermatol* 1984; **10**: 238–45.

23 Ramsey DL, Lish KM, Yalowitz CB, Soter NA. Ultraviolet-B phototherapy for early stage cutaneous T-cell lymphoma. *Arch Dermatol* 1992; **128**: 931–3.

24 Clark C, Dawe RS, Evans AT *et al.* Narrowband TL-01 phototherapy for patch stage mycosis fungoides. *Arch Dermatol* 2000; **136**: 748–52.

25 Zane C, Leali C, Airo P *et al.* 'High dose' UVA1 therapy of widespread plaque-type, nodular and erythrodermic mycosis fungoides. *J Am Acad Dermatol* 2001; **44**: 629–33.

26 Cotter GW, Baglan RJ, Wasserman TH, Mill W. Palliative radiation treatment of cutaneous mycosis fungoides: a dose response. *Int J Radiat Oncol Biol Phys* 1983; **9**: 1477–80.

27 Jones GW, Hoppe RT, Glatstein E. Electron beam treatment for cutaneous T-cell lymphoma. *Haematol Oncol Clin North Am* 1995; **9**: 1057–76.

28 Jones GW, Rosenthal D, Wilson LD. Total skin electron beam radiation for patients with erythrodermic cutaneous T-cell lymphoma (mycosis fungoides and the Sézary syndrome). *Cancer* 1999; **85**: 1985–95.

29 Hamminga B, Van Noordijk EM, Vloten WA. Treatment of mycosis fungoides: total skin electron beam irradiation vs topical mechlorethamine therapy. *Arch Dermatol* 1982; **118**: 150–3.

30 Becker M, Hoppe RT, Knox SJ. Multiple courses of high dose total skin electron beam therapy in the management of mycosis fungoides. *Int J Radiat Oncol Biol Phys* 1995; **30**: 1445–9.

31 Wilson L, Quiros PA, Kolenik SA *et al.* Additional courses of total skin electron beam therapy in the treatment of patients with recurrent cutaneous T-cell lymphoma. *J Am Acad Dermatol* 1996; **35**: 69–73.

32 Jones GW, Kacinski BM, Wilson LD *et al.* Total skin electron beam radiation in the management of mycosis fungoides: consensus of the European Organisation for Research and Treatment of Cancer (EORTC) Cutaneous Lymphoma Project Group. *J Am Acad Dermatol* 2002; **47**: 364–70.

33 Bunn PA Jr, Ihde DC, Foon KA. The role of recombinant interferon alpha-2a in the therapy of cutaneous T-cell lymphomas. *Cancer* 1986; **57**: 1689–95.

34 Olsen EA, Rosen ST, Vollmer RT *et al.* Interferon alfa-2a in the treatment of cutaneous T-cell lymphoma. *J Am Acad Dermatol* 1989; **20**: 395–407.

35 Papa G, Tura S, Mandelli F *et al.* Is interferon alpha in cutaneous T-cell lymphoma a treatment of choice? *Br J Haematol* 1991; **79**: 48–51.

36 Dreno B, Claudy A, Meynadier J *et al.* The treatment of 45 patients with cutaneous T-cell lymphoma with low doses of interferon-alpha 2a and etretinate. *Br J Dermatol* 1991; **125**: 456–9.

37 Stadler R, Otte HG, Luger T *et al.* Prospective randomized multicentre clinical trial on the use of interferon alpha-2a plus acitretin versus interferon alpha-2a plus PUVA in patients with cutaneous T-cell lymphoma stages I and II. *Blood* 1998; **10**: 3578–81.

38 Kuzel TM, Roenigk HH Jr, Samuelson E *et al.* Effectiveness of interferon alfa-2a combined with phototherapy for mycosis fungoides and the Sézary syndrome. *J Clin Oncol* 1995; **13**: 257–63.

39 Rook AH, Wood GS, Yoo EK *et al.* Interleukin-12 therapy of cutaneous T-cell lymphoma induces lesion regression and cytotoxic T-cell responses. *Blood* 1999; **94**: 902–8.

40 Kaplan EH, Rosen ST, Norris DB *et al.* Phase II study of recombinant interferon gamma for treatment of cutaneous T-cell lymphoma. *J Nat Cancer Inst* 1990; **82**: 208–12.

41 Cooper DL, Braverman IM, Sarris AH *et al.* Cyclosporine treatment of refractory T-cell lymphomas. *Cancer* 1993; **71**: 2335–41.

42 Bunn PA Jr, Hoffman SJ, Norris D *et al.* Systemic therapy of cutaneous T-cell lymphomas (mycosis fungoides and the Sézary syndrome). *Ann Intern Med* 1994; **121**: 592–602.

43 Kurzrock R, Pilat S, Duvic M. Pentostatin therapy of T-cell lymphomas with cutaneous manifestations. *J Clin Oncol* 1999; **17**: 3117–21.

44 Dearden C, Matutes E, Catovsky D. Pentostatin treatment of cutaneous T-cell lymphoma. *Oncology* 2000; **14**: 37–40.

45 Zackheim HS, Kashani-sabet M, Hwang ST. Low dose methotrexate to treat erythrodermic cutaneous T-cell lymphoma: results in twenty-nine patients. *J Am Acad Dermatol* 1996; **34**: 626–31.

46 Wollina U, Graefe T, Kaatz M. Pegylated doxorubicin for primary cutaneous T-cell lymphoma: a report on ten patients with follow-up. *J Cancer Res Clin Oncol* 2001; **127**: 128–34.

47 Zinzani PL, Baliva G, Magagnoli M *et al.* Gemcitabine treatment in pretreated cutaneous T-cell lymphoma: experience in 44 patients. *J Clin Oncol* 2000; **18**: 2603–6.

48 Olavarria E, Child F, Woolford A *et al.* T-cell depletion and autologous stem cell transplantation in the management of tumour stage mycosis fungoides with peripheral blood involvement. *Br J Haematol* 2001; **114**: 624–31.

49 Burt RK, Guitart J, Traynor A *et al.* Allogeneic hematopoietic stem cell transplantation for advanced mycosis fungoides: evidence of a graft-versus-tumour effect. *Bone Marrow Transplant* 2000; **25**: 111–13.

50 Molina A, Nademanee A, Arber DA, Forman SJ. Remission of refractory Sézary syndrome after bone marrow transplantation from a matched unrelated donor. *Biol Blood Marrow Transplant* 1999; **5**: 400–4.

51 Knox S, Hoppe RT, Maloney D *et al.* Treatment of cutaneous T-cell lymphoma with chimeric anti-CD4 monoclonal antibody. *Blood* 1996; **87**: 893–9.

52 Foss FM, Raubitscheck A, Mulshine JL *et al.* Phase I study of the pharmacokinetics of a radioimmunoconjugate, 90Y–T101, in patients with CD5-expressing leukaemia and lymphoma. *Clin Cancer Res* 1998; **4**: 2691–700.

53 Lundin J, Osterborg A, Brittinger G *et al.* CAMPATH-1H monoclonal antibody in therapy for previously treated low-grade non-Hodgkin's lymphomas: a phase II multicenter study. European Study Group of CAMPATH-1H Treatment in Low-Grade Non-Hodgkin's Lymphoma. *J Clin Oncol* 1998; **16**: 3257–63.

54 Lundin J, Hagberg H, Repp R *et al.* Phase II study of alemtuzumab (anti-CD52 monoclonal antibody, CAMPATH-1H) in patients with advanced mycosis fungoides. *Blood* 2003; **101**: 4267–72.

55 Olsen EA, Duvic M, Frankel A *et al.* Pivotal phase III trial of two dose levels of denileukin diftitox for the treatment of cutaneous T-cell lymphoma. *J Clin Oncol* 2001; **19**: 376–88.

56 Duvic M, Martin AG, Kim Y, Olsen E. Worldwide Bexarotene Study Group. Phase 2 and 3 clinical trial of oral bexarotene (Targetin capsules) for the treatment of refractory or persistent early stage cutaneous T-cell lymphoma. *Arch Dermatol* 2001; **137**: 581–93.

57 Duvic M, Hymes K, Heald P *et al.* Bexarotene is effective and safe for treatment of refractory advanced-stage cutaneous T-cell lymphoma: multinational phase II–III trial results. *J Clin Oncol* 2001; **19**: 2456–71.

58 Edelson R, Berger C, Gasparro F *et al.* Treatment of cutaneous T-cell lymphoma by extracorporeal photochemotherapy. *N Engl J Med* 1987; **316**: 297–303.

59 Heald P, Rook A, Perez M *et al.* Treatment of erythrodermic cutaneous T-cell lymphoma with extracorporeal photopheresis. *J Am Acad Dermatol* 1992; **27**: 427–33.

60 Fraser-Andrews E, Seed P, Whittaker S, Russell Jones R. Extracorporeal photopheresis in Sézary syndrome: no significant effect in the survival of 44 patients with a peripheral blood T-cell clone. *J Arch Dermatol* 1998; **134**: 1001–5.

61 Russell Jones R. Extracorporeal photopheresis in cutaneous T-cell lymphoma. Inconsistent data underline the need for randomized studies. *Br J Dermatol* 2000; **142**: 16–21.

62 Evans AV, Wood BP, Scarisbrick JJ *et al.* Extracorporeal photopheresis in Sézary syndrome: hematologic parameters as predictors of response. *Blood* 2001; **98**: 1298–301.

63 Bekkenk MW, van Geelen FA, van Voorst Vader PC *et al.* Primary and secondary cutaneous CD30+ lymphoproliferative disorders: a report from the Dutch cutaneous lymphoma group on the long term follow-up data of 219 patients and guidelines for diagnosis and treatment. *Blood* 2000; **95**: 3653–61.

64 Vonderheid EC, Sajjadian A, Kadin ME. Methotrexate is effective for lymphomatoid papulosis and other primary cutaneous CD30-positive lymphoproliferative disorders. *J Am Acad Dermatol* 1996; **34**: 470–81.

65 Van Doorn R, Scheffer E, Willemze R. Follicular mycosis fungoides, a distinct disease entity with or without associated follicular mucinosis. *Arch Dermatol* 2002; **138**: 191–8.

66 Griffiths CEM. The British Association of Dermatologists guidelines for the management of skin disease. *Br J Dermatol* 1999; **141**: 396–7.

67 Cox NH, Williams HC. The British Association of Dermatologists Therapeutic Guidelines: can we AGREE? *Br J Dermatol* 2003; **148**: 621–5.

Appendix A: WHO classification relating to primary cutaneous T-cell lymphomas

Indolent

- Mycosis fungoides (pagetoid reticulosis/follicular mucinosis)
- Primary cutaneous large cell anaplastic CD30+ lymphoma (pleomorphic/immunoblastic*)
- Lymphomatoid papulosis.

Aggressive

- Sézary syndrome
- Peripheral T-cell lymphoma (large cell CTCL CD30– pleomorphic/immunoblastic*).

Provisional

- Granulomatous slack skin
- Peripheral T-cell lymphoma (CTCL small/medium cell—pleomorphic*)
- Subcutaneous panniculitis like T-cell lymphoma.

(The EORTC classification of primary cutaneous lymphomas[1] recognizes the clinicopathological entities indicated*. Although these other entities are not clearly defined in the WHO classification, some of these primary cutaneous large cell CD30– and small/medium cell pleomorphic lymphomas may represent primary cutaneous extranodal NK-like/T-cell lymphomas (nasal type), blastic NK-cell lymphomas or uncharacterized peripheral T-cell lymphoma as described in the WHO classification.)

Appendix B: clinical staging system for cutaneous T-cell lymphoma

TNM classification

T1: Patches or plaques < 10% body surface area
T2: Patches or plaques > 10% body surface area
T3: Tumours
T4: Erythroderma
N0: No palpable nodes
N1: Palpable nodes without histological involvement (dermatopathic)
N2: Nonpalpable nodes with histological involvement
N3: Palpable nodes with histological involvement
M0: No visceral disease
M1: Visceral disease
B0: No haematological involvement

B1: Sézary count > 5% of total peripheral blood lymphocytes

Bunn & Lambert system

Stage IA: T1 N0
Stage IB: T2 N0
Stage IIA: T1/2 N1
Stage IIB: T3 N0/1
Stage III: T4 N0/1
Stage IVA: T-any N2/3
Stage IVB: T-any N-any M1

(Both staging systems are complementary. Sézary syndrome patients can be stage III, IVA or IVB. The Bunn & Lambert system does not adequately address the issue of peripheral blood involvement in CTCL.)

Appendix C

The consultation process and background details for the British Association of Dermatologists guidelines has been published elsewhere.[66,67]

Strength of recommendations

A There is good evidence to support the use of the procedure.
B There is fair evidence to support the use of the procedure.
C There is poor evidence to support the use of the procedure.
D There is fair evidence to support the rejection of the use of the procedure.
E There is good evidence to support the rejection of the use of the procedure.

Type of evidence

I Evidence obtained from at least one properly designed, randomized controlled trial.
II-i Evidence obtained from well designed controlled trials without randomization
II-ii Evidence obtained from well designed cohort or case–control analytic studies, preferably from more than one centre or research group.
II-iii Evidence obtained from multiple time series with or without the intervention. Dramatic results in uncontrolled experiments (such as the introduction of

penicillin treatment in the 1940s) could also be regarded as this type of evidence.

III Opinions of respected authorities based on clinical experience, descriptive studies or reports of expert committees.

IV Evidence inadequate owing to problems of methodology (e.g. sample size, or length or comprehensiveness of follow-up or conflicts of evidence).

Appendix D: Details of ongoing trials as at April 2003

European Organization for Research and Treatment of Cancer

1 Protocol 21011: a phase III randomized study comparing PUVA with combined PUVA and oral bexarotene in stage IB–IIA mycosis fungoides.

2 Protocol 21012: a phase II study assessing liposomal doxorubicin in stage IIB–IVA mycosis fungoides.

Multicentre studies

1 Protocol 93-04-11: a randomized study assessing two different dosage schedules for denileukin diftitox in stage IB–III CD25+ CTCL compared with placebo.

2 Protocol 93-04-14: an open study assessing denileukin diftitox (18 μg kg^{-1} day^{-1}) in stage IB–III CD25– CTCL patients.

3 Protocol Hx-CD4-007: an open study assessing a fully humanized anti-CD4 antibody in stage IB–IIA primary CTCL.

4 Protocol Hx-CD4-008: an open study assessing a fully humanized anti-CD4 antibody in stage IIB–IVB primary CTCL.

http://bad.org.uk/Portals/_Bad/Guidelines/Clinical
%20Guidelines/Cutaneous%20T%20Cell
%20Lymphoma.pdf

Comment

The management of cutaneous T-cell lymphoma (CTCL) still remains a difficult area with difficulty of making the diagnosis [1] and the heterogeneity of the different types of CTCL [2]. No one has been brave enough to embark on a systematic review of treatments for CTCL. There is a severe lack of evidence to guide us. A recently published review by Prince *et al* sums up the situation [3]:

> The most common subtypes of primary CTCL are mycosis fungoides (MF) and Sézary syndrome (SS). The majority of patients have indolent disease; and given the incurable nature of MF/SS, management should focus on improving symptoms and cosmesis while limiting toxicity. Management of MF/SS should use a 'stage-based' approach; treatment of early-stage disease (IA-IIA) typically involves skin directed therapies that include topical corticosteroids, phototherapy (psoralen plus ultraviolet A radiation or ultraviolet B radiation), topical chemotherapy, topical or systemic bexarotene [4], and radiotherapy. Systemic approaches are used for recalcitrant early-stage disease, advanced-stage disease (IIB-IV), and transformed disease and include retinoids, such as bexarotene, interferon-alpha, histone deacetylase inhibitors, the fusion toxin denileukin diftitox, systemic chemotherapy including transplantation and extracorporeal photopheresis [5]. Examples of drugs under active investigation include new histone deacetylase inhibitors, forodesine, monoclonal antibodies, proteasome inhibitors, and immunomodulatory agents, such as lenalidomide. It is appropriate to consider patients for novel agents within clinical trials if they have failed front-line therapy and before chemotherapy is used.

REFERENCES

1 Whittaker SJ, Marsden JR, Spittle M, Russell Jones R. GUIDE-LINES: Joint British Association of Dermatologists and U.K. Cutaneous Lymphoma Group guidelines for the management of primary cutaneous T-cell lymphomas. *Brit J Dermatol* 2003; 149: 1095–1107.
2 Slater DN. The new World Health Organization classification of haematopoietic and lymphoid tumours: a dermatopathological perspective. *Brit J Dermatol* 2002; 147: 633–9.
3 Prince HM, Whittaker S, Hoppe RT. How I treat mycosis fungoides and Sézary syndrome. *Blood* 2009; 114: 4337–53.
4 Abbott RA, Whittaker SJ, Morris SL, *et al*. Bexarotene therapy for mycosis fungoides and Sézary syndrome. *Brit J Dermatol* 2009; 160: 1299–307.
5 Scarisbrick JJ, Taylor P, Holtick U. U.K. consensus statement on the use of extracorporeal photopheresis for treatment of cutaneous T-cell lymphoma and chronic graft-versus-host disease. *Brit J Dermatol* 2008; 158: 659–78.

Additional professional resources

Best practice in lymphoma diagnosis and reporting. British Committee for Standards in Haematology. http://www.bcshguidelines.com/pdf/best_practice_lymphoma_diagnosis.pdf.

WHO-EORTC classification for cutaneous lymphomas. American Society of Hematology. http://bloodjournal.hematologylibrary.org/cgi/content/full/105/10/3768.

Mycosis fungoides and the Sézary syndrome treatment (PDQ®). National Cancer Institute, USA, 2008. http://www.cancer.gov/cancertopics/pdq/treatment/mycosisfungoides/healthprofessional/.

National Comprehensive Cancer Network (USA) (requires free registration) http://www.nccn.org/professionals/physician_gls/PDF/nhl.pdf (section on Mycosis Fungoides and Sézary syndrome, p 75–85, 2009).

Trautinger F, Knobler R, Willemze R, *et al*. EORTC consensus recommendations for the treatment of mycosis fungoides/Sézary syndrome. *Eur J Cancer* 2006; 42 (8): 1014–30 (http://www.dermnetnz.org/dermal-infiltrative/cutaneous-t-cell-lymphoma.html).

BAD patient information leaflet

http://www.bad.org.uk//site/841/default.aspx

Other patient resources

http://www.clfoundation.org
http://emedicine.medscape.com/article/204529-overview   http://www.dermnetnz.org/dna.CTCL/ctcl.html
http://www.cancer.gov/cancertopics/pdq/treatment/mycosisfungoides/Patient
http://www.lymphomas.org.uk/

4   Specific therapeutic agents

The overwhelming theme of the British Association of Dermatologists' (BAD) therapeutic guidelines is safety. All the drugs pose various hazards of varying severity, which are important for both the clinician and patient to be aware of. These powerful therapies are very effective and the benefit/risk ratio will usually be in favour of benefit. None the less, they all feature highly in terms of clinical governance risk. The various guidelines give clear guidance as to how to minimise that risk with careful monitoring.

British Association of Dermatologists' Management Guidelines, 1st edition. Edited by Neil Cox and John English.

British Association of Dermatologists guidelines on the efficacy and use of acitretin in dermatology

A.D. Ormerod, E. Campalani* and M.J.D. Goodfield†

Department of Dermatology, University of Aberdeen, Foresterhill, Aberdeen AB9 2ZB, U.K.
*Department of Dermatology, Royal London Hospital, Whitechapel Road, London E1 1BB, U.K.
†Department of Dermatology, Leeds General Infirmary, Great George Street, Leeds LS1 3EX, U.K.

This is a new set of guidelines prepared for the BAD Clinical Standards Unit, made up of the Therapy & Guidelines Subcommittee (T&G) and the Audit & Clinical Standards Subcommittee (A&CS). Members of the Clinical Standards Unit are: H.K. Bell (Chairman T&G), L.C. Fuller (Chairman A&CS), N.J. Levell, M.J. Tidman, P.D. Yesudian, J. Lear, J. Hughes, A.J. McDonagh, S. Punjabi, N. Morar, S. Wagle (British National Formulary), S.E. Hulley (British Dermatological Nursing Group), K.J. Lyons (BAD Scientific Administrator) and M.F. Mohd Mustapa (BAD Clinical Standards Manager).

Guidelines produced in 2010 by the British Association of Dermatologists; proposed revision in 2015.

Disclaimer

These guidelines have been prepared on behalf of the British Association of Dermatologists (BAD) and reflect the best data available at the time the report was prepared. Caution should be exercised in interpreting the data; the results of future studies may require alteration of the conclusions or recommendations in this report. It may be necessary or even desirable to depart from the guidelines in the interests of specific patients and special circumstances. Just as adherence to guidelines may not constitute defence against a claim of negligence, so deviation from them should not necessarily be deemed negligent.

DOI 10.1111/j.1365-2133.2010.09755.x

Acitretin, a synthetic retinoid, is the pharmacologically active metabolite of etretinate. It replaced etretinate in the late 1980s because of its more favourable pharmacokinetic profile, and it is an established systemic second-line therapy for severe psoriasis resistant to topical therapy. Bioavailability is enhanced by food, especially fatty food.[1] Acitretin is 50 times less lipophilic than etretinate and has a shorter elimination half-life. However, there is evidence that small amounts of acitretin are re-esterified to etretinate, which has a very long half-life, especially in the presence of alcohol.[2,3] Intracellularly, it interacts with cytosolic proteins and nuclear receptors, which are part of the steroid-thyroid hormone superfamily. We know that these nuclear receptors act as transcriptional factors for specific DNA sequences; however, their role in the retinoid pathway is largely unknown. In psoriasis and other disorders of keratinization, acitretin normalizes epidermal cell proliferation, differentiation and cornification.[4,5] It is thought to exert these effects by interfering with the expression of epidermal growth factor genes. There is also evidence that acitretin has immunomodulatory properties by inhibiting dermal microvascular endothelial cells[6] and neutrophil migration.[7,8] Acitretin is licensed for use in severe extensive psoriasis which is resistant to other forms of therapy, including topical, light and systemic; palmoplantar pustular psoriasis; severe Darier disease (keratosis follicularis) and severe congenital ichthyosis.

It is highly teratogenic and must not be used by women who are pregnant or are planning a pregnancy. Acitretin is highly bound to plasma protein and metabolized in the liver. It is excreted to an equal extent by renal and hepatic routes.

Although available for 20 years there have not been any published guidelines on the use of acitretin. Its clinical use is almost completely restricted to dermatology and it has important metabolic, skeletal and teratogenic side-effects. We felt it important to produce evidence-based guidelines on its use in dermatology.

Materials and methods

A scoping meeting decided that the guideline would include only evidence pertaining to acitretin and would not make direct inferences from studies of the parent drug etretinate. The target audience for the guideline is dermatologists.

Inclusion criteria

We included all randomized controlled trials (RCTs) testing acitretin but also needed to survey the literature on monitoring patients taking acitretin and adverse effects which could include well-designed cohort or case–control analytical studies and, for rare but significant side-effects, case reports.

We included in the search papers written in English, French, Spanish, Italian and German, and those describing adverse drug reactions, clinical monitoring and consensus statements from respected authorities based on clinical experience and consensus committees.

The following databases were searched: EMBASE, MEDLINE, CINAHL, PubMed, The Cochrane Library, RCP Guidelines Database, DARE; this gave 1325 hits. These abstracts were reviewed and, after sifting, 316 papers were reviewed by the authors. The search strategy is available separately online (see Data S1).

Stakeholder involvement and peer review

The draft guideline was made available for consultation and review by the BAD membership. The final document was peer-reviewed by the Clinical Standards Unit of the BAD (made up of the Therapy & Guidelines and Audit & Clinical Standards Subcommittees) prior to publication.

Indications and efficacy: review of the evidence

Psoriasis

We found four RCTs comparing acitretin with placebo[9–12] and four RCTs comparing acitretin with etretinate,[13–16] with one open study.[17] The types of disease in these trials and the results are heterogeneous and include generalized pustular, severe and erythrodermic variants. Acitretin is effective compared with placebo but many of these studies are poorly reported or dose ranging with small numbers in each dosage group. Higher doses of acitretin (50–75 mg daily) are more effective than low doses in these RCTs,[9–11] with lower doses of 10–25 mg daily not significantly better than placebo,[9,11,14] although one trial established efficacy at 25 mg daily.[10] Taken together, the randomized period of these studies is short, and longer-term open extensions with variable doses titrated to the patients' needs suggest greater efficacy over time with reduction in area and increasing percentage of patients cleared between 20 and 52 weeks.[12,17] Twelve-week studies are likely to underestimate the efficacy of acitretin and optimal response will be seen at 12 weeks or later with 70% showing marked improvement at 1 year in the open study.[17] Typically 75% improvement in Psoriasis Area and Severity Index (PASI) score (PASI 75) was seen at 12 weeks.[13] However, only 2–10% cleared completely.

In the comparative studies with etretinate there was a trend for acitretin to be slightly less effective and to present a higher incidence of similar side-effects. In an 8-week trial in 175 patients acitretin at 10, 25 and 50 mg daily produced a 50% improvement in psoriasis in 50%, 40·5% and 54%, respectively, compared with 61% with etretinate.[14] Anecdotal reports also suggest a differential response.[18] Side-effects, like efficacy, were dose related.

Pearce et al.[19] reanalysed retrospectively the pivotal phase three trials and found that common adverse events were two to three times more frequent in patients receiving 50 mg daily compared with patients receiving 25 mg daily. On 25 mg daily changes in liver enzymes and lipids were minimal compared with higher doses. The authors advocated use of a low dose as high doses are limited due to adverse events. Others have advocated gradual dose escalation as optimal.[20]

All studies preceded the now standardized proportion achieving PASI 75 outcome measure. However, 23% of 112 patients achieved 75% improvement in one typical study.[14] In one study 90% improvement was achieved by 10% of patients.[15] A retrospective *post hoc* analysis of the data from three studies was published using the now more widely accepted criteria of the proportion of patients achieving at least 50% improvement in PASI (PASI 50) and at least 75% improvement (PASI 75).[21] This showed 52% achieving PASI 75 and 85% achieving PASI 50 after 12 weeks in the multicentre Nordic trial on a median dose of acitretin 40 mg daily.[13] This was a per protocol analysis. In the Canadian open trial[17] patients started on acitretin 50 mg daily and were tapered to a mean of 40 mg daily. A total of 46% achieved a PASI 75 response and 76% a PASI 50 response by the end of treatment (intent to treat analysis, average duration 267 days).

There is an impression from retrospective anecdotal studies that acitretin is more effective in erythrodermic[22] and pustular psoriasis than in chronic plaque psoriasis.[23] Etretinate was the most effective agent in one study of pustular psoriasis.[24]

In an open study of 396 patients with nail psoriasis who received acitretin in doses of 0·2–0·3 mg kg^{-1} daily for 6 months, the mean improvement in Nail Psoriasis Severity Index was 41% and 25% of patients cleared or almost cleared.[25]

Combination therapy in psoriasis

Acitretin and PUVA

Four RCTs compared acitretin and PUVA (rePUVA) with placebo and PUVA, or additionally etretinate and PUVA in two.[26–28] These show the acitretin-PUVA combination to be more effective than PUVA alone, reducing the number of PUVA treatments, exposure to ultraviolet (UV) A and the clinical scores, and to be as effective as etretinate-PUVA combination. A trend was seen towards a higher incidence of side-effects in the acitretin-treated patients.[28] In considering the preventive action of acitretin against carcinogenesis and the concerns relating to the carcinogenicity of PUVA therapy there are theoretical advantages to this combination which help mitigate the more serious side-effects of PUVA. This is supported for etretinate in the American PUVA cohort[29] where the incidence of squamous cell carcinomas was reduced by retinoids. The same could be said for narrowband UVB where the carcinogenic risk is probably less.

Acitretin and ultraviolet B

One RCT, two open studies and one retrospective study compared acitretin in combination with UVB[24,30–33] with UVB alone. Better outcomes and sparing of UVB were consistently seen with acitretin-UVB in combination than with UVB alone. In a recent RCT acitretin and UVB (TL-01) cleared 55·6% of patients compared with 63·3% treated with acitretin and PUVA.[34]

Acitretin and calcipotriol ointment

Two large RCTs combining acitretin with calcipotriol ointment showed additive benefits of the combination although each relied on subjective outcome measures.[35] In one study the number of patients clear or almost clear was increased from 41% to 67% by the addition of calcipotriol[36] and the number of patients with complete clearance increased in the other from 15% to 40% after 12 weeks.[37]

Other combinations

Acitretin with hydroxycarbamide and with etanercept have anecdotally been effective for some patients with plaque psoriasis.[38] The combination of methotrexate and acitretin has been used in patients with severe psoriasis, where all other treatments have failed.[39,40] This has been based on anecdotal evidence extrapolated from etretinate.[41] Although this combination can be very effective, sporadic severe hepatotoxic responses have been reported.[42–44] The efficacy of concomitant use of acitretin with ciclosporin is not convincing[45] and, in addition, this combination carries the risk of accumulation of ciclosporin as both drugs are inactivated by the same cytochrome P-450 system.[46] A recent RCT showed similar efficacy from the combination regimen of acitretin 0·4 mg kg^{-1} daily and etanercept 25 mg once weekly to that observed with etanercept 25 mg twice weekly. Although a small study, this suggests that the addition of acitretin has an etanercept-sparing effect.[47]

Palmoplantar pustulosis

Two RCTs compared acitretin with placebo in palmoplantar pustulosis.[48,49] Acitretin was significantly more effective than placebo, acting within 4 weeks to produce a fivefold reduction in pustules. After 12 weeks the second study[49] comparing acitretin and etretinate showed a tenfold reduction in pustules which was similar for both retinoids.

Prevention of malignancy

There have been numerous reports of retinoids used as prophylaxis against skin cancer in organ transplant recipients. Three RCTs were systematically reviewed in 2005 by Chen et al.[50]

These included two parallel studies of 44 and 26 patients followed for 6 and 12 months, and a crossover study of 23 patients. Only the short study had a fixed dose of 30 mg daily. Longer-term studies had differing dose regimens. In the study by George et al.[51] acitretin was titrated from 25 mg daily up to 50 mg daily or down to 25 mg on alternate days. In the crossover study there was a 42% decrease in squamous cell carcinoma in the acitretin period compared with drug-free period. A similar trend was seen with basal cell carcinoma although numbers were small. For patients treated for 6 months and off treatment for 6 months, two of 19 patients (11%) in the acitretin group reported a total of two new squamous cell carcinomas during the treatment period, compared with nine of 19 patients (47%) in the placebo group who developed a total of 18 new carcinomas. The two trials counting premalignant lesions showed a significant reduction in these. Keratotic lesions increased by 28% in the placebo group and decreased by 13·4% in the acitretin group.[52] The third study which compared different doses of acitretin did not show a difference in tumour rate between doses of 0·4 mg kg^{-1} daily and 0·4 mg kg^{-1} daily reducing to 0·2 mg kg^{-1} for 9 months, nor a significant reduction compared with that observed in the preceding year without acitretin.[53] However, thickness of lesions was reduced and numbers of actinic keratoses were reduced. Side-effects were a limiting factor in these studies, leading to significant drop-outs, although lower doses were tolerated. Overall these were small studies with a modest reduction in cancer over a short period of observation, and further studies are required.

Other retinoids have anecdotally prevented malignancy in congenital skin cancer syndromes such as xeroderma pigmentosum (isotretinoin)[54] and basal cell naevus syndrome (etretinate)[55,56] and it may be implied that acitretin has a place here.

Congenital ichthyoses and keratoderma

Acitretin has been used in severe forms of the heterogeneous group of the ichthyoses where marked hyperkeratosis is the main pathological component. The evidence for its efficacy is based on anecdotal reports. We found five open series, one of which was prospective, describing its use in the ichthyoses.[57–60] In one, 29 children had conditions including lamellar ichthyosis (9), nonbullous ichthyosiform erythroderma (5), one of whom responded poorly, bullous ichthyosiform erythroderma (4) and Sjögren-Larsson syndrome (3).[57] A patient with Netherton syndrome experienced marked worsening. In another study, 33 patients (21 adults and 12 children) with ichthyoses, palmoplantar hyperkeratosis or Darier disease were treated for a period of 4 months. Most patients showed marked improvement or remission. The results in congenital ichthyosiform erythroderma, lamellar ichthyosis and Papillon-Lefèvre syndrome were judged by the authors empirically as better than those usually reported with etretinate.[59] Milder ichthyoses such as ichthyosis vulgaris and X-linked recessive ichthyosis should not require acitretin therapy.[61] However, six patients with severe X-linked recessive ichthyosis were successfully treated.[62]

Among the keratodermas, Vohwinkel syndrome (keratoderma mutilans with hearing loss), keratitis-ichthyosis-deafness (KID) syndrome,[63] hereditary punctate palmoplantar keratoderma,[64] type I hereditary punctate keratoderma,[65] epidermolytic hyperkeratosis (a rare form of ichthyosis sometimes associated with palmoplantar keratoderma)[66] and Papillon-Lefèvre syndrome[67,68] have all been recently reported as successfully treated with acitretin in small series. Treatment of epidermolytic palmoplantar keratoderma may result in large erosions.[61]

Darier disease

In one RCT, Christopherson et al.[69] compared acitretin with etretinate in 26 patients and found similar rates of marked improvement or remission in both groups, with 10 of 13 patients responding. An open study of five patients[70] showed marked improvement to complete clearance in four. This group found that 10–25 mg daily was sufficient, and lower doses were required in Darier disease than other diseases. This is reflected in the licence. In an open study of 13 patients,[71] three patients cleared and seven improved markedly on 30 mg daily, followed by dose reduction.

Pityriasis rubra pilaris

A single retrospective study of 14 patients, of whom nine were treated with either etretinate or acitretin 0·5 mg kg^{-1} daily for an average period of 18·8 months, achieved partial or complete clearing in seven without major side-effects. Five patients responded to methotrexate 15–25 mg daily but other treatments, including steroids and PUVA, were inconsistent.[72] Although anecdotal, the authors considered retinoids to be the first-line treatment for pityriasis rubra pilaris.

Lichen planus

In one RCT in severe lichen planus (LP), Laurberg et al.[73] showed marked improvement in 64% of patients on acitretin 30 mg daily vs. 13% on placebo. In an open 8-week extension, 83% of the placebo patients responded. A total of 17 of 23 patients with associated mucocutaneous disease improved significantly on acitretin. In a meta-analysis, Cribier et al.[74] included five open studies with 58 patients with oral LP treated with etretinate (mostly poor-quality studies), and one crossover RCT with 28 patients which showed significant improvement with etretinate over placebo. Etretinate was the favoured retinoid therapy. The authors recommend acitretin as first-line therapy in cutaneous LP and give further anecdotal evidence. Acitretin may also be preferred in the hyperkeratotic variant of LP for its modulating effect on keratinization.

Lupus erythematosus

In an RCT of 58 patients[75] comparing acitretin 50 mg daily for 8 weeks with hydroxychloroquine 400 mg daily, improvement was found in 46% and 50%, respectively, but four patients had to stop acitretin because of side-effects which were more frequent in this group. In one open trial of 20 subjects,[76] the result was unsatisfactory in five. In 15 patients, total clearing or marked reduction of all lesions was seen. Acitretin was superior to previous therapy with antimalarials and/or systemic corticosteroids in seven, and five of six patients with subacute cutaneous lupus erythematosus showed complete clearing of their lesions within 2–4 weeks. As in LP, a verrucous variant is seen where the modulation of hyperkeratosis may be an advantage favouring acitretin.

Lichen sclerosus

One RCT randomized 78 patients but only measured efficacy per protocol in 46 subjects. A total of 14 of 22 patients on acitretin responded compared with six of 24 in the placebo group.[77] However, due to the high drop-out rate the study has a high risk of bias (1−; see Appendix 1) and could not be used to make a recommendation.

Other conditions

A 51% reduction in hyperkeratotic hand eczema was seen in one RCT of 29 patients.[78] In one study of mycosis fungoides, PUVA in combination with interferon alfa-2a was superior to acitretin with interferon.[79] The evidence for the use of acitretin for the treatment of warts is sparse and insufficient to base a recommendation. An open study of etretinate in children with severe warts showed clearance in 16 of 20 patients and in four there was improvement then relapse on stopping therapy.[80] However, in this age group warts often clear spontaneously. There are a few case reports of warts clearing with acitretin,[81,82] but in one of these the warts only improved in bulk and recurred on stopping therapy.[82] Acitretin has been used anecdotally as an adjunct to therapy in giant condyloma acuminatum[83] but in this case response was arguably related to excision and imiquimod used in combination. In epidermodysplasia verruciformis acitretin has been suggested as an adjunct in combination with interferon alfa-2a[84] but as monotherapy was ineffective.[85]

Safety and side-effects

Side-effects are seen in most patients receiving acitretin. However, they usually disappear when the dosage is reduced or the medicine is withdrawn. An initial worsening of psoriasis symptoms is sometimes seen at the beginning of the treatment period.

Teratogenicity

Acitretin is teratogenic regardless of the duration of treatment or dosage used. Although since the marketing of acitretin only one report of human teratogenicity associated with acitretin has been published, acitretin is converted to etretinate, which has a much longer half-life and has been associated with several cases of retinoid-induced embryopathy.[86–88] Potential teratogenic effects associated with retinoids are characteristic of those associated with hypervitaminosis A.[89,90] Retinoid embryopathy can result in craniofacial dysmorphias such as high palate and anophthalmia, abnormalities of appendages including syndactyly and absence of terminal phalanges, malformations of the hip, meningoencephalocele, and multiple synostosis.[89–92] The teratogenic risk is particularly high for women exposed to treatment during the first trimester of pregnancy. Available data do not appear to indicate any reproductive safety risks due to paternal treatment with acitretin.[93]

Mucocutaneous effects

The most frequent side-effect is dryness of the lips, which can be alleviated by application of a fatty ointment such as Vaseline® (Unilever, Walton-on-Thames, U.K.). Mucous membranes and transitional epithelia become dried out or exhibit inflammatory lesions. This can occasionally lead to nose bleeds and rhinitis, and to ocular disturbances including photophobia, xerophthalmia and conjunctivitis sometimes resulting in intolerance of contact lenses. Cheilitis, dry mouth and thirst may also occur. Occasionally stomatitis, gingivitis and taste disturbances have been reported.

Thinning, redness and scaling of the skin may occur all over the body, particularly on the palms and soles. For many patients the increased sensitivity and fragility of the skin make walking and grasping objects difficult.

Increased hair loss, nail fragility and paronychia are sometimes observed. Hair loss can occur in up to 75% of patients, but frank alopecia is observed in < 10% of treated patients. Periungual pyogenic granuloma may occur after long-term acitretin therapy. Occasionally bullous eruption and abnormal hair texture have been reported.

Rarely, patients may experience photosensitivity reactions.

Another side-effect is the initial aggravation of psoriasis, which is sometimes seen during the first 4 weeks of treatment. A 'retinoid dermatitis', which may resemble unstable psoriasis, can also develop in up to 25% of patients receiving high-dose oral acitretin.[13,94,95] The severity of mucocutaneous side-effects was found to be dose related in some studies, with a higher incidence at doses of 50–75 mg daily.[13,94,95] However, this was not found to be the case in other studies.[9,14]

If severe mucocutaneous reactions occur during effective therapy with acitretin, dose reduction should be attempted before discontinuing the drug.

Hepatotoxicity

Transient, usually reversible, elevation of liver enzymes may occur in up to 15% of patients receiving acitretin.[22,90]

Severe hepatotoxic reactions resulting from retinoid use are rare, and reports include a severe cholestatic hepatitis occurring in a patient with a hypoplastic kidney,[11,96] and a severe hepatotoxic reaction with progression to liver cirrhosis.[90,97,98] However, data from 1877 patients receiving acitretin therapy

showed overt chemical hepatitis in only 0·26%.[90] A total of 83 patients followed by liver biopsy for 2 years showed no significant hepatotoxicity with acitretin other than mild changes.[97] Alcoholics, diabetics and obese individuals are at increased risk for hepatotoxicity and require more frequent liver function studies.

Hyperlipidaemia

Hyperlipidaemia is proportional to the dose of acitretin and usually reverses within 4–8 weeks after discontinuation.[99] The greatest increase is seen in triglycerides, which occurs in 20–40% of patients, and is associated with the very low density lipoprotein (VLDL) fraction. Hypercholesterolaemia, seen in 10–30% of patients treated with acitretin, relates to increases in both the VLDL and/or low density lipoprotein (LDL) fractions and a parallel decrease in the high density lipoprotein (HDL) fraction.[99] In addition, HDL levels have been found to be decreased in about 40% of patients taking acitretin.[100] The LDL/HDL ratio (atherogenic index) has been directly correlated to the risk of developing cardiovascular disease, and therefore fasting lipids should be regularly checked in all patients receiving treatment with acitretin. Increases of serum triglycerides to levels associated with pancreatitis are not common, although one case of fatal fulminant pancreatitis has been reported.[90]

These changes in the lipid profile are dose related and may be controlled by dietary means (including restriction of alcohol intake) and/or by reduction of dosage of acitretin. A high fish oil diet was found effective in partially reducing hypertriglyceridaemia and increasing HDL cholesterol in patients treated with etretinate and acitretin.[100] Gemfibrozil taken orally is also effective, if required.[101] Hypertriglyceridaemia is likely to occur in patients with predisposing factors such as diabetes mellitus, obesity, increased alcohol intake, or a family history of these conditions.

Skeletal abnormalities

The effects of acitretin on the skeletal system are not yet well documented; however, available data suggest similarities to etretinate.[102,103] Long-term (2–4 years) treatment with etretinate was associated with radiographic evidence of extraspinal tendon and ligament calcification. However, estimates of the incidence vary widely, the most common sites being ankles, pelvis and knees.[104,105] Diffuse idiopathic skeletal hyperostosis (DISH)-like involvement, characterized by degenerative spondylosis, vertebral arthritis, and syndesmophytes of the vertebral spine, has been reported as a side-effect of systemic retinoids. Two long-term retrospective studies involved repeated radiological surveys to detect abnormalities but no correlation with dose or duration of treatment has been shown.[105] This study in 135 patients showed no evidence of a link between hyperostosis and prolonged retinoid therapy. A prospective study of 51 patients treated with acitretin over 2 years revealed bone exostoses in only two patients (in the hip and forearm) that would not have been detected using lateral spine X-rays.[106] A further retrospective study of long-term acitretin revealed no cases of DISH.[107] Regular radiological evaluations have been suggested in the literature but the evidence does not support this practice which exposes subjects to unnecessary radiation; our consensus is that routine radiographic assessments are not required for long-term acitretin therapy. Targeted X-rays for atypical musculoskeletal pain may be informative.

Concern about the use of acitretin in children has arisen from occasional reports of bone changes, including premature epiphyseal closure,[108] skeletal hyperostosis and extraosseous calcification in children on long-term treatment with etretinate.[109] It should be noted that very high dose exposure in one case led to osteopenia and fractures in the bones that fused prematurely and in the other case premature closure was a symptomless observation on X-rays.[108] Five children treated with etretinate had periosteal thickening in the fibula, ulna, metacarpal or metatarsal bones that either developed or progressed on therapy. Compared with age- and sex-matched normal controls, the children had decreased cortical bone thickness of the second left metacarpal bone. However, prospective follow-up of 42 children treated over 11 years did not reveal any abnormalities that would significantly impede starting or continuing therapy.[110] Effects on growth have not subsequently been seen in a further 18 children treated with retinoids at Great Ormond Street Hospital (David Atherton, personal communication).

If, in the opinion of the treating physician, the child's condition is severe enough to be physically, psychologically or socially incapacitating and such therapy is undertaken because the benefits outweigh the risks, then the child should be clinically monitored for any abnormalities of growth parameters and bone development. An appropriate daily dose in children under 12 years of age is 0.5 mg kg^{-1}; occasionally this can be increased up to 1 mg kg^{-1}.

Other rheumatological manifestations that may occur during therapy with acitretin include arthralgias, arthritis, myalgia, and a few cases of vasculitis, Wegener granulomatosis and erythema nodosum. Arthralgia and myalgia represent the most frequent rheumatological sequelae, occurring in up to 25% of patients.[111]

Two previous small studies indicated a possible increased risk of osteoporosis in subjects receiving etretinate and this is a feature of the hypervitaminosis A syndrome;[112,113] however, a further study has refuted this risk[114] and in a prospective study of 30 patients treated for 3.6 years with acitretin, osteoporosis was not detected on DEXA scans.[114]

Other side-effects

Benign intracranial hypertension (pseudotumor cerebri) has occurred in very rare cases with use of systemic retinoids including one instance following acitretin use.[90,115] In some cases with isotretinoin, this effect has been associated with concurrent tetracycline or minocycline administration.[116] Patients with severe headache, nausea, vomiting and visual disturbance should discontinue acitretin immediately and be referred for neurological evaluation.

Blurred or decreased night vision has been reported occasionally.[22]

Nausea has been reported infrequently.[22]

Increased incidence of vulvovaginitis due to *Candida albicans* has been noted during treatment with acitretin.[117]

Retinoids are associated with greater insulin sensitivity and could therefore induce hypoglycaemia in patients on antidiabetic medications.[118] These patients should be advised to check their capillary glucose levels regularly, perhaps more frequently than usual, in the early stages of treatment.

Acitretin does not significantly affect wound healing. There is some evidence that healing was delayed by retinoids in diabetic rats[119] and that epidermal proliferation was reduced by acitretin in psoriasis.[120] However, in a study of 44 complex wounds in transplant recipients there were no significant effects on wound infection, dehiscence, hypertrophic scarring or hypergranulation. There is therefore no need to stop acitretin for routine surgery such as orthopaedic procedures.[121]

Overdose

Signs and symptoms of overdosage with acitretin would probably be similar to acute vitamin A toxicity and include headache, nausea, vomiting, drowsiness and vertigo. They would be expected to subside on acitretin withdrawal without need for treatment.

Recommendations

See Appendix 1 for definitions of levels of evidence and strengths of recommendation.

In which conditions should acitretin be used?

Acitretin monotherapy is recommended in the treatment of:

1 Severe psoriasis, or psoriasis with severe effects on quality of life, meriting systemic therapy, which is resistant to topical therapy, phototherapy or is unsuitable for these treatments (A, 1+).
1.1 Acitretin is recommended as a combination with PUVA therapy or narrowband phototherapy (A, 1+).
1.2 Acitretin is recommended with hydroxycarbamide (D, 3)
1.3 Acitretin is recommended in combination with calcipotriol ointment (A, 1+).
1.4 The following combinations are not recommended:
Acitretin with ciclosporin: no evidence of additive efficacy (D, 3).
Acitretin with methotrexate: potential for severe hepatic toxicity (except in exceptional cases) (D, 3).
2 Palmoplantar pustular psoriasis (A, 1+).
3 Hyperkeratotic hand eczema (A, 1+).
4 Severe Darier disease (keratosis follicularis) (A, 1+).
5 Severe congenital ichthyosis (D, 3).
6 Keratoderma (D, 3).
There is evidence that the following conditions benefit from acitretin's antimitotic and keratolytic actions:

1 Lichen planus (A, 1+)

---

2 Lichen sclerosus (A, 1+)

3 Discoid lupus erythematosus (A, 1+)

4 Prevention of cutaneous malignancies in organ transplant patients (A, 1+).

What are the contraindications to acitretin therapy?

1 Acitretin therapy is contraindicated in pregnancy and breast-feeding.

2 Acitretin therapy in the above indications should be avoided in women of childbearing potential where there is a suitable alternative.

What precautions should be taken when acitretin is prescribed for women of childbearing age?

- Strict contraception is practised 4 weeks before, during and for 3 years after treatment.
- Pregnancy has been excluded by a medically supervised negative pregnancy test within 2 weeks prior to therapy.
- Therapy should start on the second or third day of the next menstrual cycle.
- The treating physician must explain clearly and in detail what precautions must be taken. This should include the risk involved and the possible consequences of pregnancy occurring during acitretin treatment or in the 3 years following its cessation.
- The patient must be reliable and capable of understanding the risk and complying with effective contraception, and confirms that she has understood the warnings.
- The patient should be advised to abstain from alcohol which increases the metabolism of acitretin to etretinate.
- Acitretin therapy should be avoided in the presence of significant hepatic impairment (enzymes > 2 times normal), hepatitis and alcohol abuse.
- Acitretin therapy should be avoided in moderate to severe renal impairment.

What special precautions should be taken when prescribing acitretin?

- Patients should not donate blood either during or for at least 1 year following discontinuation of therapy.
- Acitretin is not recommended in children, as there have been occasional reports of bone changes, including premature epiphyseal closure, skeletal hyperostosis and extraosseous calcification in children on long-term treatment with etretinate.[108,122,123] If, in the opinion of the treating physician, the benefits significantly outweigh the risks and such therapy is undertaken, the child should be carefully monitored for any abnormalities of growth parameters and bone development including plotting growth charts.
- The effects of UV radiation are enhanced by retinoid therapy, therefore patients should avoid excessive exposure to sunlight and use of sun lamps.
- Women (and men) should refrain from waxing as a method for hair removal as retinoids cause skin fragility.

- Retinoids are associated with greater insulin sensitivity and could therefore induce hypoglycaemia in patients on antidiabetic medications.[118,124] In this subset of patients, serum glucose levels should be checked more frequently than usual in the early stages of treatment.
- People with diabetes, alcoholism and obesity need to be monitored more frequently as they have an increased risk of hypertriglyceridaemia.
- Advice against exceeding recommended daily intake of vitamin A (2400–3000 IU daily, i.e. 0·8–1 mg daily) should be given.[125]

What drugs can interact with acitretin?

Clinically significant interactions may occur with the following drugs, which should be avoided or used with caution:

- **Methotrexate**
  Increased risk of liver toxicity. Sporadic episodes of toxic hepatitis have been reported following the concomitant use of etretinate and methotrexate.[42,44]
- **Tetracycline**
  In some cases with other retinoids, benign intracranial hypertension has been associated with concurrent tetracycline or minocycline administration.[90] In the single reported case of pseudotumor cerebri occurring in a patient on acitretin, however, neither tetracycline nor minocycline was involved.[90]
- **Mini-pill**
  Acitretin decreases the anti-ovulatory effect of the progestin-only pill (mini-pill) but has no effect on the combined preparations.[126,127]
- **Phenytoin**
  Acitretin partially reduces the protein binding of phenytoin. The clinical significance of this is as yet unknown.
- **Antidiabetic agents**
  Increased risk of hypoglycaemia.
- **Corticosteroids**
  Increased risk of hyperlipidaemia.
- **Vitamin A**
  Intake should not exceed the recommended dietary allowance (2400–3000 IU daily).

What are the preliminary investigations prior to starting acitretin?

- **Teratogenicity**
  In women of childbearing age pregnancy must be excluded by negative pregnancy test within 2 weeks prior to therapy. Acitretin should be started only on the second or third day of the next menstrual cycle. Effective contraception must be practised for at least 4 weeks before and during therapy with acitretin, and for 3 years after treatment with acitretin has ceased.[128] In the U.S.A. it is recommended that contraception is practised for at least 3 years after discontinuation of acitretin therapy.[129] According to the label in Europe contraception is mandated for at least 2 years after treatment. There are no pharmacokinetic reasons for this discrepancy and the opinion of the guideline development group was to err on the side of caution and to give consistent patient advice. We have therefore recommended continuing contraceptive measures for 3 years.

- **Liver disease**
  Enquire regarding past or current history of liver disease, excess alcohol intake, and hepatotoxic drugs.
  Check alanine aminotransferase, aspartate aminotransferase, γ-glutamyltransferase, alkaline phosphatase, bilirubin.
- **Renal disease**
  Enquire regarding past or current history of renal disease, nephrotoxic drugs.
  Check urea, electrolytes and creatinine.
- **Hyperlipidaemia**
  Enquire regarding past or current history of disturbances of lipid metabolism, diabetes mellitus, obesity, alcoholism.
  Check fasting cholesterol, triglycerides.
- **Abnormal glucose tolerance**
  Enquire regarding history of diabetes mellitus, antidiabetic drugs.
  Check fasting glucose.
- **Bone changes**
  The effects of acitretin on the skeletal system are rare; however, available data[130] suggest possible similarities to etretinate. Long-term etretinate and isotretinoin treatment is associated with periosteal thickening, premature epiphyseal closure in children, osteophyte formation, extraspinal tendon and ligament calcification and DISH (diffuse idiopathic skeletal hyperostosis)-like involvement.[104,130] Routine radiography has no place in the monitoring of acitretin therapy and is potentially harmful. Musculoskeletal pain is common and only if atypical would we recommend targeted investigation with X-rays. Children taking acitretin should have their growth charted.

How should acitretin be prescribed?

Therapy should be initiated only under the responsibility of a supervising dermatologist

The capsules should be taken once daily with meals or with milk.[131] Acitretin necessitates individual adjustment of dosage in view of the fact that there is a wide variation in its absorption and rate of metabolism. In addition, both therapeutic and toxic responses to the drug are dose dependent and vary greatly among individual patients. For these reasons the following dosage recommendations can serve only as a guide.

Adults

Effective doses of acitretin as a single agent appear to be in the range of 25–50 mg daily.[20,94] Gradual dose escalation has been shown to be the most effective approach and allows gradual onset of 'tolerance' to side-effects.[94,132] The initial daily dose, 25 mg or 30 mg for 2–4 weeks, may give satisfactory therapeutic results. The maintenance dose must be based on clinical efficacy and tolerability. In general, a daily dose of 25–50 mg taken for a further 6–8 weeks achieves optimal therapeutic results. It may be necessary in some cases to increase the dose up to a maximum of 75 mg daily. Response is gradual and typically requires 3–6 months to reach a peak. Therapy can be discontinued in patients with psoriasis whose lesions have improved sufficiently. Relapses should be treated as described above.

In patients with Darier disease a starting dose of 10 mg daily may be appropriate. Patients with severe congenital ichthyosis and Darier disease are likely to require long-term treatment with acitretin, as are some patients with psoriasis; therefore the lowest effective dosage, not exceeding 50 mg daily, should be given.

How should acitretin therapy be monitored?

This is the responsibility of the supervising dermatologist; responsibility may be shared with the patient's general practitioner following mutual agreement and locally agreed protocol

- Liver enzymes every 2–4 weeks for the first 2 months of therapy and then every 3 months. If abnormal results are obtained, weekly checks should be instituted and acitretin dose adjusted accordingly. Acitretin should be discontinued if transaminases are elevated to three times their upper normal limit, and patients with bilirubin > 50 µmol L^{-1} or alanine aminotransferase > 200 IU L^{-1} should be referred to gastroenterology. In such cases it is advisable to continue monitoring hepatic function for at least 3 months. However, in those patients where the disease is particularly severe and all else has failed, therapy with acitretin could be continued in consultation with a gastroenterologist and would require a liver biopsy.
- Fasting serum cholesterol and triglycerides every 2–4 weeks for the first 2 months and then every 3 months. In the presence of a good therapeutic response to acitretin but persistently elevated lipid levels, dietary measures should be introduced before considering a lipid-lowering drug. Patients with triglycerides > 5 mmol L^{-1} should be referred to a lipidologist and investigated for other causes of hypertriglyceridaemia (e.g. alcohol, systemic lupus erythematosus, diabetes mellitus, hypothyroidism, renal and hepatic problems, hormonal dysfunction etc.). Hypertriglyceridaemia approaching or over 10 mmol L^{-1} warrants discontinuation of acitretin and urgent referral to a lipidologist, as it is a risk factor for acute pancreatitis.
- Blood sugar levels in diabetic patients on insulin or antiglycaemic agents should also be monitored at similar intervals. These patients should check their capillary glucose more frequently than usual during the first few weeks of treatment.
- Radiological investigation for skeletal changes need not be done routinely as there is a risk from exposure to radiation, the site of ossification is unpredictable and asymptomatic, and abnormal findings are common in normal individuals. However, targeted X-rays are indicated in patients becoming symptomatic.

Audit points

1 Acitretin therapy is not being used in women of childbearing potential where there is a suitable alternative.
2 Where acitretin is used in a woman of childbearing potential contraception is discussed and undertaken for 3 years.
3 Three-monthly laboratory tests are ordered including liver function and lipids, with action if limits are exceeded.

Acknowledgments

We thank Cynthia Fraser of the Health Services Research Unit, University of Aberdeen for technical assistance with literature searching.

References

1 McNamara PJ, Jewell RC, Jensen BK et al. Food increases the bio-availability of acitretin. J Clin Pharmacol 1988; 28:1051–5.

2 Larsen FG, Jakobsen P, Knudsen J et al. Conversion of acitretin to etretinate in psoriatic patients is influenced by ethanol. J Invest Dermatol 1993; 100:623–7.

3 Larsen FG, Steinkjer B, Jakobsen P et al. Acitretin is converted to etretinate only during concomitant alcohol intake. Br J Dermatol 2000; 143:1164–9.

4 Tong PS, Horowitz NN, Wheeler LA. Trans retinoic acid enhances the growth response of epidermal keratinocytes to epidermal growth factor and transforming growth factor beta. J Invest Dermatol 1990; 94:126–31.

5 Zheng ZS, Polakowska R, Johnson A et al. Transcriptional control of epidermal growth factor receptor by retinoic acid. Cell Growth Differ 1992; 3:225–32.

6 Imcke E, Ruszczak Z, Mayer-da Silva A et al. Cultivation of human dermal microvascular endothelial cells in vitro: immunocytochemical and ultrastructural characterization and effect of treatment with three synthetic retinoids. Arch Dermatol Res 1991; 283:149–57.

7 Bauer R, Schutz R, Orfanos CE. Impaired motility and random migration of vital polymorphonuclears in vitro after therapy with oral aromatic retinoid in psoriasis. Int J Dermatol 1984; 23:72–7.

8 Becherel PA, Mossalayi MD, LeGoff L et al. Mechanism of anti-inflammatory action of retinoids on keratinocytes. Lancet 1994; 344:1570–1.

9 Goldfarb MT, Ellis CN, Gupta AK et al. Acitretin improves psoriasis in a dose-dependent fashion. J Am Acad Dermatol 1988; 18:655–62.

10 Lassus A, Geiger JM, Nyblom M et al. Treatment of severe psoriasis with etretin (Ro-10-1670). Br J Dermatol 1987; 117:333–41.

11 Gupta AK, Goldfarb MT, Ellis CN et al. Side-effect profile of acitretin therapy in psoriasis. J Am Acad Dermatol 1989; 20:1088–93.

12 Olsen EA, Weed WW, Meyer CJ et al. A double-blind, placebo-controlled trial of acitretin for the treatment of psoriasis. J Am Acad Dermatol 1989; 21:681–6.

13 Kragballe K, Jansen CT, Geiger JM et al. A double-blind comparison of acitretin and etretinate in the treatment of severe psoriasis – results of a Nordic multicenter study. Acta Derm Venereol (Stockh) 1989; 69:35–40.

14 Gollnick H, Bauer R, Brindley C et al. Acitretin versus etretinate in psoriasis – clinical and pharmacokinetic results of a German multicenter study. J Am Acad Dermatol 1988; 19:458–68.

15 Meffert H, Sonnichsen N. Acitretin in the treatment of severe psoriasis: a randomized double-blind study comparing acitretin and etretinate. Acta Derm Venereol (Stockh) 1989; 146 (Suppl.):176–7.

16 Ledo A, Martin M, Geiger JM et al. Acitretin (Ro 10-1670) in the treatment of severe psoriasis – a randomized double-blind parallel study comparing acitretin and etretinate. Int J Dermatol 1988; 27:656–60.

17 Murray HE, Anhalt AW, Lessard R et al. A 12-month treatment of severe psoriasis with acitretin – results of a Canadian open multi-center study. J Am Acad Dermatol 1991; 24:598–602.

18 Bleiker TO, Bourke JF, Graham-Brown RA et al. Etretinate may work where acitretin fails. Br J Dermatol 1997; 136:368–70.

19 Pearce DJ, Klinger S, Ziel KK et al. Low-dose acitretin is associated with fewer adverse events than high-dose acitretin in the treatment of psoriasis. Arch Dermatol 2006; 142:1000–4.

20 Ling MR. Acitretin: optimal dosing strategies. J Am Acad Dermatol 1999; 41:S13–17.

21 Geiger JM. Efficacy of acitretin in severe psoriasis. Skin Ther Lett 2003; 8:1–3.

22 van de Kerkhof PC. Update on retinoid therapy of psoriasis in: an update on the use of retinoids in dermatology. Dermatol Ther 2006; 19:252–63.

23 Magis NL, Blummel JJ, van de Kerkhof PC et al. The treatment of psoriasis with etretinate and acitretin: a follow up of actual use. Eur J Dermatol 2000; 10:517–21.

24 Ozawa A, Ohkido M, Haruki Y et al. Treatments of generalized pustular psoriasis: a multicenter study in Japan. J Dermatol 1999; 26:141–9.

25 Tosti A, Ricotti C, Romanelli P et al. Evaluation of the efficacy of acitretin therapy for nail psoriasis. Arch Dermatol 2009; 145:269–71.

26 Sommerburg C, Kietzmann H, Eichelberg D et al. Acitretin in combination with PUVA: a randomized double-blind placebo-controlled study in severe psoriasis. J Eur Acad Dermatol Venereol 1993; 2:308–17.

27 Saurat JH, Geiger JM, Amblard P et al. Randomized double-blind multicenter study comparing acitretin-PUVA, etretinate-PUVA and placebo-PUVA in the treatment of severe psoriasis. Dermatologica 1988; 177:218–24.

28 Lauharanta J, Geiger JM. A double-blind comparison of acitretin and etretinate in combination with bath PUVA in the treatment of extensive psoriasis. Br J Dermatol 1989; 121:107–12.

29 Nijsten TE, Stern RS. Oral retinoid use reduces cutaneous squamous cell carcinoma risk in patients with psoriasis treated with psoralen-UVA: a nested cohort study. J Am Acad Dermatol 2003; 49:644–50.

30 Iest J, Boer J. Combined treatment of psoriasis with acitretin and UVB phototherapy compared with acitretin alone and UVB alone. Br J Dermatol 1989; 120:665–70.

31 Ruzicka T, Sommerburg C, Braun-Falco O et al. Efficiency of acitretin in combination with UV-B in the treatment of severe psoriasis. Arch Dermatol 1990; 126:482–6.

32 Lowe NJ, Prystowsky JH, Bourget T et al. Acitretin plus UVB therapy for psoriasis. Comparisons with placebo plus UVB and acitretin alone. J Am Acad Dermatol 1991; 24:591–4.

33 Kampitak T, Asawanonda P. The efficacy of combination treatment with narrowband UVB (TL-01) and acitretin vs narrowband UVB alone in plaque-type psoriasis: a retrospective study. J Med Assoc Thai 2006; 89 (Suppl. 3):S20–4.

34 Ozdemir M, Engin B, Baysal I et al. A randomized comparison of acitretin–narrow-band TL-01 phototherapy and acitretin–psoralen plus ultraviolet A for psoriasis. Acta Derm Venereol (Stockh) 2008; 88:589–93.

35 van de Kerkhof PC. Topical use of calcipotriol improves the outcome in acitretin treated patients with severe psoriasis vulgaris. Br J Dermatol 1996; 135 (Suppl. 47):30 (Abstract).

36 van de Kerkhof PC, Cambazard F, Hutchinson PE et al. The effect of addition of calcipotriol ointment (50 micrograms/g) to acitretin therapy in psoriasis. Br J Dermatol 1998; 138:84–9.

37 Rim JH, Park JY, Choe YB et al. The efficacy of calcipotriol + acitretin combination therapy for psoriasis: comparison with acitretin monotherapy. Am J Clin Dermatol 2003; 4:507–10.

38 Yamauchi PS, Ria D, Lowe NJ. Retinoid therapy for psoriasis. Dermatol Clin 2004; 22:467–76.

39 Lebwohl M, Menter A, Koo J et al. Combination therapy to treat moderate to severe psoriasis. J Am Acad Dermatol 2004; 50:416–30.

40 Roenigk HH. Acitretin combination therapy. J Am Acad Dermatol 1999; 41:S18–21.

41 Vanderveen EE, Ellis CN, Campbell JP *et al*. Methotrexate and etretinate as concurrent therapies in severe psoriasis. *Arch Dermatol* 1982; **118**:660–2.

42 Beck HI, Foged EK. Toxic hepatitis due to combination therapy with methotrexate and etretinate in psoriasis. *Dermatologica* 1983; **167**:94–6.

43 Harrison PV, Peat M, James R, Orrell D. Methotrexate and retinoids in combination for psoriasis. *Lancet* 1987; **ii**: 512.

44 Zachariae H. Methotrexate and etretinate as concurrent therapies in the treatment of psoriasis. *Arch Dermatol* 1984; **120**:155.

45 Kuijpers ALA, van Dooren-Geebe RJ, van de Kerkhof PCM. Failure of combination therapy with acitretin and cyclosporin A in 3 patients with erythrodermic psoriasis. *Dermatology* 1997; **194**:88–90.

46 Webber IR, Back DJ. Effect of etretinate on cyclosporin metabolism in vitro. *Br J Dermatol* 1993; **128**:42–4.

47 Gisondi P, Del Giglio M, Cotena C *et al*. Combining etanercept and acitretin in the therapy of chronic plaque psoriasis: a 24-week, randomized, controlled, investigator-blinded pilot trial. *Br J Dermatol* 2008; **158**:1345–9.

48 Schroder K, Zaun H, Holzmann H *et al*. Pustulosis palmo-plantaris. Clinical and histological changes during etretin (acitretin) therapy. *Acta Derm Venereol (Stockh)* 1989; **146** (Suppl.):111–16.

49 Lassus A, Geiger JM. Acitretin and etretinate in the treatment of palmoplantar pustulosis: a double-blind comparative trial. *Br J Dermatol* 1988; **119**:755–9.

50 Chen K, Craig JC, Shumack S. Oral retinoids for the prevention of skin cancers in solid organ transplant recipients: a systematic review of randomized controlled trials. *Br J Dermatol* 2005; **152**:518–23.

51 George R, Weightman W, Russ GR *et al*. Acitretin for chemoprevention of non-melanoma skin cancers in renal transplant recipients. *Australas J Dermatol* 2002; **43**:269–73.

52 Bavinck JN, Tieben LM, van der Woude FJ *et al*. Prevention of skin cancer and reduction of keratotic skin lesions during acitretin therapy in renal transplant recipients: a double-blind, placebo-controlled study. *J Clin Oncol* 1995; **13**:1933–8.

53 de Sevaux RG, Smit JV, de Jong EM *et al*. Acitretin treatment of premalignant and malignant skin disorders in renal transplant recipients: clinical effects of a randomized trial comparing two doses of acitretin. *J Am Acad Dermatol* 2003; **49**:407–12.

54 DiGiovanna JJ. Retinoid chemoprevention in patients at high risk for skin cancer. *Med Pediatr Oncol* 2001; **36**:564–7.

55 Berth-Jones J, Cole J, Lehmann AR *et al*. Xeroderma pigmentosum variant: 5 years of tumour suppression by etretinate. *J R Soc Med* 1993; **86**:355–6.

56 Berth-Jones J, Graham-Brown RA. Xeroderma pigmentosum variant: response to etretinate. *Br J Dermatol* 1990; **122**:559–61.

57 Lacour M, Mehta-Nikhar B, Atherton DJ, Harper JI. An appraisal of acitretin therapy in children with inherited disorders of keratinization. *Br J Dermatol* 1996; **134**:1023–9.

58 Katugampola RP, Finlay AY. Oral retinoid therapy for disorders of keratinization: single-centre retrospective 25 years' experience on 23 patients. *Br J Dermatol* 2006; **154**:267–76.

59 Blanchet-Bardon C, Nazzaro V, Rognin C *et al*. Acitretin in the treatment of severe disorders of keratinization. Results of an open study. *J Am Acad Dermatol* 1991; **24**:982–6.

60 Kullavanijaya P, Kulthanan K. Clinical efficacy and side effects of acitretin on the disorders of keratinization: a one-year study. *J Dermatol* 1993; **20**:501–6.

61 Happle R, van de Kerkhof PC, Traupe H. Retinoids in disorders of keratinization: their use in adults. *Dermatologica* 1987; **175** (Suppl. 1):107–24.

62 Bruckner-Tuderman L, Sigg C, Geiger JM *et al*. Acitretin in the symptomatic therapy for severe recessive X-linked ichthyosis. *Arch Dermatol* 1988; **124**:529–32.

63 Bondeson ML, Nystrom AM, Gunnarsson U *et al*. Connexin 26 (GJB2) mutations in two Swedish patients with atypical Vohwinkel (mutilating keratoderma plus deafness) and KID syndrome both extensively treated with acitretin. *Acta Derm Venereol (Stockh)* 2006; **86**:503–8.

64 Al-Mutairi N, Joshi A, Nour-Eldin O. Punctate palmoplantar keratoderma (Buschke-Fischer-Brauer disease) with psoriasis: a rare association showing excellent response to acitretin. *J Drugs Dermatol* 2005; **4**:627–34.

65 Erkek E, Erdogan S, Tuncez F *et al*. Type I hereditary punctate keratoderma associated with widespread lentigo simplex and successfully treated with low-dose oral acitretin. *Arch Dermatol* 2006; **142**:1076–7.

66 Virtanen M, Gedde-Dahl T, Mork NJ *et al*. Phenotypic/genotypic correlations in patients with epidermolytic hyperkeratosis and the effects of retinoid therapy on keratin expression. *Acta Derm Venereol (Stockh)* 2001; **81**:163–70.

67 Camacho F, Bullon P. Papillon-Lefèvre syndrome: study of three siblings. *Eur J Dermatol* 1992; **2**:421–3.

68 Lundgren T, Crossner CG, Twetman S *et al*. Systemic retinoid medication and periodontal health in patients with Papillon-Lefèvre syndrome. *J Clin Periodontol* 1996; **23**:176–9.

69 Christophersen J, Geiger JM, Danneskiold-Samsoe P *et al*. A double-blind comparison of acitretin and etretinate in the treatment of Darier's disease. *Acta Derm Venereol (Stockh)* 1992; **72**:150–2.

70 van Dooren-Greebe RJ, van de Kerkhof PC, Happle R. Acitretin monotherapy in Darier's disease. *Br J Dermatol* 1989; **121**:375–9.

71 Lauharanta J, Kanerva L, Turjanmaa K *et al*. Clinical and ultrastructural effects of acitretin in Darier's disease. *Acta Derm Venereol (Stockh)* 1988; **68**:492–8.

72 Chapalain V, Beylot-Barry M, Doutre MS *et al*. Treatment of pityriasis rubra pilaris: a retrospective study of 14 patients. *J Dermatolog Treat* 1999; **10**:113–17.

73 Laurberg G, Geiger JM, Hjorth N *et al*. Treatment of lichen planus with acitretin. A double-blind, placebo-controlled study in 65 patients. *J Am Acad Dermatol* 1991; **24**:434–7.

74 Cribier B, Frances C, Chosidow O. Treatment of lichen planus: an evidence-based medicine analysis of efficacy. *Arch Dermatol* 1998; **134**:1521–30.

75 Ruzicka T, Sommerburg C, Goerz G *et al*. Treatment of cutaneous lupus erythematosus with acitretin and hydroxychloroquine. *Br J Dermatol* 1992; **127**:513–18.

76 Ruzicka T, Meurer M, Bieber T. Efficiency of acitretin in the treatment of cutaneous lupus erythematosus. *Arch Dermatol* 1988; **124**:897–902.

77 Bousema MT, Romppanen U, Geiger JM *et al*. Acitretin in the treatment of severe lichen sclerosus et atrophicus of the vulva: a double-blind, placebo-controlled study. *J Am Acad Dermatol* 1994; **30**:225–31.

78 Thestrup-Pedersen K, Andersen KE, Menné T *et al*. Treatment of hyperkeratotic dermatitis of the palms (eczema keratoticum) with oral acitretin. A single-blind placebo-controlled study. *Acta Derm Venereol (Stockh)* 2001; **81**:353–5.

79 Stadler R, Otte HG, Luger T *et al*. Prospective randomized multicenter clinical trial on the use of interferon α-2a plus acitretin versus interferon α-2a plus PUVA in patients with cutaneous T-cell lymphoma stages I and II. *Blood* 1998; **92**:3578–81.

80 Gelmetti C, Cerri D, Schiuma AA *et al*. Treatment of extensive warts with etretinate: a clinical trial in 20 children. *Pediatr Dermatol* 1987; **4**:254–8.

81 Krupa Shankar DS, Shilpakar R. Acitretin in the management of recalcitrant warts. *Indian J Dermatol Venereol Leprol* 2008; **74**:393–5.

82 Choi YL, Lee KJ, Kim WS *et al*. Treatment of extensive and recalcitrant viral warts with acitretin. *Int J Dermatol* 2006; **45**:480–2.

83 Erkek E, Basar H, Bozdogan O, Emeksiz MC. Giant condyloma acuminata of Buschke-Löwenstein: successful treatment with a combination of surgical excision, oral acitretin and topical imiquimod. *Clin Exp Dermatol* 2009; **34**:366–8.

84 Anadolu R, Oskay T, Erdem C *et al*. Treatment of epidermodysplasia verruciformis with a combination of acitretin and interferon alfa-2a. *J Am Acad Dermatol* 2001; **45**:296–9.

85 Iraji F, Faghihi G. Epidermodysplasia verruciformis: association with isolated IgM deficiency and response to treatment with acitretin. *Clin Exp Dermatol* 2000; **25**:41–3.

86 Grote W, Harms D, Janig U *et al*. Malformation of fetus conceived 4 months after termination of maternal etretinate treatment. *Lancet* 1985; **i**:1276.

87 Kietzmann H, Schwarze I, Grote W *et al*. Embryonal malformation following etretinate therapy of Darier's disease in the mother. *Dtsch Med Wochenschr* 1986; **111**:60–2.

88 Lammer EJ. Embryopathy in infant conceived one year after termination of maternal etretinate. *Lancet* 1988; **ii**: 1080–1.

89 de Die-Smulders CE, Sturkenboom MC, Veraart J *et al*. Severe limb defects and craniofacial anomalies in a fetus conceived during acitretin therapy. *Teratology* 1995; **52**:215–19.

90 Katz HI, Waalen J, Leach EE. Acitretin in psoriasis: an overview of adverse effects. *J Am Acad Dermatol* 1999; **41**:S7–12.

91 Lammer EJ, Chen DT, Hoar RM *et al*. Retinoic acid embryopathy. *N Engl J Med* 1985; **313**:837–41.

92 Coberly S, Lammer E, Alashari M. Retinoic acid embryopathy: case report and review of literature. *Pediatr Pathol Lab Med* 1996; **16**:823–36.

93 Geiger JM, Walker M. Is there a reproductive safety risk in male patients treated with acitretin (Neotigason/Soriatane)? *Dermatology* 2002; **205**:105–7.

94 Geiger JM, Czarnetzki BM. Acitretin (Ro 10-1670, etretin): overall evaluation of clinical studies. *Dermatologica* 1988; **176**:182–90.

95 Gollnick HP. Oral retinoids – efficacy and toxicity in psoriasis. *Br J Dermatol* 1996; **135** (Suppl. 49):6–17.

96 Kreiss C, Amin S, Nalesnik MA *et al*. Severe cholestatic hepatitis in a patient taking acitretin. *Am J Gastroenterol* 2002; **97**:775–7.

97 Roenigk HH Jr, Callen JP, Guzzo CA *et al*. Effects of acitretin on the liver. *J Am Acad Dermatol* 1999; **41**:584–8.

98 Sanchez MR, Ross B, Rotterdam H *et al*. Retinoid hepatitis. *J Am Acad Dermatol* 1993; **28**:853–8.

99 Vahlquist C, Selinus I, Vessby B. Serum-lipid changes during acitretin (etretin) treatment of psoriasis and palmoplantar pustulosis. *Acta Derm Venereol (Stockh)* 1988; **68**:300–5.

100 Ashley JM, Lowe NJ, Borok ME *et al*. Fish oil supplementation results in decreased hypertriglyceridemia in patients with psoriasis undergoing etretinate or acitretin therapy. *J Am Acad Dermatol* 1988; **19**:76–82.

101 Vahlquist C, Olsson AG, Lindholm A *et al*. Effects of gemfibrozil (Lopid) on hyperlipidemia in acitretin-treated patients. Results of a double-blind cross-over study. *Acta Derm Venereol (Stockh)* 1995; **75**:377–80.

102 Rood MJ, Lavrijsen SP, Huizinga TW. Acitretin-related ossification. *J Rheumatol* 2007; **34**:837–8.

103 Mork NJ, Austad J, Kolbenstvedt A. Bamboo spine mimicking Bekhterev's disease caused by long-term acitretin treatment. *Acta Derm Venereol (Stockh)* 2006; **86**:452–3.

104 DiGiovanna JJ, Helfgott RK, Gerber LH *et al*. Extraspinal tendon and ligament calcification associated with long-term therapy with etretinate. *N Engl J Med* 1986; **315**:1177–82.

105 van Dooren-Greebe RJ, Lemmens JA, De Boo T *et al*. Prolonged treatment with oral retinoids in adults: no influence on the frequency and severity of spinal abnormalities. *Br J Dermatol* 1996; **134**:71–6.

106 Mork NJ, Kolbenstvedt A, Austad J. Efficacy and skeletal side-effects of 2 years acitretin treatment. *Acta Derm Venereol (Stockh)* 1992; **72**:445–8.

107 Lee E, Koo J. Single-center retrospective study of long-term use of low-dose acitretin (Soriatane) for psoriasis. *J Dermatolog Treat* 2004; **15**:8–13.

108 Prendiville J, Bingham EA, Burrows D. Premature epiphyseal closure – a complication of etretinate therapy in children. *J Am Acad Dermatol* 1986; **15**:1259–62.

109 Halkier-Sorensen L, Laurberg G, Andresen J. Bone changes in children on long-term treatment with etretinate. *J Am Acad Dermatol* 1987; **16**:999–1006.

110 Paige DG, Judge MR, Shaw DG *et al*. Bone changes and their significance in children with ichthyosis on long-term etretinate therapy. *Br J Dermatol* 1992; **127**:387–91.

111 Nesher G, Zuckner J. Rheumatologic complications of vitamin A and retinoids. *Semin Arthritis Rheum* 1995; **24**:291–6.

112 McClure SL, Valentine J, Gordon KB. Comparative tolerability of systemic treatments for plaque-type psoriasis. *Drug Saf* 2002; **25**:913–27.

113 McGuire J, Lawson JP. Skeletal changes associated with chronic isotretinoin and etretinate administration. *Dermatologica* 1987; **175** (Suppl. 1):169–81.

114 McMullen EA, McCarron P, Irvine AD *et al*. Association between long-term acitretin therapy and osteoporosis: no evidence of increased risk. *Clin Exp Dermatol* 2003; **28**:307–9.

115 Starling J III, Koo J. Evidence based or theoretical concern? Pseudotumor cerebri and depression as acitretin side effects. *J Drugs Dermatol* 2005; **4**:690–6.

116 Lee AG. Pseudotumor cerebri after treatment with tetracycline and isotretinoin for acne. *Cutis* 1995; **55**:165–8.

117 Sturkenboom MC, Middelbeek A, de Jong van den Berg LT *et al*. Vulvo-vaginal candidiasis associated with acitretin. *J Clin Epidemiol* 1995; **48**:991–7.

118 Hartmann D, Forgo I, Dubach UC *et al*. Effect of acitretin on the response to an intravenous glucose-tolerance test in healthy-volunteers. *Eur J Clin Pharmacol* 1992; **42**:523–8.

119 Frosch PJ, Czarnetzki BM. Effect of retinoids on wound healing in diabetic rats. *Arch Dermatol Res* 1989; **281**:424–6.

120 Gerritsen MJ, van Pelt JP, van de Kerkhof PC. Response of the clinically uninvolved skin of psoriatic patients to tape stripping during acitretin treatment. *Acta Derm Venereol (Stockh)* 1996; **76**:6–9.

121 Tan SR, Tope WD. Effect of acitretin on wound healing in organ transplant recipients. *Dermatol Surg* 2004; **30**:667–73.

122 Halkier-Sorensen L, Andresen J. A retrospective study of bone changes in adults treated with etretinate. *J Am Acad Dermatol* 1989; **20**:83–7.

123 Ruiz-Maldonado R, Tamayo L. Retinoids in disorders of keratinization: their use in children. *Dermatologica* 1987; **175** (Suppl. 1):125–32.

124 Ellis CN, Kang S, Vinik AI *et al*. Glucose and insulin responses are improved in patients with psoriasis during therapy with etretinate. *Arch Dermatol* 1987; **123**:471–5.

125 Orfanos CE, Zouboulis CC, Almond-Roesler B, Geilen CC. Current use and future potential role of retinoids in dermatology. *Drugs* 1997; **53**:358–88.

126 Mancano MA. Drug interactions with oral contraceptives. *Pharm Times* 2000; **66**:26.

127 Berbis P, Bun H, Geiger JM *et al*. Acitretin (RO10-1670) and oral contraceptives: interaction study. *Arch Dermatol Res* 1988; **280**:388–9.

128 Association of the British Pharmaceutical Industry. *Neotigason*® *Data Sheet*. London: Datapharm Publications Ltd, 2003.

129 Roche Laboratories. *Soriatane*® *Product Information*. Nutley, NJ: Roche Laboratories, 2003.

130 Mork NJ, Kolbenstvedt A, Austad J. Skeletal side-effects of 5 years' acitretin treatment. Br J Dermatol 1996; **134**:1156–7.

131 DiGiovanna JJ, Gross EG, McClean SW et al. Etretinate: effect of milk intake on absorption. J Invest Dermatol 1984; **82**:636–40.

132 Berbis P, Geiger JM, Vaisse C et al. Benefit of progressively increasing doses during the initial treatment with acitretin in psoriasis. Dermatologica 1989; **178**:88–92.

Appendix 1 Level of evidence and strength of recommendation

Level of evidence

Level of evidence	Type of evidence
1++	High-quality meta-analyses, systematic reviews of RCTs, or RCTs with a very low risk of bias
1+	Well-conducted meta-analyses, systematic reviews of RCTs, or RCTs with a low risk of bias
1−	Meta-analyses, systematic reviews of RCTs, or RCTs with a high risk of bias[a]
2++	High-quality systematic reviews of case–control or cohort studies High-quality case–control or cohort studies with a very low risk of confounding, bias or chance and a high probability that the relationship is causal
2+	Well-conducted case–control or cohort studies with a low risk of confounding, bias or chance and a moderate probability that the relationship is causal
2−	Case–control or cohort studies with a high risk of confounding, bias or chance and a significant risk that the relationship is not causal[a]
3	Nonanalytical studies (e.g. case reports, case series)
4	Expert opinion, formal consensus

RCT, randomized controlled trial. [a]Studies with a level of evidence '−' should not be used as a basis for making a recommendation.

Strength of recommendation

Once level of evidence has been derived and evidence tables drawn up, strengths of recommendation can be derived. These are the conclusions of the guideline and it is important that they stand out and stand alone. Often they can be highlighted in a box or a table. The strength of recommendation is determined by the level of evidence although the usefulness of a classification system based solely on this has been questioned because it does not take into consideration the importance of the recommendation in changing practice and it may be that more sophisticated derivations of strength of recommendation will appear in future.

Class	Evidence
A	• At least one meta-analysis, systematic review, or RCT rated as 1++, and directly applicable to the target population, **or** • A systematic review of RCTs or a body of evidence consisting principally of studies rated as 1+, directly applicable to the target population and demonstrating overall consistency of results • Evidence drawn from a NICE technology appraisal
B	• A body of evidence including studies rated as 2++, directly applicable to the target population and demonstrating overall consistency of results, **or** • Extrapolated evidence from studies rated as 1++ or 1+
C	• A body of evidence including studies rated as 2 +, directly applicable to the target population and demonstrating overall consistency of results, **or** • Extrapolated evidence from studies rated as 2++
D	• Evidence level 3 or 4, **or** • Extrapolated evidence from studies rated as 2+, **or** • Formal consensus
D (GPP)	• A good practice point (GPP) is a recommendation for best practice based on the experience of the Guideline Development Group

RCT, randomized controlled trial.

Supporting Information

Additional supporting information may be found in the online version of this article:

Data S1. Search strategy.

Please note: Wiley-Blackwell are not responsible for the content or functionality of any supporting materials supplied by the authors. Any queries (other than missing material) should be directed to the corresponding author for the article.

Comment

Acitretin is effective as mono-therapy for pustular and erythrodermic psoriasis and for chronic plaque psoriasis [1]. It can be used with other systemic agents and ultraviolet radiation. Side effects of acitretin use occur more commonly with high doses and often preclude its usefulness. There is evidence to suggest that acitretin may help prevent non-melanoma skin cancers (NMSCs) in at-risk patients such as renal transplant patients [2]. Further studies for the use of acitretin in the NMSC prophylaxis are needed. Hydroxychloroquine and acitretin appear to be of equal efficacy in discoid lupus erythematosus, although adverse effects are more frequent and more severe with acitretin [3]. There is some evidence that acitretin is effective in chronic palmar plantar pustulosis [4], but it is hoped that new retinoids such as alitretinoin will be more effective for psoriatic conditions of the hands and feet [5]. The risk of serious consequences such as pregnancy should not be underestimated but is probably less with acitretin compared with isotretinoin as the main population of patients is not adolescent females. None the less, pregnancy prevention measures must be followed with this drug.

References

1 Ormerod AD, Campalani E, Goodfield MJD. Guidelines. on the efficacy and use of acitretin in dermatology. *Brit J Dermatol* 2010; 162: 952–63.
2 Bath-Hextall FJ, Leonardi-Bee J, Somchand N, Webster AC, Delitt J, Perkins W. Interventions for preventing non-melanoma skin cancers in high-risk groups. *Cochrane Database Syst Rev* 2007; Issue 4: CD005414 (http://www.mrw.interscience.wiley.com/cochrane/clsysrev/articles/CD005414/frame.html).
3 Jessop S, Whitelaw DA, Delamere FM. Drugs for discoid lupus erythematosus. *Cochrane Database Syst Rev* 2009l; Issue 4: CD002954 (http://www.mrw.interscience.wiley.com/cochrane/clsysrev/articles/CD002954/frame.html).
4 Chalmers R, Hollis S, Leonardi-Bee J, Griffiths CEM, Marsland A. Interventions for chronic palmoplantar pustulosis. *Cochrane Database Syst Rev* 2006; Issue 1: CD001433 (http://www.mrw.interscience.wiley.com/cochrane/clsysrev/articles/CD001433/frame.html).
5 Ruzicka T, Lynde CW, Jemec GB, *et al*. Efficacy and safety of oral alitretinoin (9-*cis* retinoic acid) in patients with severe chronic hand eczema refractory to topical corticosteroids: results of a randomized, double-blind, placebo-controlled, multicentre trial. *Br J Dermatol* 2008; 158: 808–17.

Additional professional resources

Pang ML, Murase JE, Koo J. An updated review of acitretin – a systemic retinoid for the treatment of psoriasis. *Expert Opin Drug Metab Toxicol* 2008; 4: 953–64.
Menter A, Gottlieb A, Feldman SR, *et al*. Guidelines of care for the management of psoriasis and psoriatic arthritis: Section 1. Overview of psoriasis and guidelines of care for the treatment of psoriasis with biologics. *J Am Acad Dermatol* 2008; 58: 826–50.
Lee CS, Koo J. A review of acitretin, a systemic retinoid for the treatment of psoriasis. *Expert Opin Pharmacother* 2005; 1725–34.

Other patient resources

http://www.dermnetnz.org/treatments/acitretin.html

Guidelines for prescribing azathioprine in dermatology

A.V.ANSTEY, S.WAKELIN* AND N.J.REYNOLDS[†]

Department of Dermatology, Royal Gwent Hospital, Cardiff Road, Newport, Gwent NP20 2UB, U.K.
*Department of Dermatology, St Mary's Hospital, Praed Street, London W2 1NY, U.K.
[†]Department of Dermatology, School of Clinical and Laboratory Sciences, University of Newcastle upon Tyne, Framlington Place, Newcastle upon Tyne NE2 4HH, U.K.

Accepted for publication 14 May 2004

Summary

Azathioprine has been available as an immunosuppressive agent for over 40 years, and current routine usage in dermatology is not restricted to licensed indications. Advances in understanding the metabolic fate of azathioprine have led to significant changes in prescribing practice and toxicity monitoring by U.K. dermatologists. The current state of knowledge concerning the use of azathioprine in dermatology is summarized, with identification of strength of evidence. Clinical indications and contraindications for azathioprine usage in dermatology are identified. Evidence-based recommendations are made for routine safety monitoring of patients treated with azathioprine, including pretreatment assessment of red blood cell thiopurine methyltransferase activity.

Disclaimer

These guidelines have been prepared for dermatologists on behalf of the British Association of Dermatologists and reflect the best data available at the time the report was prepared. Caution should be exercised in interpreting the data; the results of future studies may require alteration of the conclusions or recommendations in this report. It may be necessary to depart from the guidelines in the interests of specific patients and in special circumstances. Just as adherence to guidelines may not constitute defence against a claim of negligence, so deviation from them should not necessarily be deemed negligent.

Introduction

Azathioprine is an immune-modulating drug that was originally developed for the control of graft rejection in transplant surgery. Since it became available in the early 1960s, azathioprine has also been prescribed for a range of autoimmune and immune-mediated dermatological conditions. Licensed indications include dermatomyositis, systemic lupus erythematosus and pemphigus vulgaris. It is used for these conditions either alone or, more commonly, in combination with corticosteroids. Therapeutic effect is typically delayed for weeks or even 2–3 months, and includes a steroid-sparing effect that reduces long-term toxicity of corticosteroids. Azathioprine is also used quite frequently as monotherapy in nonlicensed indications including atopic eczema.

Adverse drug reactions with azathioprine occur in 15–28% of patients[1–3] and include myelosuppression, nausea and vomiting, rash, pancreatitis and hypersensitivity. Polymorphism in the thiopurine methyltransferase (TPMT) gene predicts haematological adverse drug reactions in 5–10% of patients treated with thiopurine drugs.[1] The remaining adverse drug reactions are unexplained, and may be mediated by immune mechanisms or by other variables affecting the metabolic fate of the drug. It is therefore essential to continue monitoring blood counts throughout treatment with azathioprine.[4]

Methods

The aim of the search strategy was to identify recent and past publications relating to the clinical pharmacology of azathioprine that were relevant to its current usage within dermatology. The evidence gathered

These guidelines were commissioned by the British Association of Dermatologists Therapy, Guidelines and Audit Subcommittee. Members of the committee are A.D.Ormerod (Chairman), A.S.Highet, D.Mehta, R.H.Meyrick Thomas, C.H.Smith, J.C.Sterling and A.Anstey. Conflicts of interest: No additional funding was received by the authors of these guidelines to support this work. None of the authors has a conflict of interest to declare.
Correspondence: Alex Anstey.
E-mail: alex.anstey@gwent.wales.nhs.uk

includes some derived from disciplines other than dermatology, such as gastroenterology, where azathioprine usage is high and experience with TPMT-guided prescribing is established.

Types of studies

Randomized, double-blind, placebo-controlled trials; well-designed controlled trials without randomization; well-designed cohort or case–control analytical studies; evidence from multiple time series with or without intervention; opinions of respected authorities based on clinical experience, descriptive studies or reports of expert committees.

Search strategy for identification of studies

A computer-assisted search of the online bibliographic databases Medline, PubMed and Embase was carried out to identify potentially relevant papers published between 1966 and 2003. Other databases searched included the Royal College of Physicians Guidelines database, CINAHL, the Cochrane library, DARE, AMED and HMIC. The following search terms were used: azathioprine; 6-mercaptopurine; dermatology; adverse drug reactions; clinical monitoring; TPMT; thiopurine methyltransferase. Citations were limited to those in English, French, Spanish, Italian and German. Manual searches of the reference lists from the relevant papers were performed in order to identify additional studies that may have been missed by the computer-assisted strategy. These guidelines include evidence derived from the key papers identified by the search strategy.

Risks and benefits of azathioprine therapy in dermatology

Particular emphasis has been placed on assessing the risks and benefits of azathioprine therapy for patients with dermatological disease. These guidelines attempt to establish an explicit link between evidence and recommendations for clinical usage. This is sometimes difficult, as decisions in clinical medicine occur in the context of single patients and do not always relate to the context from which a guideline recommendation has been made. Finally, these guidelines have been subjected to expert review by nondermatologists (acknowledged) with recognized expertise in the prescribing of azathioprine. In line with other British Association of Dermatologists (BAD) guidelines it is the intention for these guidelines to be reviewed and updated in 5 years.

Pharmacology

Azathioprine is a prodrug with no inherent immuno-suppressive activity. Azathioprine is an imidazole derivative of 6-mercaptopurine (6-MP) and is therefore classed as a purine analogue. It was developed in an attempt to produce a drug with the same immuno-suppressive activity as 6-MP but with significantly slower metabolism. Following oral administration, azathioprine is rapidly and almost completely absorbed from the gut. No azathioprine crosses the blood–brain barrier, but there is otherwise an even distribution of the drug throughout the body. The plasma half-life is just 3 h owing to rapid nonenzymatic conversion to 6-MP, the active compound, and imidazole derivatives. 6-MP has a long half-life and is metabolized by three competing pathways (Fig. 1). Active 6-thioguanine nucleotide metabolites are generated by the action of hypoxanthine guanine phosphoribosyl transferase (HPRT). Xanthine oxidase, which is inhibited by allopurinol, metabolizes 6-MP to inactive 6-thiouric acid. The third of the competing pathways involves methylation of 6-MP to 6-methyl mercaptopurine, an inactive compound, which is catalysed by TPMT.

Azathioprine mode of action

6-MP readily crosses cell membranes, and is converted by the enzyme HPRT into a number of active purine thionucleotide metabolites. The exact mode of action of azathioprine at a cellular level remains unclear, but thionucleotide metabolites of 6-MP are believed to compete with their endogenous counterparts in many biochemical pathways. Nucleotides have a number of important roles in all cells: they are precursors of DNA and RNA, they are essential carriers of energy (e.g. adenosine triphosphate and guanosine triphosphate), and they function as cellular second messengers. These nucleotide-dependent processes endow azathioprine with both immunosuppressive and cytotoxic properties. There is also evidence that imidazole derivatives and the thiopurine intermediates have independent immunosuppressive properties.[5]

The significance of thiopurine methyltransferase in the clinical pharmacology of azathioprine

There is marked interpatient variability in the generation of immunosuppressant metabolites, resulting from

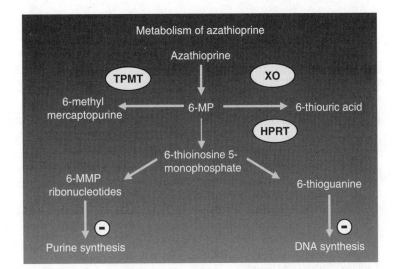

Figure 1. Metabolism of azathioprine. The first metabolite is 6-mercaptopurine (6-MP). This may be metabolized in three ways: (i) methylation to inactive 6-methyl mercaptopurine (6-MMP) catalysed by thiopurine methyl transferase (TPMT); (ii) oxidation to inactive 6-thiouric acid catalysed by xanthine oxidase (XO); and (iii) hypoxanthine guanine phosphoribosyl transferase (HPRT) catalyses the conversion of 6-MP to 6-thioinosine 5-monophosphate which is further converted to 6-thioguanine. 6-Thioguanine has an inhibitory effect on DNA synthesis.

a common genetic polymorphism in TPMT, one of three competing pathways for 6-MP metabolism (Fig. 1). Eleven per cent of the population has low TPMT activity and is vulnerable to myelosuppression with azathioprine treatment.[6] Furthermore, one in 300 individuals has undetectable TPMT activity,[6] and is susceptible to rapid-onset, prolonged, life-threatening pancytopenia if treated with conventional doses of azathioprine.[7] A recent large clinical study on patients being treated with azathioprine showed the rate of undetectable TPMT activity to be higher, at one in 200 patients;[4] however, the cases in this series were not randomly selected and there may have been some bias towards a higher rate of 'problem cases'. Inhibition of xanthine oxidase, the third enzyme in this system (Fig. 1), produces the same effect on azathioprine metabolism as deficiency in TPMT: decreased metabolism of 6-MP to inactive metabolites, and increased generation of immunosuppressant 6-thioguanine nucleotides. This explains the potentially serious drug interaction between azathioprine and allopurinol.[8,9]

Azathioprine indications in dermatology

Indications are listed in Table 1. Azathioprine is a popular drug with dermatologists, as it is perceived as an immunosuppresive drug in which the potential benefits outweigh the potential risks. The main area of use in dermatology is in the treatment of autoimmune dermatoses, in particular bullous pemphigoid[10–12] (Grade B; level IV; see Appendix 1), and pemphigus vulgaris[13,14] (Grade B; level II-iii) where azathioprine

Table 1 Licensed and unlicensed indications for azathioprine in the treatment of dermatological disorders

Licensed indications	Unlicensed indications
Systemic lupus erythematosus	Atopic dermatitis
Dermatomyositis	Psoriasis
Pemphigus vulgaris	Bullous pemphigoid
	Chronic actinic dermatitis
	Pyoderma gangrenosum
	Pityriasis rubra pilaris
	Wegener's granulomatosis
	Cutaneous vasculitis

is used as a steroid-sparing agent. Accumulating evidence also suggests a role for azathioprine as a single agent in the treatment of severe, recalcitrant atopic dermatitis[15–17] (Grade A; level I). Double-blind, placebo-controlled trials have shown azathioprine to be of benefit in chronic actinic dermatitis[18] (Grade A; level I) and Behçet's disease[19] (Grade A; level I). It may also be effective as monotherapy in the treatment of severe, recalcitrant psoriasis[20] (Grade C; level IV). Azathioprine is sometimes used in the treatment of other rare dermatological conditions including Wegener's granulomatosis,[21] pyoderma gangrenosum,[22] pityriasis rubra pilaris,[23] lupus erythematosus[24] and lichen planus,[25] but evidence to support its usage in these conditions is anecdotal[26] (Grade C; level IV).

Azathioprine contraindications

Azathioprine is contraindicated in patients with known hypersensitivity to the drug[27–29] (Grade A; level III). Evidence of teratogenicity with azathioprine in humans is equivocal,[30] but adequate contraceptive precautions are advised when either partner is taking azathioprine. Azathioprine is also contraindicated in pregnancy (except where benefit may outweigh risk such as in allograft recipients)[30–32] (Grade A; level II-ii). 6-MP has been identified in colostrum and in the breast milk of women receiving azathioprine treatment. Women on azathioprine should therefore be advised to bottle feed their babies. It is strongly recommended that azathioprine should not be used in patients whose TPMT status is unknown[4,15] (Grade A; level II-ii). Very low or absent TPMT activity is a contraindication to the usage of azathioprine because of the high risk of life-threatening pancytopenia[24] (Grade A; level II-ii). Concurrent treatment with allopurinol results in an important drug interaction which may cause significant myelosuppression, and should therefore be avoided[8,9] (Grade A; level III).

There are concerns that azathioprine treatment increases the risk of developing a malignancy. Accumulating evidence suggests that this risk is smaller than was originally feared.[33,34] Nevertheless, patients should be advised of this risk, and it is recommended that azathioprine treatment should not usually be initiated or continued in patients with known malignancy (Grade A; level III).

Contradictions to azathioprine:

- It is strongly recommended that azathioprine should not be used in patients whose TPMT status is unknown
- Known hypersensitivity to azathioprine (or 6-MP)
- Azathioprine is contraindicated in patients who may be pregnant or hope to become pregnant in the near future (except where benefit may outweigh risk)
- Women taking azathioprine should not breast feed their babies
- Very low or absent TPMT activity
- Concurrent allopurinol treatment
- Concurrent malignant disease where azathioprine treatment may increase the risk of disease progression
- Renal or hepatic insufficiency (relative contraindication)

Pretreatment thiopurine methyltransferase assessment

Azathioprine prescribing practice among U.K. dermatologists has changed in recent years, with increased demand for pretreatment assessment of TPMT activity.[4] This is explained by greater awareness of the

significance of interpatient variability in TPMT activity that coincided with availability of a National Health Service laboratory service for TPMT assay (Guy's Hospital, Purine Research Laboratory). The justification for pretreatment TPMT measurement is the presumed improvements in safety and efficacy that follow from knowing its activity. In acute lymphoblastic leukaemia (ALL) treated with 6-MP, lower TPMT activity tended to be associated with a better outcome,[35] although ALL patients with lower TPMT activity appeared to be at greater risk of developing second malignancies.[35] Although there are currently no published prospective studies for dermatological conditions which demonstrate improved prognosis, TPMT screening prior to azathioprine treatment is considered by some clinicians to be essential (Grade A; level II-ii).[4,10]

Knowledge of TPMT prevents those with very low or undetectable TPMT from receiving azathioprine, and may prevent fatal myelosuppression. This is the most important aspect of measuring TPMT. Prior TPMT assessment also identifies those with intermediate activity who would be predicted to suffer toxicity on standard doses of azathioprine but who might tolerate and respond to tailored doses of azathioprine. Other components of the azathioprine metabolic pathways may rarely be deficient or exert an immunosuppressive effect, including deficiency in purine-5′-nucleotidase and xanthine oxidase, and lethal immunosuppressive effects mediated by imidazole derivatives.[5] Dermatologists should therefore be aware that knowledge of TPMT status does not preclude the necessity for monitoring for azathioprine toxicity by regular blood tests. Genotype tests for the commonest mutations in the TPMT gene are of interest to clinicians, but do not provide the functional result which measurement of the enzyme activity provides.[36] Furthermore, the TPMT genotyping tests are not yet available in the U.K. as a routine laboratory test. Thus, dermatologists are advised to continue to use the TPMT enzymatic assay.

- Pretreatment TPMT measurement should be performed in all patients prescribed azathioprine for treatment of dermatological conditions

Azathioprine dosage

The recommended dosage of azathioprine for dermatological indications is 1–3 mg kg^{-1} daily, adjusted within these limits according to response. If no improvement occurs in the patient's condition within

3 months, consideration should be given to withdrawing azathioprine. Care should be taken when prescribing azathioprine in the elderly: it is recommended that the dosage used is at the lower end of the range. There are currently no data to support prescribing azathioprine in doses outside the above range. However, modified dosage regimens based on TPMT activity have been published for both adults[16,37] and children[38] (Grade C; level III), and are the logical progression of this pharmacogenetic assessment.

Azathioprine should not be used in patients with very low/absent TPMT activity (deficient), as the danger of severe and prolonged myelosuppression is significant[20,39] (Grade A; level II-ii). Patients with inflammatory bowel disease and low TPMT activity have been shown to be at increased risk of azathioprine toxicity.[39] Thus, for patients with low TPMT activity, alternative systemic therapies should be considered (Grade A; level II-ii). If a trial of azathioprine is deemed appropriate in this situation, a low-dosage regimen should be used (0·5–1 mg kg^{-1} daily) and extra care taken with haematological surveillance (Grade B; level III).

In patients with high TPMT activity (see Appendix 2 for laboratory ranges), the azathioprine dose should be at the higher end of the range of 1–3 mg kg^{-1} daily. It is probably safe to treat these patients from the outset with dosages of azathioprine towards the top end of this dosage range provided the usual measures are taken to monitor for myelosuppression. However, azathioprine intolerance unrelated to TPMT activity is not uncommon, and a lower initial dose of azathioprine is advocated by some authors for the first month of therapy, even in patients with high TPMT activity.[10] In patients with inflammatory bowel disease, high TPMT activity predicts treatment failure with azathioprine.[3] Thus, in dermatology patients with high TPMT activity, azathioprine dosage should be at the top of the recommended dose range of 1–3 mg kg^{-1} daily. In patients who fail to respond to 3 months of this dosage regimen, and in whom no adverse effects occur, dosage above the 1–3 mg kg^{-1} daily range might be considered for a trial period (Grade C; level III). However, if this approach is adopted, care should be taken in monitoring for myelosuppression and possible hepatotoxicity.

- If no therapeutic response is observed within 3 months of starting azathioprine, treatment should usually be withdrawn
- In patients with very low/absent TPMT activity (deficient), azathioprine is contraindicated

- In patients with low TPMT activity, azathioprine should either not be prescribed or, if used, the dose should be low (0·5–1 mg kg^{-1} daily) with careful monitoring for myelosuppression
- In patients with normal or high TPMT activity, azathioprine dosage should commence at the top of the 1–3 mg kg^{-1} daily dosage range. In patients who fail to respond, and in whom no adverse effects occur, dosage above the 1–3 mg kg^{-1} daily range might be considered for a trial period

Monitoring for azathioprine-induced toxicity

The data sheet for azathioprine recommends weekly monitoring of full blood count (FBC) for the first 8 weeks of treatment. However, the *British National Formulary* states that the 'evidence of the practical value (of weekly FBC for 8 weeks) is unsatisfactory', and recommends weekly FBCs for the first 4 weeks, followed by reduced frequency of monitoring to a minimum of once every 3 months. Routine monitoring for azathioprine toxicity should also include liver function tests (LFTs) as hepatoxicity is a recognized complication of azathioprine therapy.[10,11,40,41] Thus, it is advised that dermatologists carry out weekly blood tests (FBCs and LFTs) until maintenance dose is achieved, followed by regular monitoring reducing to a minimum of once every 3 months for the duration of therapy[42] (Grade A; level I).

For higher dosages and for patients with hepatic or renal impairment, initial blood count monitoring more frequently than once weekly is advised. Return to weekly FBCs and LFTs should also follow an increase in dosage in azathioprine in patients already established on this treatment. It is also advised that patients on azathioprine be instructed to report immediately any evidence of infection, unexpected bruising or bleeding or jaundice. In patients with low TPMT activity (3–8 nmol h^{-1} mL^{-1} red blood cells), monitoring for FBC and LFTs should be more frequent than outlined above due to the increased risk of toxicity. Acute pancreatitis is a rare but well-recognized side-effect of azathioprine treatment.[43] In azathioprine-treated patients with acute abdominal pain and/or severe vomiting, acute pancreatitis should be considered and serum amylase measured.

Monitoring for azathioprine toxicity should include:
- Weekly monitoring of FBC and LFTs for the first 4 weeks of therapy, or until the maintenance dose is achieved; reducing to a minimum of once every 3 months for the duration of therapy

- More frequent monitoring of FBC and LFTs is advised in patients with hepatic or renal impairment, in the elderly and in those treated with high doses of azathioprine
- Increase in dosage of azathioprine should be accompanied by return to weekly FBC and LFTs for 4 weeks, reducing to a minimum of once monthly or every 2 months for the duration of therapy

Azathioprine-induced susceptibility to infection

In transplant recipients, the immunosuppressive activity of azathioprine in combination with corticosteroids can lead to an increased susceptibility to viral, bacterial and fungal infections which manifest in the skin and in other body organs (azathioprine data sheet). In dermatology, azathioprine is most commonly prescribed for management of immunobullous disorders, where combination with systemic steroids is the norm. Evidence of infection in such patients is inconsistent, and in the absence of reliable information on this topic dermatologists should assume an increased rate of infection as for transplant recipients. Infection in elderly patients with bullous pemphigoid treated with azathioprine and prednisolone has been identified as a significant cause for mortality, particularly when compared with rates of such fatal infections in patients treated with prednisolone alone.[44]

The use of azathioprine monotherapy does not appear to give rise to a marked increase in susceptibility to such infections (azathioprine data sheet). However, the immunosuppressive activity of azathioprine could result in an atypical and potentially deleterious response to live vaccines. Thus, administration of live vaccines to patients receiving azathioprine is contraindicated on theoretical grounds. A diminished response to killed vaccines may occur, and has been observed with hepatitis B vaccine in patients treated with a combination of azathioprine and corticosteroids. In view of the potential severity of primary varicella zoster in the immunosuppressed, patients who have not previously had chickenpox should be identified at the outset of azathioprine prescribing and advised to seek immediate attention if they subsequently come into contact with someone who has chickenpox or shingles.[45]

- Azathioprine in combination with prednisolone is associated with an increased risk of infection,

which may be fatal in the elderly. Dermatologists are advised to use the minimum necessary doses of immunosuppressive therapies to control immunobullous diseases in the elderly[10] (Grade A; level II-ii)
- Live vaccines are contraindicated for patients receiving azathioprine (Grade A; level III)
- Killed vaccines may elicit a diminished immune response in patients receiving azathioprine (Grade B; level II-ii)

Azathioprine-related malignancy

The inhibitory effect of azathioprine on the immune surveillance system could, on theoretical grounds, lead to an increased rate of malignancy with long-term therapy. The increased incidence of neoplasms in azathioprine-taking immunosuppressed renal transplant recipients[46] cannot easily be compared with patients receiving azathioprine for other diseases due to the strong antigenic stimulation by the graft and the taking of two or more immunosuppressive drugs.[47] Importantly, there was no increase in the rate of malignancies in a large number of azathioprine-treated, nontransplant patients compared with placebo-treated controls.[48] Long-term treatment with azathioprine for inflammatory bowel disease was not associated with a significant increase in malignancy compared with matched controls.[34] However, long-term treatment with azathioprine for rheumatoid arthritis showed an increased rate of lymphoma which was estimated at one case of lymphoma per 1000 patient years of azathioprine treatment.[33] The evidence concerning mutagenicity in relation to azathioprine is unclear, and there is also no clear evidence that azathioprine *per se* is oncogenic in humans. However, the significantly increased rate of skin malignancies in transplant recipients compared with the general population is undisputed, and may in part be due to the immunosuppressive effects of azathioprine. Despite this, reports of skin malignancy in patients receiving long-term azathioprine monotherapy are rare, suggesting that the risk, if it exists, is probably small.

- Dermatologists should make patients aware of the possible increased risk of malignancy related to long-term azathioprine therapy (Grade B; level IV)
- Skin photoprotection should be advised when relevant (Grade B; level IV)

Azathioprine-induced hypersensitivity reactions

Idiosyncratic hypersensitivity reactions with azathioprine are recognized, but are rare.[49] Manifestations include nausea, diarrhoea and vomiting, malaise, dizziness, fever, rigors, rashes (urticarial, maculopapular and vasculitic) and even circulatory collapse. The drug should be discontinued immediately and circulatory support initiated if necessary. The aetiology of the reaction is unknown. Rechallenge should be avoided, as the reaction is generally more severe and occasionally life-threatening.

Management of azathioprine-induced complications

Clinical manifestations of chronic azathioprine overdosage are those of bone marrow suppression: unexplained infection, ulceration of the throat, bruising and bleeding. The most obvious aspect of management of this complication is to take the necessary measures to prevent it happening in the first place. This should include measurement of TPMT status, in combination with monitoring of the FBC as described above. Isolated lymphopenia is not uncommon with azathioprine therapy and may be due to lymphocytotoxicity induced by azathioprine-derived imidazole derivatives.[5] Dose reduction is recommended if the lymphocyte count falls below 0.5×10^9 L^{-1}.

If bone marrow suppression occurs, the earliest feature is leucopenia followed by reduction in platelet count. Early changes in these parameters with a downward trend but absolute levels within normal ranges should alert the clinician to the need for continued vigilance in haematological assessment and should raise the option of reduced dosage or withdrawal of treatment. More significant myelosuppression with blood indices below the normal ranges should be managed by immediate withdrawal of azathioprine. Regular monitoring of the FBC will indicate whether the blood count suppression is significant. Platelet count below 50×10^{-9} L^{-1} and neutrophil count below 1.0×10^9 L^{-1} should be managed jointly with a haematologist.

Azathioprine-induced hepatotoxicity should be diagnosed early (by carrying out frequent monitoring of LFTs as recommended in these guidelines) and managed by dosage reduction or withdrawal of azathioprine. Gastrointestinal upset is common with azathioprine treatment and may occasionally require dosage reduction or withdrawal of treatment. Practical suggestions on how to manage gastrointestinal upset include splitting the dose of azathioprine, starting at a lower dose and then increasing to the required dose, and taking azathioprine with, or shortly after food.

Patient information and informed consent

Because of the potential for serious adverse effects associated with azathioprine, patients should be carefully counselled before starting treatment. Patients who are unable to comply with close monitoring are unsuitable for treatment with this drug. It is recommended that the following points are discussed, an azathioprine patient information sheet is provided, and written documentation of this made in the case notes.

1 Azathioprine has a slow onset of action and benefit may not be apparent until 2–3 months after starting treatment. The importance of regular blood tests, which are particularly frequent at the start of treatment, should be reinforced. The drug should be taken once or twice daily, with or after food.
2 The prescribing physician should explain whether use of azathioprine is for a licensed indication or not.
3 Patients should be advised to seek urgent medical attention if they develop signs and symptoms of bone marrow impairment or liver impairment, such as unexplained bruising, sore throat, high fever or jaundice. It is important to explain that symptoms of azathioprine hypersensitivity may initially be mistaken for 'flu'.
4 Patients taking azathioprine who have not had chickenpox should seek immediate attention if they come into contact with someone who has chickenpox or shingles for consideration of zoster immune globulin. Patients taking azathioprine should not be given live vaccines, and due to the risk of orofaecal transmission, other members of their household should be given inactive (rather than live) polio vaccine.
5 There may be a small increase in the risk of malignancy with long-term treatment with azathioprine. The drug should be continued only when benefits outweigh the risks.
6 Patients should be warned that the following treatments may interact with azathioprine:

Allopurinol inhibits the enzyme xanthine oxidase and prolongs the action of azathioprine with potential for increased toxicity. Concomitant administration should be avoided.

Sulfasalazine inhibits TPMT activity and may potentiate azathioprine toxicity.

Warfarin. The anticoagulant effect may be impaired by azathioprine.

Myelosuppressive drugs such as penicillamine and co-trimoxazole should be avoided due to the possibility of inducing serious haematological toxicity.

Angiotensin-converting enzyme inhibitors have been reported to induce severe leucopenia in patients taking azathioprine.

Live vaccines are contraindicated on theoretical grounds in patients taking azathioprine.

7 Pregnancy should be avoided during treatment with azathioprine, and women taking this drug must ensure that they use adequate contraceptive precautions.

8 Patients should be warned that sudden onset of abdominal pain, with or without severe vomiting, may be due to pancreatitis related to the azathioprine treatment. Patients should seek urgent medical attention. Serum amylase should be checked urgently in this situation.

• Before azathioprine is prescribed, the clinician should provide the patient with an azathioprine patient information sheet, and discuss the anticipated benefits and possible side-effects

Conclusions

Better understanding of azathioprine therapeutics has resulted from its continued use for more than 40 years. Insight into the genetic basis of drug metabolism has resulted in changes in routine usage of azathioprine aimed at improving drug efficacy and safety. Measurement of TPMT activity before prescribing azathioprine combined with alterations in the routine prescribing of azathioprine is the best example to date of the evolving field of pharmacogenetics.[50,51] This is due to the unusual occurrence of a single allelic variant (i.e. that encoding low/absent TPMT activity) resulting in a significant clinical effect. Thus, the case for pre-azathioprine screening is clear-cut and is increasingly endorsed by clinician demand for this service. There is now the need to reassess azathioprine usage in the face of the change in the way it is prescribed in clinical practice, by further epidemiological research on adverse and beneficial drug effects.[52]

Audit of azathioprine prescribing

This paper includes highlighted recommendations for good practice in relation to the prescribing of azathioprine. Any one of these could be used to establish agreed local standards of care against which audit could be performed. For example, 'indications for usage of azathioprine' might be one area, taking into account the licensed indications for azathioprine and the conditions for which there is good evidence to support its use from randomized controlled trials. There is now a broad consensus among U.K. dermatologists that pretreatment TPMT measurement is necessary for improved safety and more effective dosage selection for patients treated with azathioprine. Thus, audit on usage of TPMT screening could follow the development of agreed local standards of care concerning this investigation. Routine monitoring of azathioprine toxicity is another area where recommendations are made, and locally agreed standards could precede an audit to assess compliance with that standard. Perhaps the most novel audit project concerns what we tell our patients. The recommendations for patient information in this document exceed what most dermatologists currently do. A patient information sheet has also been developed by the BAD (available on the patient section of the BAD website: http://www.bad.org.uk/patient) to be used in combination with detailed patient-focused discussion of the merits and hazards of this drug.

Acknowledgments

The authors wish to acknowledge the following contributors: Dr Alex Holme, Dr Simon Meggit, Dr Jeremy Sanderson, Dr Tony Marinaki, Dr Catherine Davies and Dr Jonathan Berg. Mrs Joanna Dundon is acknowledged for assistance with the search strategy.

References

1 Lennard L. TPMT in the treatment of Crohn's disease with azathioprine. *Gut* 2002; **51**: 143–6.
2 Sandborn W, Sutherland L, Pearson D *et al.* Azathioprine or 6-mercaptopurine for induction of remission of Crohn's disease (Cochrane Review). In: *The Cochrane Library*, Issue 2. Oxford: Update Software, 2003.
3 Ansari A, Hassan C, Duley JA *et al.* Thiopurine methyltransferase activity and the use of azathioprine in inflammatory bowel disease. *Aliment Pharmacol Ther* 2002; **16**: 1743–50.
4 Holme SA, Duley JA, Sanderson J *et al.* Erythrocyte thiopurine methyl transferase assessment prior to azathioprine use in the UK. *Q J Med* 2002; **95**: 439–44.

5 Sauer H, Hantke U, Wilmanns W. Azathioprine lymphocytotoxicity. Potentially lethal damage by its imidazole derivatives. *Arzneim-Forsch/Drug Res* 1988; **6**: 820–4.

6 Weinshilboum RM, Sladek SL. Mercaptopurine pharmacogenetics: monogenic inheritance of erythrocyte thiopurine methyltransferase activity. *Am J Hum Genet* 1980; **32**: 651–62.

7 Anstey A, Lennard L, Mayou SC, Kirby JD. Pancytopenia related to azathioprine—an enzyme deficiency caused by a common genetic polymorphism: a review. *J R Soc Med* 1992; **85**: 752–6.

8 Jeurissen MEC, Boerbooms AMT, van de Putte LBA. Pancytopenia related to azathioprine in rheumatoid arthritis. *Ann Rheum Dis* 1988; **47**: 503–5.

9 Bacon BR, Treuhaft WH, Goodman AM. Azathioprine-induced pancytopenia. Occurrence in two patients with connective-tissue disease. *Arch Intern Med* 1981; **141**: 223–6.

10 Wojnarowska F, Kirtschig G, Highet AS et al. Guidelines for the management of bullous pemphigoid. *Br J Dermatol* 2002; **147**: 214–21.

11 Khumalo N, Murrell DF, Wojnarowska F, Kirtschig G. A systematic review of treatments for bullous pemphigoid. *Arch Dermatol* 2002; **138**: 385–9.

12 Burton JL, Harman RMM, Peachey RDG, Warin RP. A controlled trial of azathioprine in the treatment of pemphigoid. *Br J Dermatol* 1978; **99** (Suppl. 16): 14.

13 Harman KE, Albert S, Black MM. Guidelines for the management of pemphigus vulgaris. *Br J Dermatol* 2003; **149**: 926–37.

14 Aberer W, Wolff-Schreiner EC, Stingl G, Wolff K. Azathioprine in the treatment of pemphigus vulgaris. *J Am Acad Dermatol* 1987; **16**: 527–33.

15 Lear JT, English JSC, Jones P, Smith AG. Retrospective review of the use of azathioprine in severe atopic dermatitis. *J Am Acad Dermatol* 1996; **35**: 642–3.

16 Meggitt SJ, Reynolds NJ. Azathioprine for atopic dermatitis. *Clin Exp Dermatol* 2001; **26**: 369–75.

17 Berth-Jones J, Takwale A, Tan E et al. Azathioprine in severe adult atopic dermatitis: a double-blind, placebo-controlled, crossover trial. *Br J Dermatol* 2002; **147**: 324–30.

18 Murphy GM, Maurice PM, Norris PG et al. Azathioprine in the treatment of chronic actinic dermatitis: a double-blind controlled trial with monitoring of exposure to ultraviolet radiation. *Br J Dermatol* 1989; **121**: 639–46.

19 Yazici H, Pazarli H, Barnes CG et al. A controlled trial of azathioprine in Behçet's syndrome. *N Engl J Med* 1990; **322**: 281–5.

20 du Vivier A, Munro DD, Verbov J. Treatment of psoriasis with azathioprine. *Br Med J* 1974; **i**: 49–51.

21 Wisehart JM. Wegener's granulomatosis—controlled by azathioprine and corticosteroids. *Br J Dermatol* 1975; **92**: 461–7.

22 Chow RK, Ho VC. Treatment of pyoderma gangrenosum. *J Am Acad Dermatol* 1996; **34**: 1047–60.

23 Hunter GA, Forbes IJ. Treatment of pityriasis rubra pilaris with azathioprine. *Br J Dermatol* 1972; **87**: 42–5.

24 Callen JP, Spencer LV, Burruss JB et al. Azathioprine: an effective, corticosteroid-sparing therapy for patients with recalcitrant cutaneous lupus erythematosus or with recalcitrant cutaneous leucocytoclastic vasculitis. *Arch Dermatol* 1991; **127**: 515–22.

25 Lear JT, English JSC. Erosive and generalised lichen planus responsive to azathioprine. *Clin Exp Dermatol* 1996; **21**: 56–7.

26 Anstey A. Azathioprine in dermatology; a review in the light of advances in the understanding of methylation pharmacogenetics. *J R Soc Med* 1995; **88**: 155–60.

27 Saway PA, Heck LW, Bonner JR et al. Azathioprine hypersensitivity. Case report and review of the literature. *Am J Med* 1988; **84**: 960–4.

28 Jones JJ, Ashworth J. Azathioprine-induced shock in dermatology patients. *J Am Acad Dermatol* 1993; **29**: 795–6.

29 Hinrichs R, Schneider LA, Ozdemir C et al. Azathioprine hypersensitivity in a patient with peripheral demyelinating polyneuropathy. *Br J Dermatol* 2003; **148**: 1076–7.

30 Bar J, Stahl B, Hod M et al. Is immunosuppression therapy in renal allograft recipients teratogenic? A single-center experience. *Am J Med Genet* 2003; **116**: 31–6.

31 The Registration Committee of the European Dialysis and Transplantation Association. Successful pregnancies in women treated by dialysis and kidney transplantation. *Br J Obstet Gynaecol* 1980; **87**: 839–45.

32 Davison JM, Dellagrammatikas H, Parkin JM. Maternal azathioprine therapy and depressed haemopoiesis in the babies of renal allograft patients. *Br J Obstet Gynaecol* 1985; **92**: 233–9.

33 Silman AJ, Petrie J, Hazleman B, Evans SJW. Lymphoproliferative cancer and other malignancy in patients with rheumatoid arthritis treated with azathioprine: a 20 year follow-up study. *Ann Rheum Dis* 1988; **47**: 988–92.

34 Connell WR, Kamm MA, Dickson M et al. Long-term neoplasia risk after azathioprine treatment in inflammatory bowel disease. *Lancet* 1994; **343**: 1249–52.

35 McLeod HL, Krynetski EY, Relling MV, Evans WE. Genetic polymorphism of thiopurine methyltransferase and its clinical relevance for childhood acute lymphoblastic leukemia. *Leukemia* 2000; **14**: 567–72.

36 Coulthard SA, Rabello C, Robson J et al. A comparison of molecular and enzyme-based assays for the detection of thiopurine methyltransferase mutations. *Br J Haematol* 2000; **110**: 599–604.

37 Snow JL, Gibson LE. The role of genetic variation in thiopurine-methyltransferase activity and the efficacy and/or side effects of azathioprine in dermatologic patients. *Arch Dermatol* 1995; **131**: 193–7.

38 Murphy L-A, Atherton D. A retrospective evaluation of azathioprine in severe childhood atopic eczema, using thiopurine methyltransferase levels to exclude patients at high risk of myelosuppression. *Br J Dermatol* 2002; **147**: 308–15.

39 Colombel J-F, Ferrari N, Debuysere H et al. Genotypic analysis of thiopurine S-methyltransferase in patients with Crohn's disease and severe myelosuppression during azathioprine therapy. *Gastroenterology* 2000; **118**: 1025–30.

40 Dubinsky MC, Yang H, Hassard PV et al. 6-MP metabolite profiles provide a biochemical explanation for 6-MP resistance in patients with inflammatory bowel disease. *Gastroenterology* 2002; **122**: 904–15.

41 Guillaume J-C, Vaillant L, Bernard P et al. Controlled trial of azathioprine and plasma exchange in addition to prednisolone in the treatment of bullous pemphigoid. *Arch Dermatol* 1993; **129**: 49–53.

42 Nielsen OH, Vainer B, Rask-Madsen J. Review article: the treatment of inflammatory bowel disease with 6-mercaptopurine or azathioprine. *Aliment Pharmacol Ther* 2001; **15**: 1699–708.

43 Sturdevant RAL, Singleton JW, Deren JJ et al. Azathioprine-related pancreatitis in patients with Crohn's disease. *Gastroenterology* 1979; **77**: 883–6.

44 Venning VA, Wojnarowska F. Lack of predictive factors for the clinical course of bullous pemphigoid. *J Am Acad Dermatol* 1992; **26**: 585–9.

45 Spencer ES, Anderson HK. Viral infections in renal allograft recipients treated with long-term immunosuppression. *Br Med J* 1979; **ii**: 829–30.

46 Hoover R, Fraumeni JF. Risk of cancer in transplant recipients. *Lancet* 1973; **ii**: 55–7.

47 Gleichmann E, Gleichmann H. Immunosuppression and neoplasia. *Klin Wochenschr* 1973; **51**: 260–5.

48 McEwan A, Petty LG. Oncogenicity of immunosuppressive drugs. *Lancet* 1972; **i**: 326–7.

49 Knowles SR, Gupta AK, Shear NH *et al*. Azathioprine hypersensitivity-like reactions—a case report and review of the literature. *Clin Exp Dermatol* 1995; **20**: 353–6.

50 Ameen M, Smith CH, Barker JNWN. Pharmacogenetics in clinical dermatology. *Br J Dermatol* 2002; **146**: 2–6.

51 Krynetski EY, Evans WE. Pharmacogenetics as a molecular basis for individualized drug therapy: the thiopurine S-methyltransferase paradigm. *Pharm Res* 1999; **16**: 342–9.

52 Jick H, Rodriguez LAG, Perez-Gutthann S. Principles of epidemiological research on adverse and beneficial drug effects. *Lancet* 1998; **352**: 1767–70.

53 Griffiths CEM. The British Association of Dermatologists guidelines for the management of skin disease. *Br J Dermatol* 1999; **141**: 396–7.

54 Cox NH, Williams HC. The British Association of Dermatologists therapeutic guidelines: can we AGREE? *Br J Dermatol* 2003; **148**: 621–5.

Appendix 1. Levels of evidence on which the guideline is based

The consultation process and background details for the British Association of Dermatologists (BAD) guidelines have been published previously.[53,54] The patient information sheet to accompany this guideline is available on the BAD website: http://www.bad.org/patient

Level	Type of evidence
I	Evidence obtained from at least one properly designed, randomized controlled trial
II-i	Evidence obtained from well-designed controlled trials without randomization
II-ii	Evidence obtained from well-designed cohort or case–control analytical studies, preferably from more than one centre or research group
II-iii	Evidence obtained from multiple time series with or without the intervention. Dramatic results in uncontrolled experiments (such as the results of the introduction of penicillin treatment in the 1940s) could also be regarded as this type of evidence
III	Opinions of respected authorities based on clinical experience, descriptive studies or reports of expert committees
IV	Evidence inadequate due to problems of methodology (e.g. sample size, or length of follow-up, or conflicts of interest)

Grade of
recommendation

A	There is good evidence to support the use of the procedure
B	There is fair evidence to support the use of the procedure
C	There is poor evidence to support the use of the procedure
D	There is fair evidence to support the rejection of the use of the procedure
E	There is good evidence to support the rejection of the use of the procedure

Appendix 2. Measurement of erythrocyte thiopurine methyltransferase (TPMT) activity

- TPMT activity should be checked before starting therapy, as azathioprine may induce TPMT enzyme activity
- In cases of doubt, clinicians should discuss the result with the testing laboratory. Genotyping may be helpful in selected cases
- Whole blood is required for analysis (4 mL in ethylenediamine tetraacetic acid)
- Turnaround time for results varies according to laboratory and demand, but is usually within 2 weeks
- The blood sample should be appropriately packaged and labelled and sent by first-class post at room temperature
- Patients who have recently received blood products can have misleading TPMT results
- The following two U.K. National Health Service laboratories provide TPMT testing. Costs of tests are available on demand from each laboratory:

The Purine Research Laboratory, 5th Floor, Thomas Guy House, Guy's Hospital, London SE1 9RT, U.K.

Department of Clinical Biochemistry, City Hospital, Dudley Road, Birmingham B18 7QH, U.K.

The details of TPMT testing by the two laboratories are as follows

	Guy's Hospital	Birmingham City Hospital
Method	Tandem mass spectrometry	High-performance liquid chromatography
Units	$pmol\ h^{-1}\ mg^{-1}$ haemoglobin	$nmol\ h^{-1}\ g^{-1}$ haemoglobin
	Very low/absent < 10	Deficient < 5
	Low 10– <25	Low 6–24
	Normal 25–50	Normal 25–55
	High > 50	High > 55

The methodology for TPMT testing used by the laboratory at Guy's Hospital measures the formation of 6-methyl mercaptopurine from the substrates 6-mercaptopurine and S-adenosylmethionine. The 6-methyl mercaptopurine product is quantified by tandem mass spectrometry relative to a deuterated 6-methyl mercaptopurine internal standard.

The methodology for TPMT testing at Birmingham City Hospital uses 6-thioguanine as substrate and measures the product 6-methylthioguanine by high-performance liquid chromatography with fluorescence detection.

http://bad.org.uk/Portals/_Bad/Guidelines/Clinical%20Guidelines/Azathioprine.pdf

Comment

Since the azathioprine guidelines were published in 2004 [1] red blood cell thiopurine methyltransferase activity (TPMT) has become much more readily available in many hospital laboratories and so is now accepted practice among most dermatologists [2]. Most of the indications dermatologists use azathioprine are still unlicensed [2] and with the introduction of a new licensed therapeutic agent for chronic hand eczema [3] and efficacy of methotrexate in atopic eczema [4] azathioprine may be used less frequently by dermatologists. Despite systemic lupus erythematous being a licensed indication for azathioprine, there appears to be insufficient evidence to recommend its use in DLE [5].

References

1 Anstey AV, Wakelin S, Reynolds NJ. Guidelines for prescribing azathioprine in dermatology. *Brit J Dermatol* 2004; 151: 1123–132.
2 Vestergaard T, Bygum A. An audit of thiopurine methyltransferase genotyping and phenotyping before intended azathioprine treatment for dermatological conditions. *Clin Exp Dermatol* 2010; 35: 140–44.
3 Ruzicka T, Lynde CW, Jemec GB, *et al.* Efficacy and safety of oral alitretinoin (9-*cis* retinoic acid) in patients with severe chronic hand eczema refractory to topical corticosteroids: results of a randomized, double-blind, placebo-controlled, multicentre trial. *Br J Dermatol* 2008; 158: 808–17.
4 Weatherhead SC, Wahie S, Reynolds NJ, Meggitt SJ. An open-label, dose-ranging study of methotrexate for moderate-to-severe adult atopic eczema. *Brit J Dermatol* 2007; 156: 346–51.
5 Jessop S, Whitelaw DA, Delamere FM. Drugs for discoid lupus erythematosus. *Cochrane Database Syst Rev* 2009; Issue 4: CD002954 (http://www.mrw.interscience.wiley.com/cochrane/clsysrev/articles/CD002954/frame.html).

Additional professional resources

Patel AA, Swerlick RA, McCall CO. Azathioprine in dermatology: the past, the present, and the future. *J Acad Am Dermatol* 2006; 55: 369–89.

DMARDs: azathioprine. Clinical Knowledge Summaries 2008. http://www.cks.nhs.uk//dmards/management/quick_answers/scenario_azathioprine#.

BAD patient information leaflet

http://www.bad.org.uk/site/799/default.aspx

Other patient resources

http://www.dermnetnz.org/treatments/azathioprine.html

British Association of Dermatologists' guidelines for biologic intervention for psoriasis 2009

C.H. Smith, A.V. Anstey,* J.N.W.N. Barker, A.D. Burden,† R.J.G. Chalmers,‡ D.A. Chandler,§ A.Y. Finlay,¶ C.E.M. Griffiths,‡ K. Jackson, N.J. McHugh,** K.E. McKenna,†† N.J. Reynolds‡‡ and A.D. Ormerod§§ (Chair of Guideline Group)

St John's Institute of Dermatology, King's College London and Guy's and St Thomas' NHS Foundation Trust, London SE1 9RT U.K.

*Department of Dermatology, Royal Gwent Hospital, Newport NP20 2UB, U.K.

†Department of Dermatology, Western Infirmary, Glasgow G11 6NT, U.K.

‡The Dermatology Centre, Salford Royal Hospital, University of Manchester, Manchester Academic Health Science Centre, Manchester M6 8HD, U.K.

§Psoriasis and Psoriatic Arthritis Alliance, PO Box 111, St Albans AL2 3JQ, U.K.

¶Department of Dermatology, Cardiff University, School of Medicine, Heath Park, Cardiff CF14 4XN, U.K.

**Royal National Hospital for Rheumatic Diseases, Bath BA1 1RL, U.K.

††Department of Dermatology, Belfast City Hospital, Belfast BT9 7AB, U.K.

‡‡Institute of Cellular Medicine, Newcastle University, Newcastle upon Tyne NE2 4HH, U.K.

§§Department of Dermatology, Aberdeen Royal Infirmary, Foresterhill, Aberdeen AB9 2ZB, U.K.

Conflicts of interest

C.H.S., invited speaker and grant/research support Abbott, Janssen-Cilag, Schering-Plough, Serono, Wyeth; A.V.A., grant/research support Abbott, Janssen-Cilag, Schering Plough, Serono, Wyeth; J.N.W.N.B., advisory boards for Abbott, Janssen-Cilag, Novartis, Schering-Plough, Wyeth; grant/research support Abbott, Janssen-Cilag, Schering-Plough, Serono, Wyeth; A.D.B., advisory boards and grant/research support Janssen-Cilag, Schering-Plough, Serono, Wyeth; R.J.G.C., none; D.A.C., none; A.Y.F., consultant for Galderma, Novartis, Schering-Plough, Serono, Wyeth, Pfizer; joint copyright owner of the DLQI; C.E.M.G., advisory boards and invited speaker for Abbott, Janssen-Cilag, Merck-Serono, Novartis, Schering-Plough, UCB Pharma, Wyeth; grant/research support Amgen, Centocor, Merck-Serono, Wyeth; K.J., advisory boards for Abbott, Schering-Plough; educational support Merck-Serono; N.J.McH., advisory boards for Janssen-Cilag, Schering-Plough; grant/research support Abbott; K.E.McK., advisory boards for Abbott, Janssen-Cilag; N.J.R., advisory boards (nonpersonal) for Abbott, Basilea Pharmaceutica, Janssen-Cilag, Merck-Serono, Schering-Plough, Succinct Healthcare; grant/research support Stiefel Laboratories, AstraZeneca; A.D.O., advisory boards for Abbott, Merck-Serono, Schering-Plough; grant/research support Abbott, Janssen-Cilag, Serono, Wyeth.

This is an updated guideline prepared for the BAD Clinical Standards Unit, made up of the Therapy & Guidelines Subcommittee (T&G) and the Audit & Clinical Standards Subcommittee (A&CS). Members of the Clinical Standards Unit are: H.K. Bell (Chairman T&G), L.C. Fuller (Chairman A&CS), N.J. Levell, M.J. Tidman, P.D. Yesudian, J. Lear, J. Hughes, A.J. McDonagh, S. Punjabi, S. Wagle, S.E. Hulley and M.F. Mohd Mustapa (BAD Clinical Standards Administrator and Information Scientist).

Guidelines produced in 2005 by the British Association of Dermatologists; reviewed and updated June 2009.

DOI 10.1111/j.1365-2133.2009.09505.x

1.0 Background

Psoriasis is a common, chronic inflammatory skin disease which typically follows a relapsing and remitting course, and is associated with joint disease in approximately 25% of patients.[1] The significant reduction in quality of life and the psychosocial disability suffered by patients underline the need for prompt, effective treatment, and long-term disease control (reviewed[2,3]). Localized, limited disease can usually be managed satisfactorily with topical agents. Those with moderate to severe disease often require systemic treatment.

Phototherapy and traditional 'standard' systemic therapies, while often effective, can be associated with long-term toxicity; some are expensive, and some patients have treatment-resistant disease.[4] Also, phototherapy is not available to many due to geographical, logistical or other constraints. Patients themselves demonstrate high levels of dissatisfaction with standard approaches to treatment.[5,6]

Biologic therapies for psoriasis utilize molecules designed to block specific molecular steps important in the pathogenesis of psoriasis and now comprise a number of well-established, licensed, treatment options for patients with severe disease. Since 2005, when the British Association of Dermatologists (BAD) first published guidance on the use of biologic therapies in psoriasis,[7] much has changed. There is a substantial body of new evidence pertinent to the clinical use of these treatments, the U.K. National Institute for Health and Clinical Excellence (NICE) has approved the use of a number of biologic therapies in severe chronic plaque psoriasis and the BAD Biologic Interventions Register (BADBIR) has been successfully launched. Despite these developments, use of biologic therapy in clinical practice remains limited in the U.K., with a shortfall in funding cited as a significant obstacle to prescribing in approximately 40% of units recently surveyed.[8]

2.0 Purpose and scope

These guidelines have been revised and updated in accordance with a predetermined scope. This is based on the original scope used in 2005, and extended to include additional areas of practice. Recommendations in this guideline supersede those in the 2005 guideline.

The overall objective of these guidelines is to provide up-to-date, evidence-based recommendations on use of biologic therapies (infliximab, adalimumab, etanercept, ustekinumab) in adults and children with all types of psoriasis and, where relevant, psoriatic arthritis, for clinical staff involved in the care of patients treated with biologic therapies. Efalizumab remains in the scope of the guideline in relation to safety only, given that the European Medicines Agency has withdrawn the marketing authorization of this drug because of concerns over the development of progressive multifocal leukoencephalopathy (PML).

3.0 Exclusions

This guidance does not cover agents licensed outside the U.K. (alefacept) or use of biologic therapies for indications other than psoriasis and psoriatic arthritis.

4.0 Stakeholder involvement

The guideline working group represents all relevant stakeholders including dermatologists, nurses, rheumatologists and patients. Draft guidance was made available for consultation and review by patients, the BAD membership and the British Dermatological Nursing Group (BDNG). Advice relating to tuberculosis was reviewed and approved by the British Thoracic Society.

5.0 Methodology

The guideline has been developed using the BAD's recommended methodology[9] and with reference to the AGREE (Appraisal of Guidelines Research and Evaluation) instrument.[10] Recommendations were developed for implementation in the National Health Service using a process of considered judgment based on the evidence and an awareness of the European product licence of the various treatments.

Cochrane, EMBASE and Medline databases were searched between 1990 and June 2009 for clinical trials involving adalimumab, efalizumab, etanercept, infliximab and ustekinumab using an agreed protocol. Two reviewers screened all titles and abstracts independently, and full papers of relevant material were obtained. In relation to efficacy, only randomized controlled trials (RCTs) of high quality (1+ or more; see Appendix 1) were included for chronic plaque psoriasis, whereas in other clinical phenotypes, given the paucity of published data, all data were included. Data from each paper were extracted by two members of the guideline group using standardized literature evaluation forms in order to create evidence tables. Evidence on safety was extracted from literature on use of biologic agents for any indication in view of the relatively limited data specifically relating to use in psoriasis. The methodological limitations of the safety analysis are detailed in section 15. The guideline was peer reviewed by the Clinical Standards Unit of the BAD (made up of the Therapy & Guidelines and Audit & Clinical Standards Subcommittees) prior to publication.

6.0 Limitations of the guideline

These guidelines have been prepared on behalf of the BAD and reflect the best data available at the time the report was prepared. Caution should be exercised in interpreting the data; the results of future studies may require alteration of the conclusions or recommendations in this report. It may be necessary or even desirable to depart from the guidelines in the interests of specific patients and special circumstances. Just as adherence to guidelines may not constitute defence against a claim of negligence, so deviation from them should not necessarily be deemed negligent.

7.0 Plans for guideline revision

This field of psoriasis biologic therapeutics is in a rapid phase of development, and revision of the scope and content of the guidelines will therefore occur on an annual basis. Where necessary, the guideline will be updated via the BAD website, and a fully revised version is planned for 2012.

8.0 Which patients should be considered eligible for treatment?

Most patients with moderate to severe disease achieve satisfactory disease control (i.e. significant or complete clearing of disease) in the short term with at least one of the systemic agents currently available.[4] Long-term disease control frequently requires some form of continuous therapy and consequent, predictable risks of toxicity. At present, the risks and benefits of biologic therapies relative to standard systemic therapy are largely unknown. Widespread use of these agents in uncomplicated moderate to severe psoriasis is inappropriate and is not supported by the licensed indications for these drugs.

Eligibility criteria should encompass both objective measures of disease severity and the impact the disease has on quality of life. All existing disease severity assessment tools are imperfect[11–13] and most require some training to complete. The Psoriasis Area and Severity Index (PASI) is a measure of disease severity in chronic plaque psoriasis[12] and has been chosen for the purposes of this guideline as it has been widely used in clinical trials including those investigating biologic therapies, and has also been adopted by NICE. A PASI score of ≥ 10 (range 0–72) has been shown to correlate with a number of indicators commonly associated with severe disease such as need for hospital admission or use of systemic therapy,[14] and reflects the minimal level of disease severity required for patient inclusion in most of the clinical trials of biologic therapies to date. Where the PASI is not applicable (e.g. pustular psoriasis), body surface area (BSA) affected should be used, with severe disease defined as > 10% BSA affected.[14]

The Dermatology Life Quality Index (DLQI) is a validated tool for the measurement of quality of life across all skin diseases, including psoriasis, and has been used in both trial and clinical practice settings.[13,15] A score of > 10 (range 0–30) has been shown to correlate with at least 'a very large effect' on an individual's quality of life.[12,14,16]

8.1 Exceptional circumstances

When using the PASI and DLQI to determine whether or not a patient should be considered for biologic therapy, clinicians should take into account the applicability of these measures to each individual patient. There are circumstances where the use of these tools fails to give a sufficiently accurate assessment of the clinical situation. With respect to the PASI, this is especially pertinent in patients with localized disease that involves special 'high-impact' sites (genitalia, hands, feet, head and neck) where highly significant functional and/or psychosocial morbidity may exist with a PASI < 10. The DLQI may be a poor indicator of emotional disabilities resulting from psoriasis and the validity of the DLQI (and of other quality of life measures) may also be undermined due to linguistic or other communication difficulties.[13]

Recommendations: Eligibility criteria for biologic therapy

Patients with psoriasis may be considered eligible to receive treatment with any of the licensed biologic interventions when they fulfil the eligibility criteria set out below. However, the decision to proceed with treatment must be made in collaboration with the patient and include a careful assessment of the associated risks and benefits[17]

Eligibility criteria

To be considered eligible for treatment, patients must have severe disease as defined in (a) **and** fulfil one of the clinical categories outlined in (b):

(a) **Severe disease** defined as a **PASI score of 10 or more** (or a BSA of 10% or greater where PASI is not applicable) *and* a **DLQI > 10**. In exceptional circumstances (for example, disease affecting high-impact sites with associated significant functional or psychological morbidity such as acral psoriasis), patients with severe disease may fall outside this definition but should be considered for treatment (*Strength of recommendation D; level of evidence 3*) **AND**

(b) **Fulfil at least one of the following clinical categories** (*Strength of recommendation D; level of evidence 3, and formal consensus*)

(i) where phototherapy[a] and alternative standard systemic therapy[b] are contraindicated or cannot be used due to the development of, or risk of developing, clinically important treatment-related toxicity.

(ii) are intolerant to standard systemic therapy

(iii) are unresponsive to standard systemic therapy[b]

(iv) have significant, coexistent, unrelated comorbidity which precludes use of systemic agents such as ciclosporin or methotrexate

(v) have severe, unstable, life-threatening disease

Eligibility criteria for patients with skin and joint disease

(i) patients with active psoriatic arthritis or skin disease that fulfils defined British Society for Rheumatology (BSR)[18] or BAD guideline criteria, respectively

(ii) patients with severe skin psoriasis and psoriatic arthritis who have failed or cannot use methotrexate may need to be considered for biologic treatment given the potential benefit of such treatment on both components of psoriatic disease

[a]Phototherapy may be inappropriate in patients (i) who have exceeded safe exposure limits (150–200 treatments for PUVA, 350 treatments for narrowband UVB[19,20]), (ii) who are non-responsive or relapse rapidly, (iii) who have a history of skin cancer or repeated episodes of severe sunburn, (iv) who are intolerant of UV exposure, especially if skin phototype I (sun-sensitive), or (v) for logistical reasons

[b]Standard systemic therapy includes ciclosporin ($2 \cdot 5$ mg kg^{-1} daily; up to 5 mg kg^{-1} daily), and in men, and women not at risk of pregnancy, methotrexate [single dose (oral, subcutaneous, intramuscular) of 15 mg weekly; max 25 mg weekly] and acitretin (25–50 mg daily)

9.0 What is the definition of a disease response?

An adequate response to treatment is defined as **either** (i) a 50% or greater reduction in baseline PASI (PASI 50 response) (or % BSA where the PASI is not applicable) and a 5-point or greater improvement in DLQI[4,21–23] **or** (ii) a 75% reduction in PASI score compared with baseline (PASI 75 response). Initial response to therapy should be assessed at time points appropriate for the drug in question (Table 1).

For patients on tumour necrosis factor (TNF) antagonist treatment with psoriasis *and* psoriatic arthritis, treatment may be continued if there has been a sufficient response in at least one of these components (see BSR guidelines[18] for definition of disease response in psoriatic arthritis).

10.0 The interventions

10.1 Tumour necrosis factor antagonists

TNF is a proinflammatory cytokine produced by a wide variety of cell types including keratinocytes. It plays a central role in the pathogenesis of psoriasis, psoriatic arthritis and a number of other disease states. TNF is released from cells as a soluble cytokine (sTNF) following cleavage from its cell surface-bound precursor (transmembrane TNF, tmTNF). Both sTNF and tmTNF are biologically active, and bind to either of two distinct receptors: TNF receptor 1 (TNFR1, p55) and TNF receptor 2 (TNFR2, p75). This leads to NF-κB activation (which promotes inflammation) and/or cell apoptosis. In addition, tmTNF can

Table 1 Summary of interventions and criteria for treatment

Intervention	Dosing schedule according to licence[a]	NICE criteria	BAD criteria	Decision to continue treatment
Infliximab[b] (Remicade®; Schering-Plough, Welwyn Garden City, U.K.)	Adults: 5 mg kg⁻¹ at weeks 0, 2, 6 and then every 8 weeks (intravenous)	Very severe plaque psoriasis, i.e. PASI ≥ 20, DLQI ≥ 18 and where CSA, MTX or PUVA has failed/cannot be used	Severe psoriasis, i.e. PASI ≥ 10, DLQI > 10 and qualifying criteria	14 weeks (licence); 10 weeks (NICE)
Etanercept[b] (Enbrel®; Wyeth, Maidenhead, U.K.)	Adults: 25 mg biweekly (50 mg once weekly up to 24 weeks); or 50 mg twice weekly up to 12 weeks reduced to once weekly thereafter (subcutaneous)	Severe plaque psoriasis, i.e. PASI ≥ 10, DLQI > 10 and where CSA, MTX or PUVA has failed/cannot be used	Severe psoriasis, i.e. PASI ≥ 10, DLQI > 10 and qualifying criteria	12 weeks (NICE, licence)
Etanercept (Enbrel®)	Children > 8 years: 0.8 mg kg⁻¹ up to max 50 mg weekly (subcutaneous)	Not applicable; proposed for Single Technology Assessment (2009)	Severe psoriasis, i.e. PASI ≥ 10, DLQI > 10 and qualifying criteria	12 weeks (licence)
Adalimumab[b] (Humira®; Abbott, Maidenhead, U.K.)	Adults: 80 mg week 0, 40 mg week 1, then every other week (subcutaneous)	Severe plaque psoriasis, i.e. PASI ≥ 10, DLQI > 10 and where CSA, MTX or PUVA has failed/cannot be used	Severe psoriasis, i.e. PASI ≥ 10, DLQI > 10 and qualifying criteria	16 weeks (NICE, licence)
Ustekinumab[b] (Stelara®; Janssen-Cilag, High Wycombe, U.K.)	Adults: 45 mg at week 0, 4 and then every 12 weeks; adults > 100 kg: 90 mg week 0, 4 and then 90 mg every 12 weeks (subcutaneous)	Severe plaque psoriasis, i.e. PASI ≥ 10, DLQI > 10 and where CSA, MTX or PUVA has failed/cannot be used.	Severe psoriasis, i.e. PASI ≥ 10, DLQI > 10 and qualifying criteria	28 weeks (licence); 16 weeks (NICE)

NICE, National Institute for Health and Clinical Excellence; BAD, British Association of Dermatologists; PASI, Psoriasis Area and Severity Index; DLQI, Dermatology Life Quality Index; CSA, ciclosporin; MTX, methotrexate; PUVA, psoralen plus ultraviolet A. [a]Licensed indication for all therapies listed is 'treatment of patients with moderate to severe chronic plaque psoriasis who have failed to respond to, or who have a contraindication to, or are intolerant to other systemic therapies including ciclosporin, methotrexate and PUVA'. [b]Also licensed for use in **psoriatic arthritis**; approved by NICE provided the person has arthritis with three or more tender joints and three or more swollen joints, and at least two other disease-modifying antirheumatic drugs, given on their own or together, have not worked.

itself act as a ligand (via a process of *reverse signalling*) to induce cell activation, cytokine suppression or apoptosis of the tmTNF-bearing cell. Soluble forms of the TNF receptors also exist and, by binding and neutralizing sTNF, may act as natural TNF antagonists.

There are currently two approved groups of biologic agents that target TNF: anti-TNF monoclonal antibodies (adalimumab and infliximab), and sTNF receptors (etanercept). **Infliximab** is a chimeric human–murine monoclonal antibody (~ 25% mouse-derived protein) whereas **adalimumab** is fully human. **Etanercept** is a genetically engineered fusion protein composed of a dimer of the extracellular portions of human TNFR2 (p75) fused to the Fc domain of human IgG1. All three agents specifically bind both soluble and transmembrane forms of TNF and act by (i) blocking TNFR-mediated mechanisms and (ii) inducing tmTNF (reverse-signalling) events. Etanercept also binds members of the lymphotoxin family [LTα3 (also known as TNF-β) and LTα2β1] although the biological significance of this is unclear. Aside from the latter, there are important differences between the three agents with respect to pharmacokinetics, immunogenicity and structure-based mechanisms of action (only some of which are completely understood).[24] It is likely that these differences, in the context of the highly complex biology of TNF, account for observed differences in the efficacy and adverse events profile of TNF antagonists.

10.2 Efalizumab (now withdrawn – see section 15.3)

Lymphocyte function-associated antigen-1 (LFA-1) is a cell surface protein that binds to intracellular adhesion molecule (ICAM) 1–3 and plays a key role in T-lymphocyte recirculation, trafficking to sites of inflammation, antigen presentation by dendritic cells and other activated cells including keratinocytes, and T-cell costimulation. **Efalizumab** is a recombinant humanized IgG1 monoclonal antibody that binds specifically to the CD11a subunit of LFA-1, which by interfering with LFA-1/ICAM binding inhibits several key steps important in the pathogenesis of psoriasis including T-cell migration into the skin and T-cell activation. More recently, *in vivo* data have shown that efalizumab induces a state of reversible T-cell 'hyporesponsiveness' including downregulation of a number of T-cell surface molecules unrelated to LFA-1 both in the circulation and in psoriatic plaques.[25,26]

10.3 Ustekinumab

Interleukin (IL)-12 and IL-23 are heterodimeric cytokines secreted by activated antigen-presenting cells, and share a common protein subunit, p40. Of relevance to psoriasis, IL-12 activates CD4 and natural killer cells to induce expression of type 1 cytokines (TNF and interferon-γ) while IL-23 stimulates survival and proliferation of a subset of T cells that produce IL-17 (Th17 cells). Recent immunological[27] and genetic studies indicate a central role for IL-23 in the pathogenesis of psoriasis.[28] **Ustekinumab** is a fully human IgG1κ monoclonal antibody which acts as an IL inhibitor by binding with high affinity and specificity to the p40 protein subunit. It thus prevents IL-12 and IL-23 from binding to their IL-12Rβ1 receptor protein expressed on the surface of immune cells.

11.0 How effective is each intervention in chronic plaque psoriasis?

11.1 Etanercept

11.11 Etanercept in chronic plaque psoriasis

Three large RCTs demonstrate that etanercept is effective in chronic plaque psoriasis.[29–31] Onset of action is slower than that seen with the monoclonal antibodies, with clinically significant improvement in disease severity scores evident between 4 and 8 weeks after initiation of treatment.[30] Response is dose related, with 34% (25 mg biweekly) and 48% (50 mg biweekly) of patients achieving PASI 75 by 12 weeks (Table 2). Continuing therapy up to 6 months improves response rates further (43% and 57% for 25 mg biweekly and 50 mg biweekly, respectively).[29,30,32] While there are no RCT data establishing efficacy beyond 6 months, data from a 2-year, open-label etanercept 50 mg biweekly extension study[32] (following the phase III study reported by Tyring *et al.*[31]) suggest that efficacy is maintained for up to 1 year, with approximately 75% of patients maintaining their PASI 75 response over the ensuing year.

Overall, continuous therapy provides better disease control and higher levels of patient satisfaction compared with interrupted therapy. When treatment is stopped, disease relapses slowly: median time to disease relapse as defined by loss of PASI 50 in those who achieved PASI 75 after 24 weeks of continuous etanercept 25 or 50 mg biweekly, was 85 and 91 days, respectively, with no evidence of disease rebound. On re-treatment, mean PASI scores were similar, with the majority of patients achieving equivalent efficacy after 12 further weeks (i.e. 56% and 60% of PASI 75 responders achieved this level of efficacy on re-treatment).[33,34] Aside from objective measures of disease improvement (PASI, physician's global assessments), studies also report associated clinically meaningful improvements in quality of life measures,[35–37] reduction in fatigue and depression,[31] and increased proportions of patients in paid employment.[38,39] Post hoc analysis of two of these RCTs demonstrated that response rates in those over 65 years were the same as those under 65 years, although numbers in the older age group were small (n = 77).[40]

The 25 mg twice weekly and 50 mg once weekly dosing regimens are probably interchangeable given that their pharmacokinetic profiles are comparable,[41] that the number of patients achieving PASI 75 at 12 weeks following etanercept 50 mg weekly (in an RCT setting compared with placebo)[42] was comparable with that seen in other RCTs investigating etanercept 25 mg biweekly and that no significant differences

Table 2 Summary of the pooled results for efficacy from all clinical trials evaluated in the systematic review

	10–16 weeks				26 weeks		48–60 weeks		Comments
	PASI 75	95% CI	PASI 90	95% CI	PASI 75	95% CI	PASI 75	95% CI	
Etanercept 25 mg biweekly	0·34[29,30]	0·28–0·38	0·11[29,30]	0·08–0·15	0·43[29,30]	0·37–0·48		–	LOCF
Etanercept 50 mg biweekly	0·48[29–31]	0·44–0·52	0·21[29,30]	0·17–0·26	0·57[29,30,32]	0·52–0·6	0·6[32]	0·52–0·67	LOCF; patients continued on unlicensed dose after 12 weeks
Infliximab 5 mg kg^{-1} at 0, 2, 6 and every 8 weeks	0·79[52–56]	0·76–0·82	0·55[53,56]	0·50–0·60	0·74[53]	0·69–0·79	0·53[53,54]	0·48–0·57	LOCF
Adalimumab 40 mg every other week	0·69[62–65]	0·66–0·79	0·43[62–65]	0·40–0·46	0·69[62,63,65,68]	0·66–0·72	0·62[62,68]	0·54–0·71	Nonresponder imputation
Ustekinumab 45 mg at 0, 4 and every 12 weeks	0·67[71,72]	0·63–0·70	0·42[71,72]	0·38–0·46	0·68[71,72]	0·65–0·72		–	Nonresponder imputation
Ustekinumab 90 mg at 0, 4 and every 12 weeks	0·72[71,72]	0·68–0·75	0·45[71,72]	0·42–0·49	0·75[71,72]	0·72–0·77		–	Nonresponder imputation

PASI, Psoriasis Area and Severity Index; PASI 75, 75% reduction in PASI score compared with baseline; PASI 90, 90% reduction in PASI score compared with baseline. [a]Continuous subgroup. For each of the outcomes the crude probability (not adjusted for the placebo response) of the biologic treatment achieving the specified endpoints is given followed by the 95% confidence interval (CI). Longer-term data are not directly comparable between studies due to differences in accounting for study drop outs. Last observation carried forward (LOCF) may overestimate efficacy whereas nonresponder imputation gives a more conservative estimate of efficacy.

were observed in mean PASI or DLQI in a cohort of patients receiving open-label etanercept 25 mg biweekly (at week 24) and etanercept 50 mg once weekly (at week 36).[43]

In the RCTs cited, the frequency of adverse events or serious adverse events in patients receiving etanercept was no greater than in the control patients, with the exception of injection site reactions.

One small (n = 20 in each treatment arm) RCT has shown superior efficacy of etanercept 25 mg *once* weekly compared with acitretin 0·4 mg kg^{-1} daily at 24 weeks (see below).[44]

Given the role of TNF in adipocyte homeostasis, elevated levels of TNF in obese patients, and the fixed (nonweight adjusted) dosing regimen used for etanercept, decreased response rates may occur in heavier patients, particularly with low-dose etanercept. This is supported, in part, by pharmacological modelling (using published RCT data)[45] and data cited in the study by de Groot *et al.*[46]

11.12 Etanercept in chronic plaque psoriasis in combination with systemic therapies

Methotrexate

The combination of etanercept and methotrexate has been shown to be more effective in rheumatoid arthritis (RA) than either agent alone, with no significant additional toxicity. Limited data suggest that the addition of methotrexate may also confer improved etanercept efficacy in psoriasis. A small RCT (n = 59) investigated the efficacy and safety of introducing etanercept (25 mg biweekly) in patients already established on methotrexate, and reported significantly increased numbers of patients 'clear or nearly clear' at 24 weeks on combination therapy, as compared with those in whom methotrexate was discontinued.[47] A retrospective case series (n = 14) reported both improved efficacy with the introduction of methotrexate in patients on etanercept and loss of efficacy on withdrawal of methotrexate from patients on combination therapy.[48]

Acitretin

Data from a small RCT (n = 60) reported that the combination of etanercept 25 mg *once* weekly with acitretin 0·4 mg kg^{-1} daily is as effective as etanercept 25 mg *twice* weekly, and that both these interventions are more effective that acitretin alone.[44] These early data would suggest that in the short term at least, the combination may offer additional efficacy but, perhaps as importantly, there is no additional associated toxicity.

11.13 Quality of evidence

The patient cohort in the cited RCTs may not be representative of patients likely to be treated in clinical practice as entry to the studies required patients only to be considered suitable for, or have previously had, PUVA or systemic therapy. However, objective disease severity criteria were the same as those currently recommended by the BAD and NICE, and mean PASI scores on entry to studies were significantly higher (ranging from 16 to 18). Prospective case cohort studies of 'real life' practice report comparable response rates in 'high-need' patients who have previously failed multiple systemic therapies, all of which suggests that data from the RCTs can be extrapolated to clinical practice.[46,49,50] There is a lack of long-term RCT data beyond 6 months, and only limited data on re-treatment (of the two published studies available,[34,51] one is open label,[34] and both report outcome following one repeat cycle of treatment only).

Existing RCT data indicate that 50 mg biweekly is more effective than 25 mg biweekly, but there are no trial data indicating whether increasing the dose to 50 mg biweekly in patients who fail to achieve or maintain adequate responses on 25 mg biweekly results in improved disease control. This is especially pertinent given NICE guidance which currently limits treatment to the 25 mg biweekly dose (see below).

11.14 Licensed indications and existing NICE guidance (Table 1)

Etanercept is licensed for use in moderate to severe psoriasis at either 50 or 25 mg biweekly for the first 3 months, and 25 mg biweekly thereafter, for up to 24 weeks. Continuous therapy beyond 24 weeks may be appropriate for some adult patients (SPC). NICE has approved use of etanercept in severe plaque psoriasis (subject to defined disease severity) at the 25 mg biweekly dose only, and did not find the 50 mg twice weekly dose cost effective, with therapy to be continued only in those patients achieving disease response at 3 months (Table 1).

Recommendations: Etanercept

- Etanercept is recommended for the treatment of patients with severe psoriasis who fulfil the stated disease severity criteria – refer to section 8.0 (*Strength of recommendation A; level of evidence 1++*)
- Etanercept therapy may be initiated at either 50 or 25 mg twice weekly and disease response assessed at 3–4 months (*Strength of recommendation A; level of evidence 1++*)
- The choice of which dose to use will depend on clinical need, disease severity, body weight and, in the U.K., the dose that will be funded (*Strength of recommendation B; level of evidence 1++*)
- Patients established on etanercept 25 mg twice weekly may wish to consider switching to etanercept 50 mg once weekly as these two dosing regimens are equivalent in terms of efficacy (*Strength of recommendation A; level of evidence 1+*)
- In patients who respond, treatment may be continued according to clinical need, although long-term data on efficacy are limited to 2 years (*Strength of recommendation C; level of evidence 2+*)
- Treatment may be discontinued without risk of disease rebound, although there may be a lower response rate on restarting therapy (*Strength of recommendation B; level of evidence 1+*)

- Methotrexate may be recommended comedication in certain clinical circumstances, e.g. where it is required for associated arthropathy, or to improve efficacy (*Strength of recommendation B; level of evidence 1+*)

11.2 Infliximab

11.21 Infliximab in chronic plaque psoriasis

Three large RCTs[52–54] indicate that infliximab therapy is highly effective in chronic plaque psoriasis (Table 2[52–56]). Onset of action is rapid, with evidence of significant improvement within the first 2 weeks of treatment and maximum benefit by week 10 when 79% of patients achieve PASI 75 (Table 2) (and mean drop in DLQI of 10[54,57]). This response is largely maintained over time with 74%[53] and 53% achieving PASI 75 at 6 and 12 months, respectively (Table 2). Loss of efficacy correlates with development of antibodies to infliximab, which occurs in 19% of patients treated.[53] One RCT[54] (n = 835) investigated continuous vs. intermittent therapy (3 and 5 mg kg^{-1}) following a standard induction course (at 0, 2 and 6 weeks); continuous therapy at 5 mg kg^{-1} every 8 weeks achieved optimal control. Time to relapse in the intermittent arm (defined by loss of PASI 75) was stated as being 'between week 14 and 22 in the majority of patients' although data were not shown.[54] An early (small) dose-finding study[58] indicated that 50% (15/30) patients relapse (loss of PASI 75) by week 26. There are no published prospective trial data beyond 1 year.

Nail disease

One study prospectively assessed nail disease during therapy[53] using the Nail Psoriasis Severity Index (NAPSI) to assess a target, worst affected, nail: a 26·8% improvement in NAPSI from baseline was observed at week 10 with a maximum of 57·2% improvement reported at week 24. This was maintained until week 50. Numbers of patients with complete clearance of nail disease (from the target nail) continued to improve between weeks 24 and 50 (26·2% and 44·7%, respectively).

11.22 Infliximab in chronic plaque psoriasis in combination with systemic therapies

There are no RCT data on use of methotrexate in combination with infliximab in psoriasis. In both RA and psoriatic arthritis, cotherapy with methotrexate is a licensed recommendation, and response rates (with and without methotrexate) are at least comparable in these disease indications. Higher serum levels of infliximab have been reported with methotrexate coadministration which may in part explain reports of improved efficacy. Methotrexate (low dose, 7·5 mg weekly) also reduces the incidence of antibodies to infliximab.[59–61]

11.23 Quality of evidence

The patient cohort in the cited RCTs may not be representative of patients likely to be treated in clinical practice. The mean PASI at baseline was ≥ 10 in all the studies cited. However, failure of previous systemic therapy was not an entry criterion, in that most studies required patients to be candidates for systemic therapy and/or failed topicals only. A subanalysis of patients in the study by Menter et al.[54] (continuous vs. intermittent) did, however, indicate that baseline PASI (< 20 vs. > 20) and the nature of previous treatments (including two or more systemic therapies, or biologic therapy) had no effect on treatment response.

The design of the study investigating continuous vs. intermittent infliximab therapy is problematic in that study visits occurred at monthly intervals: hence patients randomized to receive intermittent therapy could potentially receive infliximab at 4-weekly intervals (if PASI 75 was not maintained), and cumulative doses in both arms were reported as similar.

11.24 Licensed indications and existing NICE guidance (Table 1)

Infliximab is licensed for use (5 mg kg^{-1} every 8 weeks) in moderate to severe plaque psoriasis. NICE has approved use of infliximab in patients with 'very severe disease' (sic) (PASI ≥ 20, DLQI ≥ 18) with treatment beyond 10 weeks recommended only in those who achieve certain response criteria.

Recommendations: Infliximab

- Infliximab is recommended for the treatment of patients with severe psoriasis who fulfil the stated disease severity criteria – refer to section 8·0 (*Strength of recommendation A; level of evidence 1++*)
- Infliximab therapy should be initiated at a dose of 5 mg kg^{-1} at weeks 0, 2 and 6 and disease response assessed at 3 months (*Strength of recommendation A; level of evidence 1++*)
- In patients who respond, subsequent infusions (5 mg kg^{-1}) should be given at 8-week intervals to maintain disease control although long-term data are available only up to 1 year (*Strength of recommendation A; level of evidence 1++*)
- Interrupted therapy should be avoided given the associated increased risk of infusion reactions and poorer disease control (*Strength of recommendation A; level of evidence 1+*)
- Methotrexate may be recommended comedication in certain clinical circumstances, e.g. where it is required for associated arthropathy, to improve efficacy or to reduce the development of antibodies to infliximab (*Strength of recommendation D; level of evidence 3*)

11.3 Adalimumab

11.31 Adalimumab in chronic plaque psoriasis

Three large RCTs demonstrate that adalimumab is a highly effective treatment for chronic plaque psoriasis (Table 2).[62-64]

Onset of action is rapid, with significant improvements in disease severity evident within 2 weeks of treatment initiation[62] and maximal disease response seen between weeks 12 and 16. Response is dose related with 69% of patients achieving PASI 75 at week 12 with adalimumab 40 mg every other week[62-65] (i.e. the licensed dose for psoriasis), and 80% achieving PASI 75 with adalimumab 40 mg weekly.[62] Clinically relevant improvements in health-related quality of life indicators are also reported.[66] In one study,[62] a small subset of patients (n = 34) who had failed to achieve PASI 50 following at least 24 weeks of adalimumab every other week was escalated to the weekly dose for the remaining duration of the 60-week study (open-label); 40% of this cohort recorded PASI 50 responses, suggesting that dose escalation may further improve efficacy. Efficacy data are available up to 1 year, with no evidence of significant loss of response over time in those patients who respond and are continued on treatment.[63]

Loss of response on stopping treatment was also investigated in the third phase of the study reported by Menter et al.;[63] those who had maintained PASI 75 by week 33 were re-randomized to receive either placebo or a further 19 weeks of adalimumab (double blind). While mean time to relapse was not reported, 28% of patients receiving placebo relapsed (< PASI 50 response relative to baseline with a minimum of a 6-point increase in PASI score relative to week 33) compared with 5% relapse in those continuing on adalimumab by week 52. As part of this study, patients who lost adequate response after re-randomization to placebo could enrol into the open-label extension phase of the trial (adalimumab 40 mg every other week). Re-treatment response rates in this group are stated (only) in the summary of product characteristics (SPC), where 38% (25/66) and 55% (36/66) regained PASI 75 response after 12 and 24 weeks, respectively. These response rates are lower than those reported following first treatment, suggesting that interrupted therapy may result in loss of treatment response.

Anti-adalimumab antibodies develop in 8·4% of patients and are associated with increased clearance and reduced efficacy of adalimumab (but not specific adverse events).

11.32 Adalimumab compared with standard systemic therapy in chronic plaque psoriasis

One RCT comparing efficacy of adalimumab (40 mg every other week) vs. methotrexate (7·5 mg initial dose weekly, increasing to a maximum of 25 mg weekly as tolerated) showed adalimumab to be significantly more effective than methotrexate by week 1, with 80% of patients achieving PASI 75 by week 16. This compared with surprisingly low methotrexate (36%) and high placebo (19%) response rates.[64] The latter are considerably higher than seen in other comparable placebo-treated cohorts where PASI 75 response rates are typically 5% or less. Improvements in DLQI and a number of other quality of life measures also indicated that adalimumab was the most effective intervention.[67] Overall, the incidence of adverse events was similar in all three groups, with the exception of hepatic abnormalities which were significantly higher in patients on methotrexate.

11.33 Adalimumab in chronic plaque psoriasis in combination with systemic therapies

The addition of methotrexate to adalimumab in RA results in reduced immunogenicity (i.e. a lower rate of anti-adalimumab antibody formation) and increased effectiveness (in part due to reduced clearance of adalimumab) with no increase in adverse events. No prospective studies have investigated the potential benefit of adalimumab in combination with methotrexate in psoriasis. In the ADEPT study, a *post hoc* analysis comparing those patients who were on a stable dose of methotrexate at initiation of adalimumab, and those who were not, suggests that for both skin and joint disease the combination of adalimumab and methotrexate is more effective than adalimumab alone, although the differences were only significant between the groups for the percentage achieving PASI 50.[65,68]

11.34 Quality of evidence

The patient cohort in cited RCTs may not be representative of patients likely to be treated in clinical practice. With the exception of the first (small) RCT[62] where entry disease severity comprised BSA > 5%, and studies on psoriatic arthritis where skin disease severity criteria were not set (mean PASI on entry 7)[65,68] all studies cited required PASI of at least 10 and/or BSA 10%, and mean disease severity scores on entry to psoriasis studies[63,64] tended to be significantly higher than this.

   Previous use of systemic therapies was not an entry criterion for the RCTs cited, and of course, for the comparative study examining methotrexate vs. adalimumab, patients had to be treatment naive both to TNF antagonists and to methotrexate. One small (n = 30) open-label study evaluated the efficacy of adalimumab 40 mg *once* weekly in a cohort of patients with severe psoriasis who had failed both standard systemic therapy and other biologic therapies (including efalizumab, etanercept and infliximab).[69] By week 12, 87% of patients had achieved PASI 75, which represents a response rate comparable with that reported in the RCT by Gordon *et al.*[62] As adalimumab has only recently been licensed for use in psoriasis, few data exist on use outside clinical trials. The design of the study reported by Saurat *et al.*[64] has been criticized as favouring adalimumab, given that the maximum efficacy of methotrexate may not have been apparent by 16 weeks.

11.35 Licensed indications and existing NICE guidance (Table 1)

Adalimumab is licensed for use in moderate to severe psoriasis at 40 mg every other week (following 80 mg loading dose at week 0), with continued therapy beyond 16 weeks to be 'carefully reconsidered' in patients not responding within this time period; NICE has approved use of adalimumab (40 mg every other week) in severe plaque psoriasis (subject to defined disease severity) with continued therapy subject to adequate response at 16 weeks (Table 1).

Recommendations: Adalimumab

- Adalimumab is recommended for the treatment of patients with severe psoriasis who fulfil the stated disease severity criteria – refer to section 8.0 (*Strength of recommendation A; level of evidence 1++*)
- Adalimumab therapy should be initiated according to the licensed dosing regimen (i.e. 80 mg subcutaneously at week 0, 40 mg at week 1, and then every other week thereafter) and disease response assessed at 3–4 months (*Strength of recommendation A; level of evidence 1++*)
- Consideration may be given to increasing the dose of adalimumab to 40 mg weekly in certain clinical circumstances (e.g. in those with PASI > 10 despite achieving a response[a] to adalimumab 40 mg every other week), although this is unlicensed and not approved by NICE (and in the U.K. may not be funded) (*Strength of recommendation A; level of evidence 1+*)
- In patients who respond, treatment may be continued according to clinical need although long-term efficacy data are available only up to 1 year (*Strength of recommendation A; level of evidence 1++*)
- If necessary, treatment may be discontinued without risk of disease rebound, although there may be a lower response rate on restarting therapy (*Strength of recommendation A; level of evidence 1+*)
- Methotrexate may be recommended comedication in certain clinical circumstances, e.g. where it is required for associated arthropathy, or to increase efficacy (*Strength of recommendation B; level of evidence 3*)

[a]as defined in section 9.0 (PASI 50, DLQI −5)

11.4 Ustekinumab

11.41 Ustekinumab in chronic plaque psoriasis

Three large RCTs[70–72] demonstrate that both doses of ustekinumab (i.e. 45 mg and 90 mg) are highly effective in psoriasis (Table 2); onset of action is evident within 2 weeks, with 67% and 72% of patients achieving PASI 75 by week 12 for the 45 mg and 90 mg doses, respectively, and maximal efficacy evident between week 20 and week 24. Disease responses are maintained with continued therapy for up to 1·5 years. On cessation of therapy, median time to relapse (i.e. loss of PASI 75) is 15 weeks, with no reports of rebound psoriasis. Similar response rates are achieved on re-treatment. While there is clearly a relationship between dose (serum drug levels) and response, this is not linear, as the 90 mg dose appears to be only slightly more effective than the 45 mg dose. Further, in partial responders, increasing the frequency of dosing to every 8 weeks (as compared with every 12 weeks), while increasing serum drug levels, significantly improves response rates only in those on the 90 mg regimen [approximately 2/3 of partial responders (defined as > PASI 50, < PASI 75 at week 28) converted to responders (PASI 75) by week 52 with intensification of the 90 mg dose to 8-weekly]. Factors aside from the lower dose that are predictive of poorer response include higher body weight, previous poor response to at least one biologic therapy, longer duration of psoriasis and a history of psoriatic arthritis. While the inclusion criteria for these trials are comparable to those investigating other biologic therapies (PASI 12 and BSA 10% or greater), overall, the disease severity appears to be greater (mean PASI scores on entry around 20), with the majority of patients having received previous phototherapy and systemic therapy, and just over a third having received prior biologic therapy.

A phase II study has evaluated the use of ustekinumab in the treatment of psoriatic arthritis (n = 146, active: control allocation 1:1, dose regimen 90 mg weekly for 4 weeks). At week 12, 42% of patients achieved a clinical response [defined as a 20% improvement from baseline in the American College of Rheumatology (ACR20) core set measures].[73]

11.42 Ustekinumab compared with etanercept in chronic plaque psoriasis

A large (n = 903), phase III RCT indicates that us-tekinumab is more effective than etanercept in the short term. The percentage of patients achieving PASI 75 by week 12 with ustekinumab 90 mg and 45 mg at week 0 and 4 was 74% and 68%, respectively, compared with 57% for patients randomized to etanercept 50 mg biweekly for 12 weeks.[74]

11.43 Licensed indications and existing NICE guidance (Table 1)

Ustekinumab is licensed for use in patients with moderate to severe psoriasis at 45 mg (or 90 mg if >100 kg) at week 0, 4 and then 12 weekly thereafter with consideration given to discontinuing therapy in those who have not responded by week 28. NICE has approved the use of ustekinumab in patients with severe plaque psoriasis (subject to defined disease severity criteria) with treatment to be continued beyond 16 weeks only in those who respond (Table 1).

Recommendations: Ustekinumab

- In light of limited patient exposure, ustekinumab should be reserved for use in patients with severe psoriasis who fulfil the stated disease severity criteria AND where TNF antagonist therapy has failed or is contraindicated – refer to section 8.0 (*Strength of recommendation A; level of evidence 1+*)
- For logistical and safety reasons, drug injections should be supervised by a health care professional (*Strength of recommendation D (GPP); level of evidence 4*)

12.0 How effective are biologic therapies in pustular psoriasis and palmoplantar pustulosis?

12.1 Localized disease

There are two disabling and difficult-to-treat conditions affecting the hands and feet in which localized pustules are associated with psoriasis elsewhere on the body.

The more common of these, chronic palmoplantar pustulosis, has in the past been termed chronic palmoplantar pustular psoriasis. There is, however, evidence to suggest that, although it is associated with psoriasis in up to about 20% of cases, it is a distinct disease with a different clinical and genetic profile.[75] This evidence is strengthened by the almost complete lack of reports of benefit from TNF antagonists but, conversely, an increasing number of reports of new-onset palmoplantar pustulosis in patients with conditions other than psoriasis treated with these agents.[76,77] A recent small pilot study found no benefit over placebo of etanercept 50 mg given twice weekly for 12 weeks.[78] TNF antagonists should therefore be avoided in these patients.

The second condition is acropustulosis (acrodermatitis continua) of Hallopeau. Although uncommon, acropustulosis can result in considerable morbidity from an intense pustular inflammation centred around the terminal phalanges and often sufficiently severe to destroy the nail plate. It is commonly associated with a destructive arthritis of adjacent joints. It is recognized that patients with acropustulosis are at risk of developing generalized pustular psoriasis.

There are no controlled trials of interventions for acropustulosis. It is frequently unresponsive to conventional systemic antipsoriatic agents. There are now at least 10 case reports of significant benefit from TNF antagonists (etanercept, infliximab and adalimumab) for this rare but disabling condition. This contrasts with only two reports of failure to respond and, in one of those cases, the patient subsequently responded to a different TNF antagonist. If acropustulosis has a major impact on quality of life, it is therefore reasonable to recommend a trial of one of these agents.

12.2 Generalized pustular psoriasis

Publications concerning biologic treatments for generalized pustular psoriasis are limited to case reports and small series, reflecting the fact that these drugs are relatively new in the treatment of psoriasis, and that generalized pustular psoriasis is a very rare disorder. Infliximab has been used in the treatment of severe generalized pustular psoriasis with generally positive results. A 39-year-old man with severe generalized pustular psoriasis responded rapidly to infliximab with complete disease clearance which allowed withdrawal of all conventional systemic psoriasis treatments.[79] A follow-up study of three patients with generalized pustular psoriasis included two who cleared completely with infliximab treatment, while one was left with residual keratoderma.[80] On stopping infliximab following a variable number of infusions, two of these three relapsed, while disease remission was maintained in one. Additional case reports and a small case series (n = 3) confirm efficacy for infliximab in the treatment of generalized pustular psoriasis.[81–84] Etanercept has also been shown to be of benefit in generalized pustular psoriasis. One case series (n = 6) reports clinical efficacy of etanercept in generalized pustular psoriasis at 50 mg biweekly, but not at 25 mg biweekly, with maintenance of response for up to 48 weeks.[85] One report confirms efficacy for etanercept in a single patient with generalized pustular psoriasis following withdrawal of ciclosporin,[86] and a second, use of etanercept in generalized pustular psoriasis following induction of remission with infliximab.[87]

Reports of biologic therapies for generalized pustular psoriasis in childhood are limited to two cases: a 3-year-old child cleared rapidly with infliximab and was switched successfully to etanercept after 12 months of infliximab infusions.[88] A 15-year-old girl with severe generalized pustular psoriasis treated with ciclosporin, methotrexate and adalimumab cleared completely by 2 months.[89]

Thus, for patients with generalized pustular psoriasis, experience of treatment with biologic agents is currently limited to infliximab, etanercept and adalimumab. These initial case reports and small case series are generally positive and justify formal clinical trials to assess safety and efficacy in more detail in this difficult patient group.

13.0 How effective are biologic therapies in erythrodermic psoriasis?

TNF antagonists are reported to be of benefit in this form of psoriasis, which given that many cases evolve from chronic plaque disease is perhaps not surprising. A case series of 10 patients with erythrodermic psoriasis responded well to etanercept 25 mg twice weekly. The mean PASI decreased from 39·1 to 5·1 at 24 weeks, when 60% had achieved PASI 75.[90]

Three of five erythrodermic patients achieved PASI 75 with repeated infusions of infliximab 5 mg kg^{-1}.[80] There are also several case reports of successful treatment of erythrodermic psoriasis, including life-threatening disease, with infliximab therapy,[91–95] one clearing with a single infusion.[96] Infliximab was also successful in three patients who experienced erythrodermic flares when transitioning from efalizumab to etanercept.[97] No evidence was found concerning the efficacy of adalimumab in erythrodermic patients.

Recommendations: Use of biologic therapy for special types including pustular and erythrodermic psoriasis

• Biologic therapies cannot at present be recommended for palmoplantar pustulosis

---

• TNF antagonists may be considered for patients with severe, disabling acropustulosis (acrodermatitis continua) of Hallopeau which has failed to respond to standard systemic agents – refer to section 8.1: exceptional circumstances (*Strength of recommendation D; level of evidence 3*)
• TNF antagonists may be considered for patients with generalized pustular psoriasis (*Strength of recommendation D; level of evidence 3*)
• TNF antagonists (infliximab and etanercept) may be considered for patients with erythrodermic psoriasis (*Strength of recommendation D; level of evidence 3*)

14.0 Use of biologic therapy in combination with phototherapy

The rationale for using these two contrasting forms of treatment together is that both have differing mechanisms of action which may be synergistic when used together. However, trial data are limited to a single arm, open-label study, evaluating etanercept 50 mg twice weekly combined with narrowband UVB phototherapy given three times weekly (n = 86).[98] At week 12, 26% of patients achieved PASI 100, 58·1% achieved PASI 90, and 84·9% achieved PASI 75. It is unclear what effect each treatment had as this study failed to include a comparator group with either monotherapy or placebo.

There is currently insufficient evidence to recommend the combination of narrowband UVB phototherapy with etanercept, and no data at all on combined use of infliximab or adalimumab with phototherapy. An RCT is needed to establish whether combining UVB phototherapy with biologic therapies offers more rapid clearance of disease which is sustained when monotherapy continues with the biologic agent.

15.0 Adverse effects and toxicity

15.01 Methodological considerations

When considering the relative risks (and benefits) of biologic interventions, it is important to note that there are significant methodological limitations to published safety data. Trials are powered to detect efficacy, not adverse events, and there is therefore a high chance that low-frequency, drug-related adverse events will not be identified.[99] In addition, many of the data available in relation to psoriasis derive from clinical trials in which only the first 3 months have a comparable placebo group. Long-term extensions of these trials look at patients who remain on therapy and those lost from the cohorts may be lost because of adverse reactions (leading to under-reporting). Long-term data are also poorly reported.[100] Several high-quality meta-analyses of high-quality trials are limited by the sparsity of safety data within the original reports themselves.

Information accrued on TNF antagonist therapies used in other indications may not necessarily be applicable to the population treated for psoriasis. This may be especially relevant in relation to assessment of skin cancer risk as patients with psoriasis may already have a higher risk of skin cancer due to prior phototherapy and immunosuppressive drugs. The demographics of different diseases are also likely to influence the toxicity profile of any intervention. For example, the higher incidence of RA in women has resulted in a female bias to safety data reported to the BSR biologics register (BSRBR). This underlines the importance of ensuring that all patients are registered with the BADBIR which will assess safety issues in the relevant population.

15.02 Overview of adverse effects for all interventions

A significant body of data is now available on the adverse effects and toxicity associated with biologic therapies. Comprehensive, detailed information is available in the SPC for each drug and is regularly updated by pharmaceutical companies (and approved by the drug regulatory authorities). The U.K. versions can be accessed at http://emc.medicines. org.uk/.

Schmitt et al.[101] recently reviewed tolerability of biologic and nonbiologic therapies in a meta-analysis. Tolerability assessed by withdrawals showed monthly withdrawal rates of 1·3% (range 0·5–1·6) for infliximab, 1·2% (0·6–1·9) for efalizumab, 0·4% (0·3–1·4) for etanercept and 0·3% for adalimumab. Additionally infusion reactions occurred in 2·1% of patients per month with infliximab. Serious adverse events occurred at a monthly rate of 1·1% with infliximab, 1·2% with efalizumab and 0·5% with adalimumab. Rates for etanercept could only be computed from the data for the 50 mg biweekly dose, and were 0·6%. Brimhall et al.[102] conducted a meta-analysis of adverse events of biologic therapies based on pooled short-term trial data. They expressed a relative risk of adverse events and severe adverse events, compared with placebo. Risks for efalizumab were 1·15 (adverse events) and 1·43 (serious adverse events); for etanercept 1·05 (adverse events) and 1·17 (serious adverse events); and for infliximab 1·18 (adverse events) and 1·26 (serious adverse events). Of these, only the relative risk of adverse events with infliximab and serious adverse events with efalizumab reached an increased level of statistical significance. Adalimumab was not included in the analysis.

15.1 Tumour necrosis factor antagonist therapies

15.11 Infections: bacterial, mycobacterial, viral

Data from clinical trials indicate that infections are common, but overall rates of infection are no greater than with placebo.

Rheumatology registry data do suggest an increased risk of skin and soft tissue infections [adjusted incidence rate ratio 4·28, 95% confidence interval (CI) 1·06–17·17] compared with standard disease-modifying antirheumatic drugs (DMARDs)[100] and although these are poorly characterized,

they have included erysipelas, cellulitis, furunculosis, folliculitis, paronychia and wound infections. An increased risk of herpes zoster has also been reported in rheumatology patients on TNF monoclonal antibody therapy, but not etanercept, from the German rheumatology registry: crude incidence rate per 1000 patient-years 11·1 (95% CI 7·9–15·1) for the monoclonal antibodies, 8·9 (95% CI 5·6–13·3) for etanercept, and 5·6 (95% CI 3·6–8·3) for conventional DMARDs.[103] When rates were adjusted for age, RA severity and glucocorticoid use, a significantly increased risk was still observed for treatment with the monoclonal antibodies (hazard ratio 1·82, 95% CI 1·05–3·15), but not etanercept or TNF antagonist therapy as a class. These findings are supported by cohort and case–control studies using data from the U.K. general practice research database and a U.S. health plan claims database which showed increased risk of herpes zoster with biologic therapy (infliximab, etanercept and anakinra) compared with DMARDs in patients with RA.[104]

Serious infections, including opportunistic infections, have also been reported (see SPC and below for additional details).

15.12 Reactivation of tuberculosis

This is a major concern with all TNF antagonist therapies, as TNF plays a key role in host defence against mycobacterial infection, particularly in granuloma formation (and hence containment of mycobacteria) and inhibition of bacterial dissemination.[105,106] Early data (2003) from the BIOBADASER registry (Spanish Society of Rheumatology Database on Biologic Products) reported an estimated incidence of 1893 cases per 100 000 patient-years with infliximab[107] compared with 21 in the general population. This led to careful selection pretreatment and monitoring and greatly reduced the incidence in those complying with pretreatment testing and prophylaxis, although adherence to guidelines was poor.[108] The risk of tuberculosis may be greater with the monoclonal antibodies (infliximab and adalimumab) as compared with etanercept with incidences of tuberculosis in patients with RA reported to the BSRBR of 39 per 100 000 patient-years for etanercept, 103 per 100 000 patient-years for infliximab and 171 per 100 000 patient-years for adalimumab.[109,110] Even when latent tuberculosis is identified and treated prior to TNF antagonist therapy, patients may develop clinical evidence of infection. Thus a high index of suspicion throughout treatment is required. The clinical presentation of infection is often atypical, with at least 50% of cases associated with infliximab[111,112] and etanercept[113] being extrapulmonary. Late diagnosis, development of disseminated disease and concomitant immunosuppressive therapy may all contribute to high rates of morbidity, and associated mortality.[111,112] Onset of clinical infection varies according to the agent used, with median time between initiation of therapy and diagnosis of infection being 3 months,[111,112] 4–6 months[106] and 11·5 months[113] for infliximab, adalimumab and etanercept, respectively.

The mode of action of ustekinumab predicts that it would also facilitate reactivation of tuberculosis. All the trials conducted with this agent excluded patients with latent tuberculosis.

Although the levels of evidence and risk differ between agents the consensus of the guideline development group is to generalize the cautions and vigilance for latent or active tuberculosis to all biologic interventions.

Recommendations: Biologic therapy and infection risk

• Patients on biologic interventions should be monitored for early signs and symptoms of infection throughout treatment (*Strength of recommendation C; level of evidence 2+*)

• Patients on biologic interventions should be warned against risk factors for *Salmonella* and *Listeria* and should not consume raw or partially cooked dairy, fish or meat produce or unpasteurized milk or milk produce. Salads should be washed (*Strength of recommendation D (GPP); level of evidence 4*)

• All patients should be fully assessed for both active and latent tuberculosis before starting biologic therapy with special attention paid to those groups at high risk (*Strength of recommendation B; level of evidence 2+*)

• Patients with active or latent tuberculosis should receive treatment prior to initiating biologic therapy (*Strength of recommendation B; level of evidence 2+*)

• A high index of suspicion for tuberculosis should be maintained during therapy and for 6 months after discontinuation, with special emphasis on extrapulmonary, atypical and disseminated forms of the infection, and in those patients on additional immunosuppressant agents (*Strength of recommendation C; level of evidence 2+*)

See section 18.5 for recommendations on screening and monitoring for tuberculosis

---

Table 3 New York Heart Association classification of heart failure symptoms

Class	Symptoms[a]
I	No limitations. Ordinary activity does not cause fatigue, breathlessness or palpitations (asymptomatic left ventricular dysfunction is included in this category)
II	Slight limitation of physical activity. Such patients are comfortable at rest. Ordinary physical activity results in fatigue, breathlessness, palpitation or angina pectoris (symptomatically 'mild' heart failure)
III	Marked limitation of physical activity. Although patients are comfortable at rest, less than ordinary physical activity will lead to symptoms (symptomatically 'moderate' heart failure)
IV	Inability to carry out physical activity without discomfort. Symptoms of congestive cardiac failure are present even at rest. With any physical activity increased discomfort is experienced (symptomatically 'severe' heart failure)

[a]Patients with heart failure may have a number of symptoms, the most common being breathlessness, fatigue, exercise intolerance and fluid retention.

15.13 Cardiovascular disease

The risks of TNF antagonist therapy in the context of heart failure were first highlighted when trials in severe congestive cardiac failure [New York Heart Association (NYHA) class III and IV, left ventricular ejection fraction < 35%; Table 3] were prematurely discontinued due to an excess mortality with high-dose infliximab; a similar trial of etanercept failed to show benefit.[114] Forty-seven spontaneous reports to the U.S. Food and Drug Administration (FDA) of new onset or worsening of pre-existing heart failure following either infliximab or etanercept have been reviewed in detail with the possibility of drug-induced pathology supported by an apparent temporal association between introduction of drug and onset of symptoms (median onset 3 months with infliximab, 8·5 months with etanercept).[115] Pre-existing risk factors for heart disease were absent in 50% of cases, and complete resolution or substantial improvement of symptoms seen on withdrawal of drug in younger patients (< 50 years). Clinical trial data in psoriasis and other diseases[116] show no excess risk of heart failure although selection bias (i.e. exclusion of those at risk) may account for this.[117]

Recommendations: Cardiovascular disease and TNF antagonists

• TNF antagonist therapy should be avoided in patients with severe (NYHA class III and IV) cardiac failure (*Strength of recommendation D; level of evidence 4*)

• Patients with well-compensated (NYHA class I and II) cardiac failure should have a screening echocardiogram and those with an ejection fraction < 50% of normal should not be given TNF antagonist therapy (*Strength of recommendation D; level of evidence 4*)

• Treatment should be withdrawn at the onset of new symptoms or worsening of pre-existing heart failure (*Strength of recommendation D; level of evidence 4*)

15.14 Neurological disease

TNF antagonist therapy has been associated with the development of, or worsening of demyelinating disease although evidence for causality is inconclusive. Lenercept, a soluble p55 receptor developed for the treatment of multiple sclerosis, was withdrawn from further development due to increasing severity and duration of symptoms in clinical trial subjects. Cases of demyelination have been reported with all three TNF blockers available for psoriasis (SPC and in reference[118]). A detailed review of cases reported to the FDA in 2001 identified 17 due to etanercept and two due to infliximab, partial or complete resolution of symptoms on discontinuation and with recurrence of symptoms in at least one case following rechallenge.[118] Registry data in RA suggest that this risk is small.[119,120] Guidelines recently issued from the American Academy of Dermatology recommend that TNF antagonist therapy be avoided in patients with a personal history of, or a first-degree relative with a demyelinating disorder.[121]

> **Recommendations: Demyelination and TNF antagonists**
>
> • TNF antagonists should be avoided in patients with history of demyelinating disease and used with caution in those with a first-degree relative with such disease (*Strength of recommendation D; level of evidence 3*)
> • If neurological symptoms suggestive of demyelination develop during TNF antagonist therapy, treatment should be withdrawn and specialist advice sought (*Strength of recommendation D; level of evidence 4*)

15.15 Paradoxical events

Certain diseases, including psoriasis, that are commonly responsive to TNF antagonist therapy, have 'paradoxically' been reported, rarely, to be triggered or exacerbated by TNF antagonist therapy. Various granulomatous reactions, particularly involving the lung and including some indistinguishable from sarcoid,[122] small vessel vasculitis (predominantly in the skin)[123] and uveitis[124] have been described in patients on TNF antagonists for mainly rheumatological indications. These data derive largely from spontaneous reports or case series so it is currently unclear as to the size of any risk, and whether it is relevant to patients using TNF antagonist therapy for psoriasis.

With respect to psoriasis, more than 120 sporadic cases of both new-onset and worsening psoriasis have been reported in patients using TNF antagonist therapy for a wide spectrum of predominantly rheumatological disorders although including some cases of psoriasis (reviewed[76,77]). This association is supported by data from the BSRBR indicating a significantly increased incidence of new-onset psoriasis with TNF antagonist therapy as compared with standard DMARDs in patients with RA.[125]

15.16 Malignancy

To date, there is no robust evidence of increased risk of malignancy with TNF antagonists in patients with psoriasis. Data from clinical trials are reassuring, and there is no indication from registry data in rheumatology populations of increased risk of solid tumours and lymphoma with TNF antagonist therapy as compared with standard DMARDs to date.[126] However, uncertainty and conflicting evidence remain around the possible increased risk of lymphoma, possibly because lymphomas are more common in patients with severe RA. Bongartz *et al.*[127] carried out a meta-analysis of nine trials of patients with RA treated with infliximab or adalimumab. The data included 3493 patients who received TNF antagonist treatment and 1512 patients who received placebo and demonstrated a pooled odds ratio for malignancy of 3·3 (95% CI 1·2–9·1). This paper raised a variety of methodological concerns[128–130] which included lack of adjustment for duration of exposure to TNF antagonist therapy, inclusion of open-label extension data for biologic therapy with no comparable placebo data, infliximab induction doses exceeding labelled dose in approximately 50% of patients and an unexpectedly low rate of malignancy in the control arms. In addition, both infliximab and adalimumab have been rarely associated with hepatosplenic T-cell lymphoma.[131] This rare, aggressive, and usually fatal tumour has occurred in adolescents and young adults with Crohn's disease who were also receiving treatment with azathioprine or mercaptopurine.[132–136] There are also reports of cases of early onset of lymphoma after introduction of TNF antagonist therapy[137,138] and regression of lymphoma following withdrawal of TNF antagonist therapy.[137,139]

With respect to skin cancer, data on TNF antagonists in RA are inconsistent. Pharmacovigilance data on 1440 patients with RA treated with etanercept from clinical trials (3530 person-years total exposure time) did not show any link between squamous cell carcinoma (SCC) development and etanercept.[140] Lebwohl *et al.*[141] carried out a retrospective analysis of 1442 patients with RA treated with etanercept for up to 5 years and similarly found no increased incidence of SCC (observed four SCCs, expected 5·9–13·1). However, an increased risk of nonmelanoma skin cancer (NMSC) (odds ratio 1·5, 95% CI 1·2–1·8) and a trend towards increased risk of melanoma (odds ratio 2·3, 95% CI 0·9–5·4) has recently been reported in a large (> 13 000 patients) observational study comparing rates of malignancy in patients with RA on biologic therapies with population rates (drug-specific data from this analysis are given in the relevant section below).[139]

Leonardi *et al.*[142] evaluated the incidence of malignancy in patients receiving efalizumab in 14 clinical trials (2980 patients). One case of malignant melanoma occurred in patients treated with efalizumab (incidence rate 0·04 per 100 patient-years, 95% CI 0·00–0·22), compared with no cases in the placebo cohort and an incidence of 0·02 per 100 patient-years derived for the general population. For NMSC, 51 tumours [basal cell carcinomas (BCCs); 30 SCCs] were reported in efalizumab-treated patients (i.e. 1·2% of all efalizumab-treated patients), compared with four tumours (two BCCs, two SCCs in two patients) in placebo-treated patients, giving incidence rates of 1·38 per 100 patient-years (95% CI 0·96–1·92) for efalizumab, 1·08 per 100 person-years (95% CI 0·13–3·89) for placebo, and 0·39 per 100 patient-years in external psoriasis cohorts on oral therapy or phototherapy. This increased incidence of NMSC in both efalizumab and placebo groups was suggested to be possibly related to ascertainment bias.

Long-term registry data collated from the pertinent population are essential to address properly the question of cancer risk in patients with severe psoriasis treated with biologic therapy.

> **Recommendations: Malignancy risk and biologic therapy**
>
> • It is very strongly recommended that all patients being treated with biologic therapy should be entered into the BADBIR (subject to patient consent) in order to establish whether biologic therapy is associated with any increased risk of important side-effects such as malignancy, compared with standard systemic therapy (*Strength of recommendation D (GPP); level of evidence 4*)
> • All patients should be fully assessed prior to, and during treatment with, biologic therapy with respect to their past or current history of malignancy and/or any future risk of malignancy; the

risks and benefits of biologic therapy should be considered in this context (*Strength of recommendation D; level of evidence 4*)

• All patients should be encouraged to participate in national cancer screening programmes appropriate for their age and gender (*Strength of recommendation D (GPP); level of evidence 4*)

• Biologic therapy should be avoided in patients with a current or recent past history of malignancy *unless* the malignancy has been diagnosed and treated more than 5 years previously and/or where the likelihood of cure is high (this includes adequately treated NMSC) (*Strength of recommendation D; level of evidence 4*)

• Regular, comprehensive dermatological assessment for skin cancer, including melanoma, is recommended before and at regular intervals during therapy, especially in those patients at increased risk of skin cancer at baseline (*Strength of recommendation D; level of evidence 4*)

• Biologic therapy is relatively contraindicated in patients who have had prior therapy with > 200 PUVA and/or > 350 UVB treatments, especially when it has been followed by ciclosporin (*Strength of recommendation D; level of evidence 4*)

See Table 4 for summarized recommendations on screening and monitoring

15.2 Drug-specific details

15.21 Etanercept

The *commonest adverse events* reported are injection site reactions (14%),[143] allergic reactions, headache and upper respiratory tract infection.[102]

Injection site reactions, while common, diminish with ongoing therapy and do not relate to antibody development.

Infections constituted 21% of FDA reports of adverse effects in 2001.[144] In a short-term evaluation of 1347 patients with psoriasis these included sinusitis, upper respiratory tract infections and influenza, and were of similar rates to placebo. Skin infections occurred in 14% of patients.[145] Serious infections were rare (0·4%) and comparable with placebo rates.[143]

Aside from tuberculosis (discussed above), opportunistic infections may occur including listeriosis,[146,147] streptococcal pneumonia, aspergillosis, histoplasmosis,[148] cryptococcosis, *pneumocystis* pneumonia, *Legionella* and *Salmonella*.[144,147]

Malignancy. A long-term 3-year open-label etanercept study of 1498 patients not treated with other disease-modifying drugs revealed no change in the rate of malignancy (or severe infections) over time and malignancies were fewer than expected in the normal population.[119] An increased risk of NMSC of 1·2 (95% CI 1·0–1·5) and melanoma 2·4 (95% CI 1·0–5·8) has been reported in those patients treated with etanercept for RA.[139] Combining the results of placebo- and active comparator-controlled clinical trials of etanercept, more cases of NMSC were observed in patients receiving etanercept compared with control patients, particularly in patients with psoriasis (SPC). Other data in relation to malignancy are summarized in section 15.16.

Lupus-like syndrome with positive antibodies is reported but is rare and affected patients have not experienced systemic features.

Aplastic anaemias and pancytopenia have been reported rarely following etanercept and a neutropenia occurred in one of the long-term trials over 12 months.[144]

15.22 Infliximab

The *commonest side-effects* are upper respiratory tract infection, headache, increased hepatic enzymes and infection.

Acute infusion-related reactions with diverse symptoms occur in 3–22% of patients with psoriasis,[149] including, rarely, anaphylactic shock and delayed hypersensitivity. Antibodies to infliximab can develop which can increase the risk of immunological reactions and reduce the efficacy of therapy. Detailed information on management of infusion reactions is available in a recent comprehensive review.[149]

Hepatoxicity in the form of elevation in liver transaminases is well recognized to occur with infliximab therapy.[53] In general, these elevations are transient and asymptomatic but rare cases of severe hepatitis and acute liver failure resulting in transplantation or death have been reported.

Infections. Soft tissue infections, sepsis, candidiasis, fungal infections, pharyngitis, sinusitis and rhinitis are uncommonly reported. Serious infections have included pneumonia, bronchitis, peritonitis, septicaemia, pyelonephritis, cellulitis, systemic fungal infection and herpes zoster. Aside from tuberculosis (discussed above), opportunistic infections are also of concern and include atypical mycobacteria, histoplasmosis, coccidioidomycosis, *Pneumocystis* pneumonia, candidosis and aspergillosis.[145]

Malignancy. There is no indication from registry data of increased malignancy risk with infliximab. In a clinical trial investigating efficacy of infliximab in chronic obstructive pulmonary disease, nine of 157 patients in the active arm developed a malignancy as compared with one of 77 with placebo,[150] although this finding was not statistically significant. An increased risk of skin cancer has been reported in patients treated with infliximab: NMSC 1.7 (95% CI 1·3–2·2) and melanoma 2·6 (95% CI 1·0–6·7).[139] Other data in relation to malignancy are summarized in section 15.16.

Other adverse effects. As with etanercept, there are reports of lupus-like reactions and demyelination, but these are rare.

15.23 Adalimumab

The *commonest adverse events* reported are injection site reactions, viral, candidal and bacterial infections, dizziness, headaches, vertigo, gastrointestinal upset, musculoskeletal pain, rash, asthenia and malaise (SPC).

Injection site reactions occur in 15% of patients treated (compared with 9% of patients receiving placebo or active control) but generally do not result in discontinuing therapy.

Table 4 Recommended pretreatment and monitoring investigations

	Pretreatment[a]	Monitoring[a]	Grade of evidence; strength of recommendation[b]
BADBIR	Yes	6-monthly	D; 4
Disease severity assessment			
Skin: PASI (or BSA affected if PASI not applicable), DLQI	Yes	To establish disease response; 6-monthly thereafter	A; 1+
Joints: follow recommended BSR guidelines for psoriatic arthritis	Yes	To establish disease response; 6-monthly thereafter	A; 1+
Identification of contraindications to therapy and/or development of therapy-induced toxicity			
Thorough history, symptom enquiry, clinical examination (including full skin check; assessment for lymphadenopathy, hepatosplenomegaly)	Yes	At 3- to 6-monthly intervals	D (GPP)
Cardiovascular assessment[c]			
Echocardiogram if well-compensated NYHA class I and II	Yes	Clinical assessment at 3- to 6-monthly intervals	D; 4
Neurological assessment			
Exclude demyelination[c]	Yes	At 3- to 6-monthly intervals	D; 4
Infection			
Consider risk factors for tuberculosis; sexual history; drug abuse; history of blood transfusions; any past or current chronic infection	Yes	At 3- to 6-monthly intervals	GPP
Malignancy			
Ensure concordant with national cancer screening programmes; gynaecological review of patients with history of cervical dysplasia; any past or current malignancy	Yes	At 3- to 6-monthly intervals	GPP
Assessment for latent tuberculosis			
See Figure 1	Yes	Annually (IGRA)	A; 2+
Blood tests			
Full blood count	Yes	At 3 months, then every 6 months	A; 1+
Creatinine, urea, electrolytes	Yes	At 3 months, then every 6 months	GPP
Liver function tests	Yes	At 3 months, then every 6 months	A; 1+
Hepatitis B	Yes	Periodically in those at risk	D; 4
Hepatitis C	Yes[a]	Periodic assessment of hepatitis C viral load if positive	D; 4
Human immunodeficiency virus	Yes[d]	Periodically in those at risk	D; 4
Autoantibodies (antinuclear antibodies, antinuclear double-stranded DNA antibodies)	Yes	Only if symptoms suggest development of autoimmune phenomena, e.g. abnormal liver function tests	D; 4
Urine			
Urine analysis	Yes	Not routinely	
Urine pregnancy test	Yes	Periodically in those at risk	
Radiology			
Chest X-ray	Yes	Only if clinically indicated	

BADBIR, British Association of Dermatologists Biologic Interventions Register; PASI, Psoriasis Area and Severity Index; BSA, body surface area; DLQI, Dermatology Life Quality Index; BSR, British Society for Rheumatology; NYHA, New York Heart Association; IGRA, interferon gamma release assay. [a]Additional assessment and monitoring may be required in patients on concomitant therapy or in certain clinical circumstances. [b]See Appendix 1. [c]Applies to tumour necrosis factor blockers only. [d]In those with risk factors.

Infections. A composite of clinical trials involving 12 506 patient-years and postmarketing surveillance was reported for adalimumab in 2006.[151] The rate of serious infection was 5·1 per 100 patient-years and was not increased above those published in RA untreated with biologic therapy. Four cases of histoplasmosis occurred in endemic areas. Post-tuberculin screening, the rate of tuberculosis was 330 per 100 000 patient-years in Europe and 80 per 100 000 in

North America and 0·6% of patients receiving tuberculosis prophylaxis acquired tuberculosis. Postmarketing surveillance has revealed further cases of tuberculosis and opportunistic infections.

Malignancy. In the same analysis outlined above,[151] a standardized incidence ratio of 3·19 was reported for the rate of lymphomas but such increases are observed in severe RA without biologic interventions. A further analysis of an open-label study (REACT) with 6610 patients was published in 2007 and included patients with other concomitant disease-modifying drugs.[152] Results were similar to those in the original report,[151] with the exception of malignancy, where the standardized incidence ratio for malignancies (including lymphoma but excluding BCCs and carcinoma *in situ*) was 0·71 (95% CI 0·49–1·0). The observed number of lymphoma cases was significantly greater than the expected number only in the RA trials (standardized incidence rate 2·98; 95% CI 1·89–4·47). Other data in relation to malignancy are summarized in section 15·16.

Other adverse effects associated with TNF antagonists have also been reported with adalimumab, with incidence rates of 0·08 per 100 patient-years for demyelinating disorders, 0.1 per 100 patient-years for lupus-like syndromes and 0·28 per 100 patient-years for congestive cardiac failure.[151]

15.3 Safety and efalizumab

Safety data for efalizumab are more limited compared with TNF antagonist therapy as therapy has largely been confined to patients with psoriasis, with approximately 47 000 patient-years exposed to date. Several studies have examined safety in clinical trials with extended open observation of patients for up to 3 years[153–157] and all give a similar incidence of adverse events.

Very recently, three cases of confirmed PML have been reported in patients on efalizumab with consequent withdrawal of the European marketing licence by the European Medicines Agency. PML is a rare, progressive, demyelinating disorder of the central nervous system, associated with reactivation of John Cunningham virus (JCV) in immunosuppressed individuals. It leads to death or severe disability, and there are no known medical interventions that can reliably prevent or treat the disorder. All three of the reported cases occurred in patients on efalizumab monotherapy for 3 years or more. The occurrence of this usually fatal adverse event is of significant concern particularly given that if PML is particularly associated with protracted use of efalizumab, estimates suggest that as many as 1500 patients have been exposed to treatment for as long as 3 years. It also highlights the risk of unexpected serious adverse events that follows the introduction of any new drugs into clinical practice.

The commonest adverse events were headaches (36%), chills (11%), fever (9%), asthenia (6%) or influenza-like symptoms (9·8%), back pain (6%), diarrhoea (6%) and myalgia (6%). These commonly occur during the first few weeks of treatment but tend to resolve with continued therapy.[155]

Thrombocytopenia occurs uncommonly (between one in 500 and one in 1000 patients), so platelet counts should be monitored. Lymphocytosis and leucocytosis (up to 3·5 × upper limit of normal) is a regular finding with efalizumab therapy due to its effect of blocking their migration out of the bloodstream, and may be used to confirm patient concordance.

A transient, acute, pruritic eruption occurs commonly in previously uninvolved sites (7%).[156] The eruption may be sudden and resemble pustules joining into plaques. This eruption is self-limiting and should be treated with topical steroids and not be mistaken for a psoriasis flare. Flares of psoriasis are uncommon (2%), and tend to occur in low or nonresponders.[156]

Arthralgia and exacerbation of psoriatic arthritis have been reported in association with efalizumab. A pooled review of RCT data reported no increased incidence of joint symptoms or development of psoriatic arthritis in those patients receiving efalizumab compared with placebo.[154] However, in a 2-year follow-up study of 555 patients, the rate of arthralgia and arthritis increased over time from 1·6% to 5·6% at the end of the study with most of the affected patients having a prior history of psoriatic arthritis.[158] In addition, a multicentre, retrospective case cohort review of all patients treated with efalizumab in France identified 16 patients with new-onset, severe psoriatic arthritis, with a median time to onset of 11 weeks, and evidence of improvement in symptoms on drug withdrawal.[159]

Infection rates. There is no direct evidence of increased rates of infection with efalizumab. We are not aware of reported cases of tuberculosis. *Candida* colitis and cytomegalovirus (CMV) have been reported. However, the SPC has special warnings for infection including tuberculosis, opportunistic infection, pyelonephritis, septic arthritis and septicaemia. Opportunistic infections are reported as uncommon in the SPC.

Malignancy. There have not been increased reports of malignancy, with the overall incidence reported as 1.7 per 100 patient-years in a systematic review of safety data published in 2006.[144] Leonardi *et al.*[142] pooled data from clinical trials and reported no significant increase in solid malignancies or lymphoproliferative disease. However, as summarized in section 15.16, an increase in NMSC was noted.[142]

15.4 Safety and ustekinumab

Safety of ustekinumab in psoriasis has been evaluated in two phase III trials.[71,72] Five hundred and ten patients received up to 76 weeks of treatment in one study reported by Leonardi *et al.*[71] and 1212 received treatment for up to 52 weeks in the study reported by Papp *et al.*[72] Overall rates of adverse events were similar to placebo, and there was no consistent evidence for a relationship between dose or frequency of dosing, and the occurrence of adverse events. An RCT comparing ustekinumab and etanercept in psoriasis reported comparable rates of adverse events with both drugs through 12 weeks of therapy, with the exception of injection site reactions which were more common with etanercept.[74] Further, limited data on adverse events are available in each of three phase II studies evaluating ustekinumab in psoriatic arthritis,[73] Crohn's disease[160] and multiple sclerosis,[161] respectively, where the pattern and rates of adverse events were similar in active and placebo groups. No exacerbation of demyelinating events was reported in the study evaluating ustekinumab in multiple sclerosis (n = 150 receiving active drug).[161]

Common adverse events in both studies included upper respiratory tract infection, nasopharyngitis, arthralgia, cough and headache.

Injection site reactions were uncommon (1·5%), perhaps because of the infrequency of drug administration. Antibodies (neutralizing) develop in approximately 5% of patients and are associated with poorer responses to therapy, but do not correlate with injection site reactions.

Infection. In the study by Leonardi *et al.*[71] the incidence of serious infections was 0·4–0·8% in the different subgroups and similar to the placebo phase. There were three incident cases of noncutaneous cancers and four cutaneous cancers. Laboratory abnormalities were low in rate and were similar between treated patients and the placebo group.[71] In the study reported by Papp *et al.*,[72] serious infection occurred in 0–0·5%, similar to placebo. There were seven cutaneous cancers and one other (noncutaneous) cancer on therapy, with similar rates in the placebo arm.

No cases of tuberculosis, demyelination or lymphoma were identified. However, as discussed in section 15.1, the mode of action of ustekinumab would be expected to facilitate reactivation of tuberculosis.

16.0 How to determine the optimal choice and sequence of therapy

Given the proven efficacy of TNF antagonists in psoriasis, the substantial body of available clinical safety data (albeit not confined to patients with psoriasis) and the high proportion of patients with associated psoriatic arthropathy, TNF antagonists should be considered the first-line biologic intervention. Multiple factors will determine which of the three available TNF antagonists should be used first in a particular patient. This includes those related to the drug itself and how they relate to the clinical circumstance, patient preferences (e.g. mode of administration) and access, the latter being determined largely by local funding arrangements. In the short term, the monoclonal antibodies (infliximab and adalimumab) have a quicker onset of action, and are more effective than etanercept, although by 1 year the proportion of patients maintaining a PASI 75 may be comparable (Table 2). With respect to safety, systematic review of RCT data from short-term studies suggests that the risk of adverse events may be slightly higher with infliximab compared with etanercept[101,102] and adalimumab[101] while registry data indicate that risks of reactivation of tuberculosis and herpes zoster may be greater with adalimumab and infliximab as compared with etanercept.[103,109,110]

Ustekinumab is more effective than etanercept in the short term (based on a large RCT directly comparing the two agents)[74] and is probably of comparable efficacy to adalimumab and infliximab, but safety data are very limited. Ustekinumab should therefore be reserved for patients who have failed or cannot use TNF antagonists.

There are only limited efficacy data on use of a second biologic therapy in patients with psoriasis where the first has failed. Mechanisms underlying primary failure (i.e. inadequate response following initiation of treatment) or secondary failure (i.e. loss of response over time) are poorly understood,[24] although in the case of TNF antagonists, development of antidrug antibodies with consequent reduction in circulating drug levels is well described with both infliximab and adalimumab.[53,63] Further, while infliximab, adalimumab and etanercept all act to block TNF, they are pharmacologically distinct (see reference[24] for a detailed review). Thus failure to respond to one TNF antagonist may not preclude response to a second. This is supported by findings in a small open-label study[69] and retrospective case cohort review[162] which demonstrate efficacy of adalimumab following etanercept failure.

Of note, approximately a third of patients entered into ustekinumab RCTs had been previously treated with biologic therapy (predominantly TNF antagonists), and this did not influence therapeutic outcome.

Recommendations: How to determine the optimal choice and sequence of therapy

- TNF antagonists are recommended as first-line intervention for patients fulfilling criteria for treatment with biologic therapy – refer to section 8.0 (*Strength of recommendation B; level of evidence 1+*)
- The choice of which of the three TNF antagonists **to use first** should be based on clinical need and requires a careful assessment of risks and benefits of each agent in the context of the individual patient. With this proviso, the following additional recommendations are made:
- For patients with stable chronic plaque psoriasis, etanercept or adalimumab may be considered first choice based on the favourable risk/benefit profile and ease of administration (*Strength of recommendation D; level of evidence 4*)
- For patients requiring rapid disease control, adalimumab or infliximab may be considered first choice due to the early onset of action, and high chance of achieving PASI 75 by 3 months (*Strength of recommendation A; level of evidence 1+*)
- For patients with unstable or generalized pustular psoriasis, limited evidence indicates that infliximab is effective in these clinical situations, and may therefore be considered first choice (*Strength of recommendation D; level of evidence 3*)
- For patients who do not respond to a TNF antagonist (either primary or secondary failure), a second TNF antagonist may be considered (*Strength of recommendation D; level of evidence 3*)
- Due to the lack of patient-years exposure and long-term safety data limited to 1 year, ustekinumab should be reserved for use as a second-line biologic agent where TNF therapy has failed or cannot be used (*Strength of recommendation B; level of evidence 1+*)

17.0 How to use biologic therapy in special circumstances

17.1 Use of biologic therapy in children

One RCT[163] indicates that etanercept is effective in chronic plaque psoriasis in children. Among 106 patients aged 4–17 years (median 14 years) who received etanercept 0.8 mg kg^{-1} (up to maximum dose of 50 mg) by weekly subcutaneous injection, 57% achieved a PASI 75 at 12 weeks as against 11% in the placebo arm. Subjects had psoriasis with a baseline PASI of 12 or more and had disease that was poorly controlled with topical therapy or had prior treatment with phototherapy or systemic therapy. Improvement was noted by 4 weeks of treatment and was maintained during an open-label extension to week 36. There was no significant difference in response when the results were analysed separately for those under the age of 12 years as compared with those over the age of 12 years.

In the RCT the frequency of exposure-adjusted adverse events was low and similar to the placebo arm. Three serious infections were reported in the open-label phase in patients receiving etanercept. Longer-term safety data are needed in this patient group.

17.11 Quality of evidence

The patient cohort in the cited RCTs may not be representative of patients likely to be treated in clinical practice, in that not all patients were required to have failed or be contraindicated to systemic therapy.

17.12 Licensed indications and existing NICE guidance (Table 1)

Etanercept is licensed for treatment of chronic severe plaque psoriasis in children and adolescents from the age of 8 years who are inadequately controlled by, or are intolerant to, other systemic therapies or phototherapies. NICE is currently considering a proposal for Single Technology Assessment. Etanercept is also licensed for treating juvenile idiopathic arthritis (JIA), a term which encompasses paediatric psoriatic arthritis. NICE has approved the use of etanercept in children aged 4–17 years with five or more inflamed joints who have failed to respond to methotrexate. The long-term safety of etanercept in JIA has been demonstrated up to 8 years.[164]

> **Recommendations: Use of biologic therapy in children**
>
> • Etanercept is recommended for the treatment of severe psoriasis in children from the age of 8 years who fulfil the stated disease severity criteria – refer to section 8.0 (*Strength of recommendation A; level of evidence 1++*)
> • Etanercept therapy should be initiated at a dose of 0·8 mg kg^{-1} weekly and disease response assessed at 3–4 months (*Strength of recommendation A; level of evidence 1++*)

> • In patients who respond, treatment may be continued according to clinical need, although long-term data on efficacy are limited to 1 year (*Strength of recommendation A; level of evidence 1+*)

17.2 Use of biologic therapy in women planning pregnancy or who are pregnant

The overall question relates to the safety of biologic therapy in women who are pregnant. In practical terms this can be broken down to four main scenarios. Firstly, is it safe for women planning pregnancy or for women who are pregnant to continue with biologic therapy for psoriasis or should women established in biologic therapy come off biologic therapy prior to planning pregnancy? Secondly, is it safe for women who are pregnant and experience a flare of psoriasis during pregnancy to be initiated on biologic therapy? Thirdly, what action should women who are established on biologic therapy for psoriasis take if they discover that they are pregnant? Fourthly, is it safe for women to initiate or continue biologic therapy while breast feeding?

There are no prospective or retrospective studies that have addressed treatment of psoriasis during pregnancy with TNF antagonists. However, there are several publications concerning the outcome of pregnancy following exposure to TNF antagonists in a number of other diseases (principally Crohn's disease and arthritis) although these patients, in contrast to patients with psoriasis, are more likely to have been exposed to combination therapy.

17.21 Surveys and retrospective series: tumour necrosis factor antagonists

Mahadevan et al.[165] describe the first intentional use of infliximab during pregnancy in a retrospective review of 10 patients with Crohn's disease. Eight patients received maintenance therapy during the whole of pregnancy, one received infliximab during the first trimester and one during the third trimester. Concomitant medication included 6-mercaptopurine in five women and systemic steroids in four women. Eight of the 10 women had caesarean sections. There were no fetal congenital abnormalities; three infants were premature and one had low birth weight but these were not thought to be secondary to infliximab therapy.

Databases for monitoring safety set up by Centocor (pharmaceutical company that markets infliximab) include TREAT[166] and the Infliximab Safety Database[167] (which may in part overlap) and report 66 and 146 pregnancies,[166,167] respectively, in which exposure to infliximab occurred. No fetal abnormalities were reported in the TREAT study and rates of miscarriage and neonatal complications were not increased compared with control groups in either study. One preterm death at 24 weeks and four infants born with complications are reported in the Infliximab Safety Database[167] including one Fallot's tetralogy and one neonatal sepsis.

A report of the BSRBR includes information on 23 pregnancies in which exposure to TNF antagonists occurred at the time of conception resulting in 14 live births with no major fetal abnormalities.[168,169] There were six first-trimester spontaneous abortions and three elective first-trimester abortions.

In a retrospective study of 442 patients treated with TNF antagonists[170] three women with RA became pregnant. One patient opted for elective abortion while two patients exposed to either adalimumab or etanercept proceeded to deliver healthy infants although one was premature. Perinatal complications included neonatal jaundice, neonatal urinary *Escherichia coli* infection and adrenal congenital hyperplasia of probable hereditary origin.

Four further patients with severe arthritis were maintained on anti-TNF therapy (one etanercept, three infliximab) during pregnancy and all gave birth to healthy infants with no complications.[171]

As TNF has been hypothesized to be involved in the pathogenesis of spontaneous abortions, a recent study compared anticoagulants (group I), anticoagulants plus intravenous immunoglobulins (IVIG) (group II) or anticoagulants plus IVIG plus etanercept or adalimumab (group III; 17 patients) as treatment for women with recurrent spontaneous abortion.[172] Anti-TNF agents were administered 30 days prior to a cycle of conception and continued until fetal cardiac activity was demonstrated by ultrasound. Significant improvement in pregnancy outcome was observed in groups II and III compared with group I. No birth defects were observed in any of the babies in group III who had been exposed to anti-TNF agents.

A recent publication describes the outcome of pregnancy of 15 women receiving anti-TNF therapy (infliximab, n = 3; adalimumab, n = 2; etanercept, n = 10) at the time of conception or during pregnancy reported by French rheumatologists, through a web-based structured questionnaire.[173] The women had received anti-TNF therapy for a median of 8 months before pregnancy (range 1–48 months). Two miscarriages were reported and one woman who was also taking methotrexate opted for elective abortion. The median length of exposure to anti-TNF therapy during the 12 successful pregnancies was 6 weeks (range 3–38 weeks) with 12 of 12 women receiving anti-TNF therapy during the first trimester compared with four of 12 women during the third trimester. No complications, prematurity, malformations or neonatal illnesses were described.

In contrast to the reports above, congenital abnormalities have been associated with TNF antagonists in a recent review of the FDA database; a total of 61 congenital anomalies occurred in 41 children born to mothers taking a TNF antagonist (22 took etanercept, 19 took infliximab) in the period 1999–2005. In 24 of 41 cases, the mother was on no other medication. The most common reported congenital anomaly was some form of heart defect. Twenty-four of the 41 (59%) children had one or more congenital anomalies forming part of VACTERL (vertebral abnormalities, anal atresia, cardiac defect, tracheoesophageal, renal, and limb abnormalities). The

rate of specific anomalies was significantly higher than historical controls implicating a causal role for TNF antagonists.[174]

A survey returned by 150 American rheumatologists indicated that they were more concerned about the risks of methotrexate in pregnancy than anti-TNF biologic agents.[175] Three congenital abnormalities reported in the survey were all associated with methotrexate usage alone.

17.22 Case reports: tumour necrosis factor antagonists

A patient with psoriasis and psoriatic arthritis who continued etanercept 50 mg subcutaneously twice weekly throughout her pregnancy gave birth to a child with fetal anomalies of the VATER association (including renal dysplasia, skeletal defects and tracheoesophageal fistula).[176]

The successful use of etanercept (and IVIG) during pregnancy for flare of systemic lupus erythematosus and RA has been reported and healthy babies with no complications ensued.[177,178]

There are limited data on outcomes of pregnancies following exposure to adalimumab. There are three case reports of women with Crohn's disease who received adalimumab during pregnancy and gave birth to healthy babies with no complications.[169,179,180] A patient with Takayasu's arthritis continued adalimumab (and leflunomide) during pregnancy and delivered a healthy baby with no complications.[181]

17.23 Infliximab crosses the placenta and has a long half-life but is not detected in breast milk

High infliximab levels were detected in the serum of an infant born to a mother with refractory Crohn's disease who continued to receive infliximab (10 mg kg^{-1}) during her pregnancy.[182] The last infusion was given 2 weeks prior to labour. Infant infliximab levels were high at 6 weeks (39·5 µg mL^{-1}) and remained elevated up to 6 months of age. Infliximab was not detected in breast milk, suggesting that placental transfer results in neonatal exposure and that the half-life of infliximab is prolonged in infants.

A recent case report describes a successful pregnancy with no infant abnormalities in a mother with refractory Crohn's disease who continued to receive infliximab (10 mg kg^{-1}) during her pregnancy and while breast feeding.[183] Analysis of breast milk revealed no evidence of infliximab over 30 days.

A recent report in abstract form of a prospective study of five women receiving infliximab indicates that infliximab was detectable in infants up to 2–6 months of age depending on the date of the last infusion in relation to birth,[184] suggesting further caution over the use of infliximab in the later stages of pregnancy.

17.24 Licensing guidance and summary

Manufacturers of etanercept, infliximab and adalimumab advise avoidance during pregnancy. Although no toxicity or teratogenicity has been reported in animal studies of etanercept, caution should be exercised when considering the use of TNF antagonists during pregnancy. There are surveys and reports of successful and complication-free use of biologic therapy during pregnancy but these are limited and there are also some reports of perinatal complications including premature birth together with recent data associating VACTERL with TNF antagonists. Risk assessment is therefore difficult.

Also, these drugs may be used in combination with methotrexate which is contraindicated in pregnancy because of well-documented associations with spontaneous miscarriage, cleft palate and skeletal abnormalities.[185–187]

17.25 Use of biologic therapy in men and conception

There are very few publications that have addressed whether TNF or TNF antagonists may affect spermatogenesis, number or quality of sperm. It is therefore difficult to draw definitive conclusions. As TNF levels are elevated in infertile women with endometriosis, Eisermann et al.[188] evaluated the effects of TNF on sperm mobility and found a dose-dependent decrease that was reversed by anti-TNF antibody. On the other hand, La Montagna et al.[189] found reduced sperm mobility (although this was not quantified) in two of three patients evaluated with ankylosing spondylitis who were receiving infliximab. These data suggest that TNF/TNF antagonists may have some biological effect on sperm motility but the clinical relevance of this is presently unclear.

Recommendations: Use of biologic therapy in women planning pregnancy or who are pregnant

- Pregnancy should be avoided in patients with psoriasis receiving biologic therapy and effective contraception is strongly recommended to prevent pregnancy in women of child-bearing potential (*Strength of recommendation D; level of evidence 3*)
- In patients who are planning a pregnancy, biologic agents should be avoided (and/or stopped in advance) so the fetus is drug free during the critical developmental period of the first 12 weeks (*Strength of recommendation D; level of evidence 3*)
- If patients who are established on biologic agents discover they are pregnant, they should be referred to a specialist fetal medicine unit for further assessment and consideration should be given to stopping biologic therapy (*Strength of recommendation D; level of evidence 4*)
- Notwithstanding recommendations above, patients should be assessed on a case-by-case basis and the risks to the mother of stopping biologic therapy should be balanced against any potential harm to the fetus/infant (*Strength of recommendation D; level of evidence 4*)
- For those patients receiving infliximab during pregnancy, infusions should be avoided after 30 weeks if at all possible in view of its relatively long half-life and evidence that it crosses the placenta and may persist for several months in the fetal circulation (*Strength of recommendation D; level of evidence 3*)
- Breast feeding should be avoided in patients receiving biologic therapy although limited evidence indicates that infliximab is not excreted in breast milk (*Strength of recommendation D; level of evidence 4*)

17.3 Use of biologic therapy in the perioperative period for elective surgery

There are no prospective randomized trials comparing continuous vs. interrupted biologic therapy for patients on TNF antagonists undertaking surgery. Most published evidence comes from retrospective studies of orthopaedic procedures in RA[190–195] that have been the subject of detailed review.[196] One study found an increase in serious postoperative infection rate associated with prior TNF antagonist use,[192] whereas the other five studies did not show significant differences. However, in the largest of the latter studies[195] there was a trend towards increased early and late surgical site infection in the group who continued TNF antagonist therapy perioperatively (8·7%) vs. those who had TNF antagonist therapy interrupted perioperatively, although this did not reach significance. There was also a greater frequency of wound dehiscence in the group who continued TNF antagonist therapy (9·8%) vs. interrupted therapy (0·9%) compared with those who were TNF antagonist therapy naive (4·4%).

In a retrospective study of patients with Crohn's disease treated by intestinal resection, 40 patients on infliximab prior to surgery had no greater postoperative complication rate or prolonged hospital stay than a control group of 39 patients corrected for age, gender and type of surgery who were not exposed to infliximab.[197]

As a general rule it takes five half-lives for a product to be completely eliminated from the body. Some studies have used four half-lives to determine the interval prior to surgery for interrupting therapy. There may be additional uncertainty about tissue bioavailability. The approximate half-lives of etanercept, adalimumab, infliximab, efalizumab and ustekinumab are 3–5 days, 14–19 days, 8–9 days, 5–10 days and 21 days, respectively (in reference[196] and SPCs).

It is beyond the scope of these guidelines to address the risk of concomitant agents such as immunosuppressive drugs used with biologic therapy during surgery. However, in a well-designed randomized prospective nonblinded study, perioperative use of methotrexate was not associated with an increased risk of adverse outcomes following joint replacement.[198]

17.31 Quality of evidence

Most of the studies have been retrospective and underpowered to detect less than major risks of postoperative complications. It is also difficult to compare studies because of differences in source population, indications for surgery and underlying risk of infection due to the condition itself. From the studies available the two most robust reported[192,195] would yield grade 2+ evidence.

17.32 Existing guidance

The BSR guidelines for RA recommend that TNF antagonists (etanercept, adalimumab and infliximab) should be withheld

2–4 weeks prior to major surgical procedures and treatment restarted postoperatively if there is no evidence of infection and wound healing is satisfactory.[199] Guidelines from the Dutch Society for Rheumatology (http://www.nvr.nl/) and the French Society for Rheumatology[200] are similar and use four drug half-lives as the cut-off.

Recommendations: Use of biologic therapy in the perioperative period for elective surgery

- Until there is more evidence available concerning the risk of perioperative use of biologic therapies in psoriasis and/or psoriatic arthritis, BSR guideline recommendations on discontinuation of TNF antagonists in RA should be applied, i.e. TNF antagonists should be discontinued at least four half-lives prior to major surgery (2 weeks for etanercept, 6–8 weeks for adalimumab, 4–6 weeks for infliximab)
- Although there is no evidence for ustekinumab we would recommend ustekinumab is discontinued 12 weeks prior to major surgery (i.e. four half-lives prior to surgery) (*Strength of recommendation D (GPP); level of evidence 4*)
- Biologic therapy can be restarted postoperatively if there is no evidence of infection and wound healing is satisfactory (*Strength of recommendation D; level of evidence 3*)

17.4 Use of biologic therapy in patients with chronic viral infections (including hepatitis B and C and human immunodeficiency virus)

Patients with potentially harmful chronic viral infections have been exposed to biologic therapy either coincident to treatment for psoriasis (or other inflammatory indication) or as part of intentional adjuvant therapy, as is the case with TNF antagonist therapy in patients with hepatitis C and human immunodeficiency virus (HIV) infections. The limited data available, mainly small case series and case reports, have been subject to a recent, comprehensive review, and guidelines on screening and monitoring provided.[201]

17.41 Hepatitis C

TNF plays a role in hepatitis C-induced hepatocyte injury and treatment resistance to interferon alfa-2b. The role of TNF blockade has therefore been investigated in a phase II, randomized, placebo-controlled study, where etanercept (24 weeks, n = 19) was used as adjuvant therapy to ribavirin and interferon in treatment-naive patients.[202] Etanercept improved viral clearance rates with no significant increase in adverse events. Data from small case series and case reports[203–206] also report successful use of TNF antagonist therapy for rheumatological disease in hepatitis C virus-positive patients, with no increased rate of hepatotoxicity or viral replication.

17.42 Hepatitis B

In contrast to hepatitis C, TNF may play a role in clearing and controlling hepatitis B virus. Cases of severe (and sometimes fatal) reactivation of occult hepatitis B infections have been reported (summarized[201]).

17.43 Human immunodeficiency virus

The safety of biologic therapy in the context of HIV infection is unknown but particular caution should be exercised in this group given the risks of infection. Paradoxically, perhaps, TNF has been implicated in HIV disease progression in HIV-associated tuberculosis, and therefore the benefit of etanercept as adjunctive therapy for this indication has been investigated in a phase I study (25 mg twice weekly for 4 weeks, n = 16).[207] There was a tendency towards improved outcome in the etanercept arm and, more importantly, no increased toxicity compared with standard antituberculous therapy (n = 47). There are several case reports of successful use of TNF antagonist therapy for rheumatological indications in patients who are HIV positive.[201]

17.44 Herpesviruses

The risks of reactivation of latent herpesviruses in patients with psoriasis are unknown, although there are sporadic case reports of severe disseminated infections with both CMV and varicella-zoster[201] in the context of TNF antagonists. Registry data also indicate an increased risk of herpes zoster with adalimumab and infliximab in patients with rheumatological disease (see section 15.1).[103]

In a short-term (14-week) evaluation of 60 consecutive patients with Crohn's disease treated with infliximab, no evidence for reactivation of JCV, Epstein–Barr virus (EBV), human herpesvirus (HHV)-6, HHV-7, HHV-8 or CMV was identified in serum using polymerase chain reaction (PCR).[208] A similar study prospectively measured viral DNA in plasma and peripheral blood mononuclear cells in patients with RA (n = 15) during the first 6 weeks of infliximab treatment, and reported no evidence of reactivation of EBV, CMV or HHV-6. A further longer-term study evaluated EBV alone (measured in peripheral blood mononuclear cells using PCR) in patients with RA over a period of up to 5 years, and reported stable levels in patients using etanercept (n = 48) and infliximab (n = 68).[209]

Risks of herpes reactivation in the context of efalizumab and ustekinumab are unknown. However, with respect to efalizumab, recent reports of PML indicate that JCV reactivation can occur.

Recommendations: Use of biologic therapy in patients with chronic viral infections

- There is insufficient evidence to recommend treatment with biologic therapy in patients with known chronic, potentially harmful, viral infections and clinicians should seek specialist advice on a case-by-case basis (*Strength of recommendation D; level of evidence 4*)
- In patients who are hepatitis C carriers, there is limited evidence to support the use of etanercept provided they are appro-

---

priately evaluated and monitored during therapy (Strength of recommendation D, level of evidence 4)

• TNF antagonist therapy should be avoided in chronic carriers of hepatitis B because of the risk of reactivation (Strength of recommendation D; level of evidence 4).

See Table 4 for recommendations on screening for occult viral infections

17.5 Use of biologic therapy and vaccination

Live and live attenuated vaccinations can cause severe or fatal infections in immunosuppressed individuals due to the extensive replication of the vaccine strain and therefore are contraindicated in patients on biologic therapy.[210] Current live vaccinations available in the U.K. include bacille Calmette–Guérin (BCG), measles, mumps, rubella, yellow fever, oral polio and oral typhoid. There is no evidence available to provide recommendations on the safe time-frame from administration of a live vaccine to starting or recommencing a biologic therapy. Drug-specific advice is given only in the SPC for ustekinumab (i.e. withhold ustekinumab for 15 weeks before and 2 weeks after live vaccination). The UK's Department of Health[210] gives comprehensive guidance on vaccination, and also indications for use of human normal immunoglobulin and human varicella-zoster, for patients on immunosuppressive therapy [including cytokine inhibitors (sic)] and states that live vaccinations should not be administered until 6 months have elapsed from the withdrawal of immunosuppressive treatment.[210]

No data are available on risks for patients on biologic therapy who come into contact with individuals who have received a live vaccine (i.e. secondary transmission of infection by live vaccines) although current Department of Health guidance states that vaccination is not contraindicated in siblings/close relatives of patients who are immunosuppressed.[210]

Inactivated vaccines are safe to give to patients receiving a biologic therapy.[210] Several studies attempt to address the equally important question as to whether vaccination provides adequate protection from infection, using antibody response as a surrogate marker. Most of the evidence relates to TNF antagonists in rheumatological disease and findings differ depending on the vaccine. With respect to pneumococcal vaccination, there is no evidence to indicate that monotherapy with infliximab, etanercept or adalimumab significantly impairs humoral responses[211–215] although data on adalimumab are confined to measurement of vaccination responses following only 1 week of therapy.[215] However, in a well-designed RCT in psoriatic arthritis, methotrexate led to a significant reduction in humoral responses to pneumococcal vaccine when compared with etanercept or placebo control.[213] Findings in this study are supported by further cohort studies where methotrexate alone, or in combination with any of the three TNF antagonists, was associated with reduced antibody formation, and appeared to be a strong predictor of poor response.[211,212] Findings in relation to influenza vaccination are slightly different, in that humoral responses were found to

be reduced in patients on any of infliximab, etanercept or adalimumab[216–218] although antibody levels were still at levels predictive of clinical protection in most patients. Normal responses to influenza have also been reported in a large RCT involving adalimumab (compared with placebo) although, as outlined above, this possibly reflects the fact that vaccination occurred after only 1 week of treatment.[215]

There is little evidence available on what time period should elapse from drug discontinuation to administration of inactivated vaccines to yield an optimal immunological response.

Recommendations: Use of biologic therapy and vaccination

• Vaccination requirements should be reviewed and brought up to date prior to initiation of biologic therapy with reference to Department of Health Guidance (Strength of recommendation D (GGP); level of evidence 4)

• Patients should not receive live or live attenuated vaccinations < 2 weeks before, during, and for 6 months after discontinuation of, biologic therapy (Strength of recommendation D; level of evidence 4)

• Inactivated vaccines are safe to administer concurrently with a biologic therapy (Strength of recommendation B; level of evidence 2++)

• Where possible, inactivated vaccines should be administered 2 weeks before starting therapy to ensure optimal immune responses (Strength of recommendation D (GGP); level of evidence 4)

• Clinicians should be aware that TNF antagonist monotherapy may lead to reduced antibody responses to influenza vaccine and that TNF antagonists in combination with methotrexate (only) may lead to reduced antibody responses to pneumococcal vaccine (Strength of recommendation B; level of evidence 2++)

• Patients should be advised to receive the pneumococcal vaccine and annual influenza vaccine while on biologic therapy (Strength of recommendation D; level of evidence 4)

18.0 How to prescribe therapy

18.1 Who should prescribe biologic therapy?

These treatments should be made available to all those patients fulfilling the currently recommended eligibility criteria.

Treatment should be initiated and monitored by consultant dermatologists experienced in managing difficult psoriasis. This should include knowledge and experience of standard therapies and management of those who fail to respond. They must be familiar with, and/or have access to health care professionals trained in the use of the tools recommended for determining treatment eligibility and disease response.

In the UK, supervising consultants are responsible for ensuring that all patients receiving biologic therapies are registered with the BADBIR throughout the treatment period.

18.2 Role of the specialist nurse

The specialist nurse is a key member of the multidisciplinary team delivering a biologic therapies service. With additional training a nurse may take responsibility for a number of the tasks outlined in the patient pathway including screening, disease assessments, treatment administration, patient education, prescription coordination, patient support, patient monitoring and data collection for the BADBIR. Competencies for nurses involved in the delivery of biologic therapies are in development by the British Dermatological Nursing Group, along the lines of those already developed by the Royal College of Nursing Rheumatology Forum.[219]

Recommendations: Prescribing biologic therapy

• The specialist nurse is a key member of the multidisciplinary team delivering biologic therapy, and acts to facilitate all aspects of the patient pathway (*Strength of recommendation D (GGP); level of evidence 4*)
• In clearly defined clinical situations, suitably experienced and qualified nurse prescribers who have an expertise in the use of biologic therapies may prescribe biologic therapies under the direct supervision of a consultant dermatologist (*Strength of recommendation D (GGP); level of evidence 4*)

18.3 Patient information and consent

Patients should be fully informed of the risks and benefits of biologic therapies through detailed, collaborative discussion with the supervising consultant and clinical nurse specialist.[17] Written information should be provided (available on the BAD website) and patients given adequate time to consider their decision. Where therapies are being used outside their licensed indications, written consent should be obtained.

18.4 British Association of Dermatologists Biologic Interventions Registry

Short-term clinical trials in selected subjects do not adequately evaluate real world safety in long-term clinical usage of a drug. The potential for any new drug to result in delayed but important unexpected serious adverse effects is highlighted by recent experience with efalizumab. Voluntary reporting schemes lack the benefits of prospective follow up of a known denominator of patients in whom safety data are specifically collected. The BADBIR is now established, and collects vital long-term safety data throughout the U.K. with the intention that all patients on biologic interventions for psoriasis be registered and followed up for 5 years together with 4000 control subjects on conventional second-line drugs for psoriasis. Original NICE guidance on biologic therapies for psoriasis indicates registry participation as an important part of normal clinical care. The guideline development group very strongly recommends (above) that patients be registered in this way (see http://www.badbir.org/).

18.5 Pretreatment assessment and monitoring

All patients should undergo a full clinical history, physical examination and further investigations as indicated in recom-

mendations above, and also based on the toxicity profile of the relevant drug. Recommended pretreatment and monitoring assessments (Table 4) are summarized.

Assessment for risk of tuberculosis in patients considered for TNF antagonist therapy is outlined in Figure 1, and is based on the British Thoracic Society guideline which specifically addresses this question.[220] The British Thoracic Society guideline did not address the role of the now increasingly available in vitro interferon gamma release assay (IGRA) tests. The tests [QuantiFERON®-TB Gold (Cellestis Ltd, Carnegie, Vic., Australia) and T-SPOT®.TB (Oxford Immunotec, Abingdon, U.K.)] are both in vitro tests, based on release of interferon gamma following stimulation by *Mycobacterium tuberculosis*-specific antigens (ESAT-6, CFP-10, TB7.7). QuantiFERON is cheaper to perform than the T-SPOT.TB and can be done in batches, but may be less sensitive. These tests have some advantages in being more specific in that there is no cross-reactivity with either BCG or most (but not all) clinically relevant atypical mycobacteria. They have proven utility in identifying latent tuberculosis but their place in screening low-risk individuals is still unclear. Repeated tuberculin skin testing may lead to a boosting of the in vitro interferon gamma release, and result in a false-positive result.

The Health Protection Agency has issued an interim position statement (pending publication of the NICE Health Technology Assessment which is expected in 2010) and has provisionally approved the tests[221] in certain clinical circumstances, while also discussing the lack of evidence on which to base recommendations. It recommends that the tests may be a suitable alternative to tuberculin skin testing for screening in BCG-vaccinated individuals and also for assessment of patients who are immunosuppressed in whom tuberculin skin testing is unreliable. However, the positive predictive value and negative predictive value in these situations are unknown.

In the U.S.A., the Centers for Disease Control and Prevention advocate tuberculin skin testing in all patients irrespective of whether or not they are on immunosuppressant therapy and this is reflected in the American Academy of Dermatology guidelines on tuberculosis screening for patients considered for TNF antagonist therapy.[121]

18.51 Monitoring

Clinicians should maintain a high index of suspicion for tuberculosis throughout treatment, and for 6 months after discontinuation. Those at particular risk include recent immigrants from high-prevalence countries, injection drug users residents and employees of high-risk congregate settings (e.g. prisons, homeless shelters), mycobacteriology laboratory personnel, and persons with high-risk medical conditions (diabetes mellitus, chronic renal failure, some haematological conditions, conditions requiring prolonged high-dose corticosteroid or other immunosuppressive therapy, mastectomy/jejunoileal bypass).[222] Annual tuberculin skin testing has been recommended in the U.S.A. for both dermatology[121] and rheumatology practice,[223] although only 21–37% of U.S. rheumatologists surveyed concord with this

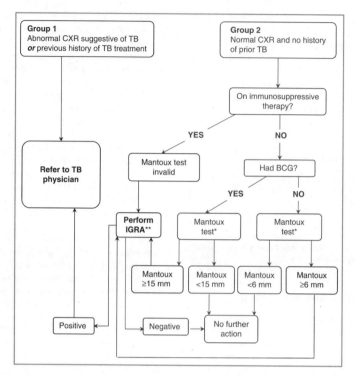

Fig 1. Algorithm for assessment and management of tuberculosis (TB) in patients scheduled for biologic therapy. Adapted from guidelines issued by the Joint Tuberculosis Committee of the British Thoracic Society.[220] CXR, chest X-ray; BCG, bacille Calmette–Guérin. *Interferon gamma release assay (IGRA) may be used in place of Mantoux testing if available. **Seek advice if uncertain how to interpret the result.

advice, and the validity of skin testing in the context of biologic therapy is unproven. Where there is a low incidence of tuberculosis in the community annual testing is unnecessary but in patients with risk factors annual checks for conversion of IGRA may be useful.

Recommendations: Assessment and monitoring for tuberculosis (Fig. 1)

• A pretreatment chest X-ray and Mantoux skin test currently remain the preferred screening tests in patients not on immunosuppression (*Strength of recommendation D; level of evidence 4*)

• Tuberculin testing is not valid in patients already established on immunosuppressive therapy (e.g. methotrexate). IGRA tests may have a role in this group and can be used if practicable, although the positive and negative predictive values are unknown. The T-SPOT.TB test may be more sensitive in patients on immunosuppressive drugs (*Strength of recommendation D; level of evidence 4*)

• Patients with signs to suggest tuberculosis or a history of previous treatment for tuberculosis should be referred to a tuberculosis physician (*Strength of recommendation D; level of evidence 4*)

• Patients with test(s) to support latent tuberculosis should be stratified for risk and considered for prophylactic antituberculous

therapy; further advice should be sought from a tuberculosis physician when necessary (*Strength of recommendation D; level of evidence 4*)

• When antituberculous therapy is indicated, patients should complete 2 months of treatment before commencing biologic therapy with either isoniazid (total treatment course 6 months) or rifampicin plus isoniazid (total treatment course 3 months) or rifampicin alone (total treatment course at least 4 months) (*Strength of recommendation D; level of evidence 4*)

• During treatment, and for 6 months following discontinuation, a high index of suspicion for tuberculosis should be maintained, especially in those at high risk (*Strength of recommendation D; level of evidence 4*)

• For patients on biologic therapies longer than 1 year who have negative screening tests for tuberculosis on initiation of therapy, annual assessment for tuberculosis may be considered in high-risk patients using whichever IGRA is locally available (*Strength of recommendation D; level of evidence 4*)

18.6 How should patients be transitioned from one therapy to another?

Patients may need to be transitioned from standard systemic therapy to biologic therapy, from one biologic therapy to another (either the same or different class) or from biologic therapy to standard systemic therapy. Ideally, there should be a washout period (the length of which is discussed below) between one drug and another so that pretreatment assessments occur off therapy (e.g. baseline disease severity, tuberculin skin tests) and so that the immunosuppressive 'burden' is minimized. However, more commonly, the transition period involves either sequential use of therapy without a 'washout' or a period of overlap between one drug and another, particularly where suddenly stopping therapy is associated with a risk of unstable disease (either treatment- or disease-related).

All the RCTs cited required patients to discontinue standard systemic therapy for at least 4 weeks, and biologic therapy (for the ustekinumab trials) for 3 months, prior to initiating biologic therapies. Given that in the short term, overall, serious adverse events were no greater than placebo, this provides evidence to support 'ideal' washout periods.

In situations where a 'washout' period is not feasible, it should be noted that safety data relating to TNF antagonists indicate additional risks of infection with concomitant use of immunosuppressive therapy. Also, even in the context of apparent treatment failure, loss of a drug's efficacy in psoriasis may not equate to loss of all pharmacological activity. This may be especially pertinent when switching from one biologic therapy to another, given that although these treatments are 'targeted', subsequent immunological events 'downstream' are complex. Standard therapies should be rationalized wherever possible and stopped (or the dose reduced) once response to the biologic treatment is achieved. Methotrexate is not associated with increased toxicity when prescribed with TNF antagonists, and limited data on combined therapy with etanercept and acitretin show no excess toxicity.

When switching from biologic therapy to biologic therapy, given the absence of data, overlap should be avoided. Traditionally, the time taken for a drug to be cleared from the body equates to four times a drug's terminal half-life and is therefore the recommended interval between therapies. Disease flares associated with discontinuation of efalizumab in low or nonresponders respond to standard systemic therapy.[224-226]

Recommendations: Transitioning from one therapy to another

• Standard systemic therapy (with the exception of methotrexate) should be discontinued for 4 weeks prior to initiation of biologic therapy whenever possible to minimize risk of infection and establish baseline disease severity. When necessary, methotrexate cotherapy may be continued at the minimal required dose (*Strength of recommendation B; level of evidence 1+*)

• Where discontinuing standard systemic therapy is associated with risk of severe or unstable disease, use of concomitant systemic therapy should be rationalized during the transition period and stopped as soon as therapeutic efficacy of the biologic therapy is established (*Strength of recommendation D; level of evidence 4*)

• When switching from one biologic therapy to another biologic therapy, overlap should be avoided with the recommended interval being four times the drug half-life (*Strength of recommendation D; level of evidence 4*)

18.7 What are the indications for stopping therapy?

Therapy should be discontinued when patients fail to achieve an adequate response following treatment initiation or when treatment response is not maintained (see section 9.0 for definition of adequate treatment response).

Withdrawal of therapy is also indicated due to the following events:

(i) a serious adverse event. Serious adverse events which may justify the withdrawal of treatment include malignancy (excluding NMSC), severe drug-related toxicity, severe intercurrent infection (temporary withdrawal)

(ii) pregnancy (temporary withdrawal)

(iii) elective surgical procedures (see section 17.3)

19.0 Recommended audit points

Dermatology teams involved in prescribing biologic interventions should use audit as a tool to monitor their service against national guidelines of care. The aim should be to ensure that the service is high in quality, safe and cost-effective. Possible topics for audit might include one or more of the following:

(i) Compliance with NICE guidance for patient selection criteria for prescribing of biologic therapies in psoriasis.

(ii) Compliance with pretreatment assessment of patients referred for biologic therapies.

(iii) Compliance with recommendation that all U.K. patients initiating biologic therapy should be registered with the BADBIR.

(iv) Compliance with withdrawal recommendations for biologic therapies in patients who fail to respond adequately or develop significant adverse events.

(v) Patient satisfaction survey of biologic therapies care.

References

1 Zachariae H. Prevalence of joint disease in patients with psoriasis: implications for therapy. *Am J Clin Dermatol* 2003; **4**:441–7.

2 Smith CH, Barker JNWN. Psoriasis and its management. *BMJ* 2006; **333**:380–4.

3 Menter A, Griffiths CE. Current and future management of psoriasis. *Lancet* 2007; **370**:272–84.

4 Griffiths CEM, Clark CM, Chalmers RJG et al. A systematic review of treatments for severe psoriasis. *Health Technol Assess* 2000; **4**:1–125.

5 Dubertret L, Mrowietz U, Ranki A et al. EUROPSO Patient Survey Group. European patient perspectives on the impact of psoriasis: the EUROPSO patient membership survey. *Br J Dermatol* 2006; **155**:729–36.

6 Nijsten T, Margolis D, Feldman SR et al. Traditional systemic treatments have not fully met the needs of psoriasis patients: results from a national survey. *J Am Acad Dermatol* 2005; **52**:434–44.

7 Smith CH, Anstey AV, Barker JNWN et al. British Association of Dermatologists guidelines for use of biological interventions in psoriasis 2005. *Br J Dermatol* 2005; **153**:486–97.

8 Eedy DJ, Griffiths CEM, Chalmers RJ et al. Care of patients with psoriasis: an audit of U.K. services in secondary care. *Br J Dermatol* 2009; **160**:557–64.

9 Bell HK, Ormerod AD. Writing a British Association of Dermatologists clinical guideline: an update on the process and guidance for authors. Br J Dermatol 2009; 160:725–8.

10 Appraisal of Guidelines Research and Evaluation. AGREE Instrument, 2004. Available at: http://www.agreecollaboration.org/instrument/ (last accessed 28 August 2009).

11 Garduno J, Bhosle MJ, Balkrishnan R et al. Measures used in specifying psoriasis lesion(s), global disease and quality of life: a systematic review. J Dermatolog Treat 2007; 18:223–42.

12 Ashcroft DM, Li Wan Po A, Williams HC et al. Clinical measures of disease severity and outcome in psoriasis: a critical appraisal of their quality. Br J Dermatol 1999; 142:185–91.

13 Both H, Essink-Bot M-L, Busschbach J et al. Critical review of generic and dermatology-specific health-related quality of life instruments. J Invest Dermatol 2007; 127:2726–39.

14 Finlay AY. Current severe psoriasis and the rule of tens. Br J Dermatol 2005; 152:861–7.

15 Basra MK, Fenech R, Gatt RM et al. The Dermatology Life Quality Index 1994–2007: a comprehensive review of validation data and clinical results. Br J Dermatol 2008; 159:997–1035.

16 Hongbo Y, Thomas CL, Harrison MA et al. Translating the science of quality of life into practice: what do Dermatology Life Quality Index scores mean? J Invest Dermatol 2005; 125:659–64.

17 NICE. Medicines Adherence: Involving Patients in Decisions about Prescribed Medicines and Supporting Adherence. NICE Clinical Guidline 76, 2009. Available at: http://www.nice.org.uk/nicemedia/pdf/CG76NICE Guideline.pdf (last accessed 28 August 2009).

18 Kyle S, Chandler D, Griffiths CE et al. Guideline for anti-TNF-alpha therapy in psoriatic arthritis [erratum appears in Rheumatology 2005; 44: 569]. Rheumatology 2005; 44:390–7.

19 Ibbotson SH, Bilsland D, Cox NH et al. An update and guidance on narrowband ultraviolet B phototherapy: a British Photodermatology Group Workshop Report. Br J Dermatol 2004; 151:283–97.

20 British Photodermatology Group guidelines for PUVA. Br J Dermatol 1994; 130:246–55.

21 Shikiar R, Willian MK, Okun MM et al. The validity and responsiveness of three quality of life measures in the assessment of psoriasis patients: results of a phase II study. Health Qual Life Outcomes 2006; 4:71.

22 Melilli L. Minimum clinically important difference in Dermatology Life Quality Index in moderate to severe plaque psoriasis patients treated with adalimumab. J Am Acad Dermatol 2006; 54:2894.

23 Khilji FA, Gonzalez M, Finlay AY. Clinical meaning of change in Dermatology Life Quality Index scores. Br J Dermatol 2002; 147 (Suppl. 62):50.

24 Tracey D, Lareskog L, Sasso E et al. Tumour necrosis factor antagonist mechanisms of action: a comprehensive review. Pharmacol Ther 2008; 117:244–79.

25 Guttman-Yassky E, Vugmeyster Y, Lowes MA et al. Blockade of CD11a by efalizumab in psoriasis patients induces a unique state of T-cell hyporesponsiveness. J Invest Dermatol 2008; 128:1182–91.

26 Joshi AB. An overview of the pharmacokinetics and pharmacodynamics of efalizumab: a monoclonal antibody approved for use in psoriasis. J Clin Pharmacol 2006; 46:10–20.

27 Wilson NJ, Boniface K, Chan JR et al. Development, cytokine profile and function of human interleukin 17-producing helper T cells. Nat Immunol 2007; 8:950–7.

28 Blauvelt A. T-helper 17 cells in psoriatic plaques and additional genetic links between IL-23 and psoriasis. J Invest Dermatol 2008; 128:1064–7.

29 Leonardi CL, Powers JL, Matheson RT et al. Etanercept as monotherapy in patients with psoriasis. N Engl J Med 2003; 349:2014–22.

30 Papp KA, Tyring S, Lahfa M et al. A global phase III randomized controlled trial of etanercept in psoriasis: safety, efficacy, and effect of dose reduction. Br J Dermatol 2005; 152:1304–12.

31 Tyring S, Gottlieb AB, Papp K et al. Etanercept and clinical outcomes, fatigue, and depression in psoriasis: double-blind placebo-controlled randomised phase III trial. Lancet 2006; 367:29–35.

32 Tyring S, Gordon KB, Poulin Y et al. Long-term safety and efficacy of 50 mg of etanercept twice weekly in patients with psoriasis. Arch Dermatol 2007; 143:719–26.

33 Gordon KB, Gottlieb AB, Leonardi CL et al. Clinical response in psoriasis patients discontinued from and then reinitiated on etanercept therapy [erratum appears in J Dermatolog Treat 2006; 17: 192]. J Dermatolog Treat 2006; 17:9–17.

34 Moore A, Gordon KB, Kang S et al. A randomized, open-label trial of continuous versus interrupted etanercept therapy in the treatment of psoriasis. J Am Acad Dermatol 2007; 56:598–603.

35 Feldman SR, Kimball AB, Krueger GG et al. Etanercept improves the health-related quality of life of patients with psoriasis: results of a phase III randomized clinical trial. J Am Acad Dermatol 2005; 53:887–9.

36 Krueger GG, Langley RG, Finlay AY et al. Patient-reported outcomes of psoriasis improvement with etanercept therapy: results of a randomized phase III trial. Br J Dermatol 2005; 153:1192–9.

37 Katugampola RP, Lewis VJ, Finlay AY et al. The Dermatology Life Quality Index: assessing the efficacy of biological therapies for psoriasis. Br J Dermatol 2007; 156:945–50.

38 Gelfand JM, Kimball AB, Mostow EN et al. Patient-reported outcomes and health-care resource utilization in patients with psoriasis treated with etanercept: continuous versus interrupted treatment. Value Health 2008; 11:400–7.

39 Krishnan R, Cella D, Leonardi C et al. Effects of etanercept therapy on fatigue and symptoms of depression in subjects treated for moderate to severe plaque psoriasis for up to 96 weeks. Br J Dermatol 2007; 157:1275–7.

40 Militello G, Xia A, Stevens SR et al. Etanercept for the treatment of psoriasis in the elderly. J Am Acad Dermatol 2006; 55:517–19.

41 Zhou H. Clinical pharmacokinetics of etanercept: a fully humanized soluble recombinant tumor necrosis factor receptor fusion protein. J Clin Pharmacol 2005; 45:490–7.

42 van de Kerkhof PCM, Segaert S, Lahfa M et al. Once weekly administration of etanercept 50 mg is efficacious and well tolerated in patients with moderate-to-severe plaque psoriasis: a randomized controlled trial with open-label extension. Br J Dermatol 2008; 159:1177–85.

43 Elewski B, Leonardi C, Gottlieb AB et al. Comparison of clinical and pharmacokinetic profiles of etanercept 25 mg twice weekly and 50 mg once weekly in patients with psoriasis. Br J Dermatol 2007; 156:138–42.

44 Gisondi P, Del Giglio M, Cotena C, Girolomoni G. Combining etanercept and acitretin in the therapy of chronic plaque psoriasis: a 24-week, randomized, controlled, investigator-blinded pilot trial. Br J Dermatol 2008; 158:1345–9.

45 Hutmacher MM, Nestorov I, Ludden T et al. Modeling the exposure-response relationship of etanercept in the treatment of patients with chronic moderate to severe plaque psoriasis. J Clin Pharmacol 2007; 47:238–48.

46 de Groot M, Appelman M, Spuls PI et al. Initial experience with routine administration of etanercept in psoriasis. Br J Dermatol 2006; 155:808–14.

47 Zachariae C, Mork NJ, Reunala T et al. The combination of etanercept and methotrexate increases the effectiveness of treatment in

active psoriasis despite inadequate effect of methotrexate therapy. *Acta Derm Venereol (Stockh)* 2008; **88**:495–501.

48 Driessen RJB, van de Kerkhof PCM, De Jong EMGJ. Etanercept combined with methotrexate for high-need psoriasis. *Br J Dermatol* 2008; **159**:460–3.

49 Berends MA, Driessen RJ, Langewouters AM *et al.* Etanercept and efalizumab treatment for high-need psoriasis. Effects and side effects in a prospective cohort study in outpatient clinical practice. *J Dermatolog Treat* 2007; **18**:76–83.

50 Ahmad K, Rogers S. Two years of experience with etanercept in recalcitrant psoriasis. *Br J Dermatol* 2007; **156**:1010–14.

51 Krueger GG, Elewski B, Papp K *et al.* Patients with psoriasis respond to continuous open-label etanercept treatment after initial incomplete response in a randomized, placebo-controlled trial. *J Am Acad Dermatol* 2006; **54**:S112–19.

52 Gottlieb AB, Evans R, Li S *et al.* Infliximab induction therapy for patients with severe plaque-type psoriasis: a randomized, double-blind, placebo-controlled trial. *J Am Acad Dermatol* 2004; **51**:534–42.

53 Reich K, Nestle FO, Papp K *et al.* Infliximab induction and maintenance therapy for moderate-to-severe psoriasis: a phase III, multicentre, double-blind trial. *Lancet* 2005; **366**:1367–74.

54 Menter A, Feldman SR, Weinstein GD *et al.* A randomized comparison of continuous vs. intermittent infliximab maintenance regimens over 1 year in the treatment of moderate-to-severe plaque psoriasis. *J Am Acad Dermatol* 2007; **56**:31.

55 Chaudhari U, Romano P, Mulcahy LD *et al.* Efficacy and safety of infliximab monotherapy for plaque-type psoriasis: a randomised trial. *Lancet* 2001; **357**:1842–7.

56 Antoni CE, Kavanaugh A, Kirkham B *et al.* Sustained benefits of infliximab therapy for dermatologic and articular manifestations of psoriatic arthritis: results from the Infliximab Multinational Psoriatic Arthritis Controlled Trial (IMPACT) [erratum appears in *Arthritis Rheum* 2005; **52**: 2951]. *Arthritis Rheum* 2005; **52**:1227–36.

57 Reich K, Nestle FO, Papp K *et al.* Improvement in quality of life with infliximab induction and maintenance therapy in patients with moderate-to-severe psoriasis: a randomized controlled trial. *Br J Dermatol* 2006; **154**:1161–8.

58 Gottlieb AB, Chaudhari U, Mulcahy LD *et al.* Infliximab monotherapy provides rapid and sustained benefit for plaque-type psoriasis. *J Am Acad Dermatol* 2003; **48**:829–35.

59 Maini RN, Breedveld FC, Kalden JR *et al.* Therapeutic efficacy of multiple intravenous infusions of anti-tumor necrosis factor monoclonal antibody combined with low-dose weekly methotrexate in rheumatoid arthritis. *Arthritis Rheum* 1998; **41**:1552–63.

60 Baert F, Noman M, Vermeire S *et al.* Influence of immunogenicity on the long-term efficacy of infliximab in Crohn's disease. *N Engl J Med* 2003; **348**:601–8.

61 Kapetanovic MC, Larsson L, Truedsson L *et al.* Predictors of infusion reactions during infliximab treatment in patients with arthritis. *Arthritis Res Ther* 2006; **8**:R131.

62 Gordon KB, Langley RG, Leonardi C *et al.* Clinical response to adalimumab treatment in patients with moderate to severe psoriasis: double-blind, randomized controlled trial and open-label extension study. *J Am Acad Dermatol* 2006; **55**:598–606.

63 Menter A, Tyring SK, Gordon K *et al.* Adalimumab therapy for moderate to severe psoriasis: a randomized, controlled phase III trial. *J Am Acad Dermatol* 2008; **58**:106–15.

64 Saurat JH, Stingl G, Dubertret L *et al.* Efficacy and safety results from the randomized controlled comparative study of adalimumab vs. methotrexate vs. placebo in patients with psoriasis (CHAMPION). *Br J Dermatol* 2008; **158**:556–66.

65 Mease PJ, Gladman DD, Ritchlin CT *et al.* Adalimumab for the treatment of patients with moderately to severely active psoriatic arthritis: results of a double-blind, randomized, placebo-controlled trial. *Arthritis Rheum* 2005; **52**:3279–89.

66 Shikiar R, Heffernan M, Langley RG *et al.* Adalimumab treatment is associated with improvement in health-related quality of life in psoriasis: patient-reported outcomes from a phase II randomized controlled trial. *J Dermatolog Treat* 2007; **18**:25–31.

67 Revicki D, Willian MK, Saurat JH *et al.* Impact of adalimumab treatment on health-related quality of life and other patient-reported outcomes: results from a 16-week randomized controlled trial in patients with moderate to severe plaque psoriasis. *Br J Dermatol* 2008; **158**:549–57.

68 Gladman DD, Mease PJ, Ritchlin CT *et al.* Adalimumab for long-term treatment of psoriatic arthritis: forty-eight week data from the adalimumab effectiveness in psoriatic arthritis trial. *Arthritis Rheum* 2007; **56**:476–88.

69 Papoutsaki M, Chimenti MS, Costanzo A *et al.* Adalimumab for severe psoriasis and psoriatic arthritis: an open-label study in 30 patients previously treated with other biologics. *J Am Acad Dermatol* 2007; **57**:269–75.

70 Krueger GG, Langley RG, Leonardi C *et al.* A human interleukin-12/23 monoclonal antibody for the treatment of psoriasis. *N Engl J Med* 2007; **356**:580–92.

71 Leonardi CL, Kimball AB, Papp K *et al.* Efficacy and safety of ustekinumab, a human interleukin-12/23 monoclonal antibody, in patients with psoriasis: 76-week results from a randomised, double-blind, placebo-controlled trial (PHOENIX 1). *Lancet* 2008; **371**:1665–74.

72 Papp K, Langley RG, Lebwohl M *et al.* Efficacy and safety of ustekinumab, a human interleukin-12/23 monoclonal antibody, in patients with psoriasis: 52-week results from a randomised, double-blind, placebo-controlled trial (PHOENIX 2). *Lancet* 2008; **371**:1675–84.

73 Gottlieb A, Menter A, Mendelsohn A *et al.* Ustekinumab, a human interleukin 12/23 monoclonal antibody, for psoriatic arthritis: randomised, double-blind, placebo-controlled, crossover trial. *Lancet* 2009; **373**:633–40.

74 Griffiths CEM, Strober BE, van de Kerkhof PC *et al.* Comparison of ustekinumab and etanercept for the treatment of moderate-to severe psoriasis. *N Engl J Med* (submitted).

75 Asumalahti K, Ameen N, Suomela S *et al.* Genetic analysis of PSORS1 distinguishes guttate psoriasis and palmoplantar pustulosis. *J Invest Dermatol* 2003; **120**:627–32.

76 Wollina U, Hansel G, Koch A *et al.* Tumor necrosis factor-alpha inhibitor-induced psoriasis or psoriasiform exanthemata: first 120 cases from the literature including a series of six new patients. *Am J Clin Dermatol* 2008; **9**:1–14.

77 Collamer AN, Guerro KT, Henning JS *et al.* Psoriatic skin lesions induced by tumor necrosis factor antagonist therapy: a literature review and potential mechanisms of action. *Arthritis Care Res* 2008; **59**:996–1001.

78 Bissonnette R, Poulin Y, Bolduc C *et al.* Etanercept in the treatment of palmoplantar pustulosis. *J Drugs Dermatol* 2008; **7**:940–6.

79 Elewski BE. Infliximab for the treatment of severe pustular psoriasis. *J Am Acad Dermatol* 2002; **47**:796–7.

80 Poulalhon N, Begon E, Lebbe C *et al.* A follow-up study in 28 patients treated with infliximab for severe recalcitrant psoriasis: evidence for efficacy and high incidence of biological autoimmunity. *Br J Dermatol* 2007; **156**:329–36.

81 Benoit S, Toksoy A, Brocker EB *et al.* Treatment of recalcitrant pustular psoriasis with infliximab: effective reduction of chemokine expression. *Br J Dermatol* 2004; **150**:1009–12.

82 Trent JT, Kerdel FA. Successful treatment of von Zumbusch pustular psoriasis with infliximab. *J Cutan Med Surg* 2004; **8**: 224–8.

83 Vieira Serrão V, Martins A, Lopes MJ. Infliximab in recalcitrant generalized pustular arthropatic psoriasis. *Eur J Dermatol* 2008; **18**:71–3.

84 Routhouska SB, Sheth PB, Korman NJ. Long-term management of generalized pustular psoriasis with infliximab: case series. *J Cutan Med Surg* 2008; **12**:184–8.

85 Esposito M, Mazzotta A, Casciello C et al. Etanercept at different dosages in the treatment of generalized pustular psoriasis: a case series. *Dermatology* 2008; **216**:355–60.

86 Kamarashev J, Lor P, Forster A et al. Generalised pustular psoriasis induced by cyclosporin A withdrawal responding to the tumour necrosis factor alpha inhibitor etanercept. *Dermatology* 2002; **205**:213–16.

87 Weisenseel P, Prinz JC, Weisenseel P et al. Sequential use of infliximab and etanercept in generalized pustular psoriasis. *Cutis* 2006; **78**:197–9.

88 Pereira TM, Vieira AP, Fernandes JC et al. Anti-TNF-alpha therapy in childhood pustular psoriasis. *Dermatology* 2006; **213**:350–2.

89 Callen JP, Jackson JH. Adalimumab effectively controlled recalcitrant generalized pustular psoriasis in an adolescent. *J Dermatolog Treat* 2005; **16**:350–2.

90 Esposito M, Mazzotta A, de Felice C et al. Treatment of erythrodermic psoriasis with etanercept. *Br J Dermatol* 2006; **155**:156–9.

91 Fiehn C, Andrassy K. Case number 29: hitting three with one strike: rapid improvement of psoriatic arthritis, psoriatic erythroderma, and secondary renal amyloidosis by treatment with infliximab (Remicade). *Ann Rheum Dis* 2004; **63**:232.

92 Lewis TG, Tuchinda C, Lim HW, Wong HK. Life-threatening pustular and erythrodermic psoriasis responding to infliximab. *J Drugs Dermatol* 2006; **5**:546–8.

93 Lisby S, Gniadecki R. Infliximab (Remicade) for acute, severe pustular and erythrodermic psoriasis. *Acta Derm Venereol (Stockh)* 2004; **84**:247–8.

94 Rongioletti F, Borenstein M, Kirsner R et al. Erythrodermic, recalcitrant psoriasis: clinical resolution with infliximab. *J Dermatolog Treat* 2003; **14**:222–5.

95 Takahashi MD, Castro LG, Romiti R. Infliximab, as sole or combined therapy, induces rapid clearing of erythrodermic psoriasis. *Br J Dermatol* 2007; **157**:828–31.

96 O'Quinn RP, Miller JL. The effectiveness of tumor necrosis factor alpha antibody (infliximab) in treating recalcitrant psoriasis: a report of 2 cases. *Arch Dermatol* 2002; **138**:644–8.

97 Yip L, Harrison S, Foley P. From biologic to biologic to biologic: lessons to learn for erythrodermic and recalcitrant chronic plaque psoriasis. *Australas J Dermatol* 2008; **49**:152–5.

98 Kircik L, Bagel J, Korman N et al. Utilization of narrow-band ultraviolet light B therapy and etanercept for the treatment of psoriasis (UNITE): efficacy, safety, and patient-reported outcomes. *J Drugs Dermatol* 2008; **7**:245–53.

99 Yazici Y, Adler NM, Yazici H. Most tumour necrosis factor inhibitor trials in rheumatology are undeservedly called 'efficacy and safety' trials: a survey of power considerations. *Rheumatology* 2008; **47**:1054–7.

100 Woolacott NF, Khadjesari ZC, Bruce IN et al. Etanercept and infliximab for the treatment of psoriatic arthritis: a systematic review. *Clin Exp Rheumatol* 2006; **24**:587–93.

101 Schmitt J, Zhang Z, Wozel G et al. Efficacy and tolerability of biologic and nonbiologic systemic treatments for moderate-to-severe psoriasis: meta-analysis of randomized controlled trials. *Br J Dermatol* 2008; **159**:513–26.

102 Brimhall AK, King LN, Licciardone JC et al. Safety and efficacy of alefacept, efalizumab, etanercept and infliximab in treating moderate to severe plaque psoriasis: a meta-analysis of randomized controlled trials. *Br J Dermatol* 2008; **159**:274–85.

103 Strangfeld A, Listing J, Herzer P et al. Risk of herpes zoster in patients with rheumatoid arthritis treated with anti-TNF-alpha agents. *JAMA* 2009; **301**:737–44.

104 Allison LS, Hyon KC, Marc CH et al. The risk of herpes zoster in patients with rheumatoid arthritis in the United States and the United Kingdom. *Arthritis Care Res* 2007; **57**:1431–8.

105 Gardam MA, Keystone E, Menzies R. Anti-tumour necrosis factor agents and tuberculosis risk: mechanisms of action and clinical management. *Lancet Infect Dis* 2003; **3**:148–55.

106 Hernandez Cruz B, Cetner AS, Jordan JE et al. Tuberculosis in the age of biologic therapy. *J Am Acad Dermatol* 2008; **59**:363–80.

107 Gomez-Reino JJ, Carmona L, Valverde VR et al. Treatment of rheumatoid arthritis with tumor necrosis factor inhibitors may predispose to significant increase in tuberculosis risk: a multicenter active-surveillance report. *Arthritis Rheum* 2003; **48**:2122–7.

108 Gomez-Reino JJ, Carmona L, Angel DM. Risk of tuberculosis in patients treated with tumor necrosis factor antagonists due to incomplete prevention of reactivation of latent infection. *Arthritis Rheum* 2007; **57**:756–61.

109 Dixon WG, Hyrich KL, Watson KD et al. Drug specific risk of tuberculosis in patients with rheumatoid arthritis treated with anti-TNF therapy; results from the BSR biologics register (BSRBR). *Rheumatology* 2008; **47**:171.

110 Dharamsi JW, Bhosle M, Balkrishnan R et al. Using 'number needed to treat' to help conceptualize the magnitude of benefit and risk of tumour necrosis factor-alpha inhibitors for patients with severe psoriasis. *Br J Dermatol* 2009; **161**:605–16.

111 Lim WS, Powell RJ, Johnston ID. Tuberculosis and treatment with infliximab. *N Engl J Med* 2002; **346**:623–6.

112 Keane J, Gershon SK, Wise R. Tuberculosis associated with infliximab, a tumor necrosis factor α-neutralizing agent. *N Engl J Med* 2001; **345**:1098–104.

113 Mohan N, Cote TR, Block JA et al. Tuberculosis following the use of etanercept, a tumour necrosis factor inhibitor. *Clin Infect Dis* 2004; **39**:295–9.

114 Mann DL, McMurray JJ, Packer M. Targeted anticytokine therapy in patients with chronic heart failure: results of the Randomized Etanercept Worldwide Evaluation (RENEWAL). *Circulation* 2004; **109**:1594–602.

115 Kwon HJ, Coté TR, Cuffe MS et al. Case reports of heart failure after therapy with a tumor necrosis factor antagonist. *Ann Intern Med* 2003; **138**:807–11.

116 Listing J, Strangfeld A, Kekow J. Does tumor necrosis factor alpha inhibition promote or prevent heart failure in patients with rheumatoid arthritis? *Arthritis Rheum* 2008; **58**:667–77.

117 Sarzi-Puttini P, Atzeni F, Shoenfeld Y et al. TNF-alpha, rheumatoid arthritis, and heart failure: a rheumatological dilemma. *Autoimmun Rev* 2005; **4**:153–61.

118 Mohan N, Edwards ET, Cupps TR et al. Demyelination occurring during anti-tumor necrosis factor alpha therapy for inflammatory arthritides. *Arthritis Rheum* 2001; **44**:2862–9.

119 Klareskog L, Gaubitz M, Rodriguez-Valverde V et al. A long-term, open-label trial of the safety and efficacy of etanercept (Enbrel) in patients with rheumatoid arthritis not treated with other disease-modifying antirheumatic drugs. *Ann Rheum Dis* 2006; **65**:1578–84.

120 Konttinen L, Honkanen V, Uotila Y et al. Biological treatment in rheumatic diseases: results from a longitudinal surveillance: adverse events. *Rheumatol Int* 2006; **26**:916–22.

121 Menter A, Gottlieb A, Feldman SR et al. Guidelines of care for the management of psoriasis and psoriatic arthritis: section 1. Overview of psoriasis and guidelines of care for the treatment of psoriasis with biologics. J Am Acad Dermatol 2008; **58**:826–50.

122 Massara A, Cavazzini L, La Corte R, Trotta F. Sarcoidosis appearing during anti-tumor necrosis factor alpha therapy: a new 'class effect' paradoxical phenomenon. Two case reports and literature review. Semin Arthritis Rheum (in press).

123 Ramos-Casals M, Brito-Zerón P, Muñoz S et al. Autoimmune diseases induced by TNF-targeted therapies: analysis of 233 cases. Medicine (Baltimore) 2007; **86**:242–51.

124 Lyndell LL, Frederick WF, James TR. Do tumor necrosis factor inhibitors cause uveitis? A registry-based study Arthritis Rheum 2007; **56**:3248–52.

125 Harrison MJ, Dixon WG, Watson KD et al. Rates of new-onset psoriasis in patients with rheumatoid arthritis receiving anti-tumour necrosis factor alpha therapy: results from the British Society for Rheumatology Biologics Register. Ann Rheum Dis 2009; **68**:209–15.

126 Zink A, Askling J, Dixon WG et al. European biologicals registers – methodology, selected results and perspectives. Ann Rheum Dis 2009; **68**:1240–6.

127 Bongartz T, Sutton AJ, Sweeting MJ et al. Anti-TNF antibody therapy in rheumatoid arthritis and the risk of serious infections and malignancies: systematic review and meta-analysis of rare harmful effects in randomized controlled trials [erratum appears in JAMA 2006; **295**: 2482]. JAMA 2006; **295**:2275–85.

128 Okada SK, Siegel JN. Risk of serious infections and malignancies with anti-TNF antibody therapy in rheumatoid arthritis. JAMA 2006; **296**:2201–2.

129 Dixon WG, Silman AJ. Is there an association between anti-TNF monoclonal antibody therapy in rheumatoid arthritis and risk of malignancy and serious infection? Commentary on the meta-analysis by Bongartz et al. Arthritis Rheum 2006; **8**:111.

130 Callegari PE, Schaible TF, Boscia JA. Risk of serious infections and malignancies with anti-TNF antibody therapy in rheumatoid arthritis. JAMA 2006; **296**:2202.

131 Rosh JR, Gross T, Mamula P et al. Hepatosplenic T-cell lymphoma in adolescents and young adults with Crohn's disease: a cautionary tale? Inflamm Bowel Dis 2007; **13**:1024–30.

132 Drini M, Prichard PJ, Brown GJ, Macrae FA. Hepatosplenic T-cell lymphoma following infliximab therapy for Crohn's disease. Med J Aust 2008; **189**:464–5.

133 Mackey AC, Green L, Liang LC et al. Hepatosplenic T cell lymphoma associated with infliximab use in young patients treated for inflammatory bowel disease. J Pediatr Gastroenterol Nutr 2007; **44**:265–7.

134 Navarro JT, Ribera JM, Mate JL et al. Hepatosplenic T-gammadelta lymphoma in a patient with Crohn's disease treated with azathioprine. Leuk Lymphoma 2003; **44**:531–3.

135 Thayu M, Markowitz JE, Mamula P et al. Hepatosplenic T-cell lymphoma in an adolescent patient after immunomodulator and biologic therapy for Crohn disease. J Pediatr Gastroenterol Nutr 2005; **40**:220–2.

136 Zeidan A, Sham R, Shapiro J et al. Hepatosplenic T-cell lymphoma in a patient with Crohn's disease who received infliximab therapy. Leuk Lymphoma 2007; **48**:1410–13.

137 Brown SL, Greene MH, Gershon SK et al. Tumor necrosis factor antagonist therapy and lymphoma development: twenty-six cases reported to the Food and Drug Administration. Arthritis Rheum 2002; **46**:3151–8.

138 Geborek P, Bladstrom A, Turesson C et al. Tumour necrosis factor blockers do not increase overall tumour risk in patients with rheumatoid arthritis, but may be associated with an increased risk of lymphomas. Ann Rheum Dis 2005; **64**:699–703.

139 Wolfe F, Michaud K. Biologic treatment of rheumatoid arthritis and the risk of malignancy: analyses from a large US observational study. Arthritis Rheum 2007; **56**:2886–95.

140 Burge D. Etanercept and squamous cell carcinoma. J Am Acad Dermatol 2003; **49**:358–9.

141 Lebwohl M, Blum R, Berkowitz E et al. No evidence for increased risk of cutaneous squamous cell carcinoma in patients with rheumatoid arthritis receiving etanercept for up to 5 years. Arch Dermatol 2005; **141**:861–4.

142 Leonardi CL, Toth D, Cather JC et al. A review of malignancies observed during efalizumab (Raptiva) clinical trials for plaque psoriasis. Dermatology 2006; **213**:204–14.

143 Gottlieb AB, Leonardi CL, Goffe BS et al. Etanercept monotherapy in patients with psoriasis: a summary of safety, based on an integrated multistudy database. J Am Acad Dermatol 2006; **54**:S92–100.

144 Woolacott N, Hawkins N, Mason A et al. Etanercept and efalizumab for the treatment of psoriasis: a systematic review. Health Technol Assess 2006; **10**:1–233, i–iv.

145 Woolacott N, Bravo Vergel Y, Hawkins N et al. Etanercept and infliximab for the treatment of psoriatic arthritis: a systematic review and economic evaluation. Health Technol Assess 2006; **10**:iii–xvi, 1–239

146 Slifman NR, Gershon SK, Lee JH et al. Listeria monocytogenes infection as a complication of treatment with tumor necrosis factor alpha-neutralizing agents. Arthritis Rheum 2003; **48**:319–24.

147 Symmons DP, Silman AJ. The world of biologics. Lupus 2006; **15**:122–6.

148 Lee JH, Slifman NR, Gershon SK et al. Life-threatening histoplasmosis complicating immunotherapy with tumor necrosis factor alpha antagonists infliximab and etanercept. Arthritis Rheum 2002; **46**:2565–70.

149 Lecluse LL, Piskin G, Mekkes JR et al. Review and expert opinion on prevention and treatment of infliximab-related infusion reactions. Br J Dermatol 2008; **159**:527–36.

150 Rennard SI, Fogarty C, Kelsen S et al. The safety and efficacy of infliximab in moderate to severe chronic obstructive pulmonary disease. Am J Respir Crit Care Med 2007; **175**:926–34.

151 Schiff MH, Burmester GR, Kent JD et al. Safety analyses of adalimumab (Humira) in global clinical trials and US postmarketing surveillance of patients with rheumatoid arthritis. Ann Rheum Dis 2006; **65**:889–94.

152 Burmester GR, Mariette X, Montecucco C et al. Adalimumab alone and in combination with disease-modifying antirheumatic drugs for the treatment of rheumatoid arthritis in clinical practice: the Research in Active Rheumatoid Arthritis (ReAct) trial. Ann Rheum Dis 2007; **66**:732–9.

153 Pariser DM, Gordon KB, Papp KA et al. Clinical efficacy of efalizumab in patients with chronic plaque psoriasis: results from three randomized placebo-controlled phase III trials: part I. J Cutan Med Surg 2005; **9**:303–12.

154 Menter A, Gordon K, Carey W et al. Efficacy and safety observed during 24 weeks of efalizumab therapy in patients with moderate to severe plaque psoriasis. Arch Dermatol 2005; **141**:31–8.

155 Gottlieb AB, Hamilton T, Caro I et al. Long-term continuous efalizumab therapy in patients with moderate to severe chronic plaque psoriasis: updated results from an ongoing trial. J Am Acad Dermatol 2006; **54**:S154–63.

156 Costanzo A, Peris K, Talamonti M et al. Long-term treatment of plaque psoriasis with efalizumab: an Italian experience. Br J Dermatol 2007; **156** (Suppl. 2):17–23.

157 Selenko-Gebauer N, Karlhofer F, Stingl G et al. Efalizumab in routine use: a clinical experience. Br J Dermatol 2007; **156** (Suppl. 2):1–6.

158 Pincelli C, Henninger E, Casset-Semanaz F et al. The incidence of arthropathy adverse events in efalizumab-treated patients is low and similar to placebo and does not increase with long-term treatment: pooled analysis of data from phase III clinical trials of efalizumab. Arch Dermatol Res 2006; **298**:329–38.

159 Viguier M, Richette P, Aubin F et al. Onset of psoriatic arthritis in patients treated with efalizumab for moderate to severe psoriasis. Arthritis Rheum 2008; **58**:1796–802.

160 Sandborn WJ, Feagan BG, Fedorak RN et al. A randomized trial of ustekinumab, a human interleukin-12/23 monoclonal antibody, in patients with moderate-to-severe Crohn's disease. Gastroenterology 2008; **135**:1130–41.

161 Segal BM, Constantinescu CS, Raychaudari A et al. Repeated subcutaneous injections of IL12/23 p40 neutralising antibody, ustekinumab, in patients with relapsing-remitting multiple sclerosis: a phase II, double-blind, placebo-controlled, randomised, dose-ranging study. Lancet Neurol 2008; **7**:796–804.

162 Ryan C, Kirby B, Collins P, Rogers S. Adalimumab treatment for severe recalcitrant chronic plaque psoriasis. Clin Exp Dermatol 2009); **34**:784–8.

163 Paller AS, Siegfried EC, Langley RG et al. Etanercept treatment for children and adolescents with plaque psoriasis. N Engl J Med 2008; **358**:241–51.

164 Lovell DJ, Giannini EH, Reiff A et al. Etanercept in children with polyarticular juvenile rheumatoid arthritis. Pediatric Rheumatology Collaborative Study Group. N Engl J Med 2000; **342**:763–9.

165 Mahadevan U, Kane S, Sandborn WJ et al. Intentional infliximab use during pregnancy for induction or maintenance of remission in Crohn's disease. Aliment Pharmacol Ther 2005; **21**:733–8.

166 Lichtenstein GR, Cohen MD, Feasel A. Safety of infliximab in Crohn's disease: data from the 5000-patient TREAT registry. Gastroenterology 2004; **126**:A54.

167 Katz JA, Antoni C, Keenan GF et al. Outcome of pregnancy in women receiving infliximab for the treatment of Crohn's disease and rheumatoid arthritis. Am J Gastroenterol 2004; **99**: 2385–92.

168 Hyrich KL, Symmons DP, Watson KD et al. Pregnancy outcome in women who were exposed to anti-tumor necrosis factor agents: results from a national population register. Arthritis Rheum 2006; **54**:2701–2.

169 Miskin DS, VanDenise W, Becker JM et al. Successful use of adalimumab for Crohn's disease in pregnancy. Inflamm Bowel Dis 2006; **12**:827–8.

170 Roux CH, Brocq O, Breuil V et al. Pregnancy in rheumatology patients exposed to anti-tumour necrosis factor (TNF)-alpha therapy. Rheumatology 2007; **46**:695–8.

171 Rosner I, Haddad A, Boulman N et al. Pregnancy in rheumatology patients exposed to anti-tumour necrosis factor (TNF)-alpha therapy. Rheumatology 2007; **46**:1508–9.

172 Winger EE, Reed JL, Ashoush S et al. Treatment with adalimumab (Humira) and intravenous immunoglobulin improves pregnancy rates in women undergoing IVF. Am J Reprod Immunol 2009; **61**:113–20.

173 Berthelot JM, DeBandt M, Goupille P et al. Exposition to anti-TNF drugs during pregnancy: outcome of 15 cases and review of the literature. Joint Bone Spine 2009; **76**:28–34.

174 Carter JD, Ladhani A, Ricca LR et al. A safety assessment of tumor necrosis factor antagonists during pregnancy: a review of the Food and Drug Administration database. J Rheumatol 2009; **36**:635–41.

175 Chakravarty EF, Sanchez-Yamamoto D, Bush TM et al. The use of disease modifying antirheumatic drugs in women with rheumatoid arthritis of childbearing age: a survey of practice patterns and pregnancy outcomes. J Rheumatol 2003; **30**:241–6.

176 Carter JD, Valeriano J, Vasey FB et al. Tumor necrosis factor-alpha inhibition and VATER association: a causal relationship. J Rheumatol 2006; **33**:1014–17.

177 Micheloud D, Nuno L, Rodriguez-Mahou M et al. Efficacy and safety of etanercept, high-dose intravenous gammaglobulin and plasmapheresis combined therapy for lupus diffuse proliferative nephritis complicating pregnancy. Lupus 2006; **15**:881–5.

178 Sinha A, Patient C. Rheumatoid arthritis in pregnancy: successful outcome with anti-TNF agent (etanercept). J Obstet Gynaecol 2006; **26**:689–91.

179 Vesga L, Terdiman JP, Mahadevan U. Adalimumab use in pregnancy. Gut 2005; **54**:890.

180 Coburn LA, Wise PE, Schwartz DA. The successful use of adalimumab to treat active Crohn's disease of an ileoanal pouch during pregnancy. Dig Dis Sci 2006; **51**:2045–7.

181 Kraemer B, Abele H, Hahn M et al. A successful pregnancy in a patient with Takayasu's arteritis. Hypertens Pregnancy 2008; **27**:247–52.

182 Vasiliauskas EA, Church JA, Silverman N et al. Case report: evidence for transplacental transfer of maternally administered infliximab to the newborn. Clin Gastroenterol Hepatol 2006; **4**:1255–8.

183 Stengel JZ, Arnold HL. Is infliximab safe to use while breastfeeding? World J Gastroenterol 2008; **14**:3085–7.

184 Mahadevan U, Terdiman JP, Church JA et al. Infliximab levels in infants born to women with inflammatory bowel disease. Gastroenterology 2007; **132**:A144 (Abstract).

185 Tauscher AEF, Fleischer AB Jr, Phelps KC, Feldman SR. Psoriasis and pregnancy. J Cutan Med Surg 2002; **6**:561–70.

186 Granzow JW, Thaller SR, Panthaki Z. Cleft palate and toe malformations in a child with fetal methotrexate exposure. J Craniofac Surg 2003; **14**:747–8.

187 Nguyen C, Duhl AJ, Escallon CS et al. Multiple anomalies in a fetus exposed to low-dose methotrexate in the first trimester. Obstet Gynecol 2002; **99**:599–602.

188 Eisermann J, Register KB, Strickler RC et al. The effect of tumor necrosis factor on human sperm motility in vitro. J Androl 1989; **10**:270–4.

189 La Montagna G, Malesci D, Buono R, Valentini G. Asthenoazoospermia in patients receiving anti-tumour necrosis factor alpha agents. Ann Rheum Dis 2005; **64**:1667.

190 Wendling D, Balblanc JC, Brousse A et al. Surgery in patients receiving anti-tumour necrosis factor alpha treatment in rheumatoid arthritis: an observational study on 50 surgical procedures. Ann Rheum Dis 2005; **64**:1378–9.

191 Talwalar SC, Grennan DM, Gray J et al. Tumour necrosis factor alpha antagonists and early postoperative complications in patients with inflammatory joint disease undergoing elective orthopaedic surgery. Ann Rheum Dis 2005; **64**:650–1.

192 Giles JT, Bartlett SJ, Gelber AC et al. Tumor necrosis factor inhibitor therapy and risk of serious postoperative orthopedic infection in rheumatoid arthritis. Arthritis Rheum 2006; **55**:333–7.

193 Bibbo C, Goldberg JW. Infectious and healing complications after elective orthopaedic foot and ankle surgery during tumor necrosis factor-alpha inhibition therapy. Foot Ankle Int 2009; **25**:331–5.

194 Ruyssen-Witrand A, Gossec L, Salliot C et al. Complication rates of 127 surgical procedures performed in rheumatic patients receiving tumor necrosis factor alpha blockers. Clin Exp Rheumatol 2007; **25**:430–6.

195 den Broeder AA, Creemers MC, Fransen J et al. Risk factors for surgical site infections and other complications in elective surgery

in patients with rheumatoid arthritis with special attention for anti-tumor necrosis factor: a large retrospective study. *J Rheumatol* 2007; **34**:689–95.

196 Pappas DA, Giles JT. Do antitumor necrosis factor agents increase the risk of postoperative orthopedic infections? *Curr Opin Rheumatol* 2008; **20**:450–6.

197 Marchal L, D'Haens G, van Assche G et al. The risk of post-operative complications associated with infliximab therapy for Crohn's disease: a controlled cohort study. *Aliment Pharmacol Ther* 2004; **19**:749–54.

198 Grennan DM, Gray J, Loudon J et al. Methotrexate and early postoperative complications in patients with rheumatoid arthritis undergoing elective orthopaedic surgery. *Ann Rheum Dis* 2001; **60**:214–17.

199 Ledingham J, Deighton C. British Society for Rheumatology Standards, Guidelines and Audit Working Group. Update on the British Society for Rheumatology guidelines for prescribing TNFalpha blockers in adults with rheumatoid arthritis (update of previous guidelines of April 2001). *Rheumatology* 2005; **44**: 157–63.

200 Pham T, Claudespierre P, Deprez X et al. Anti-TNF alpha therapy and safety monitoring. Clinical tool guide elaborated by the Club Rhumatismes et Inflammations (CRI), section of the French Society of Rheumatology (Société Française de Rhumatologie, SFR). *Joint Bone Spine* 2005; **72**:S1–58.

201 Domm S, Mrowietz U. The impact of treatment with tumour necrosis factor-alpha antagonists on the course of chronic viral infections: a review of the literature. *Br J Dermatol* 2008; **159**:1217–28.

202 Zein NN. Etanercept Study Group. Etanercept as an adjuvant to interferon and ribavirin in treatment-naive patients with chronic hepatitis C virus infection: a phase 2 randomized, double-blind, placebo-controlled study. *J Hepatol* 2005; **42**:315–22.

203 Aslanidis S, Vassiliadis T, Pyrpasopoulou A et al. Inhibition of TNFalpha does not induce viral reactivation in patients with chronic hepatitis C infection: two cases. *Clin Rheumatol* 2007; **26**:261–4.

204 Cecchi R, Bartoli L. Psoriasis and hepatitis C treated with anti-TNF alpha therapy (etanercept). *Dermatol Online J* 2006; **12**:4.

205 Marotte H, Fontanges E, Bailly F et al. Etanercept treatment for three months is safe in patients with rheumatological manifestations associated with hepatitis C virus. *Rheumatology* 2007; **46**: 97–9.

206 Peterson JR, Hsu FC, Simkin PA et al. Effect of tumour necrosis factor alpha antagonists on serum transaminases and viraemia in patients with rheumatoid arthritis and chronic hepatitis C infection. *Ann Rheum Dis* 2003; **62**:1078–82.

207 Wallis RS, Kyambadde P, Johnson JL et al. A study of the safety, immunology, virology, and microbiology of adjunctive etanercept in HIV-1-associated tuberculosis. *AIDS* 2004; **18**:257–64.

208 Lavagna A, Bergallo M, Daperno M et al. Infliximab and the risk of latent viruses reactivation in active Crohn's disease. *Inflamm Bowel Dis* 2007; **13**:896–902.

209 Balandraud N, Guis S, Meynard JB et al. Long-term treatment with methotrexate or tumor necrosis factor alpha inhibitors does not increase Epstein–Barr virus load in patients with rheumatoid arthritis. *Arthritis Rheum* 2007; **57**:762–7.

210 Department of Health. *The Green Book: Immunisation against Infectious Disease.* 2009. Available at: http://www.dh.gov.uk/en/Publichealth/Healthprotection/Immunisation/Greenbook/DH_4097254 (last accessed 28 August 2009).

211 Gelinck LB, van der Bijl AE, Visser LG et al. Synergistic immunosuppressive effect of anti-TNF combined with methotrexate on antibody responses to the 23 valent pneumococcal polysaccharide vaccine. *Ann Rheum Dis* 2006; **65**:191–4.

212 Kapetanovic MC, Saxne T, Sjoholm A et al. Influence of methotrexate, TNF blockers and prednisolone on antibody responses to pneumococcal polysaccharide vaccine in patients with rheumatoid arthritis. *Rheumatology* 2006; **45**:106–11.

213 Mease P, Ritchlin C, Martin RW et al. Pneumococcal vaccine response in psoriatic arthritis patients during treatment with etanercept. *J Rheumatol* 2004; **7**:1356–61.

214 Visanathan S, Keenan GF, Baker D et al. Response to pneumococcal vaccine in patients with early rheumatoid arthritis receiving infliximab plus methotrexate or methotrexate alone. *J Rheumatol* 2007; **34**:952–7.

215 Kaine JL, Kivitz AJ, Birbara C et al. Immune responses following administration of influenza and pneumococcal vaccines to patients with rheumatoid arthritis receiving adalimumab. *J Rheumatol* 2007; **34**:272–9.

216 Fomin I, Caspi D, Levy V et al. Vaccination against influenza in rheumatoid arthritis: the effect of disease modifying drugs, including TNF alpha blockers. *Ann Rheum Dis* 2006; **65**:191–4.

217 Gelinck LB, van der Bijl AE, Beyer WE et al. The effect of antitumour necrosis factor alpha treatment on the antibody response to influenza vaccination. *Ann Rheum Dis* 2008; **67**:713–16.

218 Kapetanovic MC, Saxne T, Nilsson JA et al. Influenza vaccination as model for testing immune modulation induced by anti-TNF and methotrexate therapy in rheumatoid arthritis patients. *Rheumatology* 2007; **46**:608–11.

219 Royal College of Nursing. *Assessing, Managing and Monitoring Biologic Therapies for Inflammatory Arthritis: Guidance for Rheumatology Practitioners.* London: Royal College of Nursing, 2003.

220 British Thoracic Society Standards of Care Committee. BTS recommendations for assessing risk and for managing *Mycobacterium tuberculosis* infection and disease in patients due to start anti-TNF-alpha treatment. *Thorax* 2005; **60**:800–5.

221 Health Protection Agency. *Position Statement on the Use of Interferon Gamma Release Assay (IGRA) Tests for Tuberculosis (TB).* 2008. Available at: http://www.hpa.org.uk/web/HPAwebFile/HPAweb_C/1214808549127 (last accessed 28 August 2009).

222 The National Collaborating Centre for Chronic Conditions. *Tuberculosis. Clinical Diagnosis and Management of Tuberculosis, and Measures for its Prevention and Control.* 2006. Available at: http://www.nice.org.uk/nicemedia/pdf/CG033FullGuideline.pdf (last accessed 28 August 2009).

223 Cush JJ. Biological drug use: US perspectives on indications and monitoring. *Ann Rheum Dis* 2005; **64**(Suppl. 4):18–23.

224 Papp KA, Toth D, Rosoph L et al. Approaches to discontinuing efalizumab: an open-label study of therapies for managing inflammatory recurrence. *BMC Dermatol* 2006; **6**:9.

225 Carey W, Glazer S, Gottlieb AB et al. Relapse, rebound, and psoriasis adverse events: an advisory group report. *J Am Acad Dermatol* 2006; **54**:S171–81.

226 Menter A, Hamilton TK, Toth DP et al. Transitioning patients from efalizumab to alternative psoriasis therapies: findings from an open-label, multicenter, phase IIIb study. *Int J Dermatol* 2007; **46**:637–48.

Appendix 1 Level of evidence and strength of recommendation

The published studies selected from the search were assessed for their methodological rigour against a number of criteria as currently recommended by the Institute for Health and Clinical Excellence (NICE) and the Scottish Intercollegiate Guidelines Network. The overall assessment of each study was graded using a code: '++', '+' or '−', based on the extent to which the potential biases have been minimized.

Level of evidence

Level of evidence	Type of evidence
1++	High-quality meta-analyses, systematic reviews of RCTs, or RCTs with a very low risk of bias
1+	Well-conducted meta-analyses, systematic reviews of RCTs, or RCTs with a low risk of bias
1−	Meta-analyses, systematic reviews of RCTs, or RCTs with a high risk of bias[a]
2++	High-quality systematic reviews of case–control or cohort studies High-quality case–control or cohort studies with a very low risk of confounding, bias or chance and a high probability that the relationship is causal
2+	Well-conducted case–control or cohort studies with a low risk of confounding, bias or chance and a moderate probability that the relationship is causal
2−	Case–control or cohort studies with a high risk of confounding, bias or chance and a significant risk that the relationship is not causal[a]
3	Nonanalytical studies (e.g. case reports, case series)
4	Expert opinion, formal consensus

RCT, randomized controlled trial. [a]Studies with a level of evidence '−' should not be used as a basis for making a recommendation.

Strength of recommendation

Class	Evidence
A	• At least one meta-analysis, systematic review, or RCT rated as 1++, and directly applicable to the target population, **or** • A systematic review of RCTs or a body of evidence consisting principally of studies rated as 1+, directly applicable to the target population and demonstrating overall consistency of results • Evidence drawn from a NICE technology appraisal
B	• A body of evidence including studies rated as 2++, directly applicable to the target population and demonstrating overall consistency of results, **or** • Extrapolated evidence from studies rated as 1++ or 1+
C	• A body of evidence including studies rated as 2+, directly applicable to the target population and demonstrating overall consistency of results, **or** • Extrapolated evidence from studies rated as 2++
D	• Evidence level 3 or 4, **or** • Extrapolated evidence from studies rated as 2+, **or** • Formal consensus
D (GPP)	• A good practice point (GPP) is a recommendation for best practice based on the experience of the guideline development group

RCT, randomized controlled trial.

http://www.bad.org.uk/Portals/_Bad/Guidelines/Clinical
Guidelines/Biologics guidelines 2009.pdf

Comment

The use of biological agents in psoriasis is an important
and evolving area. The updated guidelines are very thorough and used the 'AGREE' methodology [1]. There have
been many developments since the 2005 guideline [2].
Efalizumab was recently withdrawn following the development of progressive multifocal leucoencephalopathy
due to JC polyoma virus re-activation in three patients
[3, 4]. It is unlikely it will be reintroduced. The 2009
guidelines concern the use of etanercept, adalimumab,
infliximab and ustekunumab [1]. There still remain neurological concerns with the use of biological therapies.
Patient safety will be enhanced by national and international databases on long-term monitoring of patients
on these new therapies. Pharmacovigilance, in the form
of registries, is essential to assess the long-term safety of
these agents [5]. There is no doubt that biologic therapies
are proving to be very useful in managing patients with
very severe psoriasis. However, all systemic treatments for
psoriasis come with a cost, whether financial, clinical efficacy, toxicity or all three; the case can frequently be made
for the use of biologics [6]. Further research needs to be
undertaken into their use with other modalities such as
retinoids, methotrexate, ciclosporin and UV light. These
guidelines will be updated in 2012 as there are likely to be
newer molecules in the pipeline.

References

1 Smith CH, Anstey AV, Barker JNWN, *et al*. British Association of Dermatologists' guidelines for biologic interventions for psoriasis 2009. *Brit J Dermatol* 2009; 161:
987–1019.
2 Smith CH, Anstey AV, Barker JNWN, *et al*. British Association of Dermatologists guidelines for use of biological interventions in psoriasis 2005. *Br J Dermatol* 2005;
153:486–97.
3 Carson KR, Focosi D, Major EO, *et al*. Monoclonal
antibody-associated progressive multifocal leucoencephalopathy in patients treated with rituximab, natal-
izumab, and efalizumab: a review from the Research on
Adverse Drug Events and Reports (RADAR) Project.
Lancet Oncol 2009; 10: 816–24.
4 Berger JR, Houff SA, Major EO. Monoclonal antibodies
and progressive multifocal leukoencephalopathy. *MAbs*
2009; 1: 583–9.
5 Warren RB, Brown BC, D. Lavery D, *et al*. Biologic
therapies for psoriasis: practical experience in a U.K.
tertiary referral centre. *Brit J Dermatol* 2009; 160: 162–9.
6 Sizto S, Bansback N, Feldman SR, *et al*. Economic evaluation of systemic therapies for moderate to severe psoriasis. *Brit J Dermatol* 2009; 160: 1264–72.

Additional professional resources

Menter A, Gottlieb A, Feldman SR, *et al*. Guidelines of
care for the management of psoriasis and psoriatic
arthritis. Section 1. Overview of psoriasis and guidelines of care for the treatment of psoriasis with biologics. *J Am Acad Dermatol* 2008; 58: 826–50 (http://
www.aad.org/research/_doc/Psosection1.pdf).

BSR/BHPR guideline for disease-modifying antirheumatic drug (DMARD) therapy in consultation
with the British Association of Dermatologists. http://
www.rheumatology.org.uk/includes/documents/cm_
docs/2009/d/diseasemodifying_antirheumatic_drug_
dmard_therapy.pdf.

DMARDs: biologic agents. Clinical Knowledge Summaries 2008. http://www.cks.nhs.uk//dmards/
management/quick_answers/scenario_biologic_agents#.

Rott S, Mrowietz U. Recent developments in the use
of biologics in psoriasis and autoimmune disorders.
The role of autoantibodies. BMJ 2005; 330: 716–20
(http://www.bmj.com/cgi/content/full/330/7493/716).

Etanercept and efalizumab for the treatment of adults
with psoriasis. National Institute for Health and Clinical Excellence 2006 [note: Efalizumab now withdrawn].
http://www.nice.org.uk/nicemedia/pdf/TA103guidance.
pdf.

Adalimumab for the treatment of adults with psoriasis. National Institute for Health and Clinical Excellence 2008. http://www.nice.org.uk/nicemedia/pdf/
TA146Guidance.pdf.

Infliximab for the treatment of adults with psoriasis. National Institute for Health and Clinical Excellence 2008. http://www.nice.org.uk/nicemedia/pdf/
TA134Guidance.pdf.

Ustekinumab for the treatment of adults with moderate to severe psoriasis. National Institute for Health
and Clinical Excellence 2009. http://www.nice.org.uk/
nicemedia/pdf/TA180Guidance.pdf.

BAD patient information leaflets

Adalimumab: http://www.bad.org.uk/site/1232/Default.
aspx

Etanercept: http://www.bad.org.uk/site/818/Default.aspx
Infliximab: http://www.bad.org.uk/site/833/Default.aspx

Other patient resources

Adalimumab: http://www.humira.com/
Etanercept: http://www.enbrel.com/

Treatments for moderate to severe psoriasis: http://www.bad.org.uk/site/866/Default.aspx
Patient group: http://www.psoriasis-association.org.uk

Advice on the safe introduction and continued use of isotretinoin in acne in the U.K. 2010

M.J.D. Goodfield, N.H. Cox,* A. Bowser,† J.C. McMillan,‡ L.G. Millard,§ N.B. Simpson¶ and A.D. Ormerod**

Department of Dermatology, Leeds General Infirmary, Leeds LS1 3EX, U.K.
*Department of Dermatology, Cumberland Infirmary, Carlisle CA2 7HY, U.K.
†Independent Acne Patient Advisor, Belfast City Hospital, Belfast BT9 7AB, U.K.
‡Department of Dermatology, Belfast City Hospital, Belfast BT9 7AB, U.K.
§Department of Dermatology, The Park Hospital, Arnold, Nottingham NG5 5BX, U.K.
¶Department of Dermatology, Nuffield Health Newcastle upon Tyne Hospital, Newcastle upon Tyne NE2 1JP, U.K.
**Department of Dermatology, University of Aberdeen, Foresterhill, Aberdeen AB25 2ZN, U.K.

Introduction

Since its introduction into clinical trials in the mid 1970s, and its widespread use since the early 1980s, isotretinoin has proved a very effective therapy for severe and persistent acne.[1] The current Product Licence indications for the use of isotretinoin are severe forms of acne (such as nodular or conglobate acne or acne at risk of permanent scarring) resistant to adequate courses of standard therapy with systemic antibacterials and topical therapy. The profile of side-effects has been well described, and the need for appropriate care in its use, particularly in women at risk of pregnancy, is well understood.[2] The Medicines and Healthcare Products Regulatory Agency (MHRA) has adopted the recommendations of the European Medicines Control Agency with regard to prescribing isotretinoin for women, with the introduction of the Pregnancy Prevention Programme (PPP). The availability of generic isotretinoin has also resulted in a standardization of the Summary of Product Characteristics (SPC) across all suppliers, with resulting changes to advice for in-treatment monitoring and to the limitations of prescribing only by hospitals that had previously existed.

Other recent concerns over the potential development of mood change, particularly depression,[3,4] have led to further evaluation both of the use of isotretinoin and of the necessary pretreatment evaluation and further monitoring. As used in this document, the term 'mood change' (unless otherwise specified) implies depression, psychosis, suicidal ideation, or other deleterious effect on mood or sleep. The U.S. Food and Drug Administration (FDA) has expressed its opinion on the use of isotretinoin,[5] and updated that view recently.[6] A PPP (initially SMART, now iPLEDGE) has been implemented; compulsory registration of all patients taking isotretinoin has been introduced in the U.S.A. and is now being evaluated.

The current document expresses the view of the British Association of Dermatologists (BAD) on these issues based on current knowledge. It does not discuss the indications for use of isotretinoin or the dosage and duration of treatment.

DOI 10.1111/j.1365-2133.2010.09836.x

Overview

Most of the potential adverse effects of isotretinoin are well documented,[1-4] have been reviewed[7] and are discussed in the manufacturers' product documentation.

Contraindications and side-effects

The drug is contraindicated in patients with hypervitaminosis A, uncontrolled hyperlipidaemia, and during pregnancy or lactation. Isotretinoin is contraindicated in hepatic insufficiency and should be used with caution in patients with renal disease and diabetes. Isotretinoin is contraindicated in airline pilots and should be used with caution after counselling in patients who depend on good night vision for their employment such as coach and taxi drivers. The dose should be reduced and titrated in patients with severe renal insufficiency. Some brands contain peanut oil and are contraindicated in patients with peanut allergy.

Most adverse events are dose related and predictable in terms of the known pharmacological and physiological effects of the drug. A full and up-to-date summary of adverse events is provided in the SPC, available at http://emc.medicines.org.uk/. These include:

- Variable dryness of skin and mucous membranes including nose, eyes and lips. These symptoms are dose related, and may lead to active inflammation, e.g. cheilitis.
- Facial erythema, eczema, hair loss, photosensitivity, skin fragility, paronychia and pyogenic granuloma.
- Myalgia and arthralgia.
- Photophobia, impaired night vision, keratitis: in one study three of 50 patients had impaired night vision which can be persistent after stopping therapy. Pilots should not take isotretinoin and if exposed can return to flying only after a satisfactory eye examination. Drivers affected should declare this to the Driver and Vehicle Licensing Agency and should not drive in conditions of illumination likely to affect safe driving.[8]
- Nausea, colitis, pancreatitis (in those with hypertriglyceridaemia).
- Abnormalities of liver function including hepatitis.
- Elevation of triglyceride and cholesterol levels: these were thought to be rare, but a recent paper indicated relatively high levels of detection of abnormalities, although with little clinical relevance.[9] There are also data suggesting that routine screening tests during treatment are not worthwhile,[10,11] although they are still recommended by the manufacturers. There are also recent data indicating that the development of hyperlipidaemia during treatment may be a marker for the development of significant hyperlipidaemia in later life.[12] Full blood count, liver function tests and fasting lipids should therefore be measured before treatment and 4–6 weeks after the onset of treatment. If continuing therapy, then repeat tests every 3 months (reduce dose or discontinue if transaminase or serum lipids persistently raised).
- Bacterial overgrowth, particularly by *Staphylococcus aureus*.

- Cutaneous vasculitis.
- Acne flare.
- Benign intracranial hypertension.

While these side-effects are generally mild and reversible, occasional severe reactions occur. A full and appropriate history should be taken and recorded before isotretinoin is prescribed.

There are two specific areas for concern and care that require more specific advice: risk of teratogenicity and mood change.

Risk of teratogenicity

The consequences of taking isotretinoin while pregnant are well described.[2] A baby born to a mother who has taken isotretinoin for even a few days during pregnancy has a high risk of malformation, including facial and skull malformation, and central nervous system or cardiovascular abnormalities.

More effective pregnancy prevention measures need to be enforced. Sixteen pregnancies were reported in a BAD prospective audit in 2004, which included results from 75% of U.K. dermatologists and was performed over a 6-month period. Eight of these had unknown outcomes, one gave rise to a normal healthy baby and there were seven terminations of pregnancy. In two patients about to undergo isotretinoin treatment, unknown pregnancies were prevented from risk exposure by pretreatment pregnancy tests. As of January 2010, 105 pregnancies have been spontaneously reported to the MHRA U.K. licensing authority.

Dermatologists should take every action to ensure that all women being considered for treatment understand the risks and consequences of pregnancy. All women of childbearing potential must be fully counselled about this effect of the drug and must also receive the patient information brochure provided by the manufacturer of the brand that is being prescribed. Every prescribing physician should be obliged to follow these guidelines. If exceptions exist, refer to 'Exemption from the pregnancy prevention programme' section below.

1 Discuss and record current and predicted sexual activity/behaviour to cover the entire course of treatment in all women of childbearing potential. No assumptions can be made because of age, race or religious beliefs, although clinicians should be sensitive to such issues. It may be necessary to conduct some of this enquiry with the patient alone, in the absence of parents or partner. A patient's sexual behaviour may change during therapy, so a discussion of the risks of teratogenicity should not be limited to those who are sexually active before treatment starts.

2 A menstrual history should be taken: patients with irregular menses present a difficult management problem that may require specialist advice.

3 The prescriber should educate female patients about contraception. These patients must be provided with comprehensive information on pregnancy prevention including the manufacturers' written documentation of contraceptive measures and should be referred for contraceptive advice if they are not using effective contraception.

Ideally, the main form of contraception should be hormonal – either the combined contraceptive pill, or injectable or implantable hormonal therapy should be used. The progesterone-only pill may be less reliable in those taking isotretinoin, and may make acne worse. Female patients are advised to use at least one but ideally TWO methods of contraception for 1 month before starting treatment, including a barrier method, and to continue to use effective contraception throughout the treatment period and for at least 1 month after cessation of treatment even in patients with amenorrhoea.

4 All female patients must sign a form indicating that they fully understand the risks of pregnancy, that they are not currently pregnant, that they have been using appropriate contraception for 1 month before starting treatment, and that the responsibilities of the patient and physician have been discussed. This should include the responsibility of the patient to consult her general practitioner (GP), dermatologist or pharmacist if she has knowingly had unprotected intercourse so that the possibility of using emergency contraception can be considered. The form for signature is provided by the manufacturer and must be signed by all women who are to be prescribed isotretinoin. A woman who is prescribed isotretinoin with monthly review, pregnancy test and prescription is following the PPP (see Appendix 1).

5 All female patients of childbearing potential should have a medically supervised pregnancy test. This can be done by measurement of β-human chorionic gonadotropin in blood or in urine using a urine test with minimum sensitivity of 25 mIU mL^{-1}. This test must be performed during the consultation when isotretinoin is prescribed or in the 3 days prior to the visit, and should have been delayed until the patient has been using effective contraception for at least 1 month. The result and the date should be recorded. In patients without regular menses, the timing of this pregnancy test should reflect the sexual activity of the patient and be undertaken at least 3 weeks after the patient last had unprotected sexual intercourse.

6 Isotretinoin can only be prescribed by or under the supervision of a dermatologist with expertise in the use of systemic retinoids and with a full understanding of the risks of treatment and monitoring requirements (see Appendix 1). The definition 'physicians with expertise in the use of systemic retinoids' was chosen in the licence as the most appropriate term to describe the provision of care in all European states, which currently use many different titles. In the U.K. this refers to Consultant Dermatologists, as currently only these healthcare professionals have the required knowledge and expertise.

Isotretinoin should, therefore, be prescribed only by a consultant-led team and prescriptions should be issued, under the consultant's name, from a hospital-based pharmacy.

The consultant-led team is defined as including the following: consultants, dermatology trainees, nonconsultant career grades (Staff Grade and Associated Specialist doctors) and accredited GPs with Special Interests (GPwSIs), and Dermatology Specialist Nurses. The MHRA regards 'physicians with expertise in the use of systemic retinoids' in the licensed label as Consultant Dermatologists. Thus accreditation as a GPwSI in terms of the Department of Health guidance does not include isotretinoin prescription, and prescription by GPwSIs outwith the consultant-led team would be considered off-label. Consultant Dermatologists and experienced GPwSIs working within an integrated service may wish to develop a locally agreed care pathway including dispensing and an accreditation process to facilitate such off-label prescribing of isotretinoin.

This position was reached through discussions with the MHRA, the BAD, the Royal College of General Practitioners, the Pharmaceutical Society and the Acne Support Group.

7 Follow-up visits should be arranged at 28-day intervals. At the time of each monthly prescription, both the prescriber and the pharmacist must be aware of the result of the pregnancy test taken at the time of the prescription. Each prescription is for a maximum of 30 days and the drug must be dispensed no later than 1 week after the date of the prescription.

8 After the course of treatment, a final pregnancy test should be taken and documented, advised at 5 weeks after completion of treatment to exclude pregnancy.

Exemption from the Pregnancy Prevention Programme

Under **exceptional** circumstances, isotretinoin may be prescribed to a woman who is not at risk of pregnancy without following the rules of the PPP. Examples of such circumstances might be: a nonsexually active woman who is able to be certain that sexual activity will not start during the period of teratogenic risk, or a woman who does not have childbearing potential, e.g. following a hysterectomy.

If a woman is to be exempted from the PPP, she must:

1 Receive written information of the methods of contraception (contraceptive brochure provided by the drug supplier).

2 Receive written information of the risks of teratogenicity with isotretinoin (patient information leaflet provided by the drug supplier).

3 Sign the form (provided by the supplier of the isotretinoin) to confirm that she has received information of the teratogenic risk of the drug and the methods of contraception.

4 Agree to contact the prescriber of the isotretinoin and the GP if there is any chance of pregnancy occurring during or immediately after the course of treatment.

The prescriber of isotretinoin outside the PPP should:

1 Document the reason for exclusion from the PPP.

2 Discuss the teratogenic risks of the drug and the necessity of seeing the patient rapidly if the risk of pregnancy changes during the course of treatment.

3 Record on each prescription of isotretinoin that the patient is exempted from the PPP.

4 The prescriber may wish to take extra written documentation that the patient was aware that she was exempted from the normal PPP and was fully aware of the teratogenic risks of the treatment (e.g. BAD document: Isotretinoin – Consent for female patients not following Pregnancy Prevention Plan).

Mood change

While the evidence for the problems due to retinoids in pregnancy is clear-cut, the situation for the suggested link to mood change is less certain. Changes in mood have been reported in patients taking vitamin A,[13] etretinate[14] and isotretinoin, but not with some other retinoids such as bexarotene.[15] Such symptoms have been reported in the treatment of patients with acne, disorders of keratinization and in patients with cancer given isotretinoin.[16] Vitamin A and its metabolites do cross the blood/brain barrier, can induce benign intracranial hypertension and cause headache, and so there are no theoretical reasons why mood alteration could not occur.[17] In addition, there is evidence of alterations in functional brain imaging induced by isotretinoin, but not accompanied by changes in mood or behaviour.[18] There are limited data in animals supporting an association between the drug and depression (in mice)[19] and refuting any association (in rats)[20] with depressive behaviour characteristics. Retinoic acid is an important endogenous molecule controlling growth and differentiation of the fetal brain and remains important in maintaining neurogenesis and neuronal plasticity in the hippocampus in the adult brain and as a signalling molecule in the hippocampus and prefrontal cortex. Defects in these areas including hippocampal volume occur in depression and correlate with severity of depression, and increased neurogenesis correlates with antidepressant treatment.[21,22] Experimentally, mice treated with doses of isotretinoin giving tissue levels comparable with those used in treatment in humans display defects in learning and memory with shrinkage of the hypothalamus and diminished neurogenesis.[23] Endogenous retinoic acid also modulates the dopamine D2 receptor in the striatum in a pathway implicated in the pathogenesis of depression and schizophrenia.[21]

The clinical data in humans supporting a relationship are conflicting, with several small inconclusive studies, often with significant design faults. Larger retrospective studies have shown an association between exposure to isotretinoin and depression or use of psychiatric services. In particular it has not been possible to distinguish accurately between mood change due to the drug and to the acne itself.

The problem is not a new one. Beginning in 1983, there have been several case reports,[3,24,25] some well publicized, as well as small case studies.[24,25] These suggest that mood change, and particularly depression, can occur during or soon after the use of isotretinoin. Hard evidence is not available, but the studies in which patients with apparent mood change were rechallenged with isotretinoin and had a relapse of mood alteration are the most compelling, with 41 cases of positive dechallenge and rechallenge between 1982 and 1998 reported.[21] Of these, 28 were depressed, five were psychotic, five had an unspecified mood disorder and three had suicidal ideation. Relapse with rechallenge has also been reported with etretinate.[15] Seven of 700 isotretinoin-treated patients were described as having psychiatric symptoms in a case series by Scheinman et al.;[26] more recently, 17·2% of 1419 soldiers trea-

Table 1 Selected psychiatric events reported to Medicines and Healthcare Products Regulatory Agency with isotretinoin (January 2010)

	Number of reports
Depression	193
Anxiety	26
Mood swings	26
Aggression	21
Suicide completed	29
Suicidal ideation	39
Suicide attempted	22
Psychotic disorder	18
Schizophreniform illness	12

ted with isotretinoin, compared with 12·5% of 1102 with psoriasis, consulted the Israeli army mental health services.[27] Many other small studies have also provided limited evidence, generally against any relationship existing, but all are too small to be conclusive.[28–33] Several large reviews document the literature on this topic,[15,34,35] and a systematic review supported by the manufacturers Roche demonstrated the paucity of convincing data very effectively.[36] The most recent independent and thorough review concludes that the evidence strongly supports a link between isotretinoin and psychopathology.[21] Clinicians should be alert to the potential psychiatric side-effects which are not restricted to depression. Spontaneous reports to the MHRA list 606 psychiatric events, including those listed in Table 1,[37] in which isotretinoin was the sole agent. This does not prove a causative effect.

When symptoms have been described, they have most commonly been fatigue, irritability, poor concentration, sadness, crying spells, loss of motivation and forgetfulness. The time course of onset of mood alteration is variable, but is often later in treatment, and in some cases depressive symptoms have occurred only in second or even third courses of therapy. Resolution of symptoms is usually rapid, within days to weeks of discontinuing the drug, although there are instances of prolonged illness requiring antidepressive therapy.[20] Not all patients have stopped therapy on developing depressive symptoms; some have elected to continue with isotretinoin and have improved psychologically without additional antidepressive therapy, and others have received psychological support and/or antidepressant medication.

The frequency of suicidal behaviour appears to be small: 37 suicides in 5 million individuals exposed in the U.S.A. between 1982 and 2000.[26] This figure may be an underestimate because of under-reporting, which is a flaw inherent in spontaneous reporting, but if true, it is lower than the estimated suicide rate for a group of comparable age and sex distribution.[38] It is important to be aware that suicidal behaviour is multifactorial and is one of the commoner causes of death in young adults who constitute the group most likely to be exposed to isotretinoin.

A larger study of 7195 patients treated with isotretinoin, compared with 13 700 treated with antibiotics, drawn from

Canadian and U.K. databases,[39] examined the risk of depression and suicide in these patients with acne, and concluded that neither depression nor suicide was more common in patients treated with isotretinoin. There were some potential flaws in the study. U.K. data relied on the recording of isotretinoin therapy by GPs who are not responsible for prescribing it, and there was selection bias in the ascertainment of mental disorders. The study was not sufficiently large to detect increased suicide reliably. It was not designed to answer the question of whether there was an effect of acne itself on the development of psychiatric or psychological symptoms, although other studies have indicated this to be the case.[40,41]

However, in a recent and more powerful case–crossover retrospective study of 30 496 isotretinoin-treated subjects, a first diagnosis or hospitalization for depression or antidepressant treatment occurred in 0·4%. Exposure to isotretinoin in a 5-month risk period immediately prior to the diagnosis of depression occurred in 32·5% of cases; this is compared with 22·2% during a separate 5-month control period, at least 2 months away from exposure, to allow for a 'washout' period. A significant association with depression was shown for the first time in a controlled study, with relative risk of isotretinoin associated with depression being 2·68 (95% confidence interval 1·10–6·48).[42]

It is likely that patients with a pretreatment history of bipolar disorder or family history of psychiatric disorder are more at risk. The frequency of pretreatment anxiety and associated psychological traits both in the individual affected and in their family is strikingly high (60–70%) in those cases reported to the FDA.[26] In a recent retrospective review of a case series of 300 patients with bipolar disorder, 10 had received isotretinoin. Nine of these experienced worsening of depression, three suicidal ideation and eight had a reversal of their deteriorated mood on discontinuing isotretinoin.[43] Also, five young adults with a prior history of obsessive-compulsive disorder or neurological insult, or a family history of major psychiatric illness, developed manic psychosis within a mean of 7·6 months of exposure to isotretinoin. In three cases this was accompanied by a suicide attempt, and in three cases psychosis lasted for longer than 6 months, suggesting an association between exposure to isotretinoin and manic psychosis.[44] There are also reports of acute onset of severe spontaneous and idiosyncratic mood alteration in individuals without a preceding history of psychiatric disease;[45] thus it may be that this is an idiosyncratic effect.[37,46]

Conversely, there are data indicating an improvement in psychiatric well-being in patients with acne, as their skin disease has improved after receiving isotretinoin.[40,41] The uncertainty that still exists has led to the suggestion that isotretinoin is being over-prescribed for less severe acne.[45]

In summary, isotretinoin therapy may lead to mood change; this has been reported in patients with or without preceding psychiatric illness, although it is more likely if there has been prior psychiatric morbidity.[47] So far there are no predictive tests that allow quantification of the level of risk. It does not seem to be an effect of all retinoids or exclusive to isotretinoin. Factors that suggest it to be an idiosyncratic effect include the fact that it is rare, that it does not appear to be reliably related to pre-isotretinoin depression, that it is not dose dependent, but that it can recur in those who are rechallenged.

In the absence of a definitive prospective study large enough (requiring around 8000 subjects) to rigorously prove and assess the psychological and psychiatric effects of isotretinoin, we recommend the following (see Appendix 1):

1 A direct enquiry about previous psychiatric health should be made for all patients who are being considered for isotretinoin and the facts recorded fully in the notes. There may be a role for specific psychiatric questionnaires; self-reported questionnaires have been suggested by some authors[15] and use of the self-completion questionnaire suggested in the first edition of this document has been audited and proved acceptable to patients.[48]

2 All patients, and their families, should be made aware of the possible potential for mood change in a realistic, nonjudgmental way. It is useful to advise patients to encourage their family and close friends to offer objective, honest feedback if they notice such changes.

3 Direct enquiry about psychological symptoms should be made at each clinic visit.

4 Further research is required to study the effects of isotretinoin on cognition, learning and memory. High-resolution imaging using positron emission tomography and functional magnetic resonance imaging should be used to confirm or refute existing evidence of structural and function effects in animals. Research into biomarkers to predict risk would help avoid rare but serious idiosyncratic responses to isotretinoin.

Suggested screening questions might be:[49]

For most of the last 2 weeks, have you...

(i) been feeling unusually sad or fed up?

(ii) lost interest in things that used to interest you, or gave you pleasure?

(iii) been significantly more agitated, irritable or short-tempered?

More extensive screening using a validated questionnaire may be helpful. The Beck questionnaire,[50] the Baer HANDS questionnaire,[51] or the six-question screening tool advocated in a recent *British Medical Journal* review[52] may be useful.

1 If symptoms of depression or mood change do occur, then, ideally, isotretinoin treatment should be discontinued. However, some patients, after discussion, may wish to continue with the drug because of the benefit to their skin. In this case, specialist psychiatric support should be obtained.

2 If serious psychiatric disease is suspected, there should be an immediate referral to the psychiatric services. The Samaritan service offers immediate advice to those with suicidal thoughts.

Audit points

1 The proportion of female patients of childbearing potential receiving isotretinoin who have signed the 'acknowledgement of PPP information' form indicating that they have received appropriate information.

2 The number of patients who have had serum lipids checked at least once during treatment.

3 The frequency with which patients in PPP received pregnancy tests before treatment and at monthly intervals and at 5 weeks after treatment.

4 The number of pregnancies occurring in patients taking isotretinoin with a target of 0% pregnancies as the standard to be achieved (note these must be reported on the yellow card system).

References

1 Cunliffe WJ, Simpson N. Disorders of the sebaceous glands. In: *Rook's Textbook of Dermatology* (Burns DA, Breathnach SM, Cox NH, Griffiths CEM, eds), 7th edn. Oxford: Blackwell Science, 2004; 43.1–43.75.

2 Strauss JS, Cunningham WJ, Leyden JJ et al. Isotretinoin and teratogenicity. *J Am Acad Dermatol* 1988; **19**:353–4.

3 Hazen PG, Carney JF, Walker AE, Stewart JJ. Depression – a side effect of 13-cis-retinoic acid therapy. *J Am Acad Dermatol* 1983; **9**:278–9.

4 Hanson N, Leachman S. Safety issues in isotretinoin therapy. *Semin Cutan Med Surg* 2001; **20**:166–83.

5 Josefson D. Acne drug is linked to severe depression. *BMJ* 1998; **316**:723.

6 U.S. Food and Drug Administration. iPLEDGE 2007 Update. Available at: http://www.fda.gov/Drugs/DrugSafety/PostmarketDrugSafety InformationforPatientsandProviders/ucm094306.htm (last accessed 28 March 2010).

7 Cunliffe WJ, van de Kerkhof PCM, Caputo R et al. Roaccutane treatment guidelines: results of an international survey. *Dermatology* 1997; **194**:351–7.

8 Taibjee SM, Charles-Holmes R. Pitfalls of prescribing acne therapies including isotretinoin for pilots. *Br J Dermatol* 2007; **158**:653–5.

9 Barth JH, Macdonald-Hull SP, Mark J et al. Isotretinoin therapy for acne vulgaris: a re-evaluation of the need for measurements of plasma lipids and liver function tests. *Br J Dermatol* 1993; **129**:704–7.

10 Alcalay J, Landau M, Zucker A. Analysis of laboratory data in acne patients treated with isotretinoin: is there really a need to perform routine laboratory tests? *J Dermatolog Treat* 2001; **12**:9–12.

11 Zane LT, Leyden WA, Marqueling AL, Manos MM. A population-based analysis of laboratory abnormalities during isotretinoin therapy for acne vulgaris. *Arch Dermatol* 2006; **142**:1016–22.

12 Rodondi N, Darioli R, Ramelet A et al. High risk for hyperlipidemia and the metabolic syndrome after an episode of hypertriglyceridemia during 13-cis retinoic acid therapy for acne: a pharmacogenetic study. *Ann Intern Med* 2002; **136**:582–9.

13 Restak RM. Pseudotumor cerebri, psychosis and hypervitaminosis A. *J Nerv Ment Dis* 1972; **155**:72–5.

14 Henderson CA, Highet AS. Depression induced by etretinate. *BMJ* 1989; **298**:964.

15 Bremner JD. Does isotretinoin cause depression and suicide? *Psychopharmacol Bull* 2003; **37**:64–78.

16 Meyskens FL Jr. Short clinical reports. *J Am Acad Dermatol* 1982; **6**:732–4.

17 Krezel W, Ghyselinck N, Samad TA et al. Impaired locomotion and dopamine signaling in retinoid receptor mutant mice. *Science* 1998; **279**:863–7.

18 Bremner JD, Fani N, Ashraf A et al. Functional brain imaging alterations in acne patients treated with isotretinoin. *Am J Psychiatry* 2005; **162**:983–91.

19 O'Reilly KC, Shumake J, Gonzalez-Lima F et al. Chronic administration of 13-cis-retinoic acid increases depression-related behavior in mice. *Neuropsychopharmacology* 2006; **31**:1919–27.

20 Ferguson SA, Cisneros FJ, Gough B et al. Chronic oral treatment with 13-cis-retinoic acid (isotretinoin) or all-trans-retinoic acid does not alter depression-like behaviors in rats. *Toxicol Sci* 2005; **87**:451–9.

21 Kontaxakis VP, Skourides D, Ferentinos P et al. Isotretinoin and psychopathology: a review. *Ann Gen Psychiatry* 2009; **8**:2.

22 Bremner JD, McCaffery P. The neurobiology of retinoic acid in affective disorders. *Prog Neuropsychopharmacol Biol Psychiatry* 2008; **32**:315–31.

23 Crandall J, Sakai Y, Zhang J et al. 13-cis-retinoic acid suppresses hippocampal cell division and hippocampal-dependent learning in mice. *Proc Natl Acad Sci USA* 2004; **101**:5111–16.

24 Gatti S, Serri F. Acute depression from isotretinoin. *J Am Acad Dermatol* 1991; **25**:132.

25 Byrne A, Hnatko G. Depression associated with isotretinoin therapy. *Can J Psychiatry* 1995; **40**:567.

26 Scheinman PL, Peck GL, Rubinow DR et al. Acute depression from isotretinoin. *J Am Acad Dermatol* 1990; **22**:1112–14.

27 Friedman T, Wohl Y, Knobler HY et al. Increased use of mental health services related to isotretinoin treatment: a 5-year analysis. *Eur Neuropsychopharmacol* 2006; **16**:413–16.

28 Chia CY, Lane W, Chibnall J et al. Isotretinoin therapy and mood changes in adolescents with moderate to severe acne: a cohort study. *Arch Dermatol* 2005; **141**:557–60.

29 Rohrback JM, Fleischer AB Jr, Krowchuk DP, Feldman SR. Depression is not common in isotretinoin-treated acne patients. *J Dermatolog Treat* 2004; **15**:252.

30 Ferahbas A, Turan MT, Esel E et al. A pilot study evaluating anxiety and depressive scores in acne patients treated with isotretinoin. *J Dermatolog Treat* 2004; **15**:153–7.

31 Cohen J, Adams S, Patten S. No association found between patients receiving isotretinoin for acne and the development of depression in a Canadian prospective cohort. *Can J Clin Pharmacol* 2007; **14**:227–33.

32 Kaymak Y, Kalay M, Ilter N et al. Incidence of depression related to isotretinoin treatment in 100 acne vulgaris patients. *Psychol Rep* 2006; **99**:897–906.

33 Ng CH, Tam MM, Celi E et al. Prospective study of depressive symptoms and quality of life in acne vulgaris patients treated with isotretinoin compared to antibiotic and topical therapy. *Australas J Dermatol* 2002; **43**:262–8.

34 Strahan JE, Raimer S. Isotretinoin and the controversy of psychiatric adverse effects. *Int J Dermatol* 2006; **45**:789–99.

35 Hull PR, D'Arcy C. Isotretinoin use and subsequent depression and suicide: presenting the evidence. *Am J Clin Dermatol* 2003; **4**:493–505.

36 Marqueling AL, Zane LT. Depression and suicidal behavior in acne patients treated with isotretinoin: a systematic review. *Semin Cutan Med Surg* 2005; **24**:92–102.

37 Medicines and Healthcare Products Regulatory Agency. Download Drug Analysis Prints (DAPs). Available at: http://www.mhra.gov. uk/Onlineservices/Medicines/Druganalysisprints/index.htm (last accessed 17 December 2009).

38 Wysowski DK, Pitts M, Beitz J. An analysis of reports of depression and suicide in patients treated with isotretinoin. *J Am Acad Dermatol* 2001; **45**:515–19.

39 Jick SS, Kremers HM, Vasilakis-Scaramozza C. Isotretinoin use and risk of depression, psychotic symptoms, suicide and attempted suicide. *Arch Dermatol* 2000; **136**:1231–6.

40 Kellett SC, Gawkrodger DJ. The psychological and emotional impact of acne and the effect of treatment with isotretinoin. *Br J Dermatol* 1999; **140**:273–82.

41 Rubinow DR, Peck GL, Squillace KM, Gantt GG. Reduced anxiety and depression in cystic acne patients after successful treatment with oral isotretinoin. *J Am Acad Dermatol* 1987; **17**:25–32.

42 Azoulay L, Blais L, Koren G *et al.* Isotretinoin and the risk of depression in patients with acne vulgaris: a case–crossover study. *J Clin Psychiatry* 2008; **69**:526–32.

43 Schaffer LC, Schaffer CB, Hunter S, Miller A. Psychiatric reactions to isotretinoin in patients with bipolar disorder. *J Affect Disord* 2010; **122**:306–8.

44 Barak Y, Wohl Y, Greenberg Y *et al.* Affective psychosis following Accutane (isotretinoin) treatment. *Int Clin Psychopharmacol* 2005; **20**:39–41.

45 Millard LG. Adverse mood and behaviour change in young patients on systemic isotretinoin. *Br J Dermatol* 1999; **141** (Suppl. 55):16.

46 Ng CH, Schweitzer I. The association between depression and isotretinoin use in acne. *Aust NZ J Psychiatry* 2003; **37**:78–84.

47 O'Donnell J. Overview of existing research and information linking isotretinoin (Accutane), depression, psychosis, and suicide. *Am J Ther* 2003; **10**:148–59.

48 McMullen E, Cox NH. The British Association of Dermatologists isotretinoin questionnaire for patients: a useful clinical tool. *Clin Exp Dermatol* 2006; **31**:713–14.

49 Jacobs DG, Deutsch NL, Brewer M. Suicide, depression and isotretinoin: is there a causal link? *J Am Acad Dermatol* 2001; **45**:S168–75.

50 Beck AT, Steer RA, Brown GK. *Beck Depression Inventory Manual*, 2nd edn. San Antonio, TX: The Psychological Corporation, 1996.

51 Baer L, Jacobs DG, Meszler-Reizes J *et al.* Development of a brief screening instrument: the HANDS. *Psychother Psychosom* 2000; **69**:35–41.

52 Peveler R, Carson A, Rodin G. Depression in medical patients. *BMJ* 2002; **325**:149–52.

Appendix 1 Aids to implementation of advice on the safe introduction and continued use of isotretinoin in acne in the U.K.

Pretreatment checklist for isotretinoin treatment

Isotretinoin should be prescribed only by a consultant-led team and prescriptions should be issued, under the consultant's name, from a hospital-based pharmacy. The consultant-led team is defined as including the following: consultants, trainees, non-consultant career grades and accredited General Practitioners with Special Interests and Dermatology Specialist Nurses.

1 Take and record a full history appropriate to the known side-effects of isotretinoin.

2 The outcome of previous treatment episodes with isotretinoin should be recorded.

3 General side-effects should be discussed and written information given: for example, information leaflets produced by the manufacturers or by the Acne Support Group may be used.

4 Document the site, nature and severity of acne.

5 Take blood for liver function tests and fasting lipids.

6 For female patients for whom isotretinoin therapy is considered:

(i) Issue company-produced *patient information booklet* (explains teratogenic risk of isotretinoin, does not give information about any other potential side-effects).

(ii) Issue company-produced *contraception information booklet* (lists all methods of contraception, pros and cons).

(iii) Ensure patient has read and understood both booklets, discussed and understood the risks of isotretinoin treatment, received the information on contraception and is willing to follow the guidance and rules for treatment.

(iv) Patient to sign *acknowledgement form* that she has received, read and understood both booklets.

(v) Provide patient with any other information on isotretinoin, its uses and effects.

7 If patient is at potential risk of pregnancy start Pregnancy Prevention Plan (PPP).

(i) One and preferably TWO forms of contraception to be used from at least 1 month before, until at least 1 month after course of isotretinoin.

(ii) Medically supervised pregnancy test from blood or urine just before starting therapy.

(iii) Monthly pregnancy tests throughout therapy.

(iv) Pregnancy test 5 weeks after stopping course of therapy.

(v) Isotretinoin prescriptions – for only 1 month of therapy at a time. Prescription valid for 7 days only.

(vi) Complete the checklist for prescribing to female patients at each stage, i.e. pretreatment, each in-treatment visit and post-treatment visit.

(Pharmacists will challenge any prescriptions that deviate from PPP. In certain circumstances, e.g. foreign travel, the rule could possibly be overridden. The pharmacist will follow the guidelines in the company-produced pharmacist's guide to prescribing isotretinoin.)

8 Counsel regarding depression.

(i) Enquire and record about previous and current psychiatric health.

(ii) Specifically discuss with patients, and their carers or family where appropriate, the potential for mood change in a realistic, nonjudgmental way.

(iii) Advise that family and friends should comment if such change should occur.

9 Arrange an appropriate follow-up appointment. This will usually be within 4 weeks for female patients in the PPP.

Review checklist for isotretinoin treatment

This checklist may be used as a reminder of the steps that may be taken on return visits for patients taking isotretinoin; as with all such lists, it may be modified for individual circumstances, and is not intended to represent essential practice.

1 Check effectiveness of treatment.

2 Check compliance with both isotretinoin and contraception and ask about the risk of pregnancy. Perform pregnancy test for PPP. Remind the patient of the availability of emergency contraception.

3 Specifically enquire about common side-effects, and particularly mood change. Suggested questions might be:

For most of the last 2 weeks, have you…

(i) been feeling unusually sad or fed up?

(ii) lost interest in things that used to interest you or gave you pleasure?

(iii) been significantly more agitated, irritable or short-tempered?

Consider the use of an extended questionnaire for additional screening. If such symptoms have occurred, assess their severity and consider the need for expert psychiatric or psychological input. Discuss the need to discontinue isotretinoin with the patient and their parents if appropriate.

4 Ask an open question about other side-effects.

5 Arrange blood tests if necessary; if they are abnormal, decide whether to stop or to reduce the dose of isotretinoin.

6 In women following the PPP, do a pregnancy test and document the result. Treatment can continue only if the result is negative.

7 Prescribe the drug for an appropriate period – 30 days for women continuing in the PPP, but may be longer for men or for women exempted from the PPP.

8 Arrange a follow-up appointment as indicated by progress and the results of any investigations. This may be an open appointment in many uncomplicated cases.

Final visit checklist

This checklist may be used as a reminder of the steps that may usefully be taken at the end of an isotretinoin treatment course; as with all such lists, it may be modified for individual circumstances, and is not intended to represent essential practice.

1 Check effectiveness of treatment.

2 Check compliance with both isotretinoin and contraception. For women at risk of pregnancy (patients following the PPP), perform a pregnancy test. Arrange a final pregnancy test 5 weeks after the end of therapy.

Ensure that contraception is continued for 1 month after discontinuing isotretinoin.

3 Specifically enquire about common side-effects, and particularly mood change:

For most of the last 2 weeks, have you...

(i) been feeling unusually sad or fed up?

(ii) lost interest in things that used to interest you or gave you pleasure?

(iii) been significantly more agitated, irritable or short-tempered?

Consider the use of an extended questionnaire for additional screening. If symptoms of mood change have occurred, assess their severity and consider the need for expert psychiatric or psychological input.

4 Ask an open question about other side-effects.

5 Arrange repeat blood tests if indicated and take any necessary action.

6 Remind the patient about the need to inform the supervising consultant of any late complications.

7 Ensure that any unused isotretinoin is returned.

Possible isotretinoin side-effect checklist to be completed by patients

Name

Hospital number

Date of appointment

Have you had any of the following side-effects? (circle appropriate choices)

Dry lips	No	Mild	Moderate	Severe
Joint or muscle pain	No	Mild	Moderate	Severe
Nosebleed	No	Occasional	Frequent	
Headache different from normal	No	Yes – mild	Yes – severe	

In the last 2 weeks

Have you been feeling unusually sad or fed up?	No	Yes
Have you lost interest in things that used to interest you or gave you pleasure?	No	Yes

Any other side-effects? (please specify)

Female patients only:

Have you used reliable contraceptive measures while taking isotretinoin?

Yes   No   Not applicable

Have you any reason to believe you may have become pregnant while taking isotretinoin?

Yes   No   Not applicable

Reminder: Female patients must take effective measures to avoid pregnancy during treatment and for a month afterwards. It may be helpful to remind patients regarding the availability of emergency contraception.

Name (please print)

Signature

http://www.bad.org.uk/Portals/_Bad/Guidelines/Clinical Guidelines/Advice on the safe introduction and continued use of isotretinoin in acne.pdf

Comment

Safety of this drug is remarkable as the potential hazards are so serious. Even after 30 years of use the prescribing and monitoring has become more thorough. These guidelines are about safely prescribing and monitoring oral isotetinoin for acne vulgaris, not about the effectiveness of the drug [1]. The link with depression seems to be not proven and the risk of serious consequences due to depression extremely low, but none the less the guidance recommends screening for depressive symptoms [1–3]. The prescribing of isotretinon is about risk management, patient safety and hazard avoidance. A recently published study from Canada showed that 24% of patients needed a further course of oral isotretinoin [4]. Further research is needed to study the real life relapse rate or the percentage of patients who need further courses of oral isotretinoin.

References

1 Goodfield MJD, Cox NH, Bowser A, *et al.* Advice on the safe introduction and continued use of isotretinoin in acne in the UK. *Brit J Dermatol* 2010; 162: 1172–9.
2 Strahan JE, Raimer S. Isotretinoin and the controversy of psychiatric adverse effects. *Int J Dermatol* 2006; 45: 789–99.
3 Marqueling AL, Zane LT. Depression and suicidal behavior in acne patients treated with isotretinoin: a systematic review. *Semin Cutan Med Surg* 2007; 26: 210–20.
4 Azoulay L, Oraichi D, Bérard A. Isotretinoin therapy and the incidence of acne relapse: a nested case–control study. *Br J Dermatol* 2007; 157: 1240–48.

Additional professional resources

Strauss JS, Krowchuk DP, Leyden JJ, *et al.* Guidelines of care for acne vulgaris management. *J Am Acad Dermatol* 2007; 56: 651–63. http://www.aad.org/research/_doc/ClinicalResearch_Acne%20Vulgaris.pdf.

Isotretinoin for severe acne. Medicines and Healthcare Products Regulatory Agency 2007. http://www.mhra.gov.uk/Safetyinformation/Generalsafetyinformationand advice/Product-specificinformationandadvice/Isotretino inforsevereacne/index.htm.

http://www.library.nhs.uk/skin/SearchResults.aspx?tabID =289&catID=8229&pgIndex=0& (list of evidence sources in acne treatment)

Acne vulgaris. Clinical Knowledge Summaries 2009. http://www.cks.nhs.uk/acne_vulgaris#.

BAD acne patient information leaflet

Related to acne (includes details on isotretinoin)

http://www.bad.org.uk/site/793/default.aspx

Other patient resources (on acne generally)

http://www.aad.org/public/publications/pamphlets/common_acne.html
http://www.skincarephysicians.com/acnenet/
http://www.cks.nhs.uk/patient_information_leaflet/acne
http://www.nhs.uk/conditions/Acne/Pages/Introduction.aspx?url=Pages/what-is-it.aspx
http://www.patient.co.uk/pdf/pilsL2.pdf
http://www.dermnetnz.org/treatments/isotretinoin.html

Guidelines for dosimetry and calibration in ultraviolet radiation therapy: a report of a British Photodermatology Group workshop

D.K.TAYLOR, A.V.ANSTEY,* A.J.COLEMAN,† B.L.DIFFEY,‡ P.M.FARR,§
J.FERGUSON,¶ S.IBBOTSON,¶ K.LANGMACK,** J.J.LLOYD,‡ P.McCANN,††
C.J.MARTIN,‡‡ H.DU P.MENAGÉ,§§ H.MOSELEY,¶ G.MURPHY,¶¶ S.D.PYE,***
L.E.RHODES††† AND S.ROGERS‡‡‡

Medical Physics Department, Gloucestershire Royal Hospital, Great Western Road, Gloucester, GL1 3NN, U.K.
Dermatology Department, Royal Gwent Hospital, Newport, Gwent, U.K.
†*Medical Physics Department, St Thomas' Hospital, London, U.K.*
‡*Regional Medical Physics Department, Newcastle-upon-Tyne, U.K.*
§*Dermatology Department, Royal Victoria Infirmary, Newcastle-upon-Tyne, U.K.*
¶*Photobiology Unit, Dermatology Department, Dundee University, U.K.*
**Medical Physics Department, St George's Hospital, Lincoln, U.K.*
††*Medical Physics Department, St Luke's Hospital, Dublin, Republic of Ireland*
‡‡*Medical Physics Department, Western Infirmary, Glasgow, U.K.*
§§*Dermatology Department, University Hospital, Lewisham/St Thomas' Hospital, London, U.K.*
¶¶*Dermatology Department, Beaumont Hospital, Dublin, Republic of Ireland*
***Medical Physics Department, Western General Hospital, Edinburgh, U.K.*
†††*Photobiology Unit, Dermatology Centre, University of Manchester, U.K.*
‡‡‡*Ely Place, Dublin, Republic of Ireland*

Accepted for publication 22 October 2001

Summary

This report examines the dosimetry of ultraviolet (UV) radiation applied to dermatological treatments, and considers the definition of the radiation quantities and their measurement. Guidelines are offered for preferred measurement techniques and standard methods of dosimetry. The recommendations have been graded according to the American Joint Committee on Cancer classification of strength of recommendation and quality of evidence (summarized in Appendix 5).

Key words: dosimetry, guidelines, phototherapy, psoralen ultraviolet A, radiation, ultraviolet

Correspondence: D.K.Taylor.
E-mail: dktaylor@tiscali.co.uk

Disclaimer

These guidelines on recommendations for good practice have been prepared for medical physicists, dermatologists and phototherapists, following a Workshop meeting of the British Photodermatology Group. Caution should be exercised in interpreting the data; the results of future studies may require alteration of the conclusions or recommendations in this report. It may be necessary or desirable to depart from the guidelines in special circumstances. Just as adherence to guidelines may not constitute defence against a claim of negligence, so deviation from them should not necessarily be deemed negligent.

Optimal ultraviolet (UV) radiation therapy requires close control of the variables that may influence the clinical outcome. An essential part of control is the accurate measurement of these variables, in particular the spectral content of the UV sources employed, the UV energy applied to the patient's skin, and the psoralen administration [in psoralen UVA therapy (PUVA) therapy]. These variables are interlinked so that changing any one will lead to a change in clinical outcome, unless the others are also adjusted. These Workshop Guidelines address the importance of UV dosimetry and calibration in the delivery of effective phototherapy (used to describe both UVB and PUVA therapy, unless otherwise stated).

Background to ultraviolet radiation measurements for phototherapy

These guidelines presume that measurement and control of all therapy variables (not only UV radiation) are necessary for the safe and effective delivery of phototherapy. Variables that can influence outcomes are grouped into three main areas: (i) the UV irradiation equipment used to treat skin; (ii) the accuracy of measurements made and their practical application; and (iii) the human influences, including patient differences, treatment techniques and clinic management.

Ultraviolet irradiation equipment

An informal survey of phototherapy clinics in the U.K. and Republic of Ireland was conducted immediately prior to the workshop, to identify: (i) types of UV equipment in current use; (ii) measurement methods used to manage them; and (iii) test equipment used to make the measurements.

It is apparent that, since the survey[2] of Dootson et al. in 1993, unfiltered mercury discharge lamps have now been mostly replaced by fluorescent tube irradiators, and that broadband UVB lamps are being replaced by narrowband UVB types. Spectra of the commonest UV lamp types are given in Figure 1.

Ultraviolet radiation measurement equipment

The focus of this report concerns UV measurement in order to optimize therapy, including routine consistency checks of UV irradiation equipment and methods for measuring UV radiation in phototherapy units. Most phototherapy departments own or have access to a UV radiometer, usually hand-held, indicating a mean irradiance in mW cm^{-2} over some UV waveband.

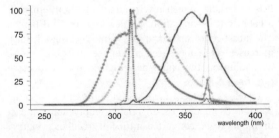

Figure 1. Spectral outputs of typical fluorescent ultraviolet (UV) therapy lamps: UVA; narrow-band TL-01; TL-12/Waldmann UV21; Waldmann UV6.

Several clinics surveyed had no meter, and relied on a manufacturer's engineer or a hospital physicist to measure irradiance. Some made no irradiance measurement, delivering treatments by exposure time only.

Those clinics with access to UV radiometers used different techniques to measure irradiance, at intervals varying from daily to annually. The pattern of UV radiometer calibration practice also showed wide variation, although a good quality meter in good condition should not require recalibration more frequently than annually. Unexpected measurement outcomes are usually the result of changes in the source (such as broken or dirty tubes and reflectors) or temperature changes. Meter malfunction is often due to failing batteries, intermittent connections or failure to configure the instrument correctly, especially where sensors, filters and diffusers can be interchanged, or a premeasurement 'zeroing' function is provided.

The irradiance of a UV therapy device measured with a hand-held meter depends upon the type of lamps fitted to the device and the calibration standard used. The device may have a UV radiometer built-in, which may be calibrated to a different standard, but which may not be readily adjustable. The international[3] and other standards in use, given in Table 1, are confusing, resulting in poor correlation between irradiance values where the calibration definitions are different or unknown. The wide range of published minimal erythemal dose (MED) values for narrow-band (TL-01) UVB radiation suggests that there are difficulties in measuring irradiance accurately, and in defining and determining MED.

Diffey's review[4] of ultraviolet dosimetry published in 1978 noted that the term 'irradiance' has been used to describe the UV intensity over all emitted wavelengths (100–400 nm), or within a restricted band (315–400 nm, for example), or 'weighted' by an action spectrum (where this is known) resulting in different numerical values for the same radiation. It is recommended that a standard definition be used for all UV radiation measurements (see Appendix 3).

Table 1. The ultraviolet (UV) radiation spectrum lies between wavelengths of 100 nm and 400 nm, by international agreement. The Commission Internationale de l'Eclairage (CIE) adopted[3] the following general definitions

Band	CIE definition	Alternative definitions in use
UVA	315–400 nm	320–400/320–410 nm
UVB	280–315 nm	280–320/290–320 nm
UVC	200–280 nm	150–280/100–280 nm

Wavelengths shorter than about 200 nm propagate only in a vacuum and are not relevant to phototherapy.

MacKenzie's review[5] of UV dosimetry in 1985 identified the factors influencing UV irradiance values, emphasizing the importance of differentiating between measurements made to demonstrate consistency or repeatability (which need not be calibrated) and those made to establish absolute values (which must be calibrated).

Factors influencing measured ultraviolet outputs from irradiation equipment

The variety of shape, size and lamp geometry of typical UV irradiation equipment implies that no single measurement method will provide a meaningful irradiance value at the patient's skin surface, which is itself not a unique value in most practical situations.

On a small panel irradiator, designed for treating palmar and plantar skin, the source–skin distance is defined by the contact glass or grille, so measurements should also be made in contact with the same surface. The value varies across the plane of the contact surface, being maximal near the centre of the panel and less towards the edges. Hands and feet usually occupy an area that includes this maximum value, but may also cover areas of reduced irradiance. It is recommended that the maximal value be used for exposure calculation, to avoid 'hot-spots' from areas that exceed the mean.

The situation is more complex for larger panels designed to treat the whole body, requiring the patient to stand in front of a lamp array. Maximum irradiance is on the skin closest to the lamp array, around the centre of the lamp length (waist height for typical patients). Irradiance on the patient's skin facing away from the array will be zero, so that uniform treatment requires rotation of the patient, and careful attention to posture and exposure times, to avoid risk of underdosing or overdosing. To minimize these risks and radiation hazards to others, it is recommended that whole-body treatments be given in enclosed cabins wherever possible.

In whole body treatment cabins, 1800-mm long fluorescent lamps line the walls, usually in front of reflective metal surfaces, surrounding the patient with radiating elements. This improves dose uniformity, but 'sanctuary sites' can still occur if the patient remains in a fixed posture with arms close to the body. The patient is not uniformly cylindrical and the intensity of the lamps is lower near the ends, so the body-surface irradiance is not a single value.

Whole-body cabin measurement methods

Two measurement methods are in common use, requiring either a cabin occupant to hold the meter, or a support on which the meter is mounted.

The Direct Method (with a cabin occupant)

A measurement protocol proposed by Moseley *et al.*[6] and summarized by Diffey and Hart[7] requires several measurements with a hand-held meter to be taken on the surface of a protected cabin occupant, at the levels of the head or shoulders, waist and knees. This is repeated for several orientations within the cabin, and the mean of all of these values is taken to be the skin irradiance. This assumes that the treatment's effectiveness is dependent only upon the quantity of energy incident on the patient's skin, and not on the rate of delivery. This reciprocity relationship has been established[8] for UV radiation on human skin over several orders of magnitude.

Alternative protocols use a simpler waist-height measurement for several orientations within the cabin to obtain a maximum value of the irradiance. This protocol gives a slightly higher value than that obtained by the previously described protocol, but reduces the risk of localized overdosing, by avoiding 'hot-spots' around the buttocks and genitalia where the irradiance exceeds the mean value.

For any whole-body treatment cabin, the skin irradiance is dependent upon the geometry of the cabin and reflectors, and the number and arrangement of the lamps inside. These influences have been described[9,10] and attempts made[11] to develop a mathematical model to calculate patient irradiance from a knowledge of the cabin characteristics.

The Indirect Method (without cabin occupant)

It is preferable to measure irradiance without entering a cabin during operation, particularly for UVB lamps. The absence of an occupant, however, significantly increases[10] the measured irradiance (by about 20%, depending on the cabin design), because of multiple internal reflections.

Moseley's protocol gives correction factors for some popular cabin designs, to enable empty cabin measurements to be converted into skin irradiance values. The factor may be readily determined for any cabin by measuring irradiance on a protected occupant and then in the empty cabin, with the meter in the same location(s), and calculating the ratio of the values. The factor should be verified periodically (annually is adequate) to take account of changes in the optical properties of the cabin components.

An alternative method of obtaining a Direct Method value, but without risking exposure to a cabin occupant, has been described by Fulljames and Welsh,[12] employing a simple phantom cabin occupant constructed of readily available materials. The meter sensor is mounted on the phantom in the same locations defined by Moseley, giving irradiance values within ± 5% of typical occupant values. Currie et al.[13] described a computer-controlled and motorized device to measure indirect irradiances automatically.

Note that the irradiance of canopies and panel units is not affected by the presence of the patient, as the radiation does not experience multiple reflections. The mean irradiance over an extended area is usually significantly less than the peak irradiance near the centre of the lamp array, so it is recommended that the highest value be used for exposure calculations, as for extremities units (above), to reduce localized overdosing.

Influences on irradiance values

Irradiances from UV therapy equipment are generally not constant. Mechanisms that can change the measured value over a treatment course include: (i) intermittent or total failure of one or more lamps; (ii) supply voltage variation (the control circuits are not regulated); (iii) intensity diminution with rising lamp operating time; (iv) dirt on lamps/reflectors or damage to reflective surfaces; and (v) temperature changes. This last is a common cause of short-term differences in irradiance, as the emission of fluorescent phosphors is strongly temperature dependent. Lamps will be cold after 15 min inactivity, and can overheat if poorly ventilated or operated in hot environments, both leading to changes in irradiance. To minimize this effect, the manufacturer's advice on ventilation and lamp warming should be followed, particularly at the beginning of a treatment session.

Built-in cabin dosimetry

To compensate for the uncontrolled effects on irradiance described above, cabins may be equipped with built-in UV dosimeters, to monitor the irradiance throughout treatment and terminate exposure after a set dose has been accumulated. This can result in more accurate dose delivery, but only if the built-in metering device closely matches Direct Method measurements made with a calibrated meter.

Users should not assume that the dose displayed on the cabin's control panel is correct, or that the cabin does not require regular performance checking. Some built-in meter devices may indicate irradiances different from those obtained directly. Measurement devices cannot be assumed to perform consistently over many years' use, especially those frequently irradiated with UV, which degrades optical and electronic components.

Any built-in device should be checked for correlation with direct body-surface measurements. If there is significant (> 10%) disagreement, the built-in dosimeter should be adjusted, or the cabin can be operated in time-exposure mode, using irradiance values obtained by the Direct or Indirect Methods described above. It is preferable to adjust built-in meter circuits to agree with a defined dosimetry standard, especially where more than one cabin may be used for successive treatments of a patient. If a correction factor is to be applied, it is probably safer to apply it to the cumulative dose at the conclusion of a treatment course, rather than at every dose calculation, which may lead to arithmetic errors.

Ultraviolet radiometry instruments

Most UV measurement devices are based on photodiode sensors having electrical characteristics varying with the radiation intensity falling on their active surfaces. For accurate and consistent performance, a meter should have adequate sensitivity to its designed spectral band but negligible sensitivity outside that band, linear operation over a useful range of irradiance values, and adequate sensitivity to radiation at all practical incident angles. Other features that may improve the flexibility and convenience of a meter, including angular response,[14] are discussed in Appendix 1.

Patient-related variables

Each patient presents a different set of skin characteristics, dependent on the skin disorder, skin type and personal life-style. These guidelines make no attempt to differentiate between different treatment protocols for all of these variables, as they are outside the scope of UV dosimetry considerations. The patient's skin type, however, does have a bearing on dosimetry, as this parameter is related to the patient's skin sensitivity and is often used to determine prescribed doses. A study[14] by Gordon *et al.* of MED measurement prior to narrow-band UVB therapy showed that skin-type assessment (a subjective value) is not always a useful predictor of erythema sensitivity obtained from testing (an objective value).

The estimation of MED [minimal phototoxic dose (MPD) in PUVA therapy] is a valuable guide to sensitivity but is not measured and reported uniformly. This subject is beyond the remit of this report, but patients' cutaneous responses to UV radiation exposure provide additional information that can inform routine radiometry practices. When skin sensitivity tests are performed and their results given in clinical reports, it is important to define all the relevant parameters and the judgement criteria. A suggested format for defining an MED/MPD test is given in Appendix 2.

Except for the photodermatoses, usually provoked by suberythemal doses, erythema defines the upper limit for most UV phototherapy treatments. The erythema action spectrum for UV is therefore critical in deter-mining the maximum dose without causing pain or burning. A proposal[16] to incorporate human skin erythemal response into UV dosimetry, by using a weighted radiometric unit, makes weighted irradiances in the UVB region numerically larger than similar intensities of UVA, which are less erythemogenic. The weighting curve for erythema in human skin has been formalized as simple mathematical functions and applied in a Commission Internationale de l'Eclairage standard.[17] The pattern of the majority of published values, however, and the recommendation of these guidelines, is that unweighted doses in SI radiometric units of J cm^{-2} (or derived units) should be used.

Defining the irradiance of broad-band UVB fluorescent lamps is particularly difficult. The peak output of these lamps falls near the boundary between UVA and UVB, so that minor changes in band width definition cause significant changes in apparent irradiance. This problem does not arise to the same extent for UVA lamps and narrow-band TL-01 lamps (Table 2).

To avoid false comparisons between irradiances defined under different calibration standards, it is recommended that spectroradiometric calibrations should include a value for the total irradiance of the source over the entire UV band from 250 to 400 nm. Other band widths may be used to match an existing meter calibration, but if the 250–400 nm value is always included in a specification of UV radiation, the differences in preferred band width become irrelevant, allowing the comparison of irradiance data from different workers.

For example, a cabin fitted with Philips TL-12 (or equivalent) fluorescent lamps might be described as having an irradiance at the skin surface of 4·5 mW cm^{-2} (UVB band defined as 280–315 nm) or 8·8 mW cm^{-2} over the whole UV band (250–400 nm). Another worker may state the irradiance of these lamps to be 5·4 mW cm^{-2} (UVB band defined as 280–320 nm) but would still find the total UV irradiance of 8·8 mW cm^{-2}.

The data in Table 2 include relative irradiance values for various band widths and the total UV band width for commonly used UV lamps, to permit this full-width irradiance to be derived, provided the lamp type and the calibrated irradiance are known.

A suggested form of defining the calibration method and traceability for UV radiometers is given in Appendix 3. The calibration laboratories identified in Appendix 4 are able to provide this total band irradiance as part of a meter calibration report. These laboratories have also agreed to collaborate with national standards agencies to align and rationalize UV calibration, to be the subject of further investigations.

Phototherapy is potentially hazardous, and successful phototherapy requires some clinical, nursing, physics and technical knowledge for optimum outcomes. The increase in published clinical trials and research into fundamental aspects of phototherapy have allowed this discipline to be practised more safely and effectively, with treatment protocols and practices that are evidence based. More needs to be done, however, to move away from clinical practice based on anecdote. UV dosimetry and calibration form a part

Table 2. Partial and total irradiances for commonly used ultraviolet (UV) lamps, normalized to 250–400 nm band width

Lamp type	280–315 nm	280–320 nm	315–400 nm	320–400 nm	320–410 nm	250–400 nm
Waldmann UV6	0·23	0·33	0·77	0·67	0·72	1·00
Waldmann UV21	0·51	0·61	0·48	0·39	0·43	1·00
Philips TL-01	0·77	0·80	0·23	0·20	0·25	1·00
Waldmann UVA	0·004	0·008	0·99	0·98	1·02	1·00
Cosmolux UVA	0·008	0·02	0·99	0·98	1·01	1·00
Arimed B	0·04	0·08	0·96	0·92	0·96	1·00

of this process, and should be considered in the context of consistent and repeatable practice and adherence to written local rules and instructions. The recommendations given here are based on the cumulative experiences of the medical physics departments and phototherapists represented by the workshop contributors, and are offered as current best practices.

Recommendations and guidelines

1 Whole-body treatments should be given in ventilated cabins surrounding the patient with radiation sources wherever possible, and it is recommended that obsolete apparatus be replaced. (American Joint Committee on Cancer classification: BIII)

2 Phototherapy clinics should use a UV radiometer to measure irradiances from all UV treatment equipment. The meter should have minimal response outside the UV band and be chosen for dynamic range, linearity and angular sensitivity. (BIII)

3 The meter should be calibrated annually for each type of UV source in use, identifying the method, its traceability to known national standards and the waveband over which irradiance is measured. Irradiance over the full UV band of 250–400 nm should also be measured, in addition to any other band width, to facilitate intercomparisons. (BIII)

4 Built-in UV dosimeters in cabins should agree closely with directly measured irradiance values. Where agreement is outside reasonable tolerance (± 10%), the built-in meter may need adjusting. The supplier or the person responsible for the equipment should be consulted for advice. (BIII)

5 Electrical equipment should be tested for compliance with electrical safety standards, and staff should be trained to operate the equipment correctly. Annual checks are acceptable, and written records should be kept. (BIII)

6 Regular consistency checks of all UV irradiation apparatus should be performed, by checking for failed lamps and measuring UV irradiance in a standard reference location to identify any changes. Failed lamps should be replaced promptly, and consistency verified at least monthly. (BIII)

7 Skin irradiances should be measured regularly by the Direct or Indirect Methods, and used to calculate exposure times and to check built-in meters. Measurement every 25–50 h of usage is acceptable, but after installing new lamps, which

degrade more quickly when new, re-measure after 10–15 h. (BIII)

8 Patient doses should be prescribed in $J\,cm^{-2}$ (or derived units), and cumulative doses calculated and recorded at the end of treatment courses, to quantify lifetime exposure to therapeutic UV. (BII-i)

9 MED/MPD techniques should be described fully, including the site(s) of test(s), the criteria used to assess erythema, the methodology of masking and exposing test sites, including any devices used for this, and the sequence of doses used (or the ratio between adjacent exposures). (BII-iii)

10 The recommendations in this report should be subject to routine audit, as part of the clinic's audit programme, to verify that objectives are being met, and to optimize clinical outcomes. (BIII)

Acknowledgments

The contributions of P.Brooks and P.Garibaldinos, and the financial support of this workshop by Leo Pharmaceuticals, are gratefully acknowledged.

References

1 Hurwitz B. Legal and political considerations of clinical practice guidelines. *Br Med J* 1999; **318**: 661–4.

2 Dootson G, Norris PG, Gibson CJ, Diffey BL. The practice of ultraviolet phototherapy in the United Kingdom. *Br J Dermatol* 1994; **131**: 873–7.

3 Commission Internationale de l'Eclairage. *Comptes Rendues (Berlin)* 1935; **9**: 596–625.

4 Diffey BL. A review of ultraviolet dosimetry. *Br J Dermatol* 1978; **98**: 703–6.

5 MacKenzie LA. UV radiometry in dermatology. *Photodermatology* 1985; **2**: 86–94.

6 Moseley H. Scottish UV dosimetry guidelines. *Photoderm Photoimmunol Photomed* 2001; **17**: 230–3.

7 Diffey BL, Hart GC. *Ultraviolet and Blue-light Phototherapy—Principles, Sources, Dosimetry and Safety*. Report 76. York: IPEM, 1997: 27.

8 Meanwell EF, Diffey BL. Reciprocity of ultraviolet erythema in human skin. *Photodermatology* 1989; **6**: 146–8.

9 Mountford PJ. Phototherapy and photochemotherapy ultraviolet irradiation equipment. *Photodermatology* 1986; **3**: 83–91.

10 Fanselow D, Crone M, Dahl MV. Dosimetry in phototherapy cabinets. *J Am Acad Dermatol* 1987; **17**: 74–7.

11 Langmack KA. An insight into the contributions of self-shielding and lamp reflectors to patient exposure in phototherapy units. *Phys Med Biol* 1998; **43**: 207–14.

12 Fulljames CA, Welsh AD. Measurement of patient dose in ultraviolet therapy using a phantom. *Br J Dermatol* 2000; **142**: 748–51.

13 Currie GD, Evans AL, Smith D *et al.* An automated dosimetry system for testing whole-body ultraviolet phototherapy cabinets. *Phys Med Biol* 2001; **46**: 333–46.

14 Martin CJ, Currie GD, Pye SD. The importance of radiometer angular response for UV therapy dosimetry. *Phys Med Biol* 1999; **44**: 843–55.

15 Gordon PM, Saunders PJ, Diffey BL, Farr PM. Phototesting prior to narrowband (TL-01) UV-B phototherapy. *Br J Dermatol* 1998; **139**: 811–14.

16 Diffey BL, Jansen CT, Urbach F, Wulf HC. The Standard Erythema Dose: a new photobiological concept. *Photoderm Photoimmunol Photomed* 1997; **13**: 64–6.

17 Commission Internationale l'Eclairage. ISO 17166/CIE S007 Joint ISO/CIE Standard. Erythema reference action spectrum and standard erythema dose. CIE Central Bureau 1999 http://www.cie.co.at/cie/framepublications.html [accessed 16/01/02].

18 Pye SD, Martin CJ. A study of the directional response of ultraviolet radiometers: I Practical evaluation and implications for ultraviolet measurement standards. *Phys Med Biol* 2000; **45**: 2701–12.

19 Martin CJ, Pye SD. A study of the directional response of ultraviolet radiometers: II Implications for ultraviolet phototherapy derived from computer simulations. *Phys Med Biol* 2000; **45**: 2713–29.

Appendix 1

Ultraviolet radiometer characteristics

UV radiometers mostly employ photodiodes sensitive to wavelengths from about 300 nm up to about 1000 nm. Wavelengths outside the UV bands are removed by filters, reducing unwanted spectral components, although not with a sharp cut-off. Some proportion of unwanted radiation may therefore be included in the measured radiation.

The meter should have a dynamic range appropriate for therapy sources (0.05–50 mW cm^{-2} is adequate) and should be linear ($< 2\%$) in that range. The meter should also respond accurately to radiation independently of its angle of incidence on the sensor ($< 5\%$ deviation from true cosine weighting).

Spectroradiometers are widely used as references for the calibration of hand-held meters. The spectra in Figure 1 were obtained from typical fluorescent UV phototherapy lamps using a spectroradiometer. The irradiance of a source is represented by the area beneath the spectral irradiance curve, so the irradiance over any chosen bandwidth is represented by the area beneath the curve in that band, permitting calibration of UV radiometers to any standard.

Hand-held meters and built-in cabin dosimeters should be calibrated regularly, by comparison with a spectroradiometer or UV radiometer with calibration traceable to recognized standards. Appendix 4 gives contact details of medical physics laboratories in the U.K. and Republic of Ireland Ireland willing to perform calibration of meters against standard UV lamp types commonly in use in phototherapy clinics.

Ultraviolet radiometer sensor characteristics

Manufacturers are encouraged to design better meter sensors and to minimize the angular sensitivity errors. The ideal sensor will have an optical diffuser that avoids specular reflection from polished flat surfaces, and accurate angular sensitivity at all incident angles.

A sensor should indicate irradiance values proportional to the cosine of the angle of incidence of the radiation. In practice, sensors often indicate significantly less than this value at angles of incidence greater than about 45° from the normal, and therefore underestimate the wide radiation field in a whole-body cabin, which arrives at a waist-height meter from nearly all angles. Inadequate angular response is identified as one of the causes of metering error.

Martin and Pye[18,19] studied the angular response of several popular UV sensors, and found that they underestimated irradiances at angles greater than about 30°. Sensors having convex or protruding diffusers usually perform better than those without a diffuser or having optical components recessed within the casing.

A UV radiometer must be calibrated for every type of UV source to be measured, typically UVA, broadband and narrowband UVB fluorescent tubes. If mercury discharge or metal halide lamps are also employed, these must also have separate calibration factors, as their spectral outputs are different from those of fluorescent tubes.

Appendix 2

Suggested form of minimal erythemal dose/ minimal phototoxic dose definition in clinical study reports

Terms in *italics* represent variables that should be modified to match the local technique employed. Each term should be identified so that all relevant details are clearly defined.

'Patient minimal erythemal dose (MED) values were determined by a sequence of *eight* trial exposures made on normal skin on *the buttocks*, using UV radiation from *a flat array of six 600 mm long fluorescent lamps (Philips TL-01)*, spectrally identical to the lamps used for treatment. A *thin opaque flexible plastic* template with *eight square* apertures *1 cm square* was placed directly in contact with the skin, and each exposure was *in a ratio of √2 (1.41) to the next* in the sequence. Erythema was judged in bright indoor lighting conditions by eye after 24 hours. The MED was taken to be the dose given to the aperture showing just perceptible erythema, with no erythema visible on the adjacent lower dose aperture. The irradiance of the test source was determined at the test distance using a meter calibrated against the lamp type being used.'

Appendix 3

Suggested form of ultraviolet calibration definition in clinical study reports

Terms in *italics* represent variables that should be modified to match the local technique employed. Each term should be identified so that all relevant details are clearly defined.

'The irradiance of the UV cabin(s) used for treatment (*manufacturer and type*) was measured directly by body surface measurements on a protected occupant of average height and build, at *shoulder, waist and knee height*, while the occupant faced each of the *four* main arrays of lamps in sequence. The *maximum/mean* of these readings was taken as the patient's skin irradiance, and used to calculate exposure times (*or was compared with the value indicated by the automatic dosemeter in the cabin control, and a correction factor derived*). The meter used for all measurements was calibrated against the lamp type used, by comparison with a *spectroradiometer measurement* of the irradiance over the wavelength intervals *280–315 nm and 250–400 nm*. The *spectroradiometer* calibration is traceable to national standards.'

Appendix 4

Contact details of medical physics departments in the U.K. and Ireland able to calibrate ultraviolet radiometers

Ms A.Bradshaw, Radiology Department, Mater Misericordiae Hospital, Eccles Street, Dublin 7, Republic of Ireland.
Tel.: +353(0)1 803 2625; e-mail: abradshaw@mater.ie
Dr A.J.Coleman, Medical Physics Department, St Thomas' Hospital, Lambeth Palace Road, London, SE1 7EH, U.K.

Tel.: +44(0)20 7922 8072; fax: +44 (0)20 7922 8279; e-mail: andrew.coleman@gstt.sthames.nhs.uk
Dr J.J.Lloyd, Regional Medical Physics Dept, Royal Victoria Infirmary, Queen Victoria Rd, Newcastle upon Tyne, NE1 4LP, U.K.
Tel.: +44(0)191 282 5173; fax: +44(0)191 233 0351; e-mail: Jim. Lloyd@nuth.northy.nhs.uk
Dr C.J.Martin, Dept of Health Physics, Western Infirmary, Dumbarton Road, Glasgow G11 6NT, U.K.
Tel.: +44(0)141 211 2951; fax: +44(0)141 211 1772; e-mail: colin.martin.wg@northglasgow.scot.nhs.uk
Dr H.Moseley, Photobiology Unit. Level 8, Dermatology Department, Ninewells Hospital, Dundee, DD1 9SY, U.K.
Tel.: +44(0)1382 632240; fax: +44(0)1382 646047; e-mail: h.moseley@dundee.ac.uk
Dr S.D.Pye, Medical Physics Department, Western General Hospital, Edinburgh, EH4 2XU, U.K.
Tel.: +44(0)131 537 2171; fax: +44(0)131 537 1026; e-mail: stephen.pye@ed.ac.uk
Mr D.K.Taylor, Medical Physics Department, Gloucestershire Royal Hospital, Great Western Road, Gloucester, GL1 3NN, U.K.
Tel.: +44(0)1452 394189; fax: +44(0)1452 394490; e-mail: dktaylor@glosrad.co.uk
Mrs A.Walker, Regional Medical Physics Department, Christie Hospital, Wilmslow Road, Withington, Manchester, M20 4BX, U.K.
Tel.: +44 (0)161 446 3544; fax: +44(0)161 446 3545; e-mail: phyaw@dalpha2.cr.man.ac.uk

Appendix 5

American Joint Committee on Cancer classification of strength of recommendation and quality of evidence.
A There is good evidence to support the use of the procedure.
B There is fair evidence to support the use of the procedure.
C There is poor evidence to support the use of the procedure.
D There is fair evidence to support the rejection of the use of the procedure.
E There is good evidence to support the rejection of the use of the procedure
I Evidence obtained from at least one properly designed, randomized control trial.
II-i Evidence obtained from well-designed control trials without randomization.

II-ii Evidence obtained from well-designed cohort or case–control analytical studies, preferably from more than one centre or research group.

II-iii Evidence obtained from multiple time series with or without the intervention. Dramatic results in uncontrolled experiments (e.g. the results of the introduction of penicillin treatment in the 1940s) could also be regarded as this type of evidence.

III Opinions of respected authorities based on clinical experience, descriptive studies or reports of expert committees.

IV Evidence inadequate owing to problems of methodology (e.g. sample size, or length or comprehensiveness of follow-up, or conflicts in evidence).

http://bad.org.uk/Portals/_Bad/Guidelines/Clinical
%20Guidelines/UV%20Radiation%20Therapy.pdf

Comment

The ultraviolet radiation guidance was a report from a workshop rather than the usual BAD method of preparing guidelines [1]. Since then equipment and techniques for dosimetry have improved and become more sophisticated [2, 3]. Accurate dosimetry is very important, as with patient litigation increasing, UV burns following light therapy are an important clinical governance risk for dermatology departments. Unfortunately, the accuracy of meters to measure NB-UVB output showed unacceptable variability the UK [4]. However, meter readings for photopatch testing lamps in 10 departments throughout Europe showed acceptable interdepartmental variation [5].

References

1 Taylor DK, Anstey AV, Coleman AJ, *et al.* Guidelines for dosimetry and calibration in ultraviolet radiation therapy: a report of a British Photodermatology Group workshop. *Brit J Dermatol* 2002; 146: 755–63.

2 Allan W, Diffey BL. A device for minimizing the risk of overexposure of patients undergoing phototherapy. *Photodermatol Photoimmunol Photomed* 2002; 18: 199–200.

3 Otman SG, Edwards C, Gambles B, Anstey AV. Validation of a semiautomated method of minimal erythema dose testing for narrowband ultraviolet B phototherapy. *Br J Dermatol* 2006; 155: 416–21.

4 Lloyd JJ. Variation in calibration of hand-held ultraviolet (UV) meters for psoralen plus UVA and narrowband UVB phototherapy. *Brit J Dermatol* 2004; 150: 1162–6.

5 Moseley H. Ultraviolet A dosimetry in photopatch test centres in Europe. *J Eur Acad Dermatol Venereol* 2005; 19: 187–90.

Additional professional resources

Diffey BL. Sources and measurement of ultraviolet radiation. *Methods* 2002; 28: 4–13.

Amatiello H, Martin CJ. Ultraviolet phototherapy: review of options for cabin dosimetry and operation. *Phys Med Biol* 2006; 51: 299–309.

Guidelines for topical PUVA: a report of a workshop of the British Photodermatology Group

S.M.HALPERN, A.V.ANSTEY,* R.S.DAWE,† B.L.DIFFEY,‡ P.M.FARR,§ J.FERGUSON,¶
J.L.M.HAWK,** S.IBBOTSON,§ J.M.McGREGOR,** G.M.MURPHY,†† S.E.THOMAS,‡‡
AND L.E.RHODES

Dermatology Unit, University Clinical Departments, University of Liverpool, Liverpool L69 3GA, U.K.
*Department of Dermatology, Royal Gwent Hospital, Newport
†Department of Dermatology, Glasgow Western Infirmary, Glasgow
‡Regional Medical Physics Department, Newcastle General Hospital, Newcastle upon Tyne
§Department of Dermatology, Royal Victoria Infirmary, Newcastle upon Tyne
¶Photobiology Unit, Department of Dermatology, Ninewells Hospital, Dundee
**Department of Photobiology, St Thomas' Hospital, London
††Department of Dermatology, Beaumont Hospital, Dublin
‡‡Dermatology Department, Barnsley General Hospital, Barnsley

Accepted for publication 20 August 1999

Summary

Psoralen photochemotherapy [psoralen ultraviolet A (PUVA)] plays an important part in dermatological therapeutics, being an effective and generally safe treatment for psoriasis and other dermatoses. In order to maintain optimal efficacy and safety, guidelines concerning best practice should be available to operators and supervisors. The British Photodermatology Group (BPG) have previously published recommendations on PUVA, including UVA dosimetry and calibration, patient pretreatment assessment, indications and contraindications, and the management of adverse reactions.[1] While most current knowledge relates to oral PUVA, the use of topical PUVA regimens is also popular and presents a number of questions peculiar to this modality, including the choice of psoralen, formulation, method of application, optimal timing of treatment, UVA regimens and relative benefits or risks as compared with oral PUVA. Bath PUVA, i.e. generalized immersion, is the most frequently used modality of topical treatment, practised by about 100 centres in the U.K., while other topical preparations tend to be used for localized diseases such as those affecting the hands and feet. This paper is the product of a recent workshop of the BPG and includes guidelines for bath, local immersion and other topical PUVA. These recommendations are based, where possible, on the results of controlled studies, or otherwise on the consensus view on current practice.

Key words: photochemotherapy, psoralens, PUVA, therapy

Pretreatment assessment

Recommendations concerning pretreatment assessment and contraindications for topical psoralen photochemotherapy [psoralen ultraviolet A (PUVA)] are largely the same as those published for oral PUVA.[1] However, topical PUVA is preferable to oral PUVA in the following circumstances.

1 In patients with hepatic dysfunction.

2 In patients with gastrointestinal disturbance and where absorption is uncertain, e.g. after ileostomy.

3 In patients with cataracts.

4 Where compliance with eye protection may be poor.

5 To permit shorter irradiation times (particularly in black patients, where very high UVA doses are otherwise needed, and in claustrophobic individuals and children).

6 Where psoralen–drug interactions are anticipated, e.g. with warfarin.

Correspondence: Dr L.E.Rhodes. E-mail: lerhod@liv.ac.uk

Table 1. (a) Generalized conditions treated with topical psoralen ultraviolet A (PUVA)[a]

Generalized dermatoses	Topical PUVA	Study methodology	No. of patients
Atopic dermatitis	8-MOP ointment	Case series[41]	114
Lichen planus	TMP bath/ointment	Case series[12]	75
	TMP bath	Case series[13]	19
	8-MOP bath	Case series[14]	4
	8-MOP bath	Retrospective case comparison[15]	13
Systemic sclerosis and generalized morphoea	8-MOP bath	Case series[16]	17
	8-MOP topical lotion	Case report[39]	1
	8-MOP bath	Case series[17]	4
Urticaria pigmentosa	8-MOP bath	Case series[18]	4
	TMP bath	Case series[13]	5
Mycosis fungoides, Sézary syndrome and parapsoriasis	TMP bath	Case series[19]	19
	8-MOP topical	Case series, within-subject control[40]	4
Vitiligo	8-MOP paint/cream	Review[38]	(review)
	8-MOP lotion/cream	Randomized comparison[37]	73
Polymorphic light eruption	TMP bath	Case series[20]	13
Nodular prurigo	TMP bath	Case series[22]	15
	TMP bath/ointment	Case series[12]	63
Prurigo simplex subacuta	8-MOP bath	Case series[21]	10
Uraemic pruritus	8-MOP ointment	Case series[42]	13
Aquagenic pruritus	8-MOP oral and bath	Case report[24]	1
	Bath	Case report[23]	1
Lymphomatoid papulosis	Bath	Case report[25]	1

[a] See text for chronic plaque psoriasis.

(b) Hand and foot dermatoses treated with topical PUVA

Hand and foot dermatoses	Topical PUVA	Study methodology	No. of patients
Hyperkeratotic eczema	8-MOP paint	Randomized double-blind comparison[28]	21
	8-MOP paint	Case series[27]	14
	Psoralen aqueous gel	Case series[31]	2
	8-MOP emulsion	Retrospective case comparison[26]	2
	8-MOP cream	Case series[29]	10
Dyshidrotic eczema	8-MOP paint	Case series[27]	14
Hyperkeratotic psoriasis	Psoralen aqueous gel	Case series[31]	7
	8-MOP ointment/lotion	Case series[30]	14
	8-MOP emulsion	Retrospective case comparison[26]	14
Palmoplantar pustulosis	8-MOP emulsion	Prospective uncontrolled (for topical psoralen)[33]	15
	8-MOP emulsion	Randomized double-blind placebo-controlled[34]	27
	8-MOP emulsion	Retrospective case comparison[26]	9
	8-MOP ointment	Case series[32]	5

TMP, trimethylpsoralen; 8-MOP, 8-methoxypsoralen.

Indications for generalized immersion bath psoralen ultraviolet A

Psoriasis

A variety of psoralen concentrations and treatment regimens have been used for generalized plaque psoriasis. Studies of 8-methoxypsoralen (8-MOP) bath PUVA with concentrations ranging from 0·5 to 4·6 mg/L and treatments given two to four times weekly, report clearance in 60–90% of patients (mean 16–21 treatments) and total UVA dose of 25–27 J/cm[2].[2–4] Treatment with 0·33 mg/L trimethylpsoralen

(TMP) bath PUVA, two to seven times weekly, resulted in a good or excellent response in 92% of patients (mean 18 treatments) and total UVA dose of about 20 J/cm[2],[5] while another study with a similar TMP regimen found good or excellent results in 67% of 51 treatment courses.[6] The use of 5-MOP bath PUVA is little reported; however, a non-randomized study of 8-MOP and 5-MOP bath PUVA in a small number of patients showed that, at the same concentration (0·0003%), there was no significant difference in efficacy, but 5-MOP appeared more phototoxic and pigmentogenic.[7] Of four comparative studies of oral and bath PUVA (one TMP, three 8-MOP),[8–11] only one is a prospective randomized trial.[10] All suggested a similar response rate, with clearance being achieved with the same number of treatments. The total UVA dose was three to six times lower with bath PUVA, but as discussed later, this does not necessarily imply reduced carcinogenicity.

Hence, bath PUVA is clearly a useful treatment for chronic plaque psoriasis, and appears equally effective to oral PUVA. In keeping with oral PUVA, however, it should be reserved for second-line therapy.[1] As the above studies have not been designed to examine the most effective protocols our recommendations are based on the consensus current practice of British Photodermatology Group (BPG) members (see later section).

Other disorders

There is a paucity of evidence concerning the efficacy of bath PUVA in other dermatoses, although there are reports (Table 1a) of its value in lichen planus,[12–15] systemic sclerosis and generalized morphoea,[16,17] urticaria pigmentosa,[13,18] mycosis fungoides,[19] polymorphic light eruption,[20] prurigo simplex subacuta,[21] nodular prurigo,[12,22] aquagenic pruritus,[23,24] and lymphomatoid papulosis.[25]

In the absence of controlled studies to examine the efficacy of bath PUVA in generalized disorders other than chronic plaque psoriasis, we suggest that a common sense approach is to try a course of bath PUVA in the above conditions if other measures have failed and oral PUVA is felt less appropriate.

Indications for topical hand and foot psoralen ultraviolet A

Topical PUVA has been extensively used and appears of value in the treatment of chronic hand and foot dermatoses, namely hyperkeratotic and dyshidrotic eczema, and hyperkeratotic and palmoplantar pustular psoriasis (PPP) (Table 1b).[26–34] However, randomized comparative studies of the efficacy of oral and topical PUVA are scarce. A retrospective review of 15 patients treated with oral 8-MOP and 25 with local immersion 8-MOP for chronic hand and foot dermatoses found the two modalities to be equally effective.[26] Using 8-MOP local immersion (1 mg/L), 93% (13 of 14) of patients with dyshidrotic eczema and 86% (12 of 14) of patients with hyperkeratotic eczema cleared or showed considerable improvement;[27] both the dyshidrotic and hyperkeratotic forms required a similar mean number of treatments (12 and 15) and total UVA dose (21 and 28 J/cm^2) for clearance.

Reports of the effect of PUVA in PPP are conflicting. In uncontrolled studies of topical 8-MOP PUVA, clearance has varied from 30% (three to 10) with local immersion or 0·1% ointment to 87% (13 of 15) with 0·15% emulsion.[32,33] In the latter study, similar response rates were found with topical and oral PUVA but maintenance treatment was noted to be required to prevent early relapse.[33] The clearance rate for oral 8-MOP PUVA in PPP has been reported as 86% (31 of 36) for palmar but only 15% (5 of 34) for plantar involvement.[35] However, a double-blind, placebo-controlled study of topical PUVA (0·75% 8-MOP emulsion, $n = 27$) for PPP, found similar improvements in both the treated and untreated groups.[34] In contrast to the findings in generalized plaque psoriasis, for palmar psoriasis local immersion with 5-MOP may be more effective than 8-MOP, when used in similar concentrations.[7] Moreover, in a comparative trial of oral and topical PUVA with etretinate, the etretinate was noted to be significantly more effective than either modality of PUVA.[36] Therefore, although local PUVA may be beneficial in other chronic hand and foot dermatoses, the case for recommending it in PPP is less convincing.

Indications for other forms of topical psoralen ultraviolet A

There are a few reported studies of the use of other topical psoralen preparations such as paints, ointments and lotions (Table 1a), these having been applied principally in chronic hand and foot dermatoses (see previous section), but also sometimes used for the treatment of other sites. Disorders treated include vitiligo,[37,38] morphoea,[39] mycosis fungoides,[40] atopic dermatitis[41] and uraemic pruritis.[42] Various products, concentrations and protocols are employed, and very little is known about their optimal use. Burning and patchy pigmentation can be a problem,[43] and the inadvertent spread of preparations on to unaffected skin can occur. Thus while they may provide a practical alternative to immersion psoralen for the treatment of localized disease, their use clearly demands greater medical supervision.

Use of adjunctive treatment

It is anticipated that adjunctive treatments of benefit in oral PUVA might also increase the efficacy of bath PUVA, but currently no controlled trials of sufficient power have been performed. However, six studies report the combination of topical PUVA regimens with oral retinoids (re-PUVA) to be beneficial in psoriasis, often with more rapid clearance and reduced total UVA dose.[44–49] Re-PUVA with either etretinate or acitretin appeared equally effective, and no differences were seen in relapse rates between topical 8-MOP alone or re-PUVA.[46,47] There are also isolated reports of the use of topical PUVA with anthralin,[50] and with tacalcitol,[51] and a single case report showing improvement of chronic actinic dermatitis with combined cyclosporin and bath PUVA therapy.[52]

Adverse effects

Skin phototoxicity

Comparative studies with oral 8-MOP PUVA have shown a far greater incidence of erythema or burning than with TMP baths[8] (40% vs. 16%) but roughly similar rates with bath 8-MOP.[9–11] In the past, difficulties with TMP solubility have led to unusual patterns of phototoxic burning due to the uneven distribution in the bath water.[53] It has also been stated that erythema is more protracted with bath than oral PUVA, lasting perhaps for 1 week even at threshold level.[54,55] Furthermore, increased sensitivity is reported to occur at about the fourth day of treatment, with the minimal phototoxic dose (MPD) decreasing by about 50%;[9,56,57] this may partly relate to the simple build-up of subclinical erythemal reactions due to the multiple PUVA treatments given per week in some studies. Additionally, it has been noted that a prolonged susceptibility to photosensitization can occur for up to 72 h after treatment (personal observation, J.Ferguson, Ninewells Hospital, Dundee, U.K.) despite the clearance of free drug from the skin.[58] A possible explanation for this might be that following the initial irradiation, psoralen DNA monoadducts occur which persist far longer in the skin than free psoralen, and with subsequent irradiation result in increased photosensitivity due to conversion to bifunctional adducts.[59] This is theoretical, however, and needs further study, and

until more information is available, it is recommended that photoprotective measures (i.e. adequate clothing, no sunbathing) are taken by patients both during the course and for up to a week after the course is completed.

Other acute effects

Pruritus appears to be equally common following oral and bath PUVA, occurring in 10–40% of patients, but bath PUVA has the advantage that gastrointestinal symptoms such as nausea are avoided. Although rare, contact dermatitis and photocontact dermatitis have been reported with TMP and 8-MOP baths.[5,60]

Eye phototoxicity

The current practice in the majority of units in the U.K. is not to recommend eye protection following bath PUVA. There is no published evidence of an increased incidence of cataract development in humans following oral or bath PUVA, and we can therefore only make an indirect judgement extrapolated from comparative information on plasma levels following oral and bath PUVA (Table 2). Both TMP and 8-MOP may be detected in plasma to variable degrees after topical administration,[6,61–69] but the concentrations of 8-MOP are generally very much lower than after oral dosing.[64,65] However, psoralen concentrations can be high with the application of paint/emulsion formulations to large areas, and comparable plasma levels with those with oral PUVA have been recorded for total body treatment with 0·15% 8-MOP emulsion;[66] on the other hand, such levels were found to be undetectable after 0·1% methoxsalen lotion to plaques covering less than 2% total surface area or to palmoplantar skin.[67,68] In contrast, TMP is poorly absorbed when given orally which explains why oral/bath concentrations are similar for this drug.[6,62,63,70] It has also been shown that psoriasis disease severity may influence psoralen absorption with greater plasma levels detected in patients with higher psoriasis area and severity index scores.[69] We therefore recommend that protective

Table 2. Comparison of plasma levels of 8-methoxypsoralen (8-MOP) and trimethylpsoralen (TMP) following oral and topical administration

No. of patients	Oral psoralen	Peak plasma levels (ng/mL)	Bath psoralen	Peak plasma levels (ng/mL)
4 oral, 8 bath[64]	8-MOP 0·5 mg/kg	108	8-MOP 1·87 mg/L	4·8
7 oral, 13 bath[65]	8-MOP 0·5 mg/kg	< 10–360	8-MOP 2·6 mg/L	< 10
21 oral, 5 bath[62]	TMP 30–40 mg	1·7–5·6	TMP 2·5 mg/L	2·3–15
11 oral[61]	TMP 30 mg	140–800	—	
11 oral, 10 bath[6]	TMP 0·6 mg/kg	0·27–12·5	TMP 0·33 mg/L	0·025–9·0
2 oral, 6 bath[63]	TMP 40 mg	All less than sensitivity of method	TMP 0·33 mg/L	2·5

spectacles are advised on the day of treatment for patients with very extensive disease (i.e. > 30% surface area), in children, and in individuals with severe atopic eczema due to their increased lifetime risk.

Skin cancer

The risk of non-melanoma skin cancer (NMSC) is now recognized following multiple treatments with oral PUVA, with an 11–13-fold relative risk of squamous cell carcinoma (SCC) and 3·7-fold relative risk of basal cell carcinoma (BCC) after more than 260 treatments.[71] No equivalent data exist for topical PUVA and there is currently insufficient evidence to conclude that this treatment is any safer.

In vitro work confirms the mutagenicity of TMP, 8-MOP and 5-MOP plus UVA, and in mice a dose relationship exists for SCC with both topical 8-MOP and 5-MOP plus UVA.[72] A melanocytic tumour has also been reported in one series of mice treated with topical PUVA.[73] Currently, there is insufficient evidence to reach a conclusion on the relative risk of topical and oral PUVA. In humans, studies to date have been limited by sample size and length of follow-up, with insufficient power to examine the long-term risk of NMSC associated with the use of topical PUVA.[74,75] It is generally held that the carcinogenic risk reflects the number of phototoxic episodes (i.e. the number of psoralen plus UVA treatments), rather than either the total UVA dose or the route of psoralen delivery. It is also likely that cancer risk is related to treatment efficacy; thus the lower cumulative UVA dose required for clearance with bath PUVA should not be interpreted as implying a lower carcinogenic risk, particularly as higher psoralen concentrations may be present in the skin thus making the overall effect of bath PUVA the same as for oral PUVA. While no excess risk of skin cancer has yet been reported in association with bath PUVA, keratoses and lentigines are common[46] and until there is good evidence to the contrary, it should probably be assumed that, for disease clearance, bath PUVA is as carcinogenic as oral PUVA. It is therefore recommended, as for oral PUVA, to keep bath PUVA treatments to a minimum.

Protocols for topical psoralen ultraviolet A

Drug protocols

It is evident from the preceding sections that many questions remain unanswered concerning the optimal protocols for topical PUVA. In the absence of studies to

address these issues, we recommend that the consensus current practice may be used for guidance. Most U.K. units use bath 8-MOP at a concentration of 2·6 mg/L (up to 3·7 mg/L), while the more phototoxic TMP is used at a concentration of 0·33 mg/L. A 15-min psoralen bath, given at a comfortably warm temperature, is then followed by immediate exposure to UVA (Appendix 2).

Some support for the above protocol is provided by diffusion theory and experimental permeability results. The lag time before a diffusing substance appears in appreciable quantity in the viable epidermis is a function of stratum corneum thickness and the diffusion coefficient. In excised normal skin *in vitro* the lag time for 8-MOP in aqueous solution at 32 °C for a stratum corneum thickness of 10 μm is 4 min, for 20 μm 15 min, and for 30 μm it would rise to 33 min.[76] However, diffusion will be influenced by factors such as vehicle characteristics[77] or the presence of emollients on the surface of the skin. Additionally, abnormalities of the stratum corneum as in psoriasis may lead to an increased permeability to psoralens when compared with unaffected skin. Further, while *in vitro* the penetration of normal epidermis by 8-MOP continues to rise in the 15–20 min after a 15-min bath,[76] MPDs *in vivo* appear to be similar for irradiation times from 0 to 20 min after bathing, prior to falling off significantly.[78–81] Using a 1% 8-MOP lotion the response to non-interval or 2 h interval PUVA on symmetrical plaques was found to be similar but with an increased risk of burning with delayed treatment.[82] Generally, the current practice of irradiating immediately after bathing therefore appears consistent with theory. In contrast, the lag time in palmoplantar skin is increased to 30–40 min,[83] implying that immediate irradiation of this site is inappropriate.

As differences in water temperature can alter the absorption kinetics of psoralens and thereby the MPD,[84,85] bath temperature should remain constant from treatment to treatment in order to reduce the risk of burning or undertreatment. A temperature of 37 °C appears optimal[85] and is comfortable for the patient. While a 15-min bathing time is generally given, it has been noted (personal observation, S.Thomas, Barnsley Hospital, U.K.) that there is no apparent loss in efficacy if the immersion time is reduced to 5 min. However, it is recommended that the 15-min bathing time is retained until further evidence is available.

In local immersion hand and foot PUVA, 8-MOP is generally used at a concentration of 3 mg/L (1·2% 8-MOP, 0·5 mL/2 L water) for a 15-min soak, and from the above evidence we now recommend that a delay of at least 30 min is allowed before irradiation (Appendix 3). Preferences in preparations for the treatment of local disease vary widely depending on individual experience (Appendix 4), and where there are problems with 8-MOP emulsion, paint or gel formulations for hand and foot dermatoses, it is appropriate to change to the standard local immersion regimen.

UVA protocols

In PUVA generally, erythema is the limiting factor with regard to the UVA dose that can be given at each treatment, and therefore basic information on the MPD, dose–response characteristics and time-course is necessary to devise an efficient treatment regimen. A number of additional variables may affect the erythemal response in bath PUVA, including the type and formulation of psoralen, skin penetration, variation with body site, duration of bath and timing of irradiation. This may explain why the MPDs reported for bath 8-MOP[9,55,86–88] and TMP[86,89] show large variations, and why erythema is more problematic during courses of bath than oral PUVA, at least for TMP.[8] Comparative studies of bath TMP and 8-MOP PUVA confirm that in equivalent concentrations, TMP is up to 30 times more phototoxic.[54,86] Studies of bath 8-MOP PUVA in chronic plaque psoriasis usually report initial UVA doses of between $0 \cdot 2$ and $0 \cdot 5$ J/cm^2, and while some studies use fixed dose increments, others report increments of 20–50% of the preceding dose, which are made every one to three visits.

In the absence of controlled trials to address optimal UVA-irradiation protocols for topical PUVA, the BPG makes recommendations based on the practice of its members (Appendices 2–4). In addition, in some areas it has been assumed that the same principles apply to bath PUVA as to oral PUVA. It is recommended first, that the initial UVA dose is based on an MPD test wherever possible, to avoid either painful erythema or, conversely, under-treatment. The determination of individual responses leads to a reduction in cumulative UVA dose and number of treatments in oral PUVA, and it is assumed that this will also occur in bath PUVA. The MPD test, defined as the lowest dose of UVA causing a perceptible erythema, should be performed on unexposed skin, and it is vital that the test site is fully immersed in psoralen prior to irradiation. Secondly, it is recommended that the initial UVA dose

should be 40–50% of the MPD, reflecting the greater tendency to burn compared with oral PUVA, where the initial dose is usually 70% of the MPD.[1] It is vital when transferring a patient from oral to bath PUVA to repeat the MPD test, in view of the generally lower UVA doses required. Thirdly, dose increments of 20–40% are recommended, with an increase every treatment. In vitiligo, however, it is appropriate to commence at a lower UVA dose of $0 \cdot 1$ J/cm^2, and increase at fixed increments of $0 \cdot 1$ J/cm^2, while higher UVA doses are recommended to treat the thicker skin of palmoplantar disorders.

Practical and financial considerations

Differences in the use of oral and topical PUVA necessitate the consideration of a number of practical issues. First, bathing facilities must be available and close nurse supervision is required throughout. The additional time taken for bathing may also reduce the throughput of patients, although this is somewhat countered by the reduction in irradiation times. The much lower exposure time required with bath PUVA can itself be problematic as there is a greater chance of error leading to accidental overtreatment, particularly if high-output machines are employed. Post-treatment bathing is unnecessary as cutaneous absorption and binding dynamics suggests that no free psoralen will remain on the skin surface, but of course exposed skin such as on the hands should still be protected from strong sunlight after local treatment.

A cost-effectiveness analysis of data collected across four centres during a Scottish phototherapy and PUVA audit in 1997 (personal communication, R.Dawe, Glasgow Western Infirmary, U.K.) revealed that courses of both bath and other topical PUVA were consistently more expensive than oral PUVA. This related predominantly to the increased nursing time required, although the greater cost of topical preparations was also a contributing factor.

Conclusions

Currently, oral PUVA is better established and studied than topical PUVA, and many questions remain concerning the efficacy, safety and optimal protocols of the latter. Thus, the carcinogenic risks of topical PUVA are unknown, and there is presently little firm evidence to suggest that the risk will be any lower than that of oral PUVA. However, advantages include shorter irradiation times and a lack of gastrointestinal and systemic side-effects, and access of phototherapy units to facilities for both modalities is therefore desirable in order to permit a wider range of patients to be treated. Finally, as for oral PUVA, it is important that PUVA units have well trained staff to perform treatments, who should work closely with the dermatologist responsible for the prescribing and supervision of treatment.

References

1 British Photodermatology Group. Guidelines for PUVA. *Br J Dermatol* 1994; **130**: 246–55.

2 Collins P, Rogers S. Bath-water delivery of 8-methoxypsoralen therapy psoriasis. *Clin Exp Dermatol* 1991; **16**: 165–7.

3 Gomez MI, Perez B, Harto A *et al.* 8-MOP bath PUVA in the treatment of psoriasis: clinical results in 42 patients. *J Dermatol Treat* 1996; **7**: 11–12.

4 Streit V, Wiedow O, Christophers E. Treatment of psoriasis with polyethylene sheet bath PUVA. *J Am Acad Dermatol* 1996; **35**: 208–10.

5 Hannuksela M, Karvonen J. Trioxsalen bath plus UVA effective and safe in the treatment of psoriasis. *Br J Dermatol* 1978; **99**: 703–7.

6 Salo OP, Lassus A, Taskinen J. Trioxsalen bath plus UVA treatment of psoriasis. *Acta Derm Venereol (Stockh)* 1981; **61**: 551–4.

7 Calzavara-Pinton PG, Zane C, Carlino A, De Panfilis G. Bath-5-methoxypsoralen-UVA therapy for psoriasis. *J Am Acad Dermatol* 1997; **36**: 945–9.

8 Turjanmaa K, Salo H, Reunala T. Comparison of trioxsalen bath and oral methoxsalen PUVA in psoriasis. *Acta Derm Venereol (Stockh)* 1985; **65**: 86–8.

9 Lowe NJ, Weingarten D, Bourget T, Moy LS. PUVA therapy for psoriasis: comparison of oral and bath-water delivery of 8-methoxypsoralen. *J Am Acad Dermatol* 1986; **14**: 754–60.

10 Collins P, Rogers S. Bath-water compared with oral delivery of 8-methoxypsoralen PUVA therapy for chronic plaque psoriasis. *Br J Dermatol* 1992; **127**: 392–5.

11 Calzavara-Pinton PG, Ortel B, Honigsmann H *et al.* Safety and effectiveness of an aggressive and individualized bath-PUVA regimen in the treatment of psoriasis. *Dermatology* 1994; **189**: 256–9.

12 Karvonen J, Hannuksela M. Long term results of topical trioxsalen PUVA in lichen planus and nodular prurigo. *Acta Derm Venereol (Suppl.) (Stockh)* 1985; **120**: 53–5.

13 Vaatainen N, Hannuksela M, Karvonen J. Trioxsalen baths plus UV-A in the treatment of lichen planus and urticaria pigmentosa. *Clin Exp Dermatol* 1981; **6**: 133–8.

14 Kerscher M, Volkenandt M, Lehmann P *et al.* PUVA-bath photochemotherapy of lichen planus. *Arch Dermatol* 1995; **131**: 1210–1.

15 Helander I, Jansen CT, Meurman L. Long-term efficacy of PUVA treatment in lichen planus: comparison of oral and external methoxsalen regimens. *Photodermatology* 1987; **4**: 265–8.

16 Kerscher M, Meurer M, Sander C *et al.* PUVA bath photochemotherapy for localized scleroderma. *Arch Dermatol* 1996; **132**: 1280–2.

17 Kanekura T, Fukumara S, Matsushita S *et al.* Successful treatment of scleroderma with PUVA therapy. *J Dermatol* 1996; **23**: 455–9.

18 Godt O, Proksh E, Streit V, Christophers E. Short and long-term effectiveness of oral and bath PUVA therapy in urticaria pigmentosa and systemic mastocytosis. *Dermatology* 1997; **195**: 35–9.

19 Fischer T, Skough M. Treatment of parapsoriasis en plaque, mycosis fungoides and Sézary's syndrome with trioxsalen baths followed by ultraviolet light. *Acta Derm Venereol (Stockh)* 1979; **59**: 171–3.

20 Jansen CT, Karvonen J, Malmiharju T. PUVA therapy for polymorphous light eruptions: comparison of systemic methoxsalen and topical trioxsalen regimens and evaluation of local protective mechanisms. *Acta Derm Venereol (Stockh)* 1982; **62**: 317–20.

21 Streit V, Thiede R, Wiedow O, Christophers E. Foil bath PUVA in the treatment of prurigo simplex subacuta. *Acta Derm Venereol (Stockh)* 1996; **76**: 319–20.

22 Vaatainen N, Hannuksela M, Karvonen J. Local photochemotherapy in nodular prurigo. *Acta Derm Venereol (Stockh)* 1979; **59**: 544–7.

23 Jahn S, von Kobyletzki G, Behrens S *et al.* Puva bath photochemotherapy successful in aquagenic pruritus. (Letter.) *H G Z Hautkr* 1997; **72**: 821–4.

24 Smith RA, Ross JS, Staughton RCD. Bath PUVA as a treatment for aquagenic pruritus. (Letter.) *Br J Dermatol* 1994; **131**: 584.

25 Volkenandt M, Kerscher M, Sander C et al. PUVA bath photochemotherapy resulting in rapid clearance of lymphomatoid papulosis in a child. *Arch Dermatol* 1995; **131**: 1094.

26 Hawk JLM, Le Grice P. The efficacy of localized PUVA therapy for chronic hand and foot dermatoses. *Clin Exp Dermatol* 1994; **19**: 479–82.

27 Schempp CM, Muller H, Czech W *et al.* Treatment of chronic palmoplantar eczema with local bath-PUVA therapy. *J Am Acad Dermatol* 1997; **36**: 733–7.

28 Sheehan-Dare RA, Goodfield MJ, Rowell NR. Topical psoralen photochemotherapy (PUVA) and superficial radiotherapy in the treatment of chronic hand eczema. *Br J Dermatol* 1989; **121**: 65–9.

29 Stege H, Berneburg M, Ruzicka T, Krutmann J. Creme-PUVA-Photochemotherapie. *Hautarzt* 1997; **48**: 89–93.

30 Abel EA, Goldberg LH, Farber EM. Treatment of palmoplantar psoriasis with topical methoxsalen plus long-wave ultraviolet light. *Arch Dermatol* 1980; **116**: 1257–61.

31 De Rie MA, Eendenburg JP, Versnick AC *et al.* A new psoralen-containing gel for topical PUVA therapy: development and treatment results in patients with palmoplantar and plaque-type psoriasis, and hyperkeratotic eczema. *Br J Dermatol* 1995; **132**: 964–9.

32 Jansen CT, Malmiharju T. Inefficacy of topical methoxalen plus UVA for palmoplantar pustulosis. *Acta Derm Venereol (Stockh)* 1981; **61**: 354–6.

33 Murray D, Corbett MF, Warin AP. A controlled trial of photochemotherapy for persistent palmoplantar pustulosis. *Br J Dermatol* 1980; **102**: 659–63.

34 Layton AM, Sheehan-Dare R, Cunliffe WJ. A double-blind, placebo-controlled trial of topical PUVA in persistent palmoplantar pustulosis. *Br J Dermatol* 1991; **124**: 581–4.

35 Agren-Jonsson S, Tegner E. PUVA therapy for palmoplantar pustulosis. *Acta Derm Venereol (Stockh)* 1985; **65**: 531–5.

36 Lassus A, Lauharanta J, Eskelinen A. The effect of etretinate compared with different regimens of PUVA in the treatment of

persistent palmoplantar pustulosis. *Br J Dermatol* 1985; **112**: 455–9.

37 Grimes PE, Minus HR, Chakrabarti SG *et al.* Determination of optimal topical photochemotherapy for vitiligo. *J Am Acad Dermatol* 1982; **7**: 771–8.

38 Halder RM. Topical PUVA therapy for vitiligo. *Dermatol Nurs* 1991; **3**: 178–98.

39 Morita A, Sakakibara S, Sakakibara N *et al.* Successful treatment of systemic sclerosis with topical PUVA. *J Rheumatol* 1995; **22**: 2361–5.

40 Nakamura M, Kobayashi S, Matsura K *et al.* The effects of non-interval PUVA therapy on the plaque stage of mycosis fungoides. *J Dermatol* 1995; **22**: 196–200.

41 Ogawa H, Yoshiike T. Atopic dermatitis: studies of skin permeability and effectiveness of topical PUVA treatment. *Pediatr Dermatol* 1992; **9**: 383–5.

42 Uesugi T, Kumasaka N, Okada Y *et al.* Topical chemotherapy (PUVA) for the relief of uremic pruritus in patients undergoing hemodialysis. *J Dermatol Treat* 1996; **7**: 247–9.

43 Petrozzi JW, Kaidbey KM, Kligmann AM. Topical methoxsalen & blacklight in the treatment of psoriasis. *Arch Dermatol* 1977; **113**: 292–6.

44 Michaelsson G, Noren P, Vahlquist A. Combined therapy with oral retinoid and PUVA baths in severe psoriasis. *Br J Dermatol* 1978; **99**: 221–2.

45 Vaatainen N, Hollmen A, Fraki JE. Trimethylpsoralen bath plus ultraviolet A combined with oral retinoid (etretinate) in the treatment of severe psoriasis. *J Am Acad Dermatol* 1985; **12**: 52–5.

46 Takashima A, Sunohara A, Matsunami E, Mizuno N. Comparison of therapeutic efficacy of topical PUVA, oral etretinate, and combined PUVA and etretinate for the treatment of psoriasis and development of PUVA lentigines and antinuclear antibodies. *J Dermatol* 1988; **15**: 471–9.

47 Lauharanta J, Geiger J-M. A double-blind comparison of acitretin and etretinate in combination with bath PUVA in the treatment of extensive psoriasis. *Br J Dermatol* 1989; **121**: 107–12.

48 Matsunami E, Takashima A, Mizuno N *et al.* Topical PUVA, etretinate, and combined PUVA and etretinate for palmoplantar pustulosis: comparison of therapeutic efficacy and the influences of tonsillar and dental focal infections. *J Dermatol* 1990; **17**: 92–6.

49 Muchenberger S, Schopf E, Simon JC. The combination of oral acitretin and bath PUVA for the treatment of severe psoriasis. *Br J Dermatol* 1997; **137**: 587–9.

50 Willis I, Harris DR. Resistant psoriasis. *Arch Dermatol* 1973; **107**: 358–62.

51 Kiriyama T, Danno K, Uehara M. Combination of topical tacalcitol and PUVA for psoriasis. *J Dermatol Treat* 1997; **8**: 62–4.

52 Marguery MC, Montazeri A, El Sayed F *et al.* Chronic actinic dermatitis: a severe case responding to cyclosporin-bath-PUVA therapy. *J Dermatol Treat* 1997; **8**: 281–3.

53 George SA, Ferguson J. Unusual pattern of phototoxic burning following trimethylpsoralen (TMP) bath photochemotherapy (PUVA). *Br J Dermatol* 1992; **127**: 444–5.

54 Koulu LM, Jansen CT. Skin photosensitizing and Langerhans' cell depleting activity of topical (bath) PUVA therapy: comparison of trimethylpsoralen and 8-methoxypsoralen. *Acta Derm Venereol (Stockh)* 1983; **63**: 137–41.

55 Calzavara-Pinton PG, Ortel B, Carlino AM *et al.* Phototesting and phototoxic side effects in bath PUVA. *J Am Acad Dermatol* 1993; **28**: 657–9.

56 Luftl M, Degitz K, Plewig G, Rocken M. Psoralen bath plus UV-A therapy. *Arch Dermatol* 1997; **133**: 1597–603.

57 Koulu LM, Jansen CT. Skin phototoxicity variations during repeated bath PUVA exposures to 8-methoxypsoralen and trimethylpsoralen. *Clin Exp Dermatol* 1984; **9**: 64–9.

58 Gold RL, Anderson RR, Natoli VD, Gange RW. An action spectrum for photoinduction of prolonged cutaneous photosensitivity by topical 8-MOP. *J Invest Dermatol* 1988; **90**: 818–22.

59 Ortel B, Gange RW. An action spectrum for the elicitation of erythema in skin persistently sensitized by photobound 8-methoxypsoralen. *J Invest Dermatol* 1990; **94**: 781–5.

60 Takashima A, Yamamoto K, Kimura S *et al.* Allergic contact and photocontact dermatitis due to psoralens in patients with psoriasis treated with topical PUVA. *Br J Dermatol* 1991; **124**: 37–42.

61 Chakrabarti SG, Grimes PE, Minus HR *et al.* Determination of trimethylpsoralen in blood, ophthalmic fluids and skin. *J Invest Dermatol* 1982; **79**: 374–7.

62 Ros A-M, Wennersten G, Wallin I, Ehrsson H. Concentration of trimethylpsoralen in blood and skin after oral administration. *Photodermatology* 1988; **9**: 121–5.

63 Fischer T, Hartvig P, Bondesson U. Plasma concentrations after bath treatment and oral administration of trioxsalen. *Acta Derm Venereol (Stockh)* 1980; **60**: 177–9.

64 David M, Lowe NJ, Halder RM, Borok M. Serum 8-methoxypsoralen (8-MOP) concentrations after bath water delivery of 8-MOP plus UVA. *J Am Acad Dermatol* 1990; **23**: 931–2.

65 Thomas SE, O'Sullivan J, Balac N. Plasma levels of 8-methoxypsoralen following oral or bath-water treatment. *Br J Dermatol* 1991; **125**: 56–8.

66 Neild VS, Scott LV. Plasma levels of 8-methoxypsoralen in psoriatic patients receiving topical 8-methoxypsoralen. *Br J Dermatol* 1982; **106**: 199–203.

67 Hallman CP, Koo JYM, Omohundro C, Lee J. Plasma levels of 8-methoxypsoralen after topical paint PUVA on nonpalmoplantar psoriatic skin. *J Am Acad Dermatol* 1994; **31**: 273–5.

68 Pham CT, Koo JYM. Plasma levels of 8-methoxypsoralen after topical paint PUVA. *J Am Acad Dermatol* 1993; **28**: 460–6.

69 Gomez MI, Azana JM, Arranz I *et al.* Plasma levels of 8-methoxypsoralen after bath-PUVA for psoriasis: relationship to disease severity. *Br J Dermatol* 1995; **133**: 37–40.

70 de Wolf FA, Thomas TV. Clinical pharmacokinetics of methoxsalen and other psoralens. *Clin Pharmacokinetics* 1986; **11**: 62–75.

71 Stern RS, Lange R. Non-melanoma skin cancer occurring in patients treated with PUVA five to ten years after first treatment. *J Invest Dermatol* 1988; **91**: 120–4.

72 Young AR. Photocarcinogenicity of psoralens used in PUVA treatment: present status in mouse and man. *J Photochem Photobiol* 1990; **6**: 237–47.

73 Alcalay J, Bucana C, Kripke ML. Cutaneous pigmented melanocytic tumour in a mouse treated with psoralen plus ultraviolet A radiation. *Photodermatol Photoimmunol Photomed* 1990; **7**: 28–31.

74 Hannuksela A, Pukkala E, Hannuksela M, Karvonen J. Cancer incidence among Finnish patients with psoriasis with trioxsalen bath PUVA. *J Am Acad Dermatol* 1996; **35**: 685–9.

75 Lindelof B, Sigurgeirsson B, Tegner E *et al.* Comparison of the carcinogenic potential of trioxsalen bath PUVA and oral methoxsalen PUVA. *Arch Dermatol* 1992; **128**: 1341–4.

76 Anigbogu ANC, Williams AC, Barry BW. Permeation characteristics of 8-methoxypsoralen through human skin; relevance to clinical treatment. *J Pharm Pharmacol* 1996; **48**: 357–66.

77 Gazith J, Schalla W, Bauer E, Schaefer H. 8-methoxypsoralen

(8-MOP) in human skin: penetration kinetics. *J Invest Dermatol* 1978; **71**: 126–30.

78 Neumann NJ, Ruzicka T, Lehmann P, Kerscher M. Rapid decrease of phototoxicity after PUVA bath therapy with 8-methoxy-psoralen. (Letter.) *Arch Dermatol* 1996; **132**: 1394.

79 Schempp CM, Schopf E, Simon JC. Phototesting in bath PUVA. marked reduction of 8-methoxypsoralen (8-MOP) activity within one hour after an 8-MOP bath. *Photodermatol Photoimmunol Photomed* 1996; **12**: 100–2.

80 Reuther T, Gruss C, Behrens S *et al.* Time course of 8-methoxy-psoralen-induced skin photosensitization in PUVA-bath photo-chemotherapy. *Photodermatol Photoimmunol Photomed* 1997; **13**: 193–6.

81 Gruss C, Behrens S, Reuther T *et al.* Kinetics of photosensitivity in bath-PUVA photochemotherapy. *J Am Acad Dermatol* 1998; **39**: 443–6.

82 Danno K, Horio T, Ozaki M, Imamura S. Topical 8-methoxy-psoralen photochemotherapy of psoriasis: a clinical study. *Br J Dermatol* 1983; **108**: 519–24.

83 Konya J, Diffey BL, Hindson TC. Time course of activity of topical 8-methoxypsoralen on palmoplantar skin. *Br J Dermatol* 1992; **127**: 654–5.

84 Jansen CT. Water temperature effect in bath-PUVA treatment. *J Am Acad Dermatol* 1988; **19**: 142–3.

85 Gruss C, Von Behrens S, Kobyletzki G *et al.* Effects of water temperature on photosensitization in bath-PUVA therapy with 8-methoxypsoralen. *Photodermatol Photoimmunol Photomed* 1998; **14**: 145–7.

86 Koulu LM, Jansen CT. Antipsoriatic, erythematogenic, and Langerhans cell marker depleting effect of bath-psoralen plus ultraviolet A treatment. *J Am Acad Dermatol* 1988; **18**: 1053–9.

87 Degitz K, Plewig G, Rocken M. Rapid decline in photosensitivity after 8-methoxypsoralen bathwater delivery. *Arch Dermatol* 1996; **132**: 1394–5.

88 Neumann NJ, Kerscher M, Ruzicka T, Lehmann P. Evaluation of PUVA bath phototoxicity. *Acta Derm Venereol (Stockh)* 1997; **77**: 385–7.

89 Rhodes LE, Friedmann PS. A comparison of the erythemal response to PUVA using oral 8-methoxypsoralen (8-MOP) and bath trimethylpsoralen (TMP). *Br J Dermatol* 1992; **127**: 420–1 (Abstr.).

Appendix 1: Psoralen formulations

All psoralens must currently be prescribed on a named patient basis, but the registration of oral 8-MOP is in progress (personal communication: M.Bedford-Stradling, Crawford Pharmaceuticals, U.K.). Topical formulations available from the main U.K. supplier (Crawford Pharmaceuticals, Milton Keynes, U.K.), include 8-MOP bath lotion (1·2%), emulsion (0·15%), paint (0·15%, 1·0%) and gel (0·005%), and TMP bath lotion (0·05%); the latter is also available from Tayside Pharmaceuticals (Dundee, U.K.). Other products which may be purchased from abroad include TMP bath lotion (50 mg/100 mL, Orion Pharmaceuticals Ltd., Espoo, Finland) and 0·75% 8-MOP paint (Promedica, Levallois-Perret, France).

Appendix 2: Protocol for bath (generalized immersion) PUVA

Bath psoralen ultraviolet A with 8-methoxypsoralen

1 Dissolve 30 mL of 1·2% 8-MOP lotion in 140 L water at 37 °C (final concentration 2·6 mg/L).
2 Bathe for 15 min, followed by immediate UVA exposure.
3 Initial UVA dose: either 40% of MPD (preferable) or 0·2–0·5 J/cm^2.
4 UVA increments: increase by 20–40% of initial dose at each treatment.
5 Frequency: twice weekly.

Bath psoralen ultraviolet A with trimethylpsoralen

1 Dissolve 50 mg TMP in 100 mL ethanol.
2 Mix in 150L water at 37 °C (final concentration 0·33 mg/L).
3 Bathe for 15 min, followed by immediate UVA exposure.
4 Initial UVA dose: either 40% of MPD (preferable) or 0·1–0·4 J/cm^2.
5 UVA increments: increase by 0·5 of initial dose at each treatment.
6 Frequency: twice weekly.

Appendix 3: Protocol for hand and foot immersion PUVA

8-methoxypsoralen lotion

1 Mix 0·5 mL of 1·2% 8-MOP lotion in 2 L water (final concentration 3 mg/L).
2 Soak for 15 min, with a delay of 30 min before UVA exposure.
3 Initial UVA dose: 1–2 J/cm^2.
4 UVA increments: 0·5–1 J/cm^2.
5 Frequency: twice weekly.

Trimethylpsoralen lotion

1 Dissolve 5 mg TMP in 10 mL ethanol.
2 Mix into 15 L water.
3 Soak for 15 min, with a delay of 30 min before UVA exposure.
4 Initial UVA dose: 1–2 J/cm^2.
5 UVA increments: 0·5–1 J/cm^2.
6 Frequency: twice weekly.
Note: If dorsa of hands or feet are affected give 50% of dose for palms and soles.

Appendix 4: Protocol for other topical 8-methoxypsoralen PUVA

8-methyoxypsoralen emulsion

1 0·15% (may be diluted 1 : 10 if erythema occurs at lowest UVA dose).
2 Apply 15 min before UVA exposure.
3 Initial UVA dose: either 40% of MPD, or (II) 0·5–1 J/cm^2 (depends on site).
4 UVA increments: 0·5–2 J/cm^2 (depends on site).
5 Frequency: twice weekly.

8-methyoxypsoralen gel

1 0·005% solution in aqueous gel.
2 Apply thin layer over diseased area using gloved hand.
3 Ensure repeated applications are given to same area.
4 Apply 15 min before UVA exposure.
5 Initial UVA dose: either 40% of MPD, or 0·5–1 J/cm^2 (depends on site).
6 UVA increments: 0·5–2 J/cm^2 (depends on site).
7 Frequency: twice weekly.

http://bad.org.uk/Portals/_Bad/Guidelines/Clinical
%20Guidelines/Topical%20PUVA%20Therapy.pdf

Comment

The 2000 topical PUVA guidelines [1] were a consensus derived from a workshop report of the British Photobiology Group. However, there has been a trend in the past 10 years to use more TL-01 narrow band UVB therapy (NB-UVB) and more local topical hand/foot PUVA rather than bath or oral PUVA. This has been driven by the likelihood that NB-UVB is less carcinogenic than PUVA. Early follow-up studies of NB-UVB treated patients would indicate it was less carcinogenic than PUVA [2]. The Dundee group found no significant association between NB-UVB treatment and BCC, SCC or melanoma. There was a small increase in BCCs amongst those also treated with PUVA. These reassuring results did not demonstrate the early increase in skin cancers that was found associated with PUVA treatment. Further long-term follow-up studies are needed to determine the safe maximum life time dose of NB-UVB.

References

1 Halpern SM, Anstey AV, Dawe RS, *et al*. Guidelines for topical PUVA: a report of a workshop of the British photodermatology Group. *Brit J Dermatol* 2000; 142: 22–31.
2 Hearn RMR, Kerr AC, Rahim KF, *et al*. Incidence of skin cancers in 3867 patients treated with narrow-band ultraviolet B phototherapy. *Brit J Dermatol* 2008; 159: 931–5.

Additional professional resources

Stern RS. Psoralen and ultraviolet a light therapy for psoriasis. *N Engl J Med* 2007; 357: 682–90.

BAD patient information leaflet

http://www.bad.org.uk/site/1223/Default.aspx

Other patient resources

http://www.dermnetnz.org/procedures/puva.html
http://www.photonet.scot.nhs.uk/publicportal.htm

NARROWBAND UVB AND PUVA

Additional professional resources and references

Menter A, Korman NJ, Elmets CA, *et al*. Guidelines of care for the management of psoriasis and psoriatic arthritis: Section 5. Guidelines of care for the treatment of psoriasis with phototherapy and photochemotherapy. *J Am Acad Dermatol* 2010; 62:114–35.
Tzaneva S, Kittler H, Holzer G, *et al*. 5-Methoxypsoralen plus ultraviolet (UV) A is superior to medium-dose UVA1 in the treatment of severe atopic dermatitis: a randomized crossover trial. *Brit J Dermatol* 2010; 162: 655–60.
Pasker-de Jong P C, Wielink G, van der Valk P G, van der Wilt G J. Treatment with UV-B for psoriasis and nonmelanoma skin cancer: a systematic review of the literature. *Arch Dermatol* 1999; 135: 834–40.
Meduri N B, Vandergriff T, Rasmussen H, Jacobe H. Phototherapy in the management of atopic dermatitis: a systematic review. *Photodermatol Photoimmunol Photomed* 2007; 23: 106–12 (http://www.ncbi.nlm.nih.gov/sites/entrez?Db=pubmed&Cmd=ShowDetailView&TermToSearch=17598862&ordinalpos=5&itool=EntrezSystem2.PEntrez.Pubmed.Pubmed_ResultsPanel.Pubmed_RVDocSum).
Gambichler T, Breuckmann F, Boms S, *et al*. Narrowband UVB phototherapy in skin conditions beyond psoriasis. *J Am Acad Dermatol* 2005; 52: 660–70.

BAD patient information leaflet

http://www.bad.org.uk/site/1223/Default.aspx

Other patient resources

http://www.dermnetnz.org/procedures/puva.html
http://www.dermnetnz.org/procedures/narrowband-uvb.html
http://www.photonet.scot.nhs.uk/publicportal.htm

Guidelines for topical photodynamic therapy: update

C.A. Morton, K.E. McKenna* and L.E. Rhodes† on behalf of the British Association of Dermatologists Therapy Guidelines and Audit Subcommittee and the British Photodermatology Group

Department of Dermatology, Stirling Royal Infirmary, Stirling FK2 8AU, U.K.

*Department of Dermatology, Belfast City Hospital, Belfast BT9 7AB, U.K.

†Photobiology Unit, Dermatological Sciences, University of Manchester, Salford Royal Foundation Hospital, Manchester M6 8HD, U.K.

Summary

Multicentre randomized controlled studies now demonstrate high efficacy of topical photodynamic therapy (PDT) for actinic keratoses, Bowen's disease (BD) and superficial basal cell carcinoma (BCC), and efficacy in thin nodular BCC, while confirming the superiority of cosmetic outcome over standard therapies. Long-term follow-up studies are also now available, indicating that PDT has recurrence rates equivalent to other standard therapies in BD and superficial BCC, but with lower sustained efficacy than surgery in nodular BCC. In contrast, current evidence does not support the use of topical PDT for squamous cell carcinoma. PDT can reduce the number of new lesions developing in patients at high risk of skin cancer and may have a role as a preventive therapy. Case reports and small series attest to the potential of PDT in a wide range of inflammatory/infective dermatoses, although recent studies indicate insufficient evidence to support its use in psoriasis. There is an accumulating evidence base for the use of PDT in acne, while detailed study of an optimized protocol is still required. In addition to high-quality treatment site cosmesis, several studies observe improvements in aspects of photoageing. Management of treatment-related pain/discomfort is a challenge in a minority of patients, and the modality is otherwise well tolerated. Long-term studies provide reassurance over the safety of repeated use of PDT.

Disclaimer

These guidelines have been prepared for dermatologists on behalf of the British Photodermatology Group and the British Association of Dermatologists and are based on the best data available at the time the report was prepared. Caution should be exercised when interpreting data where there is a limited evidence base; the results of future studies may require alteration of the conclusions or recommendations in this report. It may be necessary or even desirable to depart from the guidelines in the interests of specific patients and special circumstances. Just as adherence to guidelines may not constitute defence against a claim of negligence, so deviation from them should not necessarily be deemed negligent.

Introduction

This article represents a planned regular updating of the original guidelines for the use of topical photodynamic therapy (PDT).[1] Detailed discussion of studies evaluated in the previous paper will not be repeated except where comparison with new evidence is necessary. This may entail a disproportionate weight being given to more recent techniques and studies, but strength of evidence recommendations (see Appendix 1) take into account all available information.

Topical PDT has, to date, been approved by regulatory authorities in 18 countries worldwide, for use in at least one nonmelanoma skin cancer (NMSC) indication. Two photosensitizing agents are licensed, a formulation of 5-aminolaevulinic acid (ALA), Levulan (DUSA Pharmaceuticals, Wilmington, MA, U.S.A.) for actinic keratosis (AK), and an esterified formulation, methyl aminolaevulinate (MAL), Metvix® (Photo-Cure ASA, Oslo, Norway and Galderma, Paris, France) for AK, Bowen's disease (BD), and superficial and nodular basal cell carcinoma (BCC). Although only one formulation of ALA currently has a licence, other preparations have been used in clinical studies reviewed here. Hence, 'Levulan ALA' will be used in this update to denote when the licensed product has been used, and 'ALA' for all other formulations.

Interventional procedure guidance from The National Institute for Health and Clinical Excellence recently concluded that there was evidence of efficacy for topical PDT in AK, BD and BCC, but limited evidence for invasive squamous cell carcinoma (SCC). No major safety concerns were observed for the use of PDT in NMSC.[2]

The past 5 years has seen publication of studies of long-term response rates of topical PDT in NMSC as well as evaluation of its potential as a preventive therapy for cutaneous malignancy. Several noncancer indications have been the focus of intense study, in particular, acne and photorejuvenation. In this update, we review the evidence for the use of topical PDT in all reported dermatological indications and interpret how this modality might best be used in clinical practice, using the same validated scoring system as in the previous guidelines.[1]

Photosensitizing agents

ALA and its methylated ester MAL are prodrugs that are endogenously converted by the haem biosynthetic pathway to protoporphyrin IX (PpIX) and potentially other intermediate photosensitizing porphyrins. These agents are relatively selectively concentrated in the target tissue, possibly related to alterations in surface permeability and tumour porphyrin metabolism.[1] Initial clinical experience of topical PDT was gained through the use of ALA, largely through case series studies. However, following publication of our initial guideline report, intensive study of MAL has led to better characterization of this prodrug and publication of its use in several randomized studies.

As ALA is hydrophilic and the esterified form MAL is more lipophilic, it was anticipated that MAL may penetrate more deeply into lesions. Peng et al.[3] reported that MAL penetrated to a 2-mm depth in BCC, contrasting with more limited penetration with ALA.[4] Other investigators also found highly variable ALA uptake into nodular and infiltrating BCC.[5] However, Ahmadi et al.[6] showed in an in vitro study of human skin biopsies that ALA applied for 4 h penetrated to a depth of at least 2 mm from the lesion surface. Interestingly, using similar protocols, ALA is reported to result in higher PpIX levels than

MAL, but with less selectivity for the diseased compared with healthy tissue, in both AK[7] and inflammatory acne lesions.[8] Two recently reported small studies have attempted to compare the efficacy of MAL-PDT and ALA-PDT in diseased tissue, with application of each prodrug for 3 h.[8,9] Patients with nodular BCC were randomly assigned to either ALA-PDT (n = 22) or MAL-PDT (n = 21) (ALA/MAL 3 h, 600–730 nm, 75 J cm^{-2}, 100 mW cm^{-2}); in each group half the tumours were debulked prior to PDT.[9] On histological analysis after 8 weeks, no difference was found in lesional response. In a split-face comparison of 15 patients with inflammatory acne, no difference was found between ALA-PDT and MAL-PDT (ALA/MAL 3 h, 632 nm, 37 J cm^{-2}, 34 mW cm^{-2}) regarding treatment efficacy, whereas ALA-PDT resulted in more severe adverse effects after treatment.[8] A further randomized double-blind study compared ALA and MAL for the treatment of extensive scalp AK.[10] MAL was applied for 3 h, but ALA for 5 h (580–740 nm, 50 J cm^{-2}, 50 mW cm^{-2}). No significant difference in mean lesion count reduction was observed 1 month after treatment, although pain was more intense on the ALA side.

Recommendation: Topical application of the prodrugs ALA and MAL is effective in cutaneous PDT (*Strength of recommendation A, Quality of evidence I*).

Light sources and dosimetry

A range of light sources, reviewed in the 2002 guideline report, remains in use for topical PDT including lasers, filtered xenon arc and metal halide lamps, fluorescent lamps and light-emitting diodes (LEDs). Nonlaser light sources are popular in topical PDT, possessing the advantages over lasers of being inexpensive, stable, easy to operate, requiring little maintenance, and providing wide area illumination fields. Retrospective comparison of laser and filtered broadband sources suggests equivalent efficacy in topical PDT.[11] In the last few years, LED sources have shown considerable development, with improvements in design making these relatively inexpensive sources convenient for wide area irradiation and popular for patient use, e.g. the Aktilite 16 and 128 (Galderma) and the Omnilux (Photo Therapeutics Ltd, Altrincham, U.K.). These LED sources match the 630/635-nm activation peak of PpIX while excluding the extraneous wavelengths present in broadband sources, thus permitting shorter irradiation times. Biophysical calculations indicate that an LED source with peak emission of 631 ± 2 nm may have a deeper PDT action in tissue than a filtered halogen lamp of 560–740 nm emission, and hence LED may be more effective in treating the deeper parts of tumours.[12]

PpIX has its largest absorption peak in the blue region at 410 nm (Soret band), with smaller absorption peaks at 505, 540, 580 and 630 nm. Most light sources for PDT seek to utilize the 630-nm absorption peak in the red region, in order to improve tissue penetration. However, a blue fluorescent lamp (peak emission 417 nm) is routinely used in Levulan ALA-PDT of AK in the U.S.A. There are now several reports that blue, green and red light can each be effective in topical PDT of AK, but the more deeply penetrating red light is superior when treating BD and BCC.[1]

A report has recently described the concept of ambulatory PDT to reduce hospital attendance for PDT.[13] In a pilot study of five patients with BD, PDT was performed with ALA and a portable LED device, where low irradiance light exposure took place over 100 min (ALA 4 h, 637 nm, 75 J cm^{-2}, 12 mW cm^{-2}). Pain was minimal in most, and four of five patients were in clinical remission after a median of 9 months. In contrast, Britton et al.[14] used a pulsed dye laser (PDL) for ALA-PDT in BD, with the aim of reducing irradiation time. Overlapping 7-mm spots were applied to cover the lesions (ALA 4 h, 585 nm, 10 J cm^{-2}, 22 mW cm^{-2}), achieving high response rates and shorter average exposure time (~450 ms), but the procedure required considerable time and skill on the part of the operator for larger lesions. There was also significant post-treatment morbidity including slow healing and scarring.

Recent studies have suggested that pulsed light therapy may be useful for treatment/adjunctive treatment in topical PDT of acne, AK and photorejuvenation (see later sections). However, a recent controlled investigative study, performed in healthy human skin in vivo following microdermabrasion and acetone scrub, showed that two pulsed light sources previously reported in PDT, the PDL and a broadband flashlamp filtered intense pulsed light (IPL), produced evidence of minimal activation of photosensitizer, with a dramatically smaller photodynamic reaction than seen with a conventional continuous wave broadband source.[15] The IPL and PDL sources deliver intense light in periods < 20 ms, which might suppress oxygen consumption.[16] Inadvertent ambient light exposure may have significantly contributed to the clinical effect. On the other hand, three studies have recently addressed the possibility of using ambient light for ALA-PDT of AK, with two reports of therapeutic benefit, but with a randomized ambient light-controlled study using Levulan ALA demonstrating no significant effect on lesion ablation.[15,17,18] A randomized right/left intrapatient comparison of conventional MAL-PDT delivered with an LED device vs. daylight (for 2·5 h) for the treatment of AK of face and scalp showed an equivalent reduction in AK and significantly less pain with daylight.[19] Although ambient light exposure might achieve a therapeutically effective dose in certain circumstances, it is unlikely to offer a consistent, practical and safe approach to the delivery of PDT.

Total effective light dose or fluence is proposed as a concept for optimizing the accuracy of light dosimetry in PDT, taking into account incident spectral irradiance, optical transmission through tissue and absorption by photosensitizer.[20] In practice, light dosimetry is described as the irradiance or fluence rate (mW cm^{-2}) at the skin surface and the total dose or fluence (J cm^{-2}) delivered to the surface, the latter being a product of irradiance and time of exposure.

Experimental evidence has suggested that lower fluence rates and fractionation of light exposure could improve lesional

response by promotion of the photodynamic reaction.[21] A study of superficial BCC, illuminated with 45 J cm^{-2} at 4 h and repeated at 6 h with 633-nm laser light at 50 mW cm^{-2}, observed a complete response of 84% after a mean of 59 months.[22] More recent studies are presented in the individual indication sections later in this report. In brief, current data support superiority of the fractionation approach in BCC, although not in BD.[23,24]

Currently, a range of light sources, doses and irradiances continues to be used in ALA-PDT, whereas in MAL-PDT the standard procedure now typically involves an LED source. A range of continuous wave light sources is effective in topical PDT (Strength of recommendation A, Quality of evidence II-iii).

Protocols for delivery of photodynamic therapy

Optimization of PDT outcome requires consideration of mechanism of action and application of the most appropriate drug and light parameters. The photodynamic reaction is dependent on the presence of sufficient quantities of photosensitizer, activating light and oxygen. For utilization of this reaction, the prodrug/photosensitizer requires a high selectivity for the target vs. healthy tissue. Topically applied prodrugs are converted intracellularly to the active photosensitizer and exert direct effects on the target cells, while intravenous photosensitizers may exert a major effect on tumour vasculature, with consequent ischaemia of tumour tissue. Reactive oxygen species (ROS), principally singlet oxygen, released by the photodynamic reaction result in apoptosis of target cells, and necrosis is also reported. A vigorous inflammatory reaction usually occurs, followed by an immune response which may help eradicate residual tumour cells.[25]

In topical PDT, the first consideration is that the prodrug should be able to penetrate the skin and be delivered to the target tissue in sufficient quantities and at the required depth. As reported in the original guidelines,[1] co-application of the penetration enhancer dimethylsulphoxide and the iron chelator ethylenediamine tetraacetic acid sodium appeared to enhance the efficacy of ALA-PDT in nodular BCC, although no randomized comparison data are available. In a within-subject comparison of both healthy skin and matched skin malignancies treated with ALA-PDT alone or combined with the iron chelator desferrioxamine, significantly higher PpIX levels were seen after application of the combined agents to healthy tissue, but the lesional levels were very variable.[26] Glycolic acid may increase the tissue penetration of ALA.[27] Several papers now report the use of lesional surface preparation prior to application of prodrug;[28] this is generally a mild procedure involving the removal of surface crust or scale, producing little if any bleeding and not requiring local anaesthesia. Other investigators report perforation or even removal of the intact epithelium overlying nodular BCC; however, the impact of these procedures is unknown.[29] In a recent comparison study, each half of 16 lesions (superficial BCC or BD) was randomly assigned to surface preparation (gentle curettage or abrasion with a scalpel) or none, then treated with ALA-PDT. There was no significant difference in the response of lesions in this small study.[30]

Topical ALA-PDT has been used with a variety of protocols, apart from its defined use in solution form with blue light in AK (Levulan ALA with blue-U), whereas PDT utilizing MAL is practised according to its licensed use, based on the findings of optimization studies.[3] In nodular BCC of up to 2 mm thickness, a 3-h application of 160 mg g^{-1} MAL showed the highest selectivity for tumour, and this time interval was confirmed in a recent study;[31] this procedure is licensed in the form of two treatments 1 week apart for BCC, with the aim of reaching deeper parts of the tumour at the second treatment. It is also licensed as a double treatment for BD, but in AK only one initial treatment is recommended, with non-responders receiving a second treatment at 3 months (see AK section). In contrast to MAL, the drug–light interval applied in ALA-PDT varies widely.[1] Interestingly, whereas ALA has typically been applied for longer periods, there are now publications reporting its efficacy when applied for 3 h, as with MAL.[32] Also, while the Levulan ALA and blue-U system is licensed for a drug–light interval of 18–24 h, efficacy of this formulation when applied for 1–3 h in ALA-PDT is reported in AK and photodamage.[33] Further studies are required to optimize the drug–light interval in ALA-PDT.

The use of fluorescence spectroscopy and microscopy, to assess the time course and depth of tissue photosensitizer fluorescence, respectively, has previously been described[1] and these are applied primarily in research centres to explore methods for optimizing protocols. Illumination of a porphyrin-enriched tumour by a Wood's lamp [long wave ultraviolet (UV) A] leads to a typical brick-red fluorescence which can be utilized in detecting and delineating poorly defined tumours, and this principle can also be applied quantitatively with CCD camera systems coupled to digital imaging.[34]

The use of pulsed ultrasound to assess the depth of BCC prior to and following treatment has helped to predict treatment outcome, and could potentially be used in the future to assist decisions regarding treatment protocols.[35]

Topical photodynamic therapy in nonmelanoma skin cancer

Actinic keratoses

Previously reviewed open studies described clearance rates of 71–100% facial and scalp AKs, but a lower response of 44–73% AKs on acral sites, following a single treatment with PDT using nonlicensed ALA preparations.[1] During the past 5 years, nine randomized multicentre control/comparison studies (n = 4 ALA-PDT and n = 5 MAL-PDT), using licensed formulations, have been published for the treatment of facial and scalp AK.

The combined report of two such studies in 243 patients with multiple AKs stated that 75% or more lesions resolved in 77% of patients after one treatment with Levulan ALA-PDT (ALA 14–18 h, 417 ± 5 nm, 10 J cm^{-2}, 10 mW cm^{-2}).[36] A

second treatment at 8 weeks increased this rate to 89% (vs. 13% in placebo) with a lesion response rate, at 12 weeks, of 91% (placebo 31%). Moderate-to-severe stinging or discomfort was reported by at least 90% of patients.

A randomized two-centre study compared broad-area topical Levulan ALA-PDT (ALA 1 h, blue light 417 ± 5 nm, 10 J cm^{-2}, 10 mW cm^{-2}) with topical 5-fluorouracil (5-FU) 0·5% cream applied for 4 weeks in 36 patients with multiple face/scalp AKs. No difference in efficacy was evident 4 weeks post-treatment, with 80% and 79% lesion clearance, respectively, although PDT delivered to a third group using a 595-nm PDL cleared only 50% of lesions.[37] Additional open studies of 'short-contact' (0·5–3 h application) Levulan ALA-PDT, with prior topical 5-FU[38] or without,[32,33,39–41] achieved lesion clearance rates of 69–98% after single sessions using blue, IPL or PDL sources. Comparison of 3 h with 14–18 h Levulan ALA application demonstrated equivalent efficacy of 90% at 8 months.[32] Nonfacial AKs were included in this study with overall lower response rates of 70% for the extremities and 65% for the trunk at 4 months.

Sustainability of the response of AKs to Levulan ALA-PDT was reported in a study of 110 patients each with multiple thin or moderate thickness AKs on their face or scalp.[42] Up to two treatments (20% ALA 14–18 h, 417 ± 5 nm, 10 J cm^{-2}, 10 mW cm^{-2}) achieved a peak target lesion clearance of 86% reducing to 78% at 12 months. The histologically confirmed recurrence rate at 12 months was 19%.

Three randomized comparison/control studies of MAL-PDT using the same protocol (MAL 3 h, 570–670 nm, 75 J cm^{-2}, 50–250 mW cm^{-2}) cleared 69% of predominantly thin and moderate thickness AKs of the face or scalp after a single treatment,[43] increasing to 89–91% where two treatments were performed 7 days apart.[44,45] In comparison, clearance rates of 68% and 75% were recorded for cryotherapy in two of these studies,[43,45] with placebo responses of 30–38%.[44,45] Significant superiority of cosmetic response was observed in both studies that compared PDT with cryotherapy.[43,45]

Using a narrowband red LED light source (634 ± 3 nm, 37 J cm^{-2}, 50 mW cm^{-2}), a randomized study compared single MAL-PDT (3-h application), repeated at 3 months if required, with routine initial double therapy 7 days apart.[46] The protocols were equally effective, clearing 92% and 87% of lesions, respectively, with a single treatment clearing 93% of thin lesions and 70% of moderate thickness AKs. This study led to the European licence for MAL-PDT in AK being revised in 2006 in most countries to recommend an initial single treatment, with repeat at 3 months if required.

A large randomized intra-individual study of 1501 face/scalp AKs in 119 patients compared MAL-PDT using the same LED and MAL dosing parameters as above, with double freeze-thaw cryotherapy, repeating treatments at 3 months if required.[47] After the initial cycle of treatments, PDT resulted in a significantly higher cure rate than cryotherapy (87% vs. 76%), but with equivalent outcome after all nonresponders were re-treated (89% vs. 86%). Overall subject preference (cosmesis, efficacy and skin discomfort) significantly favoured

PDT. A recent study comparing MAL-PDT with cryotherapy for AK on the extremities demonstrated inferior efficacy with PDT, with clearance of 78% of lesions at 6 months compared with 88% for cryotherapy.[48]

Topical PDT is an effective therapy for thin and moderate thickness AK, with superiority to cryotherapy depending on protocol. Efficacy is relatively poorer for acral lesions, but PDT may still offer therapeutic benefit. Cosmetic outcome following PDT for AK is superior to cryotherapy (*Strength of recommendation A, Quality of evidence I*).

Bowen's disease

Topical ALA-PDT clears, on average, 86–93% of lesions of BD following one or two treatments.[1] Three small randomized trials using nonlicensed ALA formulations and identical protocols demonstrated PDT to be equivalent to cryotherapy,[49] superior to topical 5-FU[50] and significantly more effective when delivered using narrowband red rather than green light.[51]

Several alternative protocols have been reported since the original guidelines. A small study observed a response of BD to ALA and violet light (8 h, 400–450 nm, 10–20 J cm^{-2}, 5·4–10·8 mW cm^{-2}) in all five evaluable patients, although with recurrence in one of five by 6 months.[52] The use of low-irradiance LED light sources applied to lesions to permit ambulatory PDT has been discussed above.[13] Fractionation of light during ALA-PDT for BD (20 J cm^{-2} then 80 J cm^{-2} at 4 and 6 h) has been compared with standard single illumination (75 J cm^{-2} at 4 h) and achieved equivalent response rates of 88% and 80%, respectively, at 12 months, suggesting no current advantage to split illumination.[24]

Topical MAL-PDT has recently been compared with clinician's choice of cryotherapy or 5-FU in a multicentre randomized controlled trial of 225 patients with 275 lesions (MAL 3 h, 570–670 nm, 75 J cm^{-2}, 70–200 mW cm^{-2}).[53] Three months after last treatment, clearance rates were similar following MAL-PDT (86%), cryotherapy (82%) and 5-FU (83%). PDT gave superior cosmetic results compared with cryotherapy and 5-FU (good or excellent in 94%, 66% and 76%, respectively). After 24 months of follow up, 68% of lesions remained clear following PDT, 60% after cryotherapy and 59% after 5-FU.[54]

Topical PDT has been reported in case reports to clear BD in unusual sites (nipple, subungual)[55–57] and where it arises in a setting of poor healing (lower leg, epidermolysis bullosa and radiation dermatitis).[58–60] Topical PDT can be effective in digital lesions, with four patients treated in one study clearing to give good cosmetic and functional results (one recurrence at 8 months).[61] Complete resolution of localized bowenoid papulosis in two patients followed ALA-PDT using 6–12 h application and a same-day fractionated illumination schedule.[62]

Topical ALA-PDT has been observed to offer therapeutic benefit in erythroplasia of Queyrat.[63,64] MAL-PDT cleared residual erythroplasia following Mohs surgery for penile SCC.[65] Paoli *et al.*[66] observed that PDT (ALA/MAL) to 10 patients with penile intraepithelial neoplasia resulted in clearance in seven patients, but later recurrence in four. There was sustained clearance in the remaining patients over 46 months, including clearance of human papillomavirus (HPV) DNA.

Topical PDT is an effective therapy for BD, with equivalence to cryotherapy and equivalence or superiority to topical 5-FU. Cosmetic outcome is superior to standard therapy. Topical PDT offers particular advantages for large/multiple patch disease and for lesions at poor healing sites (*Strength of recommendation A, Quality of evidence I*).

Squamous cell carcinoma

There remain limited data on the efficacy of topical PDT for primary cutaneous invasive SCC. Clearance rates for superficial lesions of 54–100% have been observed following ALA-PDT in series of five to 35 lesions, but with recurrence rates ranging from 0% to 69% (weighted average 30%) and reduced efficacy for the few nodular lesions treated.[1,67]

Topical ALA-PDT cleared an SCC in a hospitalized patient with xeroderma pigmentosum, but produced an enhanced phototoxic reaction lasting over 2 weeks despite the absence of UV radiation.[68] Caution is advised in this indication following the report of a 5-year-old patient with DeSanctis–Cacchione syndrome, a variant of xeroderma pigmentosum, where PDT using a systemic photosensitizer to multiple eyelid SCCs was followed by a rapid extension of tumours within the treatment field.[69]

The high efficacy of topical PDT for in situ SCC, and the efficacy figures reported particularly for superficial invasive lesions limited to papillary dermis, suggest that depth of therapeutic effect is the limiting factor for PDT in invasive SCC, with further study required. Current evidence supports the potential of topical PDT for superficial, microinvasive SCC, but in view of its metastatic potential, topical PDT cannot currently be recommended for the treatment of invasive SCC (*Strength of recommendation D, Quality of evidence II-iii*).

Basal cell carcinoma

Superficial BCCs were reported to respond well to ALA-PDT with a weighted clearance rate of 87% in one review of 12 studies, compared with 53% for nodular lesions.[70] Prior debulking curettage achieved a clearance rate for nodular BCC in one study of 92% compared with 0% in the control groups (curettage or PDT alone).[71] One randomized comparison of PDT (ALA 6 h, 635 nm, 60 J cm^{-2}, 80 mW cm^{-2}) vs. cryotherapy for mixed BCC showed no difference in efficacy over 1 year but superior cosmesis with PDT.[72] The original guidelines concluded PDT to be effective in superficial BCC, but that adjunctive therapy might be required to enhance efficacy for nodular BCC.[1] However, a recent study failed to show a significant advantage of curettage followed by PDT (ALA 6 h, 630 nm, 125 J cm^{-2}, 120 mW cm^{-2}, repeated at 3 months) compared with conventional surgery for nodular BCC up to 2 cm in diameter, with clearance rates of 72% and 100%, respectively, of treatment sites reviewed at 1 year.[73]

Further approaches taken in an attempt to increase the response of BCC, particularly nodular lesions, have been to use the more lipophilic methyl ester of ALA, MAL, and to use routine double PDT treatments. In a large retrospective report of MAL-PDT for BCC, where most lesions received a single treatment (MAL 3 or 24 h, 570–670 nm, 50–200 J cm^{-2}, 100–180 mW cm^{-2}) with nodular lesions receiving prior debulking curettage, an initial complete response was observed in 310 lesions, and 277 remained clear after 35 months, with a good or excellent cosmetic response in 98%.[74] The overall cure rate for the 350 superficial and nodular BCCs was 79%, an encouraging result particularly as the population included lesions failing previous treatments. To date there has been only one small randomized study directly comparing ALA-PDT with MAL-PDT in BCC (ALA and MAL 3 h, 600–730 nm, 75 J cm^{-2}, 100 mW cm^{-2}), with no difference in lesional response on histological analysis after 8 weeks, and residual tumour in six treatment sites in each study group.[9]

Fractionation of light may enhance the efficacy of topical PDT in BCC. In an open study of ALA-PDT, 86 superficial BCCs were illuminated with red light (ALA, 633 nm, 45 J cm^{-2}, 50 mW cm^{-2}) at 4 and 6 h, with initial clearing of 76 (88%) lesions and sustained clearance of 56 of 67 (84%) evaluable lesions at 59 months.[22] The same group subsequently undertook a randomized comparison trial of 505 superficial BCCs (ALA, 630-nm diode laser or 633-nm LED or broadband light 590–650 nm, 50 mW cm^{-2}), treated with either a single illumination of 75 J cm^{-2} or twofold illumination with 20 J cm^{-2} and 80 J cm^{-2} at 4 and 6 h.[23] Twelve months after treatment, ALA-PDT with single illumination cleared 89% of tumours, while fractionated PDT produced a significantly higher response rate of 97%.

Two prospective uncontrolled multicentre studies have subsequently reported on routine double MAL-PDT treatment of 'difficult to treat' BCC (superficial and nodular) including lesions occurring on the mid-face or ear locations, of large size, and recurring after other treatments. Lesion surface preparation involved gentle scraping of superficial lesions, while nodular lesions were prepared by removing any intact overlying epidermis ± some debulking. The protocol also allowed for a second cycle of MAL-PDT (two treatment sessions) in lesions showing partial response at 3 months. In the first study [MAL 3 h, 570–670 nm (n = 106) or 580–740 nm (n = 2), 75 J cm^{-2}, 50–200 mW cm^{-2}], 87% of 108 difficult to treat lesions showed complete lesion response at 3 months when assessed clinically, falling to 77% after histological review.[29] After 2 years, the lesion recurrence rate was 22%, with recurrence rate apparently increasing with lesion diameter, while 94% of patients showed a good or excellent cosmetic outcome. Similarly, a study of 95 patients with 148 BCC lesions showed that PDT (MAL 3 h, 570–670 nm, 75 J cm^{-2}, 50–200 mW cm^{-2}) achieved a histologically confirmed lesion complete response rate of 89% at 3 months while the estimated sustained lesion complete response rate at 2 years was 78%, at which time 84% of patients were judged to have a good or excellent cosmetic response.[75] Lesions in the H-zone

and large lesions were noted to have lower sustained complete response rates.

Multicentre randomized studies have now been reported for MAL-PDT vs. standard treatment for BCC, with long-term (5 year) follow-up data becoming available. A randomized study compared double MAL-PDT with treatments 7 days apart (MAL 3 h, 570–670 nm, 75 J cm^{-2}, 50–200 mW cm^{-2}) with standard surgical excision, in 101 patients with small nodular BCC amenable to simple excision.[28] Lesions (24%) with a noncomplete response to PDT at 3 months were re-treated. Clinical complete response rates at 3 months did not differ significantly between groups, with 98% in those treated with surgery vs. 91% of lesions treated with MAL-PDT, and with total disease-free response rates at 12 months of 96% vs. 83%, respectively. A recent 5-year follow up of this study has revealed a significantly higher estimated sustained lesion response rate for surgery at 96% compared with 76% for MAL-PDT.[76] Over 5 years, 14% of lesions recurred after MAL-PDT vs. 4% for surgery, although no further recurrences with MAL-PDT were seen after the first 3 years. Cosmetic evaluation showed significantly better results for MAL-PDT, with 87% showing a good or excellent outcome at 5 years after PDT compared with 54% in the surgical group. These results imply that while surgery remains the gold standard for the treatment of nodular BCC, MAL-PDT is effective for treatment of these lesions and exhibits a more favourable cosmetic outcome.

A similar 5-year follow-up study has compared cryotherapy with PDT (MAL 3 h, 570–670 nm, 75 J cm^{-2}, 50–200 mW cm^{-2}) for the treatment of superficial BCC. The 3-month complete clinical response rates were similar for PDT (97% of 102 BCCs) and cryotherapy (95% of 98 lesions). Cosmetic outcome was superior following PDT, with an excellent or good outcome reported in 87% (PDT group) and 49% (cryotherapy). The estimated complete lesion response rate at 5 years was 75% in the MAL-PDT group vs. 74% in the cryotherapy group, with recurrence of 22% of lesions which had initially cleared following MAL-PDT, compared with 20% after cryotherapy.[77]

Topical MAL–PDT and ALA–PDT are effective treatments for superficial BCC (*Strength of recommendation A, Quality of evidence I*). Topical MAL–PDT is effective in nodular BCC, although with a lower efficacy than excision surgery, and may be considered in situations where surgery may be suboptimal (*Strength of recommendation B, Quality of evidence I*).

Cutaneous T-cell lymphoma

Several case reports[78,79] and case series successfully utilizing topical ALA-PDT and MAL-PDT for early stage localized cutaneous T-cell lymphoma (CTCL) have been published since the original guidelines, with multiple treatments usually required for clearance. One report of ALA-PDT used an incoherent red light source (ALA 5–6 h, 600–730 nm, 88–180 J cm^{-2}, 20–265 mW cm^{-2}) in 10 patients with mycosis fungoides (MF) (10 plaque lesions and two tumours) with a median number of two treatments (range 2–11 treatments).[80]

There was complete clinical clearance in seven of nine evaluable plaque lesions, but neither tumour responded. Complete remission is reported of four patients with CTCL IA–IIB treated with one to seven topical ALA-PDT treatments using an incoherent light source (ALA 6 h, 600–730 nm, 72–144 J cm^{-2}, 60–120 mW cm^{-2}).[81] These patients had varied histological types including two patients with MF, one CD30+ anaplastic large cell lymphoma and one CD8+ CTCL. Another report observed remission in four patients with unilesional MF and partial response in another following one to nine PDT treatments (MAL 3 h, 635 ± 18 nm, 37·5 J cm^{-2}, 86 mW cm^{-2}).[82]

Topical PDT using ALA (n = 2) and MAL (n = 1) has also achieved clinical and histological remission after one or two treatments in three patients with localized thin plaque cutaneous B-cell lymphoma, with clearance maintained over 8–24 months.[83]

The selective uptake of photosensitizers into lymphocytes, discussed in the original guidelines, offers an explanation for the potential of PDT in CTCL. Malignant T lymphocytes may be more susceptible than keratinocytes to PDT-induced lysis, as illustrated in a study using the novel photosensitizer silicon phthalocyanine.[84]

Topical PDT can elicit a response and has a potential role in the treatment of localized CTCL. Further studies of PDT for CTCL are required to define optimal treatment parameters (Strength of recommendation C, Quality of evidence II-iii).

Intraepithelial neoplasia of the vulva and anus

Limited data reviewed in the original guidelines suggested that topical ALA-PDT could be effective in the treatment of vulval intraepithelial neoplasia (VIN). Complete histological clearance of VIN grade III in 11 of 15 (73%) patients was achieved following PDT (ALA 2–3 h, 635 nm, 125 J cm^{-2}), with no difference in disease-free survival at 1 year compared with patients treated with laser ablation or surgery.[85] Multifocal disease was found to be a predictor of poor response to PDT. The same group also reported the histologically confirmed clearance of 57% of 22 patients with VIN II/III again following a single ALA-PDT treatment.[86] PDT was viewed as being as effective as conventional therapies, but with shorter healing times and absence of scarring. A significant post-treatment increase of cytotoxic T-cell infiltration in VIN lesions responding to ALA-PDT has been observed compared with nonresponding VIN; and the presence of high-grade dysplasia and/or high-risk HPV is associated with a poor response to PDT.[87] A retrospective review of different modalities for VIN observed a 48% relapse rate following PDT, comparable with 42% following local excision and 40% treated by laser vaporization over 54 months.[88] Topical PDT has been used to treat intraepithelial neoplasia of the anus.[89] High recurrence rates, typical of tissue-preserving therapies for these indications, necessitate close follow up of patients and more detailed comparison studies are required. Drug application remains challenging for these intraepithelial neoplasias and facilitated delivery using bioadhesive patches or systemic photosensitizers is being explored.[90–92]

Topical PDT offers therapeutic benefit in VIN, but refinement of practical aspects of delivery and optimization of protocol are required (Strength of recommendation C, Quality of evidence II-iii).

Extramammary Paget's disease

In the original guidelines, evidence for the use of topical PDT as monotherapy for extramammary Paget's disease (EMPD) was lacking. A retrospective review identified five men with 16 EMPD lesions, 11 recurrent from standard therapies, who had received Levulan ALA-PDT and red light.[93] Six months after one treatment, eight lesions were clear, but three recurred after a further 3–4 months. Although recurrence is common with conventional therapies, the authors speculate that PDT using systemic photosensitizers might be more suitable for bulky disease. A further two cases of EMPD are reported of response to ALA-PDT, and seven patients with recurrent EMPD of the vulva were treated using MAL-PDT and red light, with clearance in four.[94,95] PDT with the ALA applied via a bioadhesive patch, followed by red light illumination, cleared vulval EMPD after four treatments, with histological confirmation.[96]

Topical PDT, although potentially effective in EMPD, is currently associated with high recurrence rates in the limited cases reported (Strength of recommendation C, Quality of evidence III).

Photodynamic therapy for skin cancer prophylaxis

Repeated ALA-PDT treatments can delay the appearance of UV-induced skin cancer in mice.[97] Although an increased mortality and a greater incidence of large tumours in the PDT-treated mice were observed in the initial study, more recent studies have not concurred with this finding, with both systemic (intraperitoneal) and topical ALA-PDT in mice showing delayed appearance of UV-induced tumours in mice but no increased mortality or incidence of large tumours,[98,99] and similar findings reported for topical MAL-PDT in UV-treated mice.[100] In the study by Liu et al.,[99] a delay in large tumour appearance was observed in mice whether ALA-PDT was started concurrent with or at the end of UV exposure. Recently, a study of topical MAL-PDT in PTCH heterozygous mice exposed to UV radiation has shown significant prevention of development of microscopic BCC.[101] At 28 weeks, 19 BCCs were found in nine of 20 mice exposed to UV only whereas there were no BCCs in 15 mice additionally exposed to PDT.

The mechanism by which PDT delays the onset of UV-induced skin cancer is unknown. It is known that PpIX preferentially accumulates in neoplastic cells, and light activation may induce both necrosis and apoptosis of these cells.[102] Topical PDT may cause selective destruction of keratinocytes bearing mutated p53 induced by UV exposure.[100] Alternatively or additionally PDT may be inducing an immune response against neoplastic cells and acting as a biological response modifier.[103,104] Observed reduction in expected AK in clinical trials in organ transplant recipients (OTRs) (see section below) may in large part be due to the treatment of subclinical lesions, and evidence of a primary preventive effect of topical PDT in humans is lacking. Hence, current evidence indicates that topical PDT has the potential to provide a preventive role although further evidence is required to clarify its mechanism of action (*Strength of recommendation C, Quality of evidence IV*).

Photodynamic therapy in organ transplant recipients

OTRs are at a significantly increased risk of skin cancer.[105,106] The risk relates to the duration and degree of immunosuppression, HPV infection, and exposure to UV radiation. These tumours tend to be multiple, occurring within areas of dysplastic 'field change', and often behave in a more aggressive manner. PDT offers the potential of treating large target sites which may include multiple tumours, AK and preclinical skin cancers. In addition, it can provide a more satisfactory cosmetic outcome and, more importantly, may provide a means of preventing the development of skin cancer.

Clinical response rates for OTRs (n = 20) and immunocompetent (n = 20) individuals were compared in an open prospective trial of PDT (ALA 5 h, 600–730 nm, 75 J cm^{-2}, 80 mW cm^{-2}) for AK and BD.[107] Clinical response in both groups was similar at 4 weeks, with 86% and 94%, respectively. However, by 48 weeks the response rate in the OTRs had reduced to 48% compared with 72% in the immunocompetent patients. The reduced effectiveness of topical PDT in OTRs compared with immunocompetent individuals lends support to the importance of the role of immune response factors in its mechanism of action. The same group reported, in a randomized controlled trial, an observed clearance of AK in 13 of 17 OTRs at 16 weeks in areas treated by MAL-PDT (3 h, 600–730 nm, 75 J cm^{-2}, 80 mW cm^{-2}).[108] Another group reported complete remission of 24 tumours (75%) in five OTRs with 32 facial tumours (21 BCC, eight AK, one keratoacanthoma and two SCC), following PDT (ALA 3–5 h, 635 nm, 120 J cm^{-2}, 100 mW cm^{-2}).[109] Two tumours, both SCC, were refractory to PDT.

A recent open intrapatient randomized study of 27 renal OTRs reported a significant delay in development of new lesions at sites treated with PDT (MAL 3 h, 570–670 nm, 75 J cm^{-2}) compared with control sites (9·6 vs. 6·8 months).[110] By 12 months 62% of treated areas were free from new lesions compared with 35% in control areas. However, no significant difference in the occurrence of SCC was observed in another study of PDT (ALA 4 h, 400–450 nm, 5·5–6 J cm^{-2}) vs. no treatment after 2 years follow up in 40 OTRs.[111] A less pronounced increase in keratotic skin lesions in the PDT-treated sites was apparent but was not significant. Of note, in this latter study violet was used rather than red light and keratotic lesions were not pretreated by curettage.

A small randomized intrapatient comparison study compared PDT (MAL 3 h, 633 ± 15 nm, 75 J cm^{-2}, 80 mW cm^{-2}) with topical 5-FU for treatment of epidermal dysplasia in OTRs.[112] PDT (two treatments 7 days apart) was shown to be more effective and cosmetically acceptable than 5-FU (applied twice daily for 3 weeks) at 6-month follow up, PDT clearing eight of nine lesion areas, compared with only one of nine areas treated by 5-FU (lesional area reduction: PDT 100%, 5-FU 79%).

Current evidence suggests that topical PDT, although showing lower efficacy than in immunocompetent individuals, may provide a useful therapy for epidermal dysplasias in OTRs (*Strength of recommendation B, Quality of evidence I*).

Topical photodynamic therapy for infectious and inflammatory dermatoses

Acne and related conditions

PDT may promote improvement in acne via antibacterial activity against *Propionibacterium acnes*, selective damage to sebaceous glands, reduction in follicular obstruction by keratinocyte shedding and via secondary host responses.[113,114] *Propionibacterium acnes* naturally produces small amounts of certain porphyrins, especially coproporphyrin III, with topical ALA application promoting its accumulation.[115]

A randomized controlled trial of PDT (Levulan ALA 3 h, 550–700 nm, 150 J cm^{-2}) for acne on the back of 22 subjects demonstrated a significant reduction in inflammatory acne for 10 weeks after a single treatment and for at least 20 weeks after four treatments.[113] Sebum excretion and bacterial porphyrin fluorescence were both decreased, and sebaceous gland size was still reduced at 20 weeks after PDT, but treatment induced skin exfoliation and hyperpigmentation. A further randomized intraindividual controlled study of ALA-PDT (3 h, 635 nm, 15 J cm^{-2}, 25 mW cm^{-2}) for acne on the back demonstrated a significant reduction in inflammatory lesion counts after three weekly treatments, but without reductions in P. acnes numbers or sebum excretion. Despite the less intense regimen, postinflammatory pigmentation was observed in all patients for 1–3 months.[114]

Several open studies report a clinical benefit of topical ALA-PDT (both ALA and Levulan ALA) in facial acne using a range of application times from 0·25 to 4 h and a variety of light sources including blue light and IPL.[116] Protocol variations, some including preparatory peels, with small patient numbers and short follow-up periods, limit interpretation of these studies, with the extent of accumulation of photoactive porphyrins after very short applications yet to be determined. One intrapatient controlled study observed a 42% reduction in the inflamed lesion count 6 months following a single session of PDT (ALA 4 h, 630 ± 3 nm, 18 J cm^{-2}, 30 mW cm^{-2}) in mild-to-moderate facial acne, compared with 15% reduction in the untreated side.[117] In an open controlled study of 15 patients with a wide range of severity of facial acne, PDT (Levulan ALA 45 min, 595 nm, 7 J cm^{-2}) achieved a lesional clearance rate of 77% at 6 months (32% for the light-only controls) after a mean of 2·9 treatments (range 1–6).[118] A small study of Levulan ALA applied to half the face of 13 patients with acne followed by illumination using an IPL source to both sides resulted in improved response on the PDT treatment side, sustained at 8 weeks.[119] In a further pilot study of IPL-delivered ALA-PDT in 14 patients, lesion counts decreased by 88% after three treatments, compared with 67% following IPL alone.[120] A recent split-face comparison of ALA-PDT using blue light with blue light alone in 20 Asian patients with moderate-to-severe acne showed a greater reduction in inflamed lesions on the PDT side (71% vs. 57% at 16 weeks after four weekly sessions), but the difference was not significant.[121]

Three randomized studies have recently been reported of MAL-PDT in acne. In a randomized, controlled, investigator-blinded study of 36 patients with moderate-to-severe disease, PDT was performed with gentle lesion curettage prior to initial treatment (MAL 3 h, 635 nm, 37 J cm^{-2}, 34 mW cm^{-2}), and repeated 2 weeks later. At 3 months, a significant 69% reduction in inflammatory lesions was observed, with no change in the control group, and no reduction in noninflammatory counts.[122] All patients experienced moderate to severe pain during treatment and developed severe erythema, pustular eruptions and epithelial exfoliation. A randomized split-face comparison study of 15 patients, by the same group, of ALA- and MAL-PDT (3 h, single treatment, dosimetry as above) achieved a 59% reduction in inflammatory lesions after 3 months in both groups, but with moderate-to-severe pain and pustular reactions, more severe in the ALA-PDT-treated areas.[8] A further randomized, placebo-controlled, split-face study of PDT (MAL 3 h, 635 nm, 37 J cm^{-2}) treated 30 patients with moderate-to-severe facial acne, with PDT repeated after 2 weeks.[123] Nodular and cystic lesions were prepared using a small cannula to facilitate cream penetration. A greater reduction in inflammatory lesions was observed at 12 weeks following PDT (54% vs. 20%). A recent blinded randomized study of PDT using IPL in Asian skin, where MAL was applied for only 45 min, failed to show significant improvement of moderate inflammatory acne compared with control.[124] A small randomized split-face trial compared long-pulsed dye laser alone with the use of the laser in MAL-PDT in 15 patients. There was greater reduction in inflammatory lesions on sites receiving PDT-enhanced laser therapy (80% vs. 67% at week 12).[125] A reduction in inflammatory lesion counts (on average by 58%) has also been observed in a case series of seven patients with chronic recalcitrant folliculitis arising in areas of acne-prone skin following a single treatment of MAL-PDT.[126]

Several case reports and case series report a therapeutic benefit of topical PDT using ALA, Levulan ALA and MAL in sebaceous hyperplasia[127–130] as well as for the treatment of a sebaceous naevus although treatment of the latter was combined with curettage.[131] Further studies are required to determine longevity of effect. ALA-PDT to four patients with Fordyce spots, heterotopic sebaceous glands, produced only mild improvement after two to nine treatments.[132] One case series observed improvement in hidradenitis suppurativa,

although another series failed to confirm this, with deterioration in two patients following PDT.[133,134]

Although topical PDT can improve inflammatory acne on the face and back, optimization of protocols, to sustain response while minimizing adverse effects, is awaited (*Strength of recommendation B, Quality of evidence I*).

Viral warts

Clearance rates of 56–100% were noted in the case series and comparison trials of refractory warts and verrucas reported in the original guidelines.[1] In a subsequent controlled trial, PDT (ALA 5 h, 400–700 nm, 50 J cm^{-2}, 50 mW cm^{-2}) in 67 patients with plantar warts cleared 75% of warts (48 of 64) compared with a 22% reduction in untreated warts.[135] In another study, PDT (ALA 4–8 h, 580–720 nm, 100 mW cm^{-2}) in 31 patients with 48 plantar warts cleared 42 warts (88%), with better clearance seen in younger patients, larger warts and with longer treatment times.[136]

A study compared the treatment of verrucae by PDT using either a PDL or LED source, with the use of PDL alone (ALA 3 h, PDL at 595 nm and 20 J cm^{-2}, LED at 635 nm and 50 J cm^{-2}), with clearance rates of 100% (mean 1·96 treatments), 96% (mean 2·54 treatments) and 81% (mean 3·34 treatments), respectively.[137] Pretreatment of patients with plantar warts with 3% azone prior to ALA-PDT resulted in clearance in 67% and 100% of mosaic and myrmeci (single deep painful warts) subtypes, respectively, while clearance after ALA-PDT alone was 37·5% and 70%, respectively.[138] Success of topical ALA-PDT in a patient with multiple facial plane warts has been reported, following two treatments with ALA applied for 6 h and illumination with a metal halide lamp (peaks at 630 and 700 nm).[139] Complete clearance of periungual hand warts in 18 of 20 patients (36 of 40 warts) was achieved in a pilot study of ALA-PDT after a mean of 4·5 fortnightly treatments.[140]

Recent studies continue to support the potential of topical PDT in viral warts, particularly plantar warts, but it appears a relatively painful therapy option, with outcomes dependent on adequate paring and the use of a keratolytic agent pre-PDT (*Strength of recommendation B, Quality of evidence I*).

Genital warts

A clearance rate of 66% in 16 patients with vulval and vaginal condylomata was achieved following PDT (ALA 2–4 h, 635 nm, 80–125 J cm^{-2}, 88 ± 17 mW cm^{-2}).[86] In a further case series of 12 male patients with condylomata acuminata treated with PDT (ALA 6–11 h, 400–800 nm, 70–100 J cm^{-2}, 70 mW cm^{-2}) an overall cure rate of 73% was achieved.[141] In addition, this study showed, using *in vivo* fluorescence kinetics, that the optimal time for illumination varied from 6 to 11 h. However, in a large open study of 164 patients, between one and four treatments with PDT (ALA 3 h, 630 nm, 100 J cm^{-2}, 100 mW cm^{-2}) cleared 95% of lesions, with only 5% recurring after 6–24 months.[142] Disappointing results of PDT (ALA 5 h, 630 nm, 37 J cm^{-2}, 68 mW cm^{-2}) were seen in nine men with genital condylomata unresponsive to conventional therapies, with clearance only in three, after four treatments.[143] A recent randomized study compared ALA-PDT (ALA 3 h, 633 nm, 100 J cm^{-2}, 100 mW cm^{-2}) with conventional CO_2 laser in 65 patients with condylomata acuminata.[144] One treatment cleared 95% and 100% of lesions, respectively, with persisting lesions clearing following repeat PDT. A lower recurrence rate followed PDT (6% vs. 19%) and the authors concluded that PDT was a simpler, more effective therapy. Topical PDT may be considered as a treatment option for patients with genital warts (*Strength of recommendation B, Quality of evidence I*).

Cutaneous leishmaniasis

Recently, topical PDT has been reported to be effective in the treatment of cutaneous leishmaniasis, caused by *Leishmania major*. The challenge in treating this condition is to reduce lesion size in order to promote healing with minimal scarring, while also seeking to eradicate the amastigotes.

In a series of 11 patients (32 lesions), one or two weekly treatments with topical ALA-PDT, using broadband red light, rendered smears amastigote negative. Re-examination after 3–6 months revealed 31 of 32 lesions to remain amastigote negative with no relapses over 6 months and an average reduction in lesion size of 67%.[145] In a further series of five patients with ALA-PDT repeated weekly for 4 weeks, clearance of all lesions occurred, with eradication of amastigotes (by smear and culture), good cosmetic outcome, and no relapse over 4 months.[146]

A comparison of topical MAL-PDT, using red light, with a conventional therapy, daily topical paromomycin, in 10 lesions in the same patient, revealed that after a total of 28 PDT treatments, all five PDT-treated lesions and two of five paromomycin-treated lesions had healed and were leishmania free by histology, although cultures were not performed.[147] A recent case report found clearance of unilesional disease with MAL-PDT using red light after only three treatments.[148]

In a randomized investigator-blinded trial of 57 patients (95 lesions) receiving weekly ALA-PDT with red light, twice-daily topical paromomycin or placebo, each over 4 weeks, lesion clearance at 8 weeks was seen in 94%, 41% and 13%, respectively.[149] Parasitological cure, by smear, was demonstrated in 100%, 65% and 20%, respectively.

A recent *in vitro* and *in vivo* mechanistic study concluded that response of cutaneous leishmaniasis to PDT is likely to be due to nonspecific tissue destruction accompanied by a depopulation of macrophages rather than direct killing of parasites, although a previous study did show *in vitro* selective destruction of amastigotes in macrophages following exposure to porphyrins.[150,151]

Current evidence suggests that topical PDT is effective in clearing lesions of cutaneous leishmaniasis although further studies with culture confirmation of amastigote clearance are required (*Strength of recommendation B, Quality of evidence I*).

Psoriasis

A small study of four patients with psoriasis comparing topical PDT (ALA 4 h, 630 nm, 10 J cm^{-2}, 120 mW cm^{-2}) and narrowband UVB therapy showed the superiority of the latter.[152] Treatment with PDT was poorly tolerated by patients because of pain and resulted in early termination of the trial. A report of eight patients with psoriasis treated with ALA-PDT (ALA 4–5 h, 630 nm, 10–30 J cm^{-2}, 35–315 mW cm^{-2}) showed significant improvement of plaques but treatment was again limited by a high frequency of discomfort and pain.[153] This study also showed that PDT induced dermal neovascularization in the treated psoriatic plaques – the mechanism of this is unknown. A randomized, observer-blinded study of PDT (ALA 4–6 h, 600–740 nm, 5–20 J cm^{-2}, 60 mW cm^{-2}) for 21 patients with psoriasis showed disappointing results.[154] Complete clearance was found in only eight and substantial improvement in four of 63 plaques.

Recently, a prospective randomized, double-blind phase I/II intrapatient comparison study of 12 patients with psoriasis treated by topical PDT (ALA 4–6 h, 600–740 nm, 20 J cm^{-2}, 60 mW cm^{-2}) has also shown limited mean improvement of 37·5%, 45·6% and 51·2% in the 0·1%, 1% and 5% ALA-treated groups, respectively.[155] Part of this improvement was related to the effects of prior use of salicylic acid. In addition, treatment was frequently interrupted by severe pain.

A single case of recalcitrant palmoplantar pustular psoriasis refractory to both acitretin and methotrexate has been reported showing significant benefit from topical ALA-PDT using a diode laser.[156] The same group reported marked improvement in two patients with intractable palmoplantar pustulosis and mild change in a third, following ALA-PDT with the diode laser, but seven to 10 weekly treatments were required.[157]

Overall, current evidence, combined with studies reviewed in our previous guidelines, does not support the use of topical ALA-PDT as a practical therapy for psoriasis (*Strength of recommendation D, Quality of evidence I*).

Photodynamic photorejuvenation

Chronic actinic damage, or photoageing, clinically comprises wrinkling, rough elastotic skin, dyschromia, lentigines, and telangiectases.[158] IPL (500–1200 nm) has been applied with the aim of reversing the features of photoageing. As AKs frequently coexist with other features of photoageing, there has been recent interest in exploring the potential merits of firstly combining the ALA with IPL (ALA-IPL) and secondly of using standard PDT, for treatment of both chronic photodamage and AK.

In a case series of 17 subjects, 33 of 38 (87%) AKs resolved after two sessions of ALA-IPL, but the ALA was applied only to the sites of the AK and therefore the effects of ALA-IPL on photodamage were not explored.[159] In a further case series of 17 subjects it was reported that ALA-IPL was effective in both AK and photodamage.[41] Levulan ALA was applied to the entire face for 1 h, with subsequent illumination from an IPL source (560-nm filter), clearing 68% of AKs and achieving improvement in telangiectasia, pigmentary irregularities and skin texture. The treatment was reported to be well tolerated. PDT using blue light has also been studied (ALA 1, 2 or 3 h, 400–410 nm, 10 J cm^{-2}, 10 mW cm^{-2}), in a case series of 18 patients with a combination of nonhypertrophic facial AKs and mild to moderate diffuse facial photodamage.[33] A clearance rate for AKs of 85–96% was observed after 1 month, with no difference between ALA incubation times. Regarding photodamage, modest but significant improvements were seen in the Griffiths score,[160] fine wrinkling and degree of sallowness, with borderline improvement of mottled pigmentation. All patients reported discomfort during the procedure, with moderately severe phototoxic reactions observed on day 1 in all patients.

In a split-face study, all 20 subjects with a moderate or higher degree of photoageing received a course of five full-face treatments with IPL (515–1200 nm, 23–26 J cm^{-2}), but with ALA applied as adjunctive treatment for 0·5–1 h to a randomly assigned hemiface before the first three IPL treatments.[161] A significantly greater improvement was reported for the ALA-treated side 1 month after the final (IPL) treatment, with respect to global score for photoageing, mottled pigmentation, and fine lines. The authors stressed the importance of good photoprotective measures, including physical sun blocks, in the 48 h following treatment, and felt that this may have contributed significantly to the high tolerability of the procedure.

A further split-face study compared ALA-IPL with IPL alone, given three times at 1-monthly intervals in 13 subjects.[162] The ALA-pretreated side reportedly showed enhanced improvement of fine lines, skin roughness, mottled hyperpigmentation and telangiectases, compared with the side treated with IPL alone, although it is not clear whether randomization was performed and no statistical analysis is presented.

In a small randomized split-face study of PDT (MAL 1 and 3 h, 630 nm, 37 J cm^{-2}) in 10 patients with moderate photodamage, the authors noted an improvement in skin quality and fine wrinkling, although details on methodology and again, statistical analysis, are not provided.[163]

Interest is clearly gathering in this area, although at present there is a need for well-designed randomized, controlled, adequately powered studies with a longer follow up and ideally histological confirmation of clinical findings. The relative roles of PDT and IPL as treatment/adjunctive treatment are anticipated to undergo further exploration. Standard topical PDT (continuous wave light source) and ALA-IPL appear effective in photorejuvenation (*Strength of recommendation* B, *Quality of evidence* II-iii).

Other indications

Topical ALA-PDT has been reported to be effective in the treatment of localized scleroderma in five patients, with the same group demonstrating induction of the collagen-degrad-ing matrix metalloproteinase (MMP)-1 and MMP-3 by fibroblasts following PDT.[164,165] In addition, interleukin-1 released by keratinocytes following PDT triggers MMP production in dermal fibroblasts in a paracrine manner.[166] Other photosensitizers used for PDT may be more effective in modifying collagen metabolism.[167]

Case series and individual reports describe the potential of topical PDT in a variety of other indications[168–194] (Table 1). In addition to the limited evidence, several reports detail pain and inflammatory responses that potentially limit the practicality of using this modality outwith the setting of disease unresponsive to conventional therapies. However, it is possible that optimization of protocols could broaden the indication for topical PDT in inflammatory and infectious dermatoses.

Adverse effects

Acute

The most common and troublesome acute adverse event of topical PDT is the burning or stinging pain that occurs during light exposure, and may continue postexposure in a minority. Pain is restricted to the illuminated area and may reflect nerve stimulation and/or tissue damage by ROS, possibly aggravated by hyperthermia.[1] Treatment of psoriasis and viral warts in particular is frequently limited by pain.[1,155] Pain appears more intense in large area lesions, with AK, BD and BCC covering an area of > 130 mm^2 significantly more painful to treat.[195] The latter study also found a positive association of pain intensity with AK, lesions located on the head, and in the male sex, although these factors could not be dissociated. A further study of 94 patients, all with AK, found a clear dose–response relationship for lesion size and intensity of pain, but no significant difference between genders.[196] A large interindividual variation in pain experienced was noted in both studies, with approximately 20% of patients experiencing severe pain.[195,196]

The above studies were performed with the prodrug ALA. As ALA but not MAL is transported by γ-aminobutyric acid carriers, it has been speculated that MAL might provoke less nerve fibre stimulation and subsequent pain.[197] In a double-blind randomized study in tape-stripped healthy skin of the forearm, pain was found to be significantly higher in the ALA- than the MAL-treated sites, both during and immediately after PDT (ALA and MAL 3 h, 570–670 nm, 70 J cm^{-2}, 90 mW cm^{-2}).[198] The ALA-treated skin showed a higher PpIX fluorescence peak than MAL-treated skin, and a greater decrease in peak PpIX fluorescence was seen during illumination in ALA-PDT. No correlation was found between pain and peak PpIX fluorescence, nor absolute decrease in peak PpIX fluorescence; however, the high intersubject variability could potentially obscure any relationship in this small subject group. In a recent comparison study of pain during MAL-PDT for acne and AK, pain was shown to be greater with more intense PpIX fluorescence and also with higher fluence rate.[199] Two comparison studies have observed that MAL-PDT was less painful than ALA-PDT for the treatment of scalp AK, although

Table 1 Topical photodynamic therapy (PDT) beyond nonmelanoma skin cancer: applications suggested on the basis of case reports and case series

Condition	Study	No. patients	Treatments	PDT	Outcome
Actinic cheilitis[168–170]	CS + CS + CS	3 + 3 + 15	ALA-PDT: 1–3 / MAL-PDT: 2 / MAL-PDT: 2	ALA, broadband (n = 3) / MAL, red (n = 3) / MAL, red (n = 15)	All sites cleared, good cosmesis, no recurrence 6–12 months. In large series, complete clearance in 47%, partial clearance in 47%
Disseminated superficial actinic porokeratoses[171,172]	CS + CR	3 + 1	2 (CS), 2 (CR)	ALA, red (n = 3) / MAL, red (n = 1)	CS: Initial response in one of three only at 4 weeks CR: Marked improvement, no recurrence at 1 year
Localized pagetoid reticulosis[173]	CR	1	3	ALA, red	Histological clearance, no recurrence at 1 year
Nephrogenic fibrosing dermopathy[174]	CR	1	2	MAL, red	Normal texture by 4 weeks, no recurrence at 1 year
Hailey–Hailey disease[175]	CS	2	2	ALA, red	Histological clearance, no recurrences at 19–25 months
Darier disease[176,177]	CS + CR	6 + 1	1	ALA, red (n = 6) / ALA, blue (n = 1)	Four cleared/improved, one exacerbated
Lichen planus (penile)[178]	CR	1	2	ALA, red	Complete clearance, no recurrence at 6 months
Vulval lichen sclerosus[179]	CS	12	1–3	ALA, red	Improved pruritus (10 of 12) for mean of 6 months
Extragenital lichen sclerosus[180]	CR	1	3	ALA, red	Complete clearance, no recurrence at 2 years
Sarcoidosis[181]	CR	1	22	3% ALA gel + DMSO, red	Histological clearance, no recurrence at 18 months
Necrobiosis lipoidica[182]	CR	1	6	MAL, red	Histological clearance, no recurrence at 2 years
Granulation in Goltz syndrome[183]	CR	1	1	MAL, red	Followed curettage, clearance for 8 months
Rosacea[184,185]	CS + CR	4 + 1	1 (CS), 6 (CR)	MAL + red (n = 4) / Levulan ALA + PDT at 595 nm (n = 1)	CS: Response in three, sustained in one to 9 months CR: Excellent response, only 1 month review
Perioral dermatitis[186]	SFC	21	4	Levulan ALA, blue	92% lesions clear (vs. 81% on clindamycin); seven of 21 did not complete due to photosensitivity reactions
Radiodermatitis[187]	CS	5	2–8	ALA, red (+ near infrared)	Remission in two, partial clearing in three
Venous leg ulcer[188]	CR	1	8	ALA, red	Significant improvement, clearance of MRSA
Molluscum contagiosum[189,190]	CS + CR	6 + 1	3–5 (CS), 4 (CR)	Levulan ALA, blue	Reduced lesion counts (all patients HIV positive)
Epidermodysplasia verruciformis[191]	CR	1	1	ALA, red	Histological clearance, but HPV not eradicated, new lesions at 1 year
Erythrasma[192]	CS	13	1	Endogenous porphyrins, red	Clearance in three, 30% reduction in other cases
Interdigital mycoses[193]	CS	9	1–4	ALA, red	Clinical and mycological clearance in six, but recurrence in four by 1 month
Mycobacterium marinum[194]	CR	1	3	MAL, red	Clearance of lesion unresponsive to light alone, no recurrence at 7 months

CS, case series; CR, case report; SFC, split-face comparison (nonrandomized); ALA, 5-aminolaevulinic acid; MAL, methyl aminolaevulinate; DMSO, dimethyl sulphoxide; MRSA, methicillin-resistant *Staphylococcus aureus*; HIV, human immunodeficiency virus; HPV, human papillomavirus.

ALA was applied for 6 and 5 h, respectively, compared with the shorter application time of 3 h for MAL.[10,200] Two recently reported small studies comparing MAL- and ALA-PDT in the indications of nodular BCC and acne, with application of each prodrug for 3 h, found no significant difference between the agents in pain experienced during treatment, although in the acne study the ALA-PDT side was significantly more painful 24 h after treatment.[8,9] Degree of pain also appears related to intensity of light delivery; fractionated light doses increase tolerance of the procedure, and may at the same time increase cure rates.[201] A recent split-face randomized study compared variable pulse light (VPL) with LED for MAL-PDT of face and scalp AK (MAL 3 h; VPL 610–950 nm, 80 J cm^{-2} vs. LED 635 ± 3 nm, 37 J cm^{-2}, 50 mW cm^{-2}). Pain score was significantly lower on the VPL side (visual analogue score 4·3 vs. 6·4), with similar, although relatively low, remission rates at 3 months (47% for VPL vs. 57% for LED) for both light sources.[202]

A range of techniques has been used in an attempt to reduce PDT-related pain, including local anaesthesia and cooling the skin with fans or sprayed water.[1] No significant difference was seen between patients receiving topical anaesthesia with amethocaine or control in a randomized double-blind study in 42 patients with superficial NMSC (ALA 3–5 h, 630 nm, 125 J cm^{-2}, 20–125 mW cm^{-2}).[203] Due to high intersubject variability in pain experienced, and the differing diagnoses and sites, it is conceivable that a significant effect could have been obscured. However, the effect of a topical mixture of lignocaine and prilocaine (EMLA®; AstraZeneca, Luton, U.K.) vs. control was also studied in 14 men with extensive scalp AK and again no significant alleviation of pain with the use of topical anaesthesia was observed.[204]

Cold air analgesia may be effective in topical PDT.[205] Two matched superficial skin cancers were treated either with or without cold air analgesia (−35 °C) at the time of irradiation. While no significant difference was seen in pain score at the first session, the score was significantly lower during the second treatment session of the cold air-treated lesion. The investigators also found that level of skin erythema was reduced after treatment. It is conceivable that the profound cooling induced by this device could result in a significant vasoconstriction, theoretically making less oxygen available for the photodynamic reaction.

Other than pain, topical PDT has a low morbidity, and few significant acute adverse effects occur. An acute inflammatory response is observed, sometimes followed by erosion and crust formation. Complete healing usually occurs within 2 weeks but is reported occasionally to take up to 6 weeks.[1] A small minority of patients shows a heightened acute inflammatory response, during or immediately after PDT, typically when wide areas of the face/scalp are treated. Recent investigations have shown that the erythema and oedema seen immediately postirradiation are attributable to a dose-related urticarial response mediated by histamine, and that this occurs to some degree in all subjects.[206] Caution has been advised in treating large skin fields by PDT in case of pronounced photo-

toxic reaction, with the option to consider initial small-area PDT prior to large-field exposure.[207] The skin inflammation induced by PDT might contribute to its therapeutic effect, acting as an optimizing event for the development of specific antitumour immunity and long-term suppression of tumour growth after PDT.[21] Interestingly, it was found in a study of ALA-PDT for AK that pretreatment lesional erythema was significantly related to both PDT-induced pain and the cure rate.[196] The pretreatment erythema is likely to reflect degree of vasodilatation and inflammation in the lesions, and may indicate the amount of oxygen locally available. Further clinical studies are clearly required, to determine whether interventions that reduce pretreatment erythema or the PDT-induced inflammatory response may impact adversely on therapeutic effect.

Pain is a common feature during light exposure in PDT, but topical PDT is overall a well-tolerated treatment modality with a low rate of serious acute adverse events (*Strength of recommendation A, Quality of evidence I*).

Application of topical anaesthetics is of limited use for pain relief during light exposure of AK (*Strength of recommendation D, Quality of evidence II-i*).

Chronic

The incidence of scarring associated with topical PDT is very low and is reflected in the good or excellent cosmetic outcome widely reported, including in the randomized comparison trials of PDT in NMSC indications reported above and in the original guidelines.[1] In vivo studies of the effect of haematoporphyrin-mediated PDT compared with hyperthermia on mouse skin compliance have found the former not to produce a fibrotic response.[208] The levels of collagen measured in vitro are elevated in modalities associated with scarring in vivo (e.g. ionizing radiation, hyperthermia and bleomycin) but not after exposure to haematoporphyrin ester-mediated PDT.[209]

Postinflammatory hypopigmentation or hyperpigmentation can occur following PDT.[1] Studies on healthy skin showed that hyperpigmentation following PDT is dependent on ALA dose, occurs after 48–72 h and increases during the 2 weeks following treatment.[26,210] Hyperpigmentation of psoriatic lesions following PDT appears to be common. Mild to moderate pigmentation was seen in all PDT-treated lesions in a study of 21 patients with psoriasis and in seven of eight patients in a further study.[153,154] However, pigmentary disturbance appears only occasionally to be more than a minor complication of skin tumour PDT. Pigmentary change was observed in only 1% of lesions (mild/moderate scarring: 0·8%) from a centre reporting on PDT for 762 patients with NMSC.[211] Hair loss is a potential side-effect of PDT as concomitant sensitization of the pilosebaceous unit takes place.[212] Permanent localized hair loss following PDT is uncommon but has occurred more frequently after treatment of BCC rather than BD, presumably determined by the extent of involvement of pilosebaceous units by the primary disease.[213]

Carcinogenicity

As PDT does not induce covalent modifications of DNA, treatment-related carcinogenesis is expected to be low or absent compared with UV therapy.[214] In addition, porphyrin-like molecules also possess antioxidant and antimutagenic properties.[215] PDT has the potential of promoting genotoxic effects from the generation of ROS, but with effects limited to the vicinity of their site of generation, and ROS liberated by ALA- and MAL-PDT mediate their effects in the mitochondria as opposed to the nucleus.[216] Recent research has shown that PDT induces low levels of p53 and generated ROS do not induce DNA damage via p53 phosphorylation pathways as seen with PUVA.[217] PDT does not induce cyclobutane pyrimidine dimers or (6–4) photoproducts, as induced by UV radiation: these are DNA lesions that are associated with characteristic p53 mutations at dipyrimidine sites in NMSC.[218]

Two cases of skin cancer possibly related to PDT have previously been reported in the original guidelines.[64,219] One was a melanoma arising in the scalp of a patient receiving PDT for AK, the other an SCC arising in an area of erythroplasia of Queyrat treated by PDT. In the past 5 years, only one further lesion possibly induced by topical PDT has been reported, in a patient who developed a keratoacanthoma after ALA-PDT for treatment of AK.[220]

Topical PDT has a low risk of carcinogenicity and reported cases of skin cancer occurring in relation to this therapy are rare (*Strength of recommendation A, Quality of evidence II-iii*).

Safety aspects of topical photodynamic therapy

Contraindications to PDT include a history of porphyria and allergy/photoallergy to active ingredients of the applied photosensitizer.[221–223] Blue light can pose a hazard to the retina, potentially causing irreversible damage to the photosensitive neurotransmitters in the macula.[1] However, most PDT is carried out using red light which is not phototoxic to the retina. Nevertheless, the wearing of goggles for both patient and staff is recommended to limit the transmission of high-intensity light and to avoid discomfort and disturbance of colour perception.

Following topical PDT, localized photosensitivity can remain for up to 48 h, ALA degrading with a half-life of about 24 h, and MAL-induced PpIX clearing from normal skin within 24–48 h.[224,225]

Photodynamic therapy: cost assessment

The original guidelines provided a detailed cost-comparison of ALA-PDT with standard therapy derived from two studies of BD.[1] Estimated costs for ALA-PDT were comparable with cryotherapy and topical 5-FU when morbidity costs were included, but reflected the use of a nonlicensed ALA preparation and light sources no longer in routine use. A cost-minimization study of six treatments commonly used for BD in the U.K. National Health Service concluded that ALA-PDT

was the most expensive option for treating a single lesion, but considered average costs for three light sources now rarely used, including laser, making extrapolation difficult to current practice of PDT.[226] The cost of topical PDT will be influenced by clinic set-up, opportunities for safe multiple use of the same package for more than one lesion/patient, nurse/technician- vs. doctor-led therapy, use of relatively low-cost LED sources, etc. A discrete choice survey of members of the general public in Australia demonstrated that preference for avoidance of scarring was considered to be more important even than lesion response, with a willingness to pay more for MAL-PDT over simple excision for BCC.[227]

A recent detailed economic evaluation of topical MAL-PDT, based on multicentre comparison trials for AK,[45] superficial and nodular BCC,[28,77] calculated the cost per full responder, defined as clearance of all lesions in a patient and an excellent cosmetic outcome. The authors concluded that PDT is a cost-effective intervention in AK when compared with cryotherapy over 1 year, and better value for money than excision in BCC when compared over 5 years (to allow time for recurrences).[228] This industry-sponsored study took into account response rates, possible recurrence and cosmesis as well as estimating the costs of managing nonresponse, recurrence and nonexcellent cosmetic outcome, and represents the most detailed consideration, to date, of the relative cost of PDT when a value on cosmetic outcome benefit is included.

Novel methods of delivering topical PDT could improve its cost-effectiveness. The cost-effectiveness of delivering topical PDT in a community setting was demonstrated in a small randomized study using a portable PDT light source, with therapy delivered by a nurse, permitting a more convenient service for typically elderly patients presenting with BD and BCC.[229] Ambulatory PDT could minimize hospital resources as well as offer treatment at/closer to home using portable LED devices.[13] Further studies are required to update cost-effectiveness analysis for topical PDT as currently used in the U.K. National Health Service, with particular consideration to its use in multiple and/or large lesions/field treatments.

Overview

These updated guidelines provide strong evidence confirming the high efficacy of topical PDT in AK, BD and superficial BCC. Randomized comparison studies also support the efficacy of topical PDT, following lesion preparation, in thin nodular BCC, with recurrence rates over 5 years recently published. Licensed products and convenient light sources with short irradiation times are now available for topical PDT in NMSC.

The response of OTRs to PDT appears reduced compared with immunocompetent controls, but this modality may still be useful for the treatment and possible prevention of NMSC in this challenging situation. Current evidence demonstrates reductions in anticipated lesion numbers following PDT; the relative contribution of primary prevention of *de-novo* lesions and treatment of preclinical lesions requires study. The lack of additional studies of PDT in SCC cautions practitioners not to use topical PDT where invasive malignancy is suspected. Small patient numbers of individual reports continue to limit the evidence for PDT in localized CTCL, although available data are encouraging.

Since the original guidelines a large number of additional applications for topical PDT has been described in the literature (Table 1). It appears that efficacy as well as greater patient tolerance of PDT can be achieved in infective and inflammatory indications through lower dose, less intense treatment regimens, although multiple treatments are usually required. A variety of protocols, including several randomized studies, results in clinical response of acne to PDT, but a narrow therapeutic window may exist between clinical and phototoxic responses, potentially limiting patient tolerance. Further study data indicate disappointing outcomes of PDT for psoriasis. In contrast, several reports now describe the clearance of cutaneous leishmaniasis lesions by topical PDT, an interesting novel indication.

During the past 5 years, considerable interest has been shown in the potential of PDT to promote photorejuvenation with observed improvements of fine lines, skin roughness and mottled hyperpigmentation. Further well-designed studies are required.

Topical PDT is well tolerated, while treatment-associated pain remains problematic for certain indications. To date, the use of topical anaesthesia appears ineffective, and alternative therapies, including cold air analgesia, offer scope for pain reduction when required. Reports of possible secondary skin malignancy remain very low, and high-quality cosmesis following PDT is consistently observed.

Tools for guideline users

Presented in this update:
1 Summary of the evidence for PDT in its principal approved and emerging indications.
2 A tabular summary of possible applications of topical PDT where evidence is currently restricted to case reports and series (Table 1).
3 A summary of the main recommendations from this comprehensive update (Table 2).
4 Suggestions for audit.

Possible audit points

1 Initial clearance rates of AK, BD and superficial BCC at 3 months after last treatment of at least 75% lesions.
2 Sustained clearance rates of AK, BD and superficial BCC at 12 months after last treatment of at least 75% lesions.
3 Recurrence rates at 24 months post-treatment in BD and at 24–36 months in superficial BCC of no more than 20% lesions.
4 Demonstration of an effective protocol for pain management with severe pain in < 10% of patients treated for individual BD/BCC lesions by standard technique.

Table 2 Clinical indications for topical photodynamic therapy in dermatology: recommendations and evidence assessment

Strength of recommendation	Quality of evidence	Indication
A	I	Thin and moderate thickness actinic keratoses
		Bowen's disease
		Superficial basal cell carcinoma
B	I	Thin nodular basal cell carcinoma
		Epidermal dysplasias in organ transplant recipients
		Inflammatory acne on the face and back
		Viral warts, particularly plantar warts
		Genital warts
		Cutaneous leishmaniasis
B	II-iii	Photorejuvenation
C	II-iii	Localized cutaneous T-cell lymphoma
		Vaginal intraepithelial neoplasia
C	III	Extramammary Paget's disease
C	IV	Skin cancer prevention
D	I	Psoriasis
D	II-iii	Invasive squamous cell carcinoma

5 Cosmetic outcome at 1 year – demonstrate satisfaction (good-excellent) with cosmesis in a minimum of 80% of patients.

References

1 Morton CA, Brown SB, Collins S et al. Guidelines for topical photodynamic therapy: report of a workshop of the British Photodermatology Group. Br J Dermatol 2002; **146**:552–67.
2 National Institute for Health and Clinical Excellence. IPG155. *Photodynamic Therapy for Non-Melanoma Skin Tumours (Including Premalignant and Primary Non-Metastatic Skin Lesions)*. 2006. Available at: http://www.nice.org.uk/page.aspx?o=IPG155guidance (last accessed 29 August 2008).
3 Peng Q, Soler AM, Warloe T et al. Selective distribution of porphyrins in thick basal cell carcinoma after topical application of methyl 5-aminolevulinate. J Photochem Photobiol B 2001; **62**:140–5.
4 Peng Q, Warloe T, Moan J et al. Distribution of 5-aminolevulinic acid-induced porphyrins in noduloulcerative basal cell carcinoma. Photochem Photobiol 1995; **62**:906–13.
5 Martin A, Tope WD, Grevelink JM et al. Lack of selectivity of protoporphyrin IX fluorescence for basal cell carcinoma after topical application of 5-aminolevulinic acid: implications for photodynamic treatment. Arch Dermatol 1995; **287**:665–74.
6 Ahmadi S, McCarron PA, Donnelly RF et al. Evaluation of the penetration of 5-aminolevulinic acid through basal cell carcinoma: a pilot study. Exp Dermatol 2004; **13**:445–51.

7 Fritsch C, Homey B, Stahl W *et al.* Preferential relative porphyrin enrichment in solar keratoses upon topical application of delta-aminolevulinic acid methylester. *Photochem Photobiol* 1998; **68**:218–21.

8 Wiegell S, Wulf HC. Photodynamic therapy of acne vulgaris using 5-aminolevulinic acid versus methyl aminolevulinate. *J Am Acad Dermatol* 2006; **54**:647–51.

9 Kuijpers D, Thissen MR, Thissen CA, Neumann MH. Similar effectiveness of methyl aminolevulinate and 5-aminolevulinate in topical photodynamic therapy for nodular basal cell carcinoma. *J Drugs Dermatol* 2006; **5**:642–5.

10 Moloney FJ, Collins P. Randomized, double-blind, prospective study to compare topical 5-aminolaevulinic acid methylester with topical 5-aminolaevulinic acid photodynamic therapy for extensive scalp actinic keratosis. *Br J Dermatol* 2007; **157**:87–91.

11 Clark C, Bryden A, Dawe R *et al.* Topical 5-aminolaevulinic acid photodynamic therapy for cutaneous lesions: outcome and comparison of light sources. *Photodermatol Photoimmunol Photomed* 2003; **19**:134–41.

12 Juzeniene A, Juzenas P, Ma LW *et al.* Effectiveness of different light sources for 5-aminolevulinic acid photodynamic therapy. *Lasers Med Sci* 2004; **19**:139–49.

13 Moseley H, Allen JW, Ibbotson S *et al.* Ambulatory photodynamic therapy: a new concept in delivering photodynamic therapy. *Br J Dermatol* 2006; **154**:747–50.

14 Britton JER, Goulden V, Stables G *et al.* Investigation of the use of the pulsed dye laser in the treatment of Bowen's disease using 5-aminolaevulinic acid phototherapy. *Br J Dermatol* 2005; **153**:780–4.

15 Strasswimmer J, Grande DJ. Do pulsed lasers produce an effective photodynamic therapy response? *Lasers Surg Med* 2006; **38**:22–5.

16 Kawauchi S, Morimoto Y, Sato S *et al.* Differences between cytotoxicity in photodynamic therapy using a pulsed laser and a continuous wave laser: study of oxygen consumption and photobleaching. *Lasers Med Sci* 2004; **18**:179–83.

17 Marcus SL, Houlihan A, Lundahl S, Ferdon ME. Does ambient light contribute to the therapeutic effects of topical photodynamic therapy (PDT) using aminolevulinic acid (ALA)? *Lasers Surg Med* 2007; **39**:201–2.

18 Batchelor RJ, Stables GI, Stringer MR. Successful treatment of scalp actinic keratoses with photodynamic therapy using ambient light. *Br J Dermatol* 2007; **156**:779–81.

19 Wiegell SR, Haedersdal M, Philipsen PA *et al.* Continuous activation of PpIX by daylight is as effective as and less painful than conventional photodynamic therapy for actinic keratoses; a randomized, controlled, single-blinded study. *Br J Dermatol* 2008; **158**:740–6.

20 Moseley H. Total effective fluence: a useful concept in photodynamic therapy. *Lasers Med Sci* 1996; **11**:139–43.

21 Henderson B, Gollnick SO, Snyder JW *et al.* Choice of oxygen-conserving treatment regimen determines the inflammatory response and outcome of photodynamic therapy of tumours. *Cancer Res* 2004; **64**:2120–6.

22 Star WM, van't Veen AJ, Robinson DJ *et al.* Topical 5-aminolevulinic acid mediated photodynamic therapy of superficial basal cell carcinoma using two light fractions with a two-hour interval: long-term follow-up. *Acta Derm Venereol (Stockh)* 2006; **86**:412–7.

23 de Haas ER, Kruijt B, Sterenborg HJ *et al.* Fractionated illumination significantly improves the response of superficial basal cell carcinoma to aminolevulinic acid photodynamic therapy. *J Invest Dermatol* 2006; **126**:2679–86.

24 de Haas ER, Sterenborg HJ, Neumann HA, Robinson DJ. Response of Bowen disease to ALA-PDT using a single and a 2-fold illumination scheme. *Arch Dermatol* 2007; **143**:264–5.

25 Castano A, Mroz P, Hamblin MR. Photodynamic therapy and anti-tumour immunity. *Nat Rev Cancer* 2006; **6**:535–45.

26 Choudry K, Brooke RC, Farrar W, Rhodes LE. The effect of an iron chelating agent on protoporphyrin IX levels and phototoxicity in topical 5-aminolaevulinic acid photodynamic therapy. *Br J Dermatol* 2003; **149**:124–30.

27 Ziolkowski P, Osiecka BJ, Oremek G *et al.* Enhancement of photodynamic therapy by use of aminolevulinic acid/glycolic acid drug mixture. *J Exp Ther Oncol* 2004; **4**:121–9.

28 Rhodes LE, de Rie M, Enström Y *et al.* Photodynamic therapy using topical methyl aminolevulinate vs. surgery for nodular basal cell carcinoma: results of a multicenter randomized prospective trial. *Arch Dermatol* 2004; **140**:17–23.

29 Horn M, Wolf P, Wulf HC *et al.* Topical methyl aminolaevulinate photodynamic therapy in patients with basal cell carcinoma prone to complications and poor cosmetic outcome with conventional treatment. *Br J Dermatol* 2003; **149**:1242–9.

30 Moseley H, Brancaleon L, Lesar AE *et al.* Does surface preparation alter ALA uptake in superficial non-melanoma skin cancer *in vivo*? *Photodermatol Photoimmunol Photomed* 2008; **24**:72–5.

31 Angell-Petersen E, Sørenson R, Warloe T *et al.* Porphyrin formation in actinic keratosis and basal cell carcinoma after topical application of methyl 5-aminolevulinate. *J Invest Dermatol* 2006; **126**:265–71.

32 Alexiades-Armenakas MR, Geronemus RG. Laser-mediated photodynamic therapy of actinic keratoses. *Arch Dermatol* 2003; **139**:1313–20.

33 Touma D, Yaar M, Whitehead S *et al.* A trial of short incubation, broad-area photodynamic therapy for facial actinic keratoses and diffuse photodamage. *Arch Dermatol* 2004; **140**:33–40.

34 Fritsch C, Lang K, Schulte KW *et al.* Fluorescence diagnosis and photodynamic therapy in dermatology: an overview. In: *Photodynamic Therapy* (Patrice T, ed.). Cambridge: Royal Society of Chemistry, 2003; 177–212.

35 Moore J, Allan E. Pulsed ultrasound measurements of depth and regression of basal cell carcinomas after photodynamic therapy: relationship to probability of 1-year local control. *Br J Dermatol* 2003; **149**:1035–40.

36 Piacquadio DJ, Chen DM, Farber HF *et al.* Photodynamic therapy with aminolevulinic acid topical solution and visible blue light in the treatment of multiple actinic keratoses of the face and scalp: investigator-blinded, phase 3, multicenter trials. *Arch Dermatol* 2004; **140**:41–6.

37 Smith S, Piacquadio D, Morhenn V *et al.* Short incubation PDT versus 5-FU in treating actinic keratoses. *J Drugs Dermatol* 2003; **2**:629–35.

38 Gilbert DJ. Treatment of actinic keratoses with sequential combination of 5-fluorouracil and photodynamic therapy. *J Drugs Dermatol* 2005; **4**:161–3.

39 Goldman M, Atkin D. ALA/PDT in the treatment of actinic keratosis: spot versus confluent therapy. *J Cosmet Laser Ther* 2003; **5**:107–10.

40 Gold MH. Intense pulsed light therapy for photorejuvenation enhanced with 20% aminolevulinic acid photodynamic therapy. *J Lasers Med Surg* 2003; **15** (Suppl.):47.

41 Avram DK, Goldman MP. Effectiveness and safety of ALA-IPL in treating actinic keratoses and photodamage. *J Drugs Dermatol* 2004; **3** (Suppl.):S36–9.

42 Tschen EH, Wong DS, Pariser DM *et al.* The Phase IV ALA-PDT Actinic Keratosis Study Group. Photodynamic therapy using

aminolaevulinic acid for patients with nonhyperkeratotic actinic keratoses of the face and scalp: phase IV multicentre clinical trial with 12-month follow up. Br J Dermatol 2006; **155**:1262–9.

43 Szeimies RM, Karrer S, Radakovic-Fijan S et al. Photodynamic therapy using topical methyl 5-aminolevulinate compared with cryotherapy for actinic keratosis: a prospective, randomized study. J Am Acad Dermatol 2002; **47**:258–62.

44 Pariser DM, Lowe NJ, Stewart DM et al. Photodynamic therapy with topical methyl aminolevulinate for actinic keratosis: results of a prospective randomized multicenter trial. J Am Acad Dermatol 2003; **48**:227–32.

45 Freeman M, Vinciullo C, Francis D et al. A comparison of photodynamic therapy using topical methyl aminolevulinate (Metvix®) with single cycle cryotherapy in patients with actinic keratosis: a prospective, randomized study. J Dermatolog Treat 2003; **14**:99–106.

46 Tarstedt M, Rosdahl I, Berne B et al. A randomized multicenter study to compare two treatment regimens of topical methyl aminolevulinate (Metvix®)-PDT in actinic keratosis of the face and scalp. Acta Derm Venereol (Stockh) 2005; **85**:424–8.

47 Morton CA, Campbell S, Gupta G et al. Intraindividual, right-left comparison of topical methyl aminolaevulinate-photodynamic therapy and cryotherapy in subjects with actinic keratoses: a multicentre, randomized controlled study. Br J Dermatol 2006; **155**:1029–36.

48 Kaufmann R, Spelman L, Weightman W et al. Multicentre intra-individual randomized trial of topical methyl aminolaevulinate-photodynamic therapy vs. cryotherapy for multiple actinic keratoses on the extremities. Br J Dermatol 2008; **158**:994–9.

49 Morton CA, Whitehurst C, Moseley H et al. Comparison of photodynamic therapy with cryotherapy in the treatment of Bowen's disease. Br J Dermatol 1996; **135**:766–71.

50 Salim A, Leman JA, McColl JH et al. Randomized comparison of photodynamic therapy with topical 5-fluorouracil in Bowen's disease. Br J Dermatol 2003; **148**:539–43.

51 Morton CA, Whitehurst C, Moore JV, MacKie RM. Comparison of red and green light in the treatment of Bowen's disease by photodynamic therapy. Br J Dermatol 2000; **143**:767–72.

52 Dijkstra AT, Majoie IM, van Dongen JW et al. Photodynamic therapy with violet light and topical 6-aminolaevulinic acid in the treatment of actinic keratosis, Bowen's disease and basal cell carcinoma. J Eur Acad Dermatol Venereol 2001; **15**:550–4.

53 Morton CA, Horn M, Leman J et al. Comparison of topical methyl aminolevulinate photodynamic therapy with cryotherapy or fluorouracil for treatment of squamous cell carcinoma in situ: results of a multicenter randomized trial. Arch Dermatol 2006; **142**:729–35.

54 Lehmann P. Methyl aminolevulinate-photodynamic therapy: a review of clinical trials in the treatment of actinic keratoses and nonmelanoma skin cancer. Br J Dermatol 2007; **156**:793–801.

55 Brookes PT, Jhawar S, Hinton CP et al. Bowen's disease of the nipple – a new method of treatment. Breast 2005; **14**:65–7.

56 Tan B, Sinclair R, Foley P. Photodynamic therapy for subungual Bowen's disease. Australas J Dermatol 2004; **45**:172–4.

57 Usmani N, Stables GI, Telfer NR, Stringer MR. Subungual Bowen's disease treated by topical aminolevulinic acid-photodynamic therapy. J Am Acad Dermatol 2005; **53**:S273–6.

58 Ball SB, Dawber RPR. Treatment of cutaneous Bowen's disease with particular emphasis on the problem of lower leg lesions. Australas J Dermatol 1998; **39**:63–70.

59 Souza CS, Felicio LB, Bentley MV et al. Topical photodynamic therapy for Bowen's disease of the digit in epidermolysis bullosa. Br J Dermatol 2005; **153**:672–4.

60 Guillen C, Sanmartin O, Escudero A et al. Photodynamic therapy for in situ squamous cell carcinoma on chronic radiation dermatitis after photosensitization with 5-aminolaevulinic acid. J Eur Acad Dermatol Venereol 2000; **14**:298–300.

61 Wong TW, Sheu HM, Lee JY, Fletcher RJ. Photodynamic therapy for Bowen's disease (squamous cell carcinoma in situ) of the digit. Dermatol Surg 2001; **27**:452–6.

62 Yang CH, Lee JC, Chen CH et al. Photodynamic therapy for bowenoid papulosis using a novel incoherent light-emitting diode device. Br J Dermatol 2003; **149**:1297–9.

63 Stables GI, Stringer MR, Robinson DJ, Ash DV. Erythroplasia of Queyrat treated by topical aminolaevulinic acid photodynamic therapy. Br J Dermatol 1999; **140**:514–17.

64 Varma S, Holt PJ, Anstey AV. Erythroplasia of Queyrat treated by topical aminolaevulinic acid photodynamic therapy: a cautionary tale. Br J Dermatol 2000; **142**:825–6.

65 Lee MR, Ryman W. Erythroplasia of Queyrat treated with topical methyl aminolevulinate photodynamic therapy. Australas J Dermatol 2005; **46**:196–8.

66 Paoli J, Ternesten Bratel A, Lowhagen G-B et al. Penile intraepithelial neoplasia: results of photodynamic therapy. Acta Derm Venereol (Stockh) 2006; **86**:418–21.

67 Wolf P, Rieger E, Kerl H. An alternative treatment modality for solar keratoses, superficial squamous cell carcinomas and basal cell carcinomas? J Am Acad Dermatol 1993; **28**:17–21.

68 Wolf P, Kerl H. Photodynamic therapy in patient with xeroderma pigmentosum. Lancet 1991; **337**:1613–14.

69 Procianoy F, Cruz A, Baccega A et al. Aggravation of eyelid and conjunctival malignancies following photodynamic therapy in DeSanctis–Cacchione syndrome. Ophthal Plast Reconstr Surg 2006; **22**:498–9.

70 Peng Q, Warloe T, Berg K et al. 5-Aminolevulinic acid-based photodynamic therapy. Clinical research and future challenges. Cancer 1997; **79**:2282–308.

71 Thissen MR, Schroeter CA, Neumann HA. Photodynamic therapy with delta-aminolaevulinic acid for nodular basal cell carcinomas using a prior debulking technique. Br J Dermatol 2000; **142**:338–9.

72 Wang I, Bendsoe N, Klinteberg CA et al. Photodynamic therapy vs. cryosurgery of basal cell carcinomas: results of a phase III clinical trial. Br J Dermatol 2001; **144**:832–40.

73 Berroeta L, Clark C, Dawe RS et al. A randomized study of minimal curettage followed by topical photodynamic therapy compared with surgical excision for low-risk nodular basal cell carcinoma. Br J Dermatol 2007; **157**:401–3.

74 Soler AM, Warloe T, Berner A, Giercksky KE. A follow-up study of recurrence and cosmesis in completely responding superficial and nodular basal cell carcinomas treated with methyl 5-aminolaevulinate-based photodynamic therapy alone and with prior curettage. Br J Dermatol 2001; **145**:467–71.

75 Vinciullo C, Elliott T, Francis D et al. Photodynamic therapy with topical methyl aminolaevulinate for 'difficult-to-treat' basal cell carcinoma. Br J Dermatol 2005; **152**:765–72.

76 Rhodes LE, de Rie MA, Leifsdottir R et al. Five-year follow-up of a randomized, prospective trial of topical methyl aminolevulinate photodynamic therapy vs surgery for nodular basal cell carcinoma. Arch Dermatol 2007; **143**:1131–6.

77 Basset-Séguin N, Ibbotson SH, Emtestam L et al. Topical methyl aminolaevulinate photodynamic therapy versus cryotherapy for superficial basal cell carcinoma: a 5 year randomized trial. Eur J Dermatol 2008; **18**:547–53.

78 Leman JA, Dick DC, Morton CA. Topical 5-ALA photodynamic therapy for the treatment of cutaneous T-cell lymphoma. Clin Exp Dermatol 2002; **27**:516–18.

79 Paech V, Lorenzen T, Stoehr A et al. Remission of cutaneous mycosis fungoides after topical 5-ALA sensitisation and photodynamic therapy in a patient with advanced HIV-infection. Eur J Med Res 2002; **7**:477–9.

80 Edström DW, Porwit A, Ros AM. Photodynamic therapy with topical 5-aminolevulinic acid for mycosis fungoides: clinical and histological response. Acta Derm Venereol (Stockh) 2001; **81**:184–8.

81 Coors EA, von den Driesch P. Topical photodynamic therapy for patients with therapy-resistant lesions of cutaneous T cell lymphoma. J Am Acad Dermatol 2004; **50**:363–7.

82 Zane C, Venturini M, Sala R, Calzavara-Pinton P. Photodynamic therapy with methyl aminolevulinate as a valuable treatment option for unilesional cutaneous T-cell lymphoma. Photodermatol Photoimmunol Photomed 2006; **22**:254–8.

83 Mori M, Campolmi P, Mavilia L et al. Topical photodynamic therapy for primary cutaneous B-cell lymphoma: a pilot study. J Am Acad Dermatol 2006; **54**:524–6.

84 Garcia-Zuazaga J, Cooper K, Baron ED. Photodynamic therapy in dermatology: current concepts in the treatment of skin cancer. Expert Rev Anticancer Ther 2005; **5**:791–800.

85 Fehr MK, Hornung R, Schwarz VA et al. Photodynamic therapy of vulvar intraepithelial neoplasia III using topically applied 5-aminolevulinic acid. Gynecol Oncol 2001; **80**:62–6.

86 Fehr MK, Hornung R, Degen A et al. Photodynamic therapy of vulvar and vaginal condyloma and intraepithelial neoplasia using topically applied 5-aminolevulinic acid. Lasers Surg Med 2002; **30**:273–9.

87 Abdel-Hady E-S, Martin-Hirsch P, Duggan-Keen M et al. Immunological and viral factors associated with the response of vulval intraepithelial neoplasia to photodynamic therapy. Cancer Res 2001; **61**:192–6.

88 Hillemanns P, Wang X, Staehle S et al. Evaluation of different treatment modalities for vulvar intraepithelial neoplasia (VIN): CO_2 laser vaporization, photodynamic therapy, excision and vulvectomy. Gynecol Oncol 2006; **100**:271–5.

89 Hamdan KA, Tait IS, Nadeau V et al. Treatment of grade III anal intraepithelial neoplasia with PDT. Dis Colon Rectum 2003; **46**:1555–9.

90 McCarron PA, Ma LW, Juzenas P et al. Facilitated delivery of ALA to inaccessible regions via bioadhesive patch systems. J Environ Pathol Toxicol Oncol 2006; **25**:389–402.

91 Webber J, Fromm D. PDT for carcinoma in situ of the anus. Arch Surg 2004; **139**:259–61.

92 Campbell SM, Gould DJ, Salter L et al. Photodynamic therapy using meta-tetrahydroxyphenylchlorin (Foscan) for the treatment of vulval intraepithelial neoplasia. Br J Dermatol 2004; **151**:1076–80.

93 Shieh S, Dee AS, Cheney RT et al. Photodynamic therapy for the treatment of extramammary Paget's disease. Br J Dermatol 2002; **146**:1000–5.

94 Mikasa K, Watanabe D, Kondo C et al. 5-Aminolevulinic acid-based photodynamic therapy for the treatment of two patients with extramammary Paget's disease. J Dermatol 2005; **32**:97–101.

95 Raspagliesi F, Fontanelli R, Rossi G et al. Photodynamic therapy using a methyl ester of 5-aminolevulinic acid in recurrent Paget's disease of the vulva: a pilot study. Gynecol Oncol 2006; **103**:581–6.

96 Zawislak AA, McCarron PA, McCluggage WG et al. Successful photodynamic therapy of vulval Paget's disease using a novel patch-based delivery system containing 5-aminolevulinic acid. Br J Obstet Gynaecol 2004; **111**:1143–5.

97 Stender IM, Bech-Thomsen N, Poulsen T, Wulf HC. Photodynamic therapy with topical delta-aminolevulinic acid delays UV photocarcinogenesis in hairless mice. Photochem Photobiol 1997; **66**:493–6.

98 Sharfaei S, Viau G, Lui H et al. Systemic photodynamic therapy with aminolaevulinic acid delays the appearance of ultraviolet-induced skin tumours in mice. Br J Dermatol 2001; **144**:1207–14.

99 Liu Y, Viau G, Bissonnette R. Multiple large-surface photodynamic therapy sessions with topical or systemic aminolevulinic acid and blue light in UV-exposed hairless mice. J Cutan Med Surg 2004; **8**:131–9.

100 Sharfaei S, Juzenas P, Moan J, Bissonnette R. Weekly topical application of methyl aminolevulinate followed by light exposure delays the appearance of UV-induced skin tumours in mice. Arch Dermatol Res 2002; **294**:237–42.

101 Caty V, Liu Y, Viau G, Bissonnette R. Multiple large surface photodynamic therapy sessions with topical methyl aminolaevulinate in PTCH heterozygous mice. Br J Dermatol 2006; **154**:740–2.

102 Noodt BB, Berg K, Stokke T et al. Apoptosis and necrosis induced with light and 5-aminolaevulinic acid-derived protoporphyrin IX. Br J Cancer 1996; **74**:22–9.

103 Korbelik M, Dougherty GJ. Photodynamic therapy-mediated immune response against subcutaneous mouse tumours. Cancer Res 1999; **59**:1941–6.

104 Oseroff A. PDT as a cytotoxic agent and biological response modifier: implications for cancer prevention and treatment in immunosuppressed and immunocompetent patients. J Invest Dermatol 2006; **126**:542–4.

105 Berg D, Otley CC. Skin cancer in organ transplant recipients: epidemiology, pathogenesis, and management. J Am Acad Dermatol 2002; **47**:1–17.

106 Euvrard S, Kanitakis J, Claudy A. Skin cancers after organ transplantation. N Engl J Med 2003; **348**:1881–91.

107 Dragieva G, Hafner J, Dummer R et al. Topical photodynamic therapy in the treatment of actinic keratoses and Bowen's disease in transplant recipients. Transplantation 2004; **77**:115–21.

108 Dragieva G, Prinz BM, Hafner J et al. A randomized controlled clinical trial of topical photodynamic therapy with methyl aminolaevulinate in the treatment of actinic keratoses in transplant recipients. Br J Dermatol 2004; **151**:196–200.

109 Schleier P, Hyckel P, Berndt A et al. Photodynamic therapy of virus-associated epithelial tumours of the face in organ transplant recipients. J Cancer Res Clin Oncol 2004; **130**:279–84.

110 Wulf HC, Pavel S, Stender I, Bakker-Wensveen CAHB. Topical photodynamic therapy for prevention of new skin lesions in renal transplant recipients. Acta Derm Venereol (Stockh) 2006; **86**:25–8.

111 de Graaf YGL, Kennedy C, Wolterbeek R et al. Photodynamic therapy does not prevent cutaneous squamous-cell carcinoma in organ-transplant recipients: results of a randomized-controlled trial. J Invest Dermatol 2006; **126**:569–74.

112 Perrett CM, McGregor JM, Warwick J et al. Treatment of post-transplant premalignant skin disease: a randomized intrapatient comparative study of 5-fluorouracil cream and topical photodynamic therapy. Br J Dermatol 2007; **156**:320–8.

113 Hongcharu W, Taylor CR, Chang Y et al. Topical ALA-photodynamic therapy for the treatment of acne vulgaris. J Invest Dermatol 2000; **115**:183–92.

114 Pollock B, Turner D, Stringer MR et al. Topical aminolaevulinic acid-photodynamic therapy for the treatment of acne vulgaris: a study of clinical efficacy and mechanism of action. Br J Dermatol 2004; **151**:616–22.

115 Ramstad S, Futsaether CM, Johnsson A. Porphyrin sensitization and intracellular calcium changes in the prokaryote, *Propionibacterium acnes*. J Photochem Photobiol B 1997; **40**:141–8.

116 Nester MS, Gold MH, Kauvar ANB et al. The use of photodynamic therapy in dermatology: results of a consensus conference. J Drugs Dermatol 2006; **5**:140–54.

117 Hong SB, Lee MH. Topical aminolevulinic acid-photodynamic therapy for the treatment of acne vulgaris. Photodermatol Photoimmunol Photomed 2005; **21**:322–5.

118 Alexiades-Armenakas M. Long-pulsed dye laser-mediated photodynamic therapy combined with topical aminolevulinic acid for mild to severe comedonal, inflammatory, or cystic acne. J Drugs Dermatol 2006; **5**:45–55.

119 Santos MA, Belo VG, Santos G. Effectiveness of photodynamic therapy with topical 5-aminolevulinic acid and intense pulsed light versus intense pulsed light alone in the treatment of acne vulgaris: comparative study. Dermatol Surg 2005; **31**:910–15.

120 Rojanamatin J, Choawawanich P. Treatment of inflammatory facial acne vulgaris with intense pulsed light and short contact of topical 5-aminolevulinic acid: a pilot study. Dermatol Surg 2006; **32**:991–6.

121 Akaraphanth R, Kananawanitchkul W, Gritiyarangsan P. Efficacy of ALA-PDT vs. blue light in the treatment of acne. Photodermatol Photoimmunol Photomed 2007; **23**:186–90.

122 Wiegell SR, Wulf HC. Photodynamic therapy of acne vulgaris using methyl aminolaevulinate: a blinded, randomized, controlled trial. Br J Dermatol 2006; **154**:969–76.

123 Hörfelt C, Funk J, Frohm-Nilsson M et al. Topical methyl aminolaevulinate photodynamic therapy for treatment of facial acne vulgaris: results of a randomized, controlled study. Br J Dermatol 2006; **155**:608–13.

124 Yeung CK, Shek SY, Bjerring P et al. A comparative study of intense pulse light alone and its combination with photodynamic therapy for the treatment of facial acne in Asian skin. Lasers Surg Med 2007; **39**:1–6.

125 Haedersdal M, Togsverd-Bo K, Wiegell SR, Wulf HC. Long-pulsed dye laser versus long-pulsed dye laser-assisted photodynamic therapy for acne vulgaris: a randomized controlled trial. J Am Acad Dermatol 2008; **58**:387–94.

126 Horn M, Wolf P. Topical methyl aminolevulinate photodynamic therapy for the treatment of folliculitis. Photodermatol Photoimmunol Photomed 2007; **23**:145–7.

127 Horio T, Horio O, Miyauchi-Hashimoto H et al. Photodynamic therapy of sebaceous hyperplasia with topical 5-aminolaevulinic acid and slide projector. Br J Dermatol 2003; **148**:1274–6.

128 Alster TS, Tanzi EL. Photodynamic therapy with topical aminolevulinic acid and pulsed dye laser irradiation for sebaceous hyperplasia. J Drugs Dermatol 2003; **2**:501–4.

129 Gold MH, Bradshaw VL, Boring MM et al. Treatment of sebaceous gland hyperplasia by photodynamic therapy with 5-aminolevulinic acid and a blue light source or intense pulsed light source. J Drugs Dermatol 2004; **3** (Suppl. 6):S6–9.

130 Perrett CM, McGregor J, Barlow RJ et al. Topical photodynamic therapy with methyl aminolevulinate to treat sebaceous hyperplasia in an organ transplant recipient. Arch Dermatol 2006; **142**:781–2.

131 Dierickx CC, Goldenhersh M, Dwyer P et al. Photodynamic therapy for nevus sebaceus with topical delta-aminolevulinic acid. Arch Dermatol 1999; **135**:637–40.

132 Kim YJ, Kang HY, Lee E-S, Kim YC. Treatment of Fordyce spots with 5-aminolevulinic acid photodynamic therapy. Br J Dermatol 2007; **156**:399–400.

133 Gold MH, Bridges NM, Bradshaw VL, Boring M. ALA-PDT and blue light therapy for hidradenitis suppurativa. J Drugs Dermatol 2004; **3**:S32–5.

134 Strauss RM, Pollock B, Stables GI et al. Photodynamic therapy using aminolaevulinic acid does not lead to clinical improvement in hidradenitis suppurativa. Br J Dermatol 2005; **152**:803–4.

135 Fabbrocini G, Di Costanzo MP, Riccardo AM et al. Photodynamic therapy with topical delta-aminolaevulinic acid for the treatment of plantar warts. J Photochem Photobiol B 2001; **61**:30–4.

136 Schroeter CA, Pleunis J, van Nispen tot Pannerden C et al. Photodynamic therapy: new treatment for therapy-resistant plantar warts. Dermatol Surg 2005; **31**:71–5.

137 Smucler R, Jatsová E. Comparative study of aminolevulinic acid photodynamic therapy plus pulsed dye laser versus pulsed dye laser alone in treatment of viral warts. Photomed Laser Surg 2005; **31**:51–3.

138 Ziolkowski P, Osiecka BJ, Siewinski M et al. Pretreatment of plantar warts with azone enhances the effect of 5-aminolevulinic acid photodynamic therapy. J Environ Pathol Toxicol Oncol 2006; **25**:403–10.

139 Mizuki D, Kaneko T, Hanada K. Successful treatment of topical photodynamic therapy using 5-aminolaevulinic acid for plane warts. Br J Dermatol 2003; **149**:1087–8.

140 Schroeter CA, Kaas L, Waterval JJ et al. Successful treatment of periungual warts using photodynamic therapy: a pilot study. J Eur Acad Dermatol Venereol 2007; **21**:1170–4.

141 Stefanaki IM, Georgiou S, Themelis GC et al. In vivo fluorescence kinetics and photodynamic therapy in condylomata acuminata. Br J Dermatol 2003; **149**:972–6.

142 Wang XL, Wang HW, Wang HS et al. Topical 5-aminolaevulinic acid-photodynamic therapy for the treatment of urethral condylomata acuminata. Br J Dermatol 2004; **151**:880–5.

143 Herzinger T, Wienecke R, Weisenseel P et al. Photodynamic therapy of genital condyloma in men. Clin Exp Dermatol 2005; **31**:51–3.

144 Chen K, Chang BZ, Ju M et al. Comparative study of photodynamic therapy vs. CO_2 laser vaporization in treatment of condylomata acuminata: a randomized clinical trial. Br J Dermatol 2007; **156**:516–20.

145 Enk CD, Fritsch C, Jonas F et al. Treatment of cutaneous leishmaniasis with photodynamic therapy. Arch Dermatol 2003; **139**:432–4.

146 Ghaffarifar F, Jorjani O, Mirshams M et al. Photodynamic therapy as a new treatment of cutaneous leishmaniasis. East Mediterr Health J 2006; **12**:902–8.

147 Gardlo K, Horska Z, Enk CD et al. Treatment of cutaneous leishmaniasis by photodynamic therapy. J Am Acad Dermatol 2003; **48**:893–6.

148 Sohl S, Kauer F, Paasch U, Simon JC. Photodynamic treatment of cutaneous leishmaniasis. J Dtsch Dermatol Ges 2007; **5**:128–30.

149 Asilian A, Davami M. Comparison between the efficacy of photodynamic therapy and topical paromomycin in the treatment of Old World cutaneous leishmaniasis: a placebo-controlled, randomized clinical trial. Clin Exp Dermatol 2006; **31**:634–7.

150 Kosaka S, Akilov OE, O'Riordan K, Hasan T. A mechanistic study of delta-aminolevulinic acid-based photodynamic therapy for cutaneous leishmaniasis. J Invest Dermatol 2007; **127**:1546–9.

151 Abok K, Cadelas E, Brunk U. An experimental model system for leishmaniasis. Effects of porphyrin-compounds and menadione on leishmania parasites engulfed by cultured macrophages. APMIS 1998; **96**:543–51.

152 Beattie PE, Dawe RS, Ferguson J, Ibbotson SH. Lack of efficacy and tolerability of topical PDT for psoriasis in comparison with narrowband UVB phototherapy. Clin Exp Dermatol 2004; **29**:560–2.

153 Fransson J, Ros AM. Clinical and immunohistochemical evaluation of psoriatic plaques treated with topical 5-aminolaevulinic acid photodynamic therapy. *Photodermatol Photoimmunol Photomed* 2005; **21**:326–32.

154 Radakovic-Fijan S, Blecha-Thalhammer U, Schleyer V et al. Topical aminolaevulinic acid-based photodynamic therapy as a treatment option for psoriasis? Results of a randomized, observer-blinded study. *Br J Dermatol* 2005; **152**:279–83.

155 Schleyer V, Radakovic-Fijan S, Kerrer S et al. Disappointing results and low tolerability of photodynamic therapy with topical 5-aminolaevulinic acid in psoriasis A randomized, double-blind phase I/II study. *J Eur Acad Dermatol Venereol* 2006; **20**:823–8.

156 Yim YC, Lee ES, Chung PS, Rhee CK. Recalcitrant palmoplantar pustular psoriasis successfully treated with topical 5-aminolaevulinic acid photodynamic therapy. *Clin Exp Dermatol* 2005; **30**:723–4.

157 Kim JY, Kang HY, Lee ES, Kim YC. Topical 5-aminolaevulinic acid photodynamic therapy for intractable palmoplantar psoriasis. *J Dermatol* 2007; **34**:37–40.

158 Fisher G, Kang S, Varani J et al. Mechanisms of photoaging and chronological skin aging. *Arch Dermatol* 2002; **138**:1462–70.

159 Ruiz-Rodriguez R, SanzSanchez T, Cordoba S. Photodynamic photorejuvenation. *Dermatol Surg* 2002; **28**:742–4.

160 Griffiths C, Wang TS, Hamilton TA et al. A photonumeric scale for the assessment of cutaneous photodamage. *Arch Dermatol* 1992; **128**:347–51.

161 Dover J, Bhatia AC, Stewart B, Arndt KA. Topical 5-aminolevulinic acid combined with intense pulsed light in the treatment of photoaging. *Arch Dermatol* 2005; **141**:1247–52.

162 Gold M, Bradshaw VL, Boring MM et al. Split-face comparison of photodynamic therapy with 5-aminolevulinic acid and intense pulsed light versus intense pulsed light alone for photodamage. *Dermatol Surg* 2006; **32**:795–801.

163 Ruiz-Rodriguez R, Lopez-Rodriguez L. Nonablative skin resurfacing: the role of PDT. *J Drugs Dermatol* 2006; **5**:756–62.

164 Karrer S, Abels C, Landthaler M, Szeimies RM. Topical photodynamic therapy for localized scleroderma. *Acta Derm Venereol* (Stockh) 2000; **80**:26–7.

165 Karrer S, Bosserhoff AK, Weiderer P et al. Influence of 5-aminolevulinic acid and red light on collagen metabolism of human dermal fibroblasts. *J Invest Dermatol* 2003; **120**:325–31.

166 Karrer S, Bosserhoff AK, Weiderer P et al. Keratinocyte-derived cytokines after photodynamic therapy and their paracrine induction of metalloproteinases in fibroblasts. *Br J Dermatol* 2004; **151**:776–83.

167 Takahashi H, Komatsu S, Ibe M et al. ATX-S10(Na)-PDT shows more potent effect on collagen metabolism of human normal and scleroderma dermal fibroblasts than ALA-PDT. *Arch Dermatol Res* 2006; **298**:257–63.

168 Stender IM, Wulf HC. Photodynamic therapy with 5-aminolaevulinic acid in the treatment of actinic cheilitis. *Br J Dermatol* 1996; **135**:454–6.

169 Hauschild A, Lischner S, Lange-Asschenfeldt B, Egberts F. Treatment of actinic cheilitis using photodynamic therapy with methyl aminolevulinate: report of three cases. *Dermatol Surg* 2005; **31**:1344–7.

170 Berking C, Herzinger T, Flaig MJ et al. The efficacy of photodynamic therapy in actinic cheilitis of the lower lip: a prospective study in 15 patients. *Dermatol Surg* 2007; **33**:825–30.

171 Nayeemuddin FA, Wong M, Yell J, Rhodes LE. Topical photodynamic therapy in disseminated superficial actinic porokeratosis. *Clin Exp Dermatol* 2002; **27**:703–6.

172 Cavicchini S, Tourlaki A. Successful treatment of disseminated superficial actinic porokeratosis with methyl aminolevulinate-photodynamic therapy. *J Dermatolog Treat* 2006; **17**:190–1.

173 Berroeta L, Lewis-Jones MS, Evans AT, Ibbotson SH. Woringer–Kolopp (localized pagetoid reticulosis) treated with topical photodynamic therapy (PDT). *Clin Exp Dermatol* 2005; **30**:446–7.

174 Schmook T, Budde K, Ulrich C et al. Successful treatment of nephrogenic fibrosing dermopathy in a kidney transplant recipient with photodynamic therapy. *Nephrol Dial Transplant* 2005; **20**:220–2.

175 Ruiz-Rodriguez R, Alvarez JG, Jaén P et al. Photodynamic therapy with 5-aminolevulinic acid for recalcitrant familial benign pemphigus (Hailey–Hailey disease). *J Am Acad Dermatol* 2002; **45**:740–2.

176 Exadaktylou D, Kurwa HA, Calonje E, Barlow RJ. Treatment of Darier's disease with photodynamic therapy. *Br J Dermatol* 2003; **149**:606–10.

177 van't Westeinde SC, Sanders CJ, van Weelden H. Photodynamic therapy in a patient with Darier's disease. *J Eur Acad Dermatol Venereol* 2006; **20**:870–2.

178 Kirby B, Whitehurst C, Moore JV, Yates VM. Treatment of lichen planus of the penis with photodynamic therapy. *Br J Dermatol* 1999; **141**:765–6.

179 Hillemanns P, Untch M, Pröve F et al. Photodynamic therapy of vulvar lichen sclerosus with 5-aminolevulinic acid. *Obstet Gynecol* 1999; **93**:71–4.

180 Alexiades-Armenakas M. Laser-mediated photodynamic therapy of lichen sclerosus. *J Drugs Dermatol* 2004; **3**:S25–7.

181 Karrer S, Abels C, Wimmershoff MB et al. Successful treatment of cutaneous sarcoidosis using topical photodynamic therapy. *Arch Dermatol* 2002; **138**:581–4.

182 Heidenheim M, Jemec GBE. Successful treatment of necrobiosis lipoidica diabeticorum with photodynamic therapy. *Arch Dermatol* 2006; **142**:1548–50.

183 Mallipeddi R, Chaudhry SI, Darley CR, Kurwa HA. A case of focal dermal hypoplasia (Goltz) syndrome with exophytic granulation tissue treated by curettage and photodynamic therapy. *Clin Exp Dermatol* 2006; **31**:228–31.

184 Nybaek H, Jemec GB. Photodynamic therapy in the treatment of rosacea. *Dermatology* 2005; **211**:135–8.

185 Katz B, Patel V. Photodynamic therapy for the treatment of erythema, papules, pustules, and severe flushing consistent with rosacea. *J Drugs Dermatol* 2006; **5** (Suppl. 2):6–8.

186 Richey DF, Hopson B. Photodynamic therapy for perioral dermatitis. *J Drugs Dermatol* 2006; **5** (Suppl. 2):12–16.

187 Escudero A, Nagore E, Sevila A et al. Chronic X-ray dermatitis treated by topical 5-aminolaevulinic acid photodynamic therapy. *Br J Dermatol* 2002; **147**:394–5.

188 Clayton TH, Harrison PV. Photodynamic therapy for infected leg ulcers. *Br J Dermatol* 2007; **156**:384–5.

189 Moiin A. Photodynamic therapy for molluscum contagiosum infection in HIV-co-infected patients: review of 6 patients. *J Drugs Dermatol* 2003; **2**:637–9.

190 Gold MH, Boring MM, Bridges TM et al. The successful use of ALA-PDT in the treatment of recalcitrant molluscum contagiosum. *J Drugs Dermatol* 2004; **3**:187–90.

191 Karrer S, Szeimies RM, Abels C et al. Epidermodysplasia verruciformis treated using topical 5-aminolaevulinic acid photodynamic therapy. *Br J Dermatol* 1999; **140**:935–8.

192 Darras-Vercambre S, Carpentier O, Vincent P et al. Photodynamic action of red light for treatment of erythrasma: preliminary results. *Photodermatol Photoimmunol Photomed* 2006; **22**:153–6.

193 Calzavara-Pinton PG, Venturini M, Capezzera R et al. Photo-dynamic therapy of interdigital mycoses of the feet with topical application of 5-aminolevulinic acid. *Photodermatol Photoimmunol Photomed* 2004; **20**:144–7.

194 Wiegell SR, Kongshoj B, Wulf HC. *Mycobacterium marinum* infection cured by photodynamic therapy. *Arch Dermatol* 2006; **142**:1241–2.

195 Grapengiesser S, Ericson M, Gudmundsson F et al. Pain caused by photodynamic therapy of skin cancer. *Clin Exp Dermatol* 2002; **27**:493–7.

196 Sandberg C, Stenquist B, Rosdahl I et al. Important factors for pain during photodynamic therapy for actinic keratosis. *Acta Derm Venereol (Stockh)* 2006; **86**:404–8.

197 Rud E, Gederaas O, Høgset A, Berg K. 5-Aminolevulinic acid, but not 5-aminolevulinic acid esters, is transported into adenocarcinoma cells by system BETA transporters. *Photochem Photobiol* 2000; **71**:640–7.

198 Wiegell S, Stender IM, Na R, Wulf HC. Pain associated with photodynamic therapy using 5-aminolevulinic acid or 5-aminolevulinic acid methylester on tape-stripped normal skin. *Arch Dermatol* 2003; **139**:1173–7.

199 Wiegell SR, Skiveren PA, Philipsen PA, Wulf HC. Pain during photodynamic therapy is associated with protoporphyrin IX fluorescence and fluence rate. *Br J Dermatol* 2008; **158**:727–33.

200 Kasche A, Luderschmidt S, Ring J, Hein R. Photodynamic therapy induces less pain in patients treated with methyl aminolevulinate compared to aminolevulinic acid. *J Drugs Dermatol* 2006; **5**:353–6.

201 Ericson M, Sandberg C, Stenquist B et al. Photodynamic therapy of actinic keratosis at varying fluence rates: assessment of photobleaching, pain and primary clinical outcome. *Br J Dermatol* 2004; **151**:1204–12.

202 Babilas P, Knobler R, Hummel S et al. Variable pulse light is less painful than light-emitting diodes for topical photodynamic therapy of actinic keratoses: a prospective randomized controlled trial. *Br J Dermatol* 2007; **157**:111–17.

203 Holmes M, Dawe RS, Ferguson J, Ibbotson SH. A randomized, double-blind, placebo-controlled study of the efficacy of tetracaine gel (Ametop) for pain relief during topical photodynamic therapy. *Br J Dermatol* 2004; **150**:337–40.

204 Langan SM, Collins P. Randomized, double-blind, placebo-controlled prospective study of the efficacy of topical anaesthesia with a eutectic mixture of lignocaine 2·5% and prilocaine 2·5% for topical 5-aminolaevulinic acid-photodynamic therapy for extensive scalp actinic keratoses. *Br J Dermatol* 2006; **154**:146–9.

205 Pagliaro J, Elliott T, Bulsara M et al. Cold air analgesia in photodynamic therapy of basal cell carcinomas and Bowen's disease: an effective addition to treatment: a pilot study. *Dermatol Surg* 2004; **30**:63–6.

206 Brooke RCC, Sinha A, Sidhu MK et al. Histamine is released following aminolevulinic acid-photodynamic therapy of human skin and mediates an aminolevulinic acid dose-related immediate inflammatory response. *J Invest Dermatol* 2006; **126**:2296–301.

207 Kerr AC, Ferguson J, Ibbotson SH. Acute phototoxicity with urticarial features during topical 5-aminolaevulinic acid photodynamic therapy. *Clin Exp Dermatol* 2007; **32**:201–2.

208 Verrico AK, Haylett AK, Moore JV. *In vivo* expression of the collagen-related heat shock protein HSP47, following hyperthermia or photodynamic therapy. *Lasers Med Sci* 2001; **16**:192–8.

209 Haylett AK, Higley K, Chiu M et al. Collagen secretion after photodynamic therapy versus scar-inducing anticancer modalities: an *in vitro* study. *Photochem Photobiol Sci* 2002; **1**:673–7.

210 Monfrecola G, Procaccini EM, d'Onofrio D et al. Hyperpigmentation induced by topical 5-aminolevulinic acid plus visible light. *J Photochem Photobiol B* 2002; **68**:147–55.

211 Moseley H, Ibbotson I, Woods J et al. Clinical and research applications of photodynamic therapy in dermatology: experience of the Scottish PDT centre. *Lasers Surg Med* 2006; **38**:403–16.

212 Babilas P, Landthaler M, Szeimies RM. Photodynamic therapy in dermatology. *Eur J Dermatol* 2006; **16**:340–8.

213 Morton CA, Whitehurst C, McColl JH et al. Photodynamic therapy for large or multiple patches of Bowen's disease and basal cell carcinoma. *Arch Dermatol* 2001; **137**:319–24.

214 Fritsch C, Goerz G, Ruzicka T. Photodynamic therapy in dermatology. *Arch Dermatol* 1998; **134**:207–14.

215 Chung WY, Lee JM, Lee WY et al. Protective effects of hemin and tetrakis (4-benzoic acid) porphyrin on bacterial mutagenesis and mouse skin carcinogenesis induced by 7,12-dimethylbenz[a]anthracene. *Mutat Res* 2000; **472**:139–45.

216 Fuchs J, Weber S, Kaufmann R. Genotoxic potential of porphyrin type photosensitizers with particular emphasis on 5-aminolevulinic acid: implications for clinical photodynamic therapy. *Free Radic Biol Med* 2000; **28**:537–48.

217 Finlan LE, Kernhan NM, Thomson G et al. Differential effects of 5-aminolaevulinic acid photodynamic therapy and psoralen + ultraviolet A therapy on p53 phosphorylation in normal skin *in vivo*. *Br J Dermatol* 2005; **153**:1001–10.

218 Takahashi H, Nakajima S, Sakata I et al. ATX-S10(Na)-photodynamic therapy is less carcinogenic for mouse skin compared with ultraviolet B irradiation. *Br J Dermatol* 2005; **153**:1182–6.

219 Wolf P, Fink-Puches R, Reimann-Weber A, Kerl H. Development of malignant melanoma after repeated topical photodynamic therapy with 5-aminolevulinic acid at the exposed site. *Dermatology* 1997; **194**:53–4.

220 Maydan E, Nootheti PK, Goldman MP. Development of a keratoacanthoma after topical photodynamic therapy with 5-aminolevulinic acid. *J Drugs Dermatol* 2006; **5**:804–6.

221 Wulf HC, Philipsen P. Allergic contact dermatitis to 5-aminolaevulinic acid methylester but not to 5-aminolaevulinic acid after photodynamic therapy. *Br J Dermatol* 2004; **150**:143–5.

222 Harries MJ, Street G, Gilmour E et al. Allergic contact dermatitis to methyl aminolevulinate (Metvix®) cream used in photodynamic therapy. *Photodermatol Photoimmunol Photomed* 2007; **23**:35–6.

223 Hohwy T, Andersen KE, Sølvsten H, Sommerlund M. Allergic contact dermatitis to methyl aminolevulinate after photodynamic therapy in 9 patients. *Contact Dermatitis* 2007; **57**:321–3.

224 Golub AL, Gudgin DE, Kennedy JC et al. The monitoring of ALA-induced protoporphyrin IX accumulation and clearance in patients with skin lesions by *in vivo* surface-detected fluorescence spectroscopy. *Lasers Med Sci* 1999; **14**:112–22.

225 Angell-Peterson E, Christensen C, Mullet CR, Warloe T. Phototoxic reaction and porphyrin fluorescence in skin after topical application of methyl aminolaevulinate. *Br J Dermatol* 2006; **156**:301–7.

226 Ramrakha-Jones VS, Herd RM. Treating Bowen's disease: a cost-minimization study. *Br J Dermatol* 2003; **148**:1167–72.

227 Weston A, FitzGerald P. Discrete choice experiment to derive willingness to pay for methyl aminolevulinate photodynamic therapy versus simple excision in basal cell carcinoma. *Pharmacoeconomics* 2004; **22**:1195–209.

228 Caekelbergh K, Annemans L, Lambert J, Roelands R. Economic evaluation of methyl aminolaevulinate photodynamic therapy in the management of actinic keratoses and basal cell carcinoma. *Br J Dermatol* 2006; **155**:784–90.

229 Clayton TH, Tait J, Whitehurst C, Yates VM. Photodynamic therapy for superficial basal cell carcinoma and Bowen's disease. *Eur J Dermatol* 2006; **16**:39–41.

Appendix 1

Strength of recommendations and quality of evidence.

Strength of recommendations	
A	There is good evidence to support the use of the procedure
B	There is fair evidence to support the use of the procedure
C	There is poor evidence to support the use of the procedure
D	There is fair evidence to support the rejection of the use of the procedure
E	There is good evidence to support the rejection of the use of the procedure
Quality of evidence	
I	Evidence obtained from at least one properly designed, randomized controlled trial
II-i	Evidence obtained from well-designed controlled trials without randomization
II-ii	Evidence obtained from well-designed cohort or case–control analytical studies, preferably from more than one centre or research group
II-iii	Evidence obtained from multiple time series with or without the intervention. Dramatic results in uncontrolled experiments could also be regarded as this type of evidence
III	Opinions of respected authorities based on clinical experience, descriptive studies or reports of expert committees
IV	Evidence inadequate owing to problems of methodology (e.g. sample size, or length of comprehensiveness of follow-up or conflicts in evidence)

http://bad.org.uk/Portals/_Bad/Guidelines/Clinical
%20Guidelines/PDTguideline%20BJD%20Dec
%202008.pdf

Comment

The main differences between the updated topical photo-dynamic therapy guidelines [1] and the 2002 guidelines [2] are the emphasis on newer irradiation techniques [3], other indications and the established indications. Other indications include acne, lichen sclerosus, psoriasis, leishmaniasis, but are based on case reports and case series [1]. Further research is needed to improve pain control during PDT [4, 5] and its efficacy in other conditions.

References

1 Morton CA, McKenna KE, Rhodes LE, *et al.* Guidelines for topical photodynamic therapy: update. *Brit J Dermatol* 2008; 159: 1245–66.

2 Morton CA, Brown SB, Collins S, *et al.* Guidelines for topical photodynamic therapy: report of a workshop of the British Photodermatology Group. *Br J Dermatol* 2002; 146: 552–67.

3 Hauschild A, Stockfleth E, Popp G, *et al.* Optimization of photodynamic therapy with a novel self-adhesive 5-aminolaevulinic acid patch: results of two randomized controlled phase III studies. *Brit J Dermatol* 2009; 160: 1066–74.

4 Halldin CB, Paoli J, Sandberg C. Nerve blocks enable adequate pain relief during topical photodynamic therapy of field cancerization on the forehead and scalp. *Brit J Dermatol* 2009; 160: 795–800.

5 Mikolajewska P, Iani V, Juzeniene A, Moan J. Topical aminolaevulinic acid- and aminolaevulinic acid methyl ester-based photodynamic therapy with red and violet light: influence of wavelength on pain and erythema. *Brit J Dermatol* 2010; 161: 1173–9.

Additional professional resources

Photodynamic therapy for non-melanoma skin tumours (including premalignant and primary non-metastatic skin lesions). NICE 2006. http://www.nice.org.uk/nicemedia/pdf/ip/IPG155guidance.pdf.

BAD patient information leaflet

http://www.bad.org.uk//site/1275/default.aspx

Other patient resources

http://www.cancerbackup.org.uk/Treatments/Othertreatments/Photodynamictherapy
http://www.cancerhelp.org.uk
http://dermnetnz.org/procedures/photodynamic-therapy.html
http://www.nice.org.uk/IPG155publicinfo

Index

Note: Italicized f's and t's refer to figures and tables